AF327123

New Macrolides, Azalides, and Streptogramins in Clinical Practice

INFECTIOUS DISEASE AND THERAPY

Series Editors

Brian E. Scully, M.B., B.Ch.
Harold C. Neu, M.D.

College of Physicians & Surgeons
Columbia University
New York, New York

1. Parasitic Infections in the Compromised Host, *edited by Peter D. Walzer and Robert M. Genta*
2. Nucleic Acid and Monoclonal Antibody Probes: Applications in Diagnostic Methodology, *edited by Bala Swaminathan and Gyan Prakash*
3. Opportunistic Infections in Patients with the Acquired Immunodeficiency Syndrome, *edited by Gifford Leoung and John Mills*
4. Acyclovir Therapy for Herpesvirus Infections, *edited by David A. Baker*
5. The New Generation of Quinolones, *edited by Clifford Siporin, Carl L. Heifetz, and John M. Domagala*
6. Methicillin-Resistant *Staphylococcus aureus*: Clinical Management and Laboratory Aspects, *edited by Mary T. Cafferkey*
7. Hepatitis B Vaccines in Clinical Practice, *edited by Ronald W. Ellis*
8. The New Macrolides, Azalides, and Streptogramins: Pharmacology and Clinical Applications, *edited by Harold C. Neu, Lowell S. Young, and Stephen H. Zinner*
9. Antimicrobial Therapy in the Elderly Patient, *edited by Thomas T. Yoshikawa and Dean C. Norman*
10. Viral Infections of the Gastrointestinal Tract: Second Edition, Revised and Expanded, *edited by Albert Z. Kapikian*
11. Development and Clinical Uses of Haemophilus b Conjugate Vaccines, *edited by Ronald W. Ellis and Dan M. Granoff*

12. *Pseudomonas aeruginosa* Infections and Treatment, *edited by Aldona L. Baltch and Raymond P. Smith*

13. Herpesvirus Infections, *edited by Ronald Glaser and James F. Jones*

14. Chronic Fatigue Syndrome, *edited by Stephen E. Straus*

15. Immunotherapy of Infections, *edited by K. Noel Masihi*

16. Diagnosis and Management of Bone Infections, *edited by Luis E. Jauregui*

17. Drug Transport in Antimicrobial and Anticancer Chemotherapy, *edited by Nafsika H. Georgopapadakou*

18. New Macrolides, Azalides, and Streptogramins in Clinical Practice, *edited by Harold C. Neu, Lowell S. Young, Stephen H. Zinner, and Jacques F. Acar*

Additional Volumes in Production

Novel Therapeutic Strategies in the Treatment of Sepsis, *edited by David C. Morrison and John L. Ryan*

New Macrolides, Azalides, and Streptogramins in Clinical Practice

edited by

Harold C. Neu
College of Physicians & Surgeons
Columbia University
New York, New York

Lowell S. Young
Kuzell Institute for Arthritis and Infectious Diseases
California Pacific Medical Center
San Francisco, California

Stephen H. Zinner
Brown University
Rhode Island Hospital
Roger Williams Medical Center
Providence, Rhode Island

Jacques F. Acar
Hôpital Saint-Joseph
Paris, France

Marcel Dekker, Inc. New York•Basel•Hong Kong

Library of Congress Cataloging-in-Publication Data

New macrolides, azalides, and streptogramins in clinical practice / edited by
    Harold C. Neu ... [et al.].
        p.   cm. — (Infectious disease and therapy ; 18)
    "Second International Conference on the Macrolides, Azalides, and
Streptogramins (ICMAS II)"—Pref.
        Conference was held in Venice, Italy in January 1994.
        Includes index.
        ISBN 0-8247-9311-0 (hardcover : alk. paper)
        1. Macrolide antibiotics—Congresses. 2. Antibiotics—Congresses.
    I. Neu, Harold C. II. International Conference on the Macrolides, Azalides,
    and Streptogramins (2nd : 1994 : Venice, Italy) III. Series.
        [DNLM: 1. Antibiotics, Macrolide—pharmacology—congresses. 2.
    Antibiotics, Macrolide—therapeutic use—congresses. 3. Aza
    Compounds—pharmacology—congresses. 4. Streptomyces—metabolism—
    congresses. W1 IN406HMN v.18 1995 / QV 350 N5323 1995]
    RM666.M25N478   1995
    615'.329—dc20
    DNLM/DLC
    for Library of Congress   95-22123
                                                                          CIP

The publisher offers discounts on this book when ordered in bulk quantities. For
more information, write to Special Sales/Professional Marketing at the address
below.

This book is printed on acid-free paper.

Marcel Dekker, Inc.
270 Madison Avenue, New York, New York 10016

Current printing (last digit):

10 9 8 7 6 5 4 3 2 1

PRINTED IN THE UNITED STATES OF AMERICA

Series Introduction

Marcel Dekker, Inc., has for many years specialized in the publication of high-quality monographs in tightly focused areas in a variety of medical disciplines. These have been of great value to both the practicing physician and the research scientist as sources of detailed and up-to-date information presented in an attractive format. During the last decade, there has been a veritable explosion in knowledge in the various fields related to infectious diseases and clinical microbiology. Antimicrobial resistance, antibacterial and antiviral agents, AIDS, Lyme disease, infections in immunocompromised patients, and parasitic diseases are but a few of the areas in which an enormous amount of significant work has been published. The Infectious Disease and Therapy series covers carefully chosen topics that should be of interest and value to the practicing physician, the clinical microbiologist, and the research scientist.

Brian E. Scully, M.B., B.Ch.
Harold C. Neu, M.D.

Preface

The macrolides were discovered in the Philippines in 1952 and, at that time, multiple esters were made. Subsequently, erythromycin and then spiramycin, roxithromycin, azithromycin, and clarithromycin became available. The problems with the early drugs included their minimal activity against many organisms and the small number of diseases for which they could be used.

Some of the special features of erythromycin are its derivatives, which we examine in this book and which include low toxicity and the lowest incidence of sensitization of any antimicrobial class. Although some gram-positive cocci are resistant to erythromycin, this is not a clinical problem in all countries. On the other hand, you will see from some of the posters that erythromycin (macrolide) resistance is a real problem in France and Spain. Nonetheless, the macrolides are excellent choices for the treatment of outpatient infections. Treatment of common bacterial infections is primarily by the oral route, although intramuscular and intravenous preparations are used in serious respiratory tract infections. The streptogramins in current development are parenteral agents, and these agents are of considerable importance, for they may overcome some of the resistance to other macrolides.

The clinical indications for the macrolide (and azalide) drugs have primarily been staphylococcal soft-tissue infections, *Mycoplasma pneumoniae* and chlamydial infections, diphtheria, pertussis, *Legionella* sp. infections, and pustular acne. In day care centers in the United States, campylobacter enteritis has been treated with erythromycin. The macrolides provide an alternative to penicillin in the treatment of streptococcal pharyngitis, tonsillitis, and pyoderma, and also pneumococcal pneumonia in the United States and some other parts of the world. Erythromycin, josamycin, and spiramycin have proved to be effective therapy of bacterial exacerbations of bronchitis caused by *Streptococcus pneumoniae* in many parts of the world. The macrolides certainly have been effective in the treatment and prevention of rheumatic fever. In this book we discuss the role of the new derivatives in the treatment and prophylaxis of many infections, especially those of the upper respiratory tract.

With the modest activity of erythromycin against *Haemophilus influenzae*, there has been concern about macrolide efficacy, and that is one of the reasons they have not been used extensively in these infections. However, the new macrolides have been effective in treatment of *S. pneumoniae*, *Moraxella*, and *H. influenzae* infections, and they compare well with the oral penicillins. We have just published a paper in *Chest* comparing cefixime with clarithromycin in a multicenter study of respiratory infections and have shown similar results for the two treatment groups.

The new macrolides also have activity against *Corynebacterium diphtheriae*, *Corynebacterium minitissimum*, *Listeria monocytogenes*, *Neisseria gonorrhoeae*, and in many infections caused by these organisms. Moreover, *Bordetella pertussis*, which is reappearing because of a decline in vaccination, and legionnaires' disease, are also effectively treated with the macrolide drugs.

The macrolides are also available for the topical treatment of acne, and many anaerobic infections have been treated with erythromycin when used as part of prophylaxis regimens at the time of surgery.

The structure–activity relations and pharmacokinetics of the new macrolides azalides, and streptogramins are discussed in some detail because they are obviously very important. Most of these new drugs show a postantibiotic effect against gram-positive organisms.

The importance of localization of antimicrobial agents within cells is particularly critical to a discussion of the new macrolides, as these agents accumulate within cells, including polymorphonuclear leukocytes, peritoneal macrophages, and Kupfer cells in the liver. Moreover, localization within the phagosome, the cytoplasms or the lysosomal packets may also be important. We present more about these issues in this volume.

In most studies of the therapy of respiratory infections (for which these drugs have been used most often), the number of patients with culture-proved infections approaches only 30–40%. Interpretation of studies of new antibiotics in this context is very difficult. Nonetheless, results with the new macrolides compare favorably with those obtained with β-lactam antibiotics. One of the major advantages of the new macrolides, in addition to improvements in their dosing regimen, is better patient tolerance relative to erythromycin.

The new streptogramin compound RP 59500, Synercid, is a combination of two pristinamycins. This agent may find particular use in the treatment of resistant staphylococcal, streptococcal, and enterococcal infections. Its in vitro activity against these organisms is excellent, and clinical studies will be of great interest.

The problem with erythromycin is that its antibacterial spectrum is incomplete. Streptogramins and some of the 16-membered macrolides will extend this spectrum of activity. Resistance to the macrolides is a difficulty in some parts of the world, and as is discussed here, resistance to these drugs may be spreading around the world. Also there is poor gastrointestinal tolerance of erythromycin compounds and poor compliance with multiple-dose regimens, which has probably contributed to the resistance problem. We hope that a better toleration of the new derivatives by patients will minimize this problem in the future. The convenience of once- or twice-daily dosing is also a major advantage of the new drugs. This book provides updates on the pharmacology, microbiology, toxicology, and clinical usefulness of the new macrolide, azalide, and streptogramin antibiotics. We were gratified by the response to the first International Conference on the Macrolides, Azalides, and Streptogramins (ICMAS) held 2 years ago in Santa Fe, New Mexico, with 300 attendees. The second conference, had 800 colleagues in attendance.

We hope that this book will open the door to further research in and development of these important new drugs.

Harold C. Neu
Lowell S. Young
Stephen H. Zinner
Jacques F. Acar

Contents

Series Introduction *iii*
Preface *v*
Contributors *xi*

BIOLOGY AND PHARMACOLOGY

1. New Insights into the Structure–Activity Relationship of
   Macrolides and Azalides 3
   André Bryskier, Constantin Agouridas, and Jean-Francois Chantot

2. Resistance to Macrolides, Azalides, and Streptogramins 31
   Roland Leclercq and Patrice Courvalin

3. Clinical Epidemiology of Resistance to Macrolides 41
   Jacques F. Acar and Fred W. Goldstein

4. Pharmacokinetics of Newer Macrolides 51
   Tom Bergan

5. Safety and Drug–Drug Interactions of Macrolides, Azalides,
   and Streptogramins 61
   S. Ragnar Norrby

Biology and Pharmacology: Discussion 71

ix

CLINICAL APPLICATIONS

6. Macrolides, Azalides, and Streptogramins in Staphylococcal
    and Other Gram-Positive Infections   83
    Stephen H. Zinner

7. Clinical Application of Macrolides and Azalides in *Legionella*,
    Mycoplasma, and *Chlamydia* Respiratory Infections   95
    Giuliana Gialdroni Grassi and Carlo Grassi

8. Macrolides as Antimycobacterial Agents   121
    Lowell S. Young

9. Macrolides in Toxoplasmosis   131
    Hernan R. Chang and Jean-Claude Pechère

10. Treatment of Early Lyme Borreliosis with Macrolide Antibiotics   141
    Benjamin J. Luft and Elizabeth M. Bosler

11. Chlamydia and Other Sexually Transmitted Diseases   147
    Geoffrey L. Ridgway

Clinical Applications: *Discussion*   155

POSTER RAPPORTEURS' SUMMARIES

Biology and Pharmacology   167
Kenneth H. Mayer and Fernando Baquero

Clinical Applications   177
Dieter Adam and Vincent T. Andriole

POSTERS

Index   529

Contributors

Jacques F. Acar Laboratoire de Microbiologie Médicale, Hôpital Saint-Joseph, Paris, France

Dieter Adam Children's Hospital of the University of Munich, Munich, Germany

Constantin Agouridas Domaine Antibiothérapie, Roussel-Uclaf, Romainville, France

Vincent T. Andriole Yale University School of Medicine, New Haven, Connecticut

Fernando Baquero Ramon E. Cajal Hospital, Madrid, Spain

Tom Bergan Institute of Medical Microbiology, Rikshospitalet, Oslo, Norway

Elizabeth M. Bosler State University of New York at Stony Brook, Stony Brook, New York

André Bryskier Domaine Antibiothérapie, Roussel-Uclaf, Romainville, France

Hernan R. Chang National University of Singapore, Lower Kent Ridge, Singapore

Jean-Francois Chantot Domaine Antibiothérapie, Roussel-Uclaf, Romainville, France

Patrice Courvalin Institut Pasteur, Paris, France

Fred W. Goldstein Laboratoire de Microbiologie Médicale, Hôpital Saint-Joseph, Paris, France

Carlo Grassi Pavia University, Pavia, Italy

Giuliana Gialdroni Grassi Pavia University, Pavia, Italy

Roland Leclercq Hôpital Henri Mondor, Créteil, France

Benjamin J. Luft State University of New York at Stony Brook, Stony Brook, New York

Kenneth H. Mayer Brown University AIDS Program, Providence, and Memorial Hospital of Rhode Island, Pawtucket, Rhode Island

S. Ragnar Norrby Chinese University of Hong Kong, Prince of Wales Hospital, Sha Tin, Hong Kong

Jean-Claude Pechère University of Geneva School of Medicine, Geneva, Switzerland

Geoffrey L. Ridgway University College London Hospitals, London, England

Lowell S. Young Kuzell Institute for Arthritis and Infectious Diseases, California Pacific Medical Center, San Francisco, California

Stephen H. Zinner Brown University, Rhode Island Hospital, and Roger Williams Medical Center, Providence, Rhode Island

BIOLOGY AND PHARMACOLOGY

1

New Insights into the Structure–Activity Relationship of Macrolides and Azalides

André Bryskier, Constantin Agouridas, and Jean-Francois Chantot

Domaine Antibiothérapie
Roussel-Uclaf
Romainville, France

INTRODUCTION

Macrolide antibiotics have been used for almost 40 years and are considered to be among the best-tolerated anti-infectives. Macrolides show a fairly uniform degree of activity against common pyogens (e.g., *Streptococcus* spp. and *Staphylococcus* spp.), but some variation in activity against *Legionella* spp., *Chlamydia* spp., *Mycoplasma* spp., and *Haemophilus influenzae* have been described with new drugs (38).

The major problem with earlier macrolides was their poor pharmacokinetics, with wide inter- and intraindividual variations in their intestinal absorption, plus the gastrointestinal intolerance of erythromycin. Many of the problems with older compounds, such as acid instability and poor pharmacokinetics, have now been solved with the new drugs. The main goals for future macrolide development will most probably be to expand the antibacterial spectrum and to increase the antibacterial activity against generally susceptible bacteria; to develop new compounds showing little if any cross-resistance with existing macrolides; and to increase intracellular concentration and bioactivity within various cellular compartments in which pathogens are found (3).

Evidence has accumulated in recent years that macrolide antibiotics have a wide variety of pharmacological effects. Some adverse effects might be used in a positive way in other fields, such as gastroenterology, rheumatology, or cardiology. This review deals with the antibacterial activity of macrolides and also their unexpected actions and potential clinical indications.

DEFINITIONS

Macrolides

By slightly modifying the definition proposed by Woodward, it can be said that *macrolides* are lipophilic molecules with a characteristic central lactone ring bearing 12–16 atoms, few if any double bonds, and no nitrogen atoms. Several amino or neutral sugars are fixed to the aglycone (5).

Azalides

Azalides are not included in the Woodward definition because they have an endogenous nitrogen in the aglycone ring (6). The question arises "are azalides a new medicinal chemical family?" Various chemical modifications have been proposed to prevent inactivation of erythromycin A under acidic conditions, and one of them leads to azalides. Azalides derive from a Beckman rearrangement of the C-9 oxime intermediate obtained from erythromycin A. Azalides were prepared to improve the pharmacokinetic properties of erythromycin A and to expand the antibacterial spectrum to cover gram-negative bacteria.

Two categories of azalides have been described: 14- and 15-membered–ring azalides.

The 15-Membered Ring Azalides

The 15-membered azalides can be divided into two subgroups: 9a- and 8a-azalides (Fig. 1). The first series synthesized showed an interesting improvement in minimum inhibitory concentration (MIC) over erythromycin A against gram-negative bacteria (13). Other series of azalides have been prepared; semisynthetic

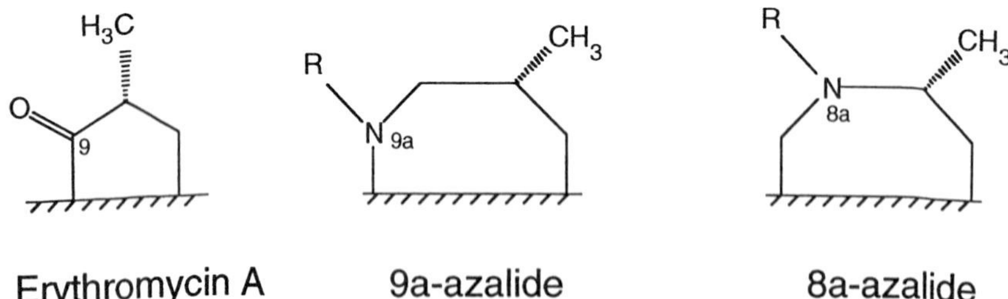

Figure 1   The 15-membered ring azalides are divided into two subgroups: 9a- and 8a-azalides.

Table 1 Comparative Activities (MIC; mg/L) Various 15-Membered Ring Azalides

Drug	*Staphylococcus aureus*	*Enterococcus faecalis*	*Escherichia coli*
Azithromycin	0.39	0.05	0.78
6-*O*-Methylazithromycin	0.78	0.05	3.1
11-*O*-Methylazithromycin	0.10	0.05	0.78
6,11-Di-*O*-Methylazithromycin	0.78	0.78	6.25
6,11,4″-Tri-*O*-Methylazithromycin	3.1	0.78	6.25

modifications focused on various substitutions on the macrocyclic ring nitrogen and epimerization or amine substitution at the C-4″ hydroxyl site within the L-cladinose sugar. 4″-Aminoazithromycin, the most basic analogue, demonstrated the greatest increase in anti–gram-negative activity. 6-*O*-Methylazithromycin was prepared, by analogy with clarithromycin, but is less active than azithromycin (Table 1).

In a series of patents, Merck lists the novel 15-membered ring azalides containing a nitrogen atom at position 8a. The essential step in the synthesis of these ring-expanded erythromycins is the isomerization of the *E*-oxime of erythromycin A to its *Z*-isomer, followed by the standard Beckman rearrangement. The 8a-azalides were used to produce cyclic iminoether, modifications at positions 4″ and 8a, and cyclic lactam derivatives (37); (Fig. 2).

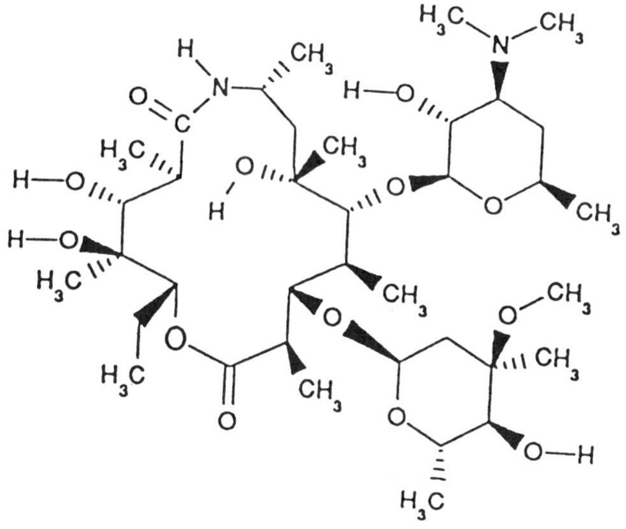

Figure 2 Some 8a-aza-8a-homoerythromycin lactams.

Table 2 Comparative Activities (MIC; mg/L) of 15-Membered Azalides: 8a-Azalide Cyclic Imino Ethers

	Staphylococcus aureus	*Streptococcus pneumoniae*	*Streptococcus pyogenes*	*Escherichia coli*	*Pseudomonas stutzeri*
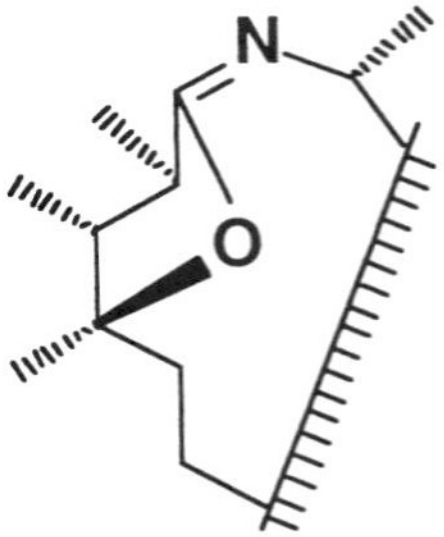	0.5	1.0	8.0	0.5	0.5
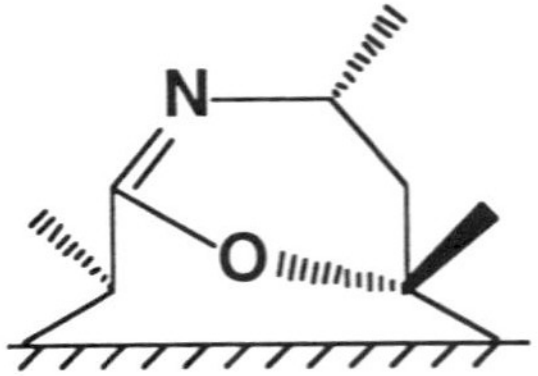	16.0	4.0	2.0	32	2.0

Wilkening et al. (37) have prepared a series of 8a-alkyl-substituted azalides. Selected compounds were further converted to the corresponding 4''-deoxy-4''-amino analogues. Many of the 8a-alkyl derivatives exhibit in vitro activity comparable with that of azithromycin. In general, addition of polar groups to the alkyl side chain results in a decrease in overall activity. Replacement of the 4''-hydroxy substituent with an amino group leads to a two- to eightfold increase in activity against gram-negative bacilli and two- to fourfold decrease in activity against gram-positive organisms (Table 2). For each pair of 4'' (*R*) and 4'' (*S*) amino isomers, the overall activities of each isomer are nearly equivalent. The most active compounds are the 4''-amino-8a fluoroethyl analogues, L-738629 and L-738630.

The 14-Membered Ring Azalides

The 14-membered ring azalides (Fig. 3) show a pattern of antibacterial activity similar to 15-membered-ring azalides (Table 3). The 10-aza compound is approximately twofold less active against gram-positive organisms and four- to eightfold less active against gram-negative organisms than azithromycin. Relative to erythromycin A, this corresponds to an approximate twofold increase in activity against gram-negative isolates.

CLASSIFICATIONS

Several classifications have been proposed for this family of antibiotics (2). A simpler classification based on the lactone structure and the natural or semisynthetic origin has also been put forward. Three main groups have been distinguished 14-, 15-, and 16-membered ring macrolides. Within each group,

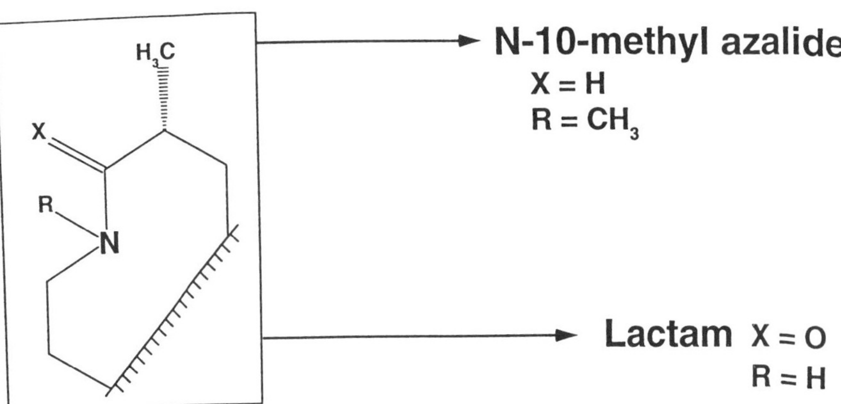

Figure 3   Some 14-membered ring azalides.

Table 3 Comparative Activities (MIC; mg/L) of 14-Membered Azalides

	Staph. aureus	Strep. pyogenes	E. coli	Klebsiella pneumoniae	Haemophilus influenzae
Erythromycin	0.25	0.015	32	32	2
Azithromycin	0.5–1	0.03	1–2	2	0.25–1
10-*N*-Methylazalide	2–4	0.125	4–8	8	2–8
10-*N*-Azalide lactam	>128	>128	>128	>128	>128
10-*N*-Methyl-4'' aminoazalide	4	0.125	4	2	1

Source: From Ref. 40.

compounds are classified according to their natural or semisynthetic origin. A third subgroup might be added for the azalide derivatives (Fig. 4).

MACROLIDES AS ANTIBACTERIAL AGENTS

The chemical modifications of erythromycin A began with considerable efforts to solve the acid instability of this agent, to eliminate bitterness, and to increase water solubility. Recent developments in the macrolide field have concentrated on modifications to erythromycin A, with the objective of achieving pharmaco-kinetic improvements, while retaining an antibacterial spectrum and potency close to that of erythromycin. New goals are to expand the antibacterial spectrum, to enhance activity against susceptible organisms, and to overcome bacterial resistance.

Conformational studies on erythromycins have shown that the orientation of the hydrophilic groups (the lactone carbonyl, ketone carbonyl, and hydroxyl groups at C-6 and C-11) and the hydrophobic groups (the methyl groups at C-4, C-8, and C-12, and the ethyl chain at C-13) in the aglycone ring and the D-desosamine moiety play a very important role in the antibacterial activity of erythromycin A. Mao et al. (27) have proposed the model of erythromycin–ribosome complex; the 2′-hydroxyl and 3′-dimethylamino groups of D-desosamine form two pairs of hydrogen bonds with the nitrogenous base of the nucleotide.

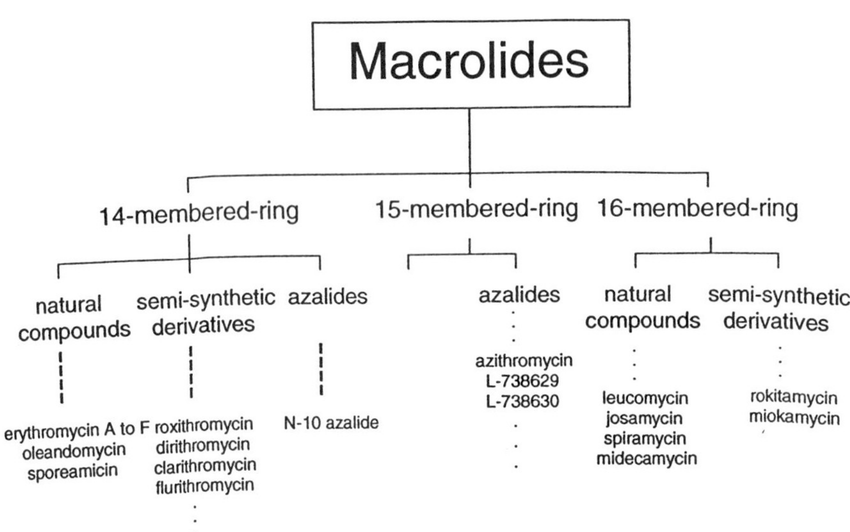

Figure 4 Some 14-, 15-, and 16-membered-ring macrolides.

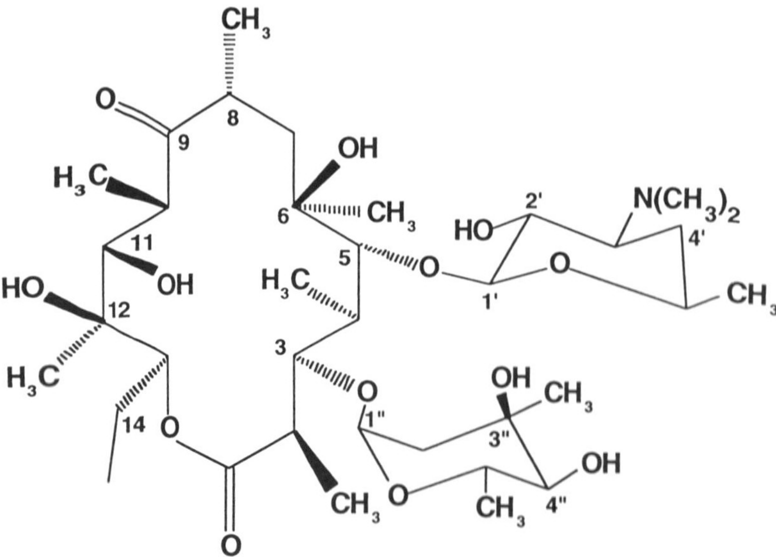

Figure 5   Erythromycin A.

With adjacent nucleotides, the 11, 12-hydroxyl, 9-carbonyl, and 3″-methoxyl and probably 6-hydroxyl group form additional hydrogen bonds.

Numerous modifications of erythromycin A have been made on erythronolide A and on the two sugars: L-cladinose and D-desosamine (Fig. 5).

Chemical Modifications on the Aglycone Ring

Chemical alterations can involve a direct modification of the lactone ring (Fig. 6), or modifications of the various substituents.

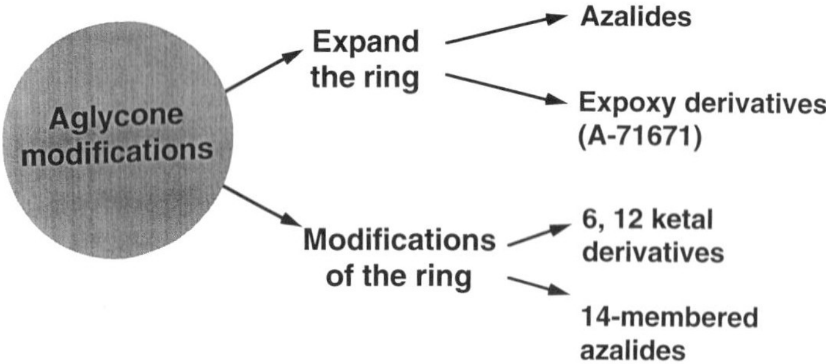

Figure 6   Chemical modifications on the aglycone ring.

Modifications of the Aglycone

Erythromycin A rapidly loses its antibacterial activity in acidic media because of decomposition. The degradation products (8,9-anhydroerythromycin-6,9-hemiketal and 6,9;9,12-erythromycin spiroketal) are inactive and show low ribosomal binding. 10,11-Anhydroerythromycin A and 11,12-epoxyerythromycin A are poorly active. The introduction of a double bond or an epoxy group to erythronolide A reduced the overall antibacterial activity. Introduction of a nitrogen in position 10 gives rise to N^{10} 14-membered ring azalides. Expanding the lactone ring is another way to modify the aglycone. Two examples are the 15-membered azalides, with an introduction of a nitrogen atom at C-8 or C-9, and 9,12-epoxyerythromycin A such as A-69334 (Fig. 7, 8). These compounds are more stable in acidic media, and some of them display better anti–gram-negative activity.

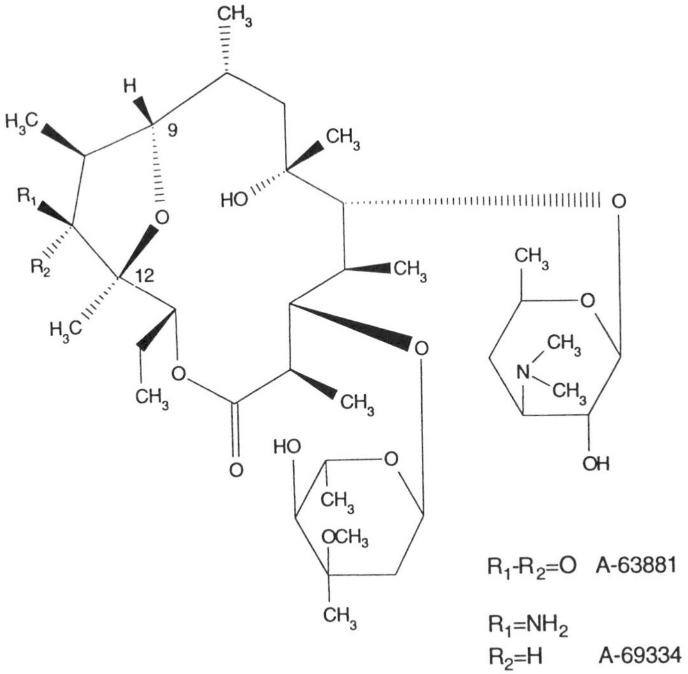

Figure 7 Chemical modifications of the aglycone that give more acid-stable compounds.

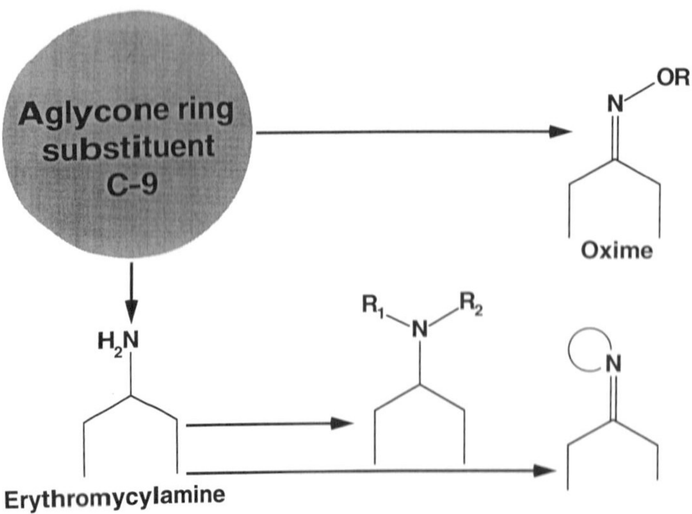

Figure 8   Modifications at position-9.

Modifications of the Substituents

Modifications in Position 6

The weak point of erythronolide A is the 9-keto group. The anchorage points enabling the formation of hemicetal and spiroketal derivatives are the 6- and 12-hydroxyl groups on the aglycone.

Clarithromycin is the 6-*O*-methyl derivative (a noncleavable ether). Clarithromycin has antibacterial activity equal or superior to that of erythromycin A (Table 4). One of its metabolites is 14-hydroxyclarithromycin. The 14(*R*)-hydroxy epimer is as active as clarithromycin, whereas the 14(*S*)-hydroxy epimer is poorly active (Table 5).

A series of 6-deoxoerythromycins have been prepared. Those compounds are acid-stable. They are less active than erythromycin A.

Modifications in Position 9

Various chemical modifications have been proposed to prevent inactivation, including blockade or transformation of the 9-keto group into another functional group. Three series of derivatives have been prepared: 9(*S*)-erythromycylamine, ether-oxime derivatives, and 15-membered ring azalides (Fig. 8).

9-Ether Oxime Derivatives   Various ether oxime derivatives of erythromycin have been prepared (Fig. 9; 14). Five series of compounds were synthesized according to the chemical nature of the ether chain; aliphatic ether chain, aromatic

Table 4 Comparative Activities of Macrolides: Aglycone Ring Substituent C-6 Erythromycin A Modifications

	MIC$_{90}$(mg/L)	
	Clarithromycin	Erythromycin
Strep. pneumoniae	0.03	0.03
Strep. pyogenes	0.06	0.06
Moraxella catarrhalis	0.25	0.25
Haemophilus influenzae	4.0	8.0

Source: From Ref. 41.

ether chain, nitrogen-, oxygen-, or sulfur ether chain. Among 65 oxime ether derivatives of erythromycin A, 5 were selected for investigation. Two nitrogen-containing oxime ether derivatives were very active in vitro, but were toxic after repeated doses in dogs and rats. The oxygen- and sulfur-containing oxime ether analogues were less active than roxithromycin (Table 6). Roxithromycin possesses a spectrum and antibacterial activity similar to those of erythromycin, but it is two- to tenfold more active in vivo (7). Roxithromycin is far more stable in acid media than erythromycin base and 2′-esters, such as erythromycin 2′-propionate (14).

Erythromycylamine Derivatives 9(*S*)-Erythromycylamine is almost as active as erythromycin A and more active than the 9(*R*)-epimer, but it is poorly absorbed. Several synthetic modifications of erythromycylamine have been reported. These are designed to expand its antibacterial activity to gram-negative bacilli, especially *H. influenzae*. The introduction of an additional amino group increases the overall hydrophilicity of the macrolide, which probably influences bacterial outer membrane penetration and the anti–gram-negative activity of these compounds.

Table 5 Comparative Activities of Macrolides: Aglycone Ring Substituent Erythromycin A Modifications

	MIC$_{50}$(mg/L)	
	Clarithromycin	14-OH-Clarithromycin (A-62671)
Streptococcus pneumoniae	0.12	0.12
Streptococcus pyogenes	0.06	0.06
Moraxella catarrhalis	0.06	0.06
Haemophilus influenzae	4	4

Source: From Ref. 42.

Table 6 Comparative Activities of 9-Ether Oxime Derivatives

Oxime ether R =	In vivo activity (mouse)			Pharmacokinetic data (rat)		
	In vitro activity MIC (mg/L)	Staphylococcal infection ED_{50} (mg/kg)	Streptococcal infection ED_{50} (mg/kg)	T_{max} (h)	C_{max} (μg/ml)	C at 7 h (μg/ml)
$-CH_2-CH_2-N(CH_3)_2$ RU 29065	0.126	2.36	20	2	1.9	1
$-CH_2-CH_2-N(C_2H_5)_2$ RU 29702	0.118	1.55	12	1	3.8	0.3
$-CH_2-O-CH_3$ RU 38482	0.118	2.78	5	0.5	1.60	0.15
$CH_2-O-CH_2-CH_2-OCH_3$ RU 28965 (roxithromycin)	0.296	3.84	2.3	0.25	3.8	0.44
$-CH_2-S$ RU 40403	0.334	2.5	1.98	1	4.2	0.47
Erythromycin	0.151	1	1		0.25	Not detect.

Source: Adapted from Ref. 14.

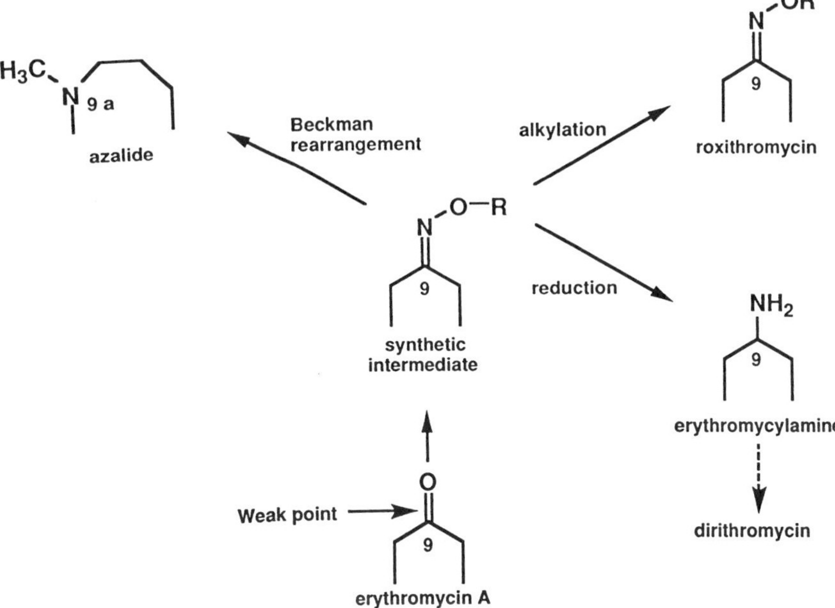

Figure 9   Some 9-ether oxime derivatives.

N-Aryldene derivatives show reduced antibacterial activity compared with erythromycin A, but somewhat enhanced in vivo activities, in particular *N*-benzyldene and *N*-salicylidene. In humans, blood levels of these derivatives are lower than those of erythromycin A. *N*-Acyl derivatives are less active than 9(*S*)-erythromycylamine. The most active compound is the phenylacylamino analogue.

Tertiary amine derivatives of erythromycylamine (morpholino, piperidino, piperazino analogues) have been synthesized (Fig. 10). The 9(*R*)-derivatives are more active than their 9(*S*)-counterparts. The 9(*R*)-piperidino derivatives are the most active in vitro, and the *O*-alkyl piperidine show the best activity. All these compounds are active against gram-positive cocci, but failed to exert any antibacterial activity against *Escherichia coli* (28).

Lartey et al. (26) introduced polar functions at C-21 (moiety pending at C-12) on 9(*R*)-amino-9-deoxoerythromycin A. The C-21 amino analogues show slightly improved activity against gram-negative bacilli (Table 7).

Modifications in Position 8

If we consider the stereochemistry of the methyl group on the lactone ring, 8-epierythromycin B possesses only one-tenth the antibacterial activity of

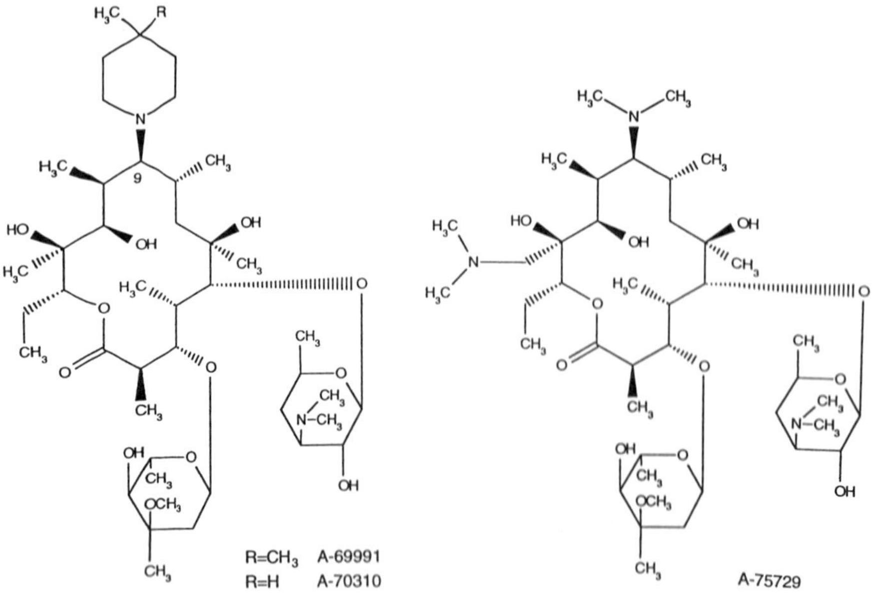

- 9-methylpiperidino derivatives.   - (9R)-erythromycylamino derivatives.

Figure 10 Tertiary amine derivatives of erythromycylamine.

erythromycin B. This might illustrate the importance of the orientation of each methyl group of the erythronolide. A hydroxyl group has been introduced on the C-8 of the lactone ring. Two epimers have been also prepared. The antibacterial activity of the 8(*S*)-epimer and 8(*R*)-epimer against *Staphylococcus aureus* Smith was $\frac{1}{8}$ and $\frac{1}{30}$ that of erythromycin A, respectively. Introduction of a fluorine at C-8 gave flurithromycin (Fig. 11). Replacement of the hydrogen at position 8 by a fluorine, which is almost isosteric, was aimed at increasing the stability of the 9-keto group. In vitro flurithromycin is less active than erythromycin A, but in vivo it is two to three times more active (Table 8).

Modifications in Position 11,12

Erythromycin A is twice as active as erythromycin B. They differ by the lack of a 12-group in erythromycin B. A number of 11,12-modified erythromycin A compounds have been synthesized. Davercin, the 11,12-cyclic carbonate derivative of erythromycin A (Fig. 12), is at least twice as active as erythromycin A (Table 9). A number of 11,12-cyclic derivatives of erythromycin A have been described. For example, erythromycin 11,12-cyclic methylene acetal shows better antistaphylococcal activity than erythromycin A.

Table 7 Comparative Activities (MIC; mg/L) OF C-21 Substituents of Erythromycylamine C-21 Substituents

Compounds C-21 Substituents	A-67180 Methyl	A-75412 *N*-Benzyl-*N*- methylamino	A-75611 *N*-Methylamino	A-75729 *N,N*-Dimethylamino
Strep. pyogenes EES 6	0.05	0.78	0.78	0.10
Staph. aureus ATTC 6538P	0.39	12.5	12.5	1.56
Staph. epidermidis 3519	0.39	6.2	12.5	1.56
Micrococcus luteus ATCC 4698	0.10	3.1	1.56	0.78
Enterococcus faecium ATCC 8043	0.20	1.56	3.1	0.39
E. coli H 560	25	50	12.5	3.1
K. pneumoniae ATCC 8045	50	100	50	6.2
P. aeruginosa K 799/WT	>100	12.5	3.1	1.56
H. influenzae 1177	2	2	4	0.5

Source: Adapted From Ref. 26.

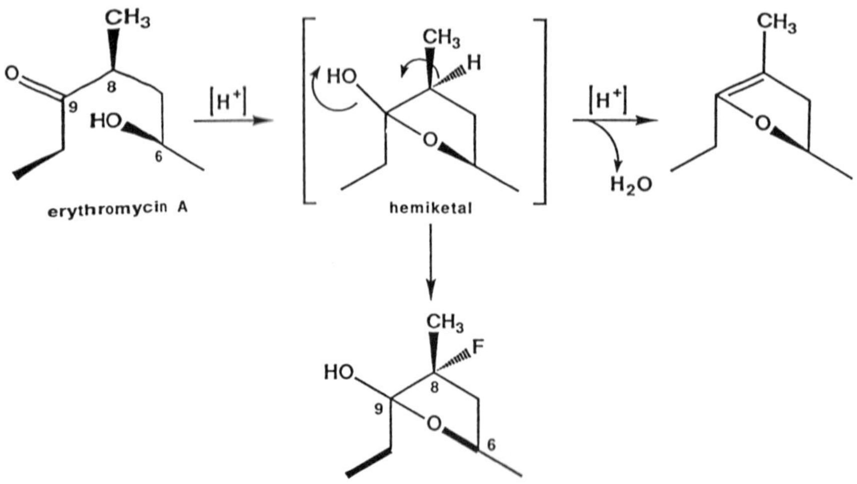

Figure 11   Introduction of a fluorine at C-8 gives flurithromycin.

ER-42859 is a 9-methoxime erythromycin A derivative (Fig. 13), with an 11-ether side chain (2-dimethylaminoethyloxymethyl). It is two- to fourfold more potent than erythromycin A against *S. aureus* and *Streptococcus pyogenes*.

A series of *O*-alkyl erythromycin A derivatives have been synthesized. 6,12-di-*O*-methylerythromycin A (TE-032) and 11-*O*-methylerythromycin A have close antibacterial activity, but they are less active than erythromycin A. In vitro, TE-032 is less active than clarithromycin, but it is several times more active than erythromycin A in vivo.

Modifications of D-Desosamine

Various modifications have been proposed on the D-desosamine moiety, (Fig. 14). The *N*-oxide and dedimethylamino derivatives showed poor antibacterial

Table 8   Comparative Activities of Macrolides: Aglycone Ring Substituent C-8 Erythromycin A Modifications

	MIC_{90}(mg/L)	
	Flurithromycin	Erythromycin
S. pneumoniae	0.25	0.03
S. pyogenes	0.06	0.06
M. catarrhalis	0.25	0.25
H. influenzae	8.0	8.0

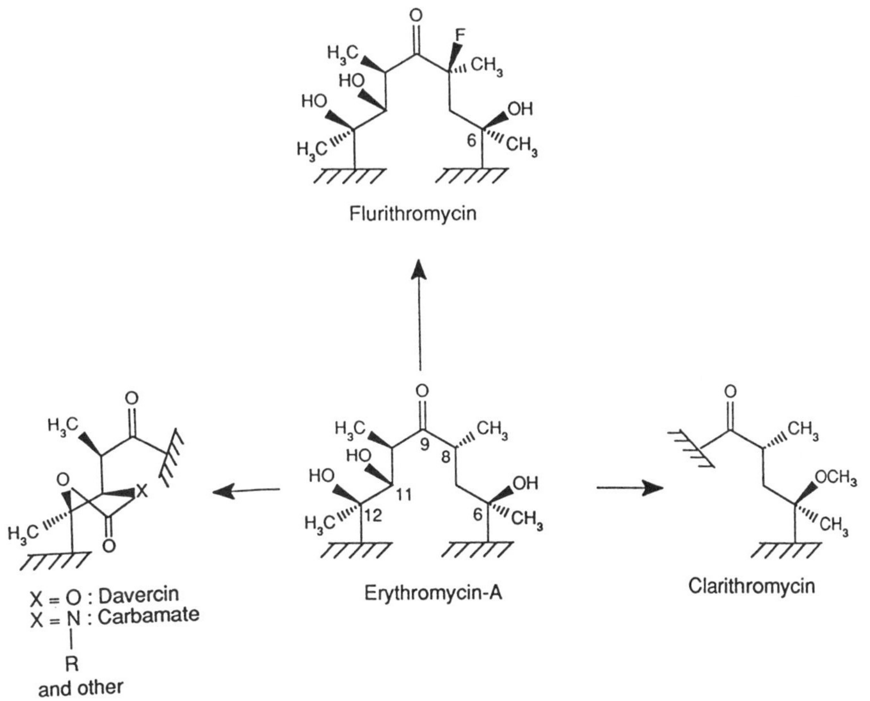

Figure 12 Modified 11,12-erythromycin A derivatives.

activity and no ribosomal binding. It was subsequently suggested that the dimethylamino group should be considered an important functional group for the antibacterial activity of erythromycin A. *N*-Alkyl derivatives produced by reductive alkylation of de-*N*-methylerythromycin were inactive. It was stated that any changes involving the dimethylamino function resulted in decreased antibacterial activity. The 4′-dimethylamino isomer of erythromycin A is inactive.

Table 9 Comparative Activities of Macrolides: Aglycone Ring C-11, C-12 Substituent Modification of Erythromycin A

	Erythromycin A (mg/L)	Davercin (mg/L)
S. aureus	0.25	0.12
E. faecalis	1	0.5
S. pyogenes	0.03	≤0.015
H. influenzae	2.0	—

Source: From Ref. 43.

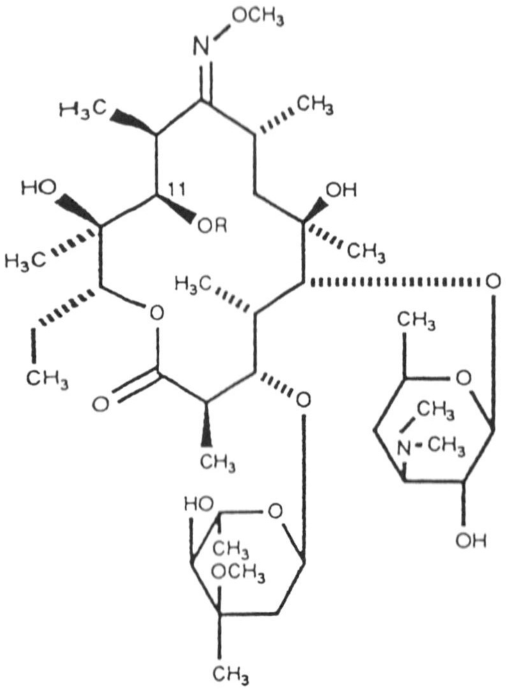

$$R = CH_2\text{-}O\text{-}CH_2\text{-}CH_2\text{-}N(CH_3)_2$$

Figure 13 ER-42859. A 9-methoxime erythromycin A derivative with an 11-ether side chain.

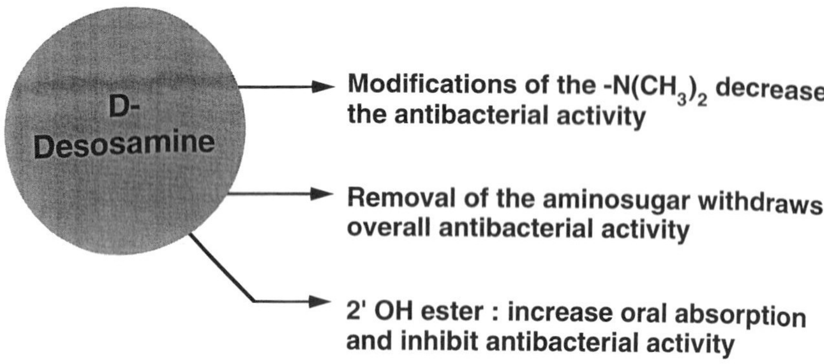

Figure 14 Modifications of D-desosamine.

A large number of 2'-esters have been synthesized, and nearly all are poorly active, probably because of reduced affinity for ribosomes. The presence of a hydroxyl group at C-4' decreases antibacterial activity by 50%. It was hypothesized that the 4'-hydroxyl group adjacent to the dimethylamino group, or a small change in the orientation of the dimethylamino group caused by intramolecular hydrogen bonding between the 4'-hydroxyl group and the nitrogen atom of the dimethylamino group, modified ribosomal linking.

Modifications of L-Cladinose

The antibacterial activity of erythromycin C, in which the methoxyl at C-3'' position of erythromycin A is replaced by a hydroxyl group (Fig. 15), is one-third that of erythromycin A, and its ribosomal binding is reduced. The 3''-methoxy group on L-cladinose in erythromycin A is the only polar group located in proximity to the 3'-dimethylamino group or the 2'-hydroxyl group of D-desosamine, and it has significant influence on the antibacterial activity of erythromycin A.

4''-oxime, 4''-amino, and 4''-*O*-sulfonyl derivatives of erythromycin A or their 9-oximes were 25–100% more active than erythromycin A and showed enhanced activity against erythromycin-resistant strains. 4''-Acyl and 4''-*O*-carbamoyl derivatives of clarithromycin have been prepared. 4''-*O*-carbamoylclarithromycin (A-63075) is more active than the parent compound. The introduction of a methoxy group at C-4'' in addition to that at C-6, results in a further increase in acid stability, but the methylation of this secondary hydroxyl group results in a decrease in in vitro activity.

MACROLIDES AS ANTIFUNGAL AGENTS?

Desmycosin and lactonecin (desmycarosyl tylosin compounds) exhibit greater activity against gram-negative bacteria than do the analogous derivatives of tylosin and macrocin. Some C-20-modified derivatives unexpectedly show antifungal activity in vitro. One compound bearing a C-20-deoxo-20-(3,5 dimethylpiperidin-1-yl) group displays moderate activity against *Candida al-*

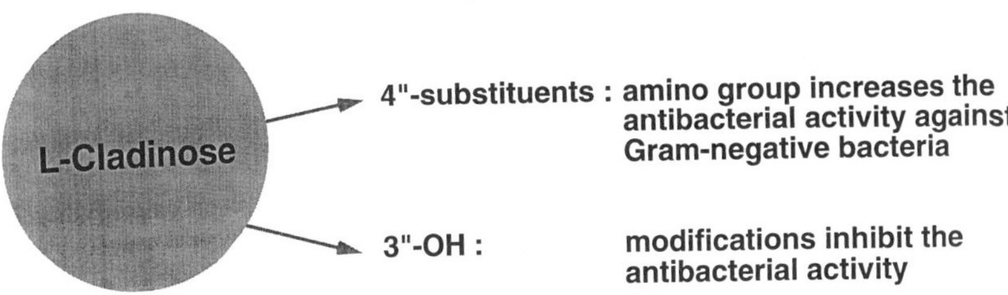

Figure 15 Modifications of L-cladinose.

bicans and *Trichophyton mentagrophytes*. The MIC values were, respectively, 5.0 and 2.5 mg/L.

Another strategy was to replace the mycinose sugar by nonsaccharide substituents. 5-*O*-mycanosyl tylonolide (OMT) was used as starting material. The hydroxyl group of OMT was converted into *O*-acyl, *O*-sulfonyl, *O*-tetrahydropyranyl, or *O*-aryl derivatives. Other modifications at C-23 included the replacement of oxygen as heteroatom by sulfur (*S*-aryl or *S*-alky), nitrogen (tertiary amine), or a halogen (iodine; Table 10). Despite good in vitro activity, all the compounds failed to cure *C. albicans* infections in mice (18).

MACROLIDES AS ANTIPARASITIC AGENTS

Since the initial recognition of acquired immunodeficiency syndrome (AIDS), a disorder that leaves the host exposed to normally controlled infections, several organisms have emerged as severe pathogens in this setting (e.g., *Pneumocystis carinii*, *Cryptosporidium* spp., and *Isospora belli*). Macrolides also could be a therapeutic alternative in patients with *Giardia lamblia intestinalis*) and *Entamoeba histolytica* infections. Macrolides in combination with antimalarial drugs might be an alternative in therapy for *Plasmodium falciparum* malaria (3,4). Antitoxoplasmosis activity in AIDS patients is controversial. No structure–activity relations have been defined in this setting.

MACROLIDES AS ANTI-INFLAMMATORY AGENTS?

Macrolide antibiotics have been reported to exert anti-inflammatory activity in both humans and different animal models (11,33). Topically applied erythromycin proved to be very effective in preventing acute inflammatory reactions produced in the mouse ear by croton oil, cantharidin, or picryl chloride. These effects were unrelated to the blockade of the prostanoid pathway (35). Recently, it has been reported that erythromycin decreased the inflammatory process associated with zymosan-induced peritonitis in mice (30).

Erythromycin possesses antioxidant activity. This pharmacological property might be beneficial for the reduction of inflammation associated with bacterial infections of the skin. The antioxidant properties have been documented for roxithromycin (23), dirithromycin, and erythromycylamine (22). The strongest impairment occurred with C-9-modified macrolides, whereas alteration at C-6 (clarithromycin) did not seem to inhibit this phagocyte function (24). The 16-membered ring macrolides do not decrease the phagocyte oxidative burst. Josamycin and rokitamycin have been reported to increase the neutrophil oxidative burst (25; Table 11).

The influence of macrolides on the production of various cytokine mediators by monocytes has been investigated in humans and animals. A significant increase in interleukin-6 (IL-6) production by spiramycin and, to a lesser extent, crythromycin has been reported. Human IL-4 possesses anti-in-

Table 10 In Vitro Antifungal Activity (MIC; (μg/ml) of Macrolides

C-23 substituent (X)	C. albicans	T. mentagrophytes	A. flavus
O-(Tetrahydropyranyl)	1.25	5	20
O-Phenylsulfonyl	1.25	5	20
O-Phenyl	1.25	1.25	10
S-Phenyl	0.312	0.625	5
S-(2-Pyridyl)	2.5	2.5	2.5
S-(2-Pyrimidinyl)	10	10	40
S-(Cyclohexyl)	5	2.5	2.5
N-(3,5-Dimethylpiperidinyl)	0.312	2.5	2.5
N-(Octahydroindolyl)	0.625	1.25	5

Source: From Ref. 18.

flammatory properties. It suppresses production of tumor necrosis factor-α (TNF-α), IL-1, and prostaglandin (PG)E$_2$ by stimulated monocytes–macrophages (15). After repeated doses (28 days) of roxithromycin in mice, IL-1, IL-2, and TNF-α production are significantly increased. Supernatants of mouse splenocytes cultured in the presence of roxithromycin suppressed the production of TNF-α and PGE$_2$ by stimulated monocytes, and this suppressive activity was impaired by a monoclonal antibody to murine IL-4 (20). Roxithromycin is active in reducing the acute inflammatory reaction in rat models through mechanisms different from conventional nonsteroidal anti-inflammatory agents, which exert their action through inhibition of cyclooxygenase or lipooxygenase activities (1).

MACROLIDES AS CARDIOVASCULAR AGENTS?

Rare cardiovascular effects have been reported with macrolide antibodies. Hypotension has been described with josamycin (9). Erythromycin has been reported to produce ventricular tachycardia (29).

Are Macrolides Potential Class III Antiarrhythmic Agents?

Erythromycin is known to produce a long QTU interval in the electrocardiogram and to be associated with the development of torsades de pointes. Recent studies have implicated M cells in the deep subepicardial and midmyocardial layers of the ventricle in these effects. Erythromycin (10–100 mg/L) induced a much more pronounced prolongation of action potential in M cells. Erythromycin acts as a potassium channel blocker (39).

Hypotensive Activity of Macrolides

9-*N*-Propylerythromycylamine (LY 281389; Fig. 16) was examined for autonomic activity in isolated smooth and cardiac muscle preparations and for cardiac effects, by intravenous infusion in anesthetized beagle dogs (10). In isolated

Table 11 Macrolides as Anti-Inflammatory Agents?

| | Antioxidant Properties (PMN oxidative burst) | | |
	Reduce	Increase	No effect
14-Membered ring macrolides	Erythromycin Roxithromycin Dirithromycin Erythromycylamine		Clarithromycin Oleandomycin
15-Membered ring azalides			Azithromycin
16-Membered ring macrolides		Rokitamycin Josamycin	Spiramycin

Source: From Ref. 24.

tissues, LY 281389 antagonized the cell receptor agonists tested (acetylcholine, angiotensin I, isoproterenol, norepinephrine, and oxytocin) at concentrations of 10^{-3} and $10^{-4}M$. The concentrations achieved in heart tissue are in the range of those tested in isolated tissue. The nonselective nature of these effects of LY 281389 indicate that, at concentrations of $\geq 10^{-4}\ M$, the compound may exert its effects directly on smooth and cardiac muscle tissues. Similar findings have been described with josamycin (34).

MACROLIDES: GASTROINTESTINAL PROKINETIC AGENTS

Erythromycin A has side effects, such as anorexia, nausea, vomiting, abdominal pain, and diarrhea. These side effects are caused by the gastrointestinal motor-stimulating activity of erythromycin A.

Migrating Motor Complex in Human Gastrointestinal Tract

Cyclic caudally migrating bands of strong contractions in the small bowel, or migrating motor complex (MMC), were first reported by Vantrappen et al. (36) in fasted volunteers: MMC is made up of three distinct phases:

Phase I: few intermittent contractions during a period of relative quiescence
Phase II: frequency of contractions increases
Phase III: intense activity period

In humans, the MMC cycling time is about 1.5 h.

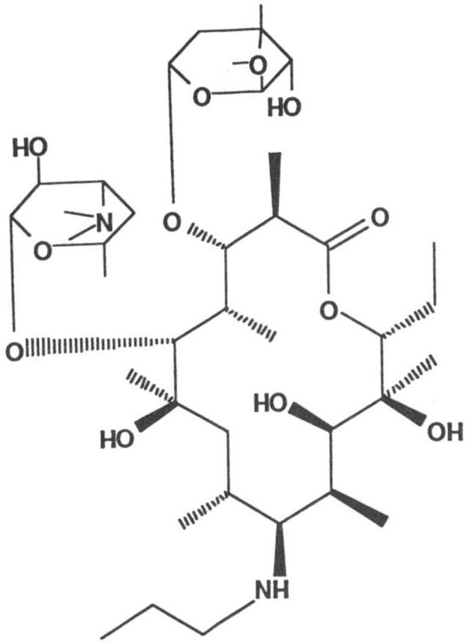

Figure 16 9-*N*-Propylerythromycylamine (LY 281389).

Motilin

Motilin is an endogenous peptide hormone that controls the MMC, and peaks of plasma motilin coincide with the occurrence of phase III activities in MMC in the duodenum. The action of erythromycin A resembles that of motilin. Erythromycin A mimics the physiological action of motilin by acting as an agonist of a motilin receptor (21). The motility effects of erythromycin are accompanied by a release of motilin.

Rationale to Develop Prokinetic Macrolidelike Agents

Janssens et al. (17) were the first to increase the gastric emptying rate of patients suffering from diabetes mellitus-related gastroparesis, with a single intravenous dose of erythromycin. Gastric emptying of solids and liquids improved significantly with 200 mg of erythromycin intravenously, thereby relieving symptoms that usually accompany food retention in the stomach.

Motilides

Itoh et al. (16) examined many compounds and named those mimicking in vitro effect of motilin, motilides. Chemical modifications of 8,9-anhydroerythromycin A, 6,9 hemicetal (32), which showed gastrointestinal motor-stimulating (GMS) activity ten times more potent (3 μg/kg) than erythromycin A (30 μg/kg), were undertaken to search for derivatives with stronger GMS activity and no antibacterial activity.

EM-523

EM-523 (Fig. 17) was selected from a series of O-substituted and tertiary-N-substituted derivatives of 8,9-anhydroerythromycin-6,9-hemicetal. In dogs and healthy volunteers, EM-523 induced motilinlike contractile responses in the gastrointestinal tract and gallbladder.

LY 267108

Scientists at Eli Lilly reported the synthesis of derivatives of 8,9-anhydroerythromycin-6,9-hemicetal in which the 14-membered ring macrolide was contracted to a 12-membered ring compound by intramolecular transacylation. One compound, LY 267108 (Fig. 18), was more potent than erythromycin A in stimulating gastrointestinal motility in guinea pigs and dogs and was devoid of antibacterial activity (18,19).

Structure–Activity Relations

The strongest effect on gastrointestinal motility was observed with 14-membered ring macrolides such as erythromycin. The 16-membered ring macrolides, such

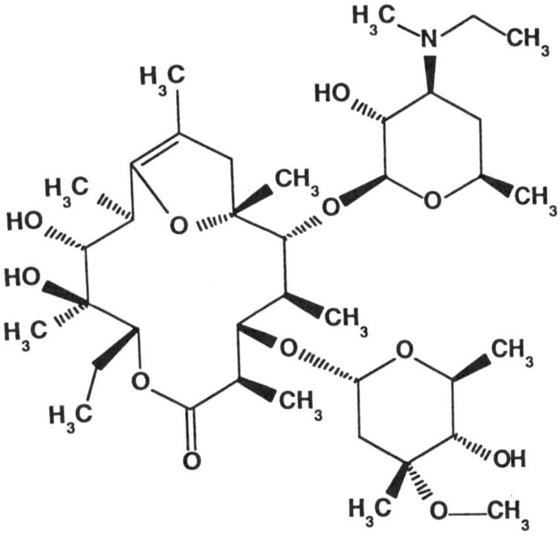

Figure 17 EM-523.

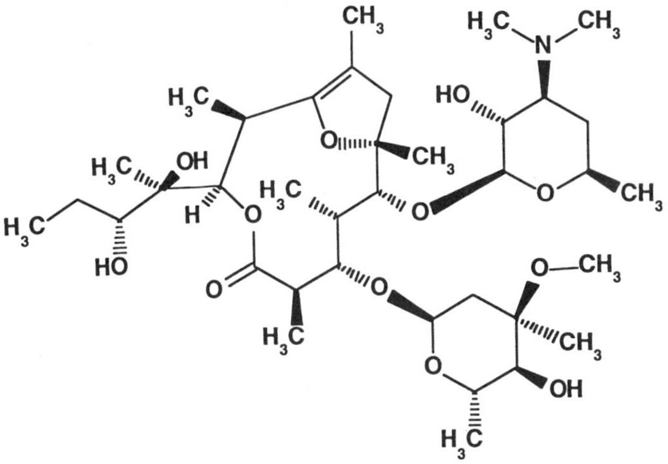

Figure 18 LY 267108.

as josamycin, midecamycin, spiramycin, tylosin, and miokamycin, did not affect gastrointestinal motility.

Glycosidic linkages of the lactone ring were necessary for a structure to exhibit strong contractile activity. Descladinosylerythromycin induces weak and short contractions. Aglycone does not affect gastrointestinal motility (31). The presence of the dimethylamino group on the D-desosamine appeared to be necessary for MMC activity (12). Depoortere et al. (12) have stressed the importance of the configuration at C-6 through C-9 for MMC.

REFERENCES

1. Agen C, Danesi R, Blandizzi C, Costa M, Stacchini B, Favini P, Del Taca M. Macrolide antibiotics as antiinflammatory agents: roxithromycin in an unexpected role. Agents Action 1993; 38:85–90.

2. Bryskier A, Agouridas C, Gasc J-C. Classification of macrolide antibiotic. In: Bryskier AJ, Butzler J-P, Neu HC, Tulkens PM, eds. Macrolides, Chemistry, Pharmacology and Clinical Uses. Paris: Arnette-Blackwell, 1993:5–66.

3. Bryskier A. Newer macrolides and their potential target organisms. Curr Opin Infect Dis 1992; 5:764–772.

4. Bryskier A, Labro MT. Antiparasitic activity of macrolide antibiotics. In: Bryskier AJ, Butzler J-P, Neu HC, Tulkens PM, eds., Macrolides, Chemistry, Pharmacology and Clinical Uses. Paris: Arnette-Blackwell, 1993:307–320.

5. Bryskier A, Agouridas C, Chantot J-F. Macrolides, azalides and streptogramins: structure and activity. In: Neu HC, Young LS, Zinner SH, eds. The New Macrolides, Azalides and Streptogramins, Pharmacology and Clinical Applications. New York: Marcel Dekker, 1993:3–11.

6. Bryskier A, Agouridas C. Azalides: a new medicinal chemical family? Curr Opin Invest Drugs 1993; 2:687–694.

7. Chantot J-F, Bryskier A, Gasc J-C. Antibacterial activity of roxithromycin, a laboratory evaluation. J Antibiot 1986; 39:660–668.

8. Clement JJ, Shipkowitz NL, Swanson PA, Lartey PA, Alder JD. Efficacy of a 9,R,epoxy erythromycin derivative, A-69334 in *Haemophilus influenzae* induced otitis media in gerbils. 30th Interscience Conference on Antimicrobiol Agents and Chemotherapy. Atlanta, 1990: abstr 814.

9. Cohen LS, Wechsler AS, Mitchell JH, Glick G. Depression of cardiac function by streptomycin and other antimicrobial agents. Am J Cardiol 1970; 26:505–511.

10. Colbert WE, Turk JA, Williams PD, Buening MK. Cardiovascular and autonomic pharmacology of the macrolide antibiotic LY 281389 in anesthetized beagles and in isolated smooth and cardiac muscles. Antimicrob Agents Chemother 1991; 35:1365–1369.

11. Dalziel K, Dykes PS, Marks R. The effect of tetracycline and erythromycin in a model of acne-type inflammation. Br J Exp Pathol 1987; 68:67–70.

12. Depoortere I, Peeters TL, Matthijs G, Cachet T, Hoogmartens J, Vantrappen G. Structure activity relation of erythromycin-related macrolides in inducing contractions and in displacing bound motilin in rabbit duodenum. J Gastrointest Motil 1989; 1:150–159.

13. Djokic S, Kobrehel G, Lazarevski G. Antibacterial in vitro evaluation of 10-dihydro-10-deoxo-11-azaerythromycin A:synthesis and structure activity relationship of its acyl derivatives. J Antibiot 1987; 40:1006–1015.

14. Gasc J-C, Gouin d'Ambrières S, Lutz A, Chantot J-F. New ether oxime derivatives of erythromycin A—a structure activity relationship study. J Antibiot 1991; 44:313–330.

15. Hart PH, Whitty GA, Burgess DR, Croatto M, Hamilton J. Augmentation of glucocorticoid action on human monocytes by interleukin-4. Lymphokines Res 1990; 9:147–153.

16. Itoh Z, Ohmura S. Motilide, a new family of macrolide compounds mimicking motilin. Dig Dis Sci 1987; 32:915.

17. Janssens J, Peeters TL, Vantrappen G, Tack J, Urbain JL, De Roo M, Muls E, Bouillon R. Improvement of gastric emptying in diabetic gastroparesis by erythromycin. N Engl J Med 1990; 322:1028–1031.

18. Kirst HA. Expanding the therapeutic potential of macrolide compounds. In: Krohn K, Kirst HA, Maag H, eds. Antibiotics and Antiviral Compounds, Chemical Synthesis and Modifications. New York: VCH, 1993:143–151.

19. Kirst HA. New macrolides: expanded horizons for an old class of antibiotics. J Antimicrob Chemother 1991; 28:787–790.

20. Kita E, Sawaki M, Misaka K, Hamada K, Takeuchi S, Maeda K, Narita N. Alterations of host response by a long-term treatment of roxithromycin. J Antimicrob Chemother 1993; 32:285–294.

21. Kondo Y, Torii K, Omura S, Itoh Z. Erythromycin and its derivatives with motilin-like biological activities inhibit the specific binding of ^{125}I-motilin to duodenal muscle. Biochem Biophys Res Commun 1988; 150:877–882.

22. Labro MT, El Benna J, Abdelghaffar H. Modulation of human polymorphonuclear neutrophil function by macrolides: preliminary data concerning dirithromycin. J Antimicrob Chemother 1993; 31 (suppl C): 51–64.

23. Labro MT, El Benna J, Babin-Chevaye C. Comparison of the in vitro effect of several macrolides on the oxidative burst of human neutrophils. J Antimicrob Chemother 1989; 24:561–572.

24. Labro MT. Interaction of macrolides and quinolones with the host defence system. Eur Bull Drug Res 1993; 2 (suppl 1):7–13.

25. Labro MT, Babin-Chevaye C. Synergistic interaction of josamycin with human neutrophils bactericidal function in vitro. J Antimicrob Chemother 1989; 24:731–740.

26. Lartey PA, De Nino SL, Faghih R, Hardy DJ, Clement JJ, Plattner JJ, Stephens RL. Synthesis and antibacterial activities of C-21 functionalized derivatives of 9(R)-9-amino-9-deoxoerythromycin A. J Med Chem 1991; 34:3390–3395.

27. Mao CH, Putterman M. Intermolecular complex of erythromycin and ribosome. J Mol Biol 1969; 44:347–361.

28. Maring CJ, Klein LL, Pariza RJ, Lartey PA, Grampovnick DJ, Yeung CM, Buytendorp M, Hardy DJ. Synthesis and structure–activity relationships of derivatives of 9(R)-erythromycylamine. 29th Interscience Conference on Antimicrobial Agents and Chemotherapy, Houston. 1989: abstr 1023.

29. McComb JM, Campbell NPS, Cleland J. Recurrent ventricullar tachycardia associated with QT prolongation after mitral valve replacement and its association with intravenous administration of erythromycin. Am J Cardiol 1984; 54:922–923.

30. Misaka K, Kita E, Sawaki M, et al. The antiinflammatory effect of erythromycin in zymozan induced peritonitis of mice. J Antimicrob Chemother 1992; 30:339–348.

31. Nakayashi T, Izumi M, Tatsuta K. Comparison of effects of 14- and 16-membered macrolides on gastrointestinal contractile activity in dogs. 17th International Congress of Chemotherapy, Berlin. 1991.

32. Ohmura S, Tzuzuki K, Sunazuka T, Marui S, Toyoda H, Inatomi N, Itoh Z. Macrolides with gastrointestinal motor stimulating activity. J Med Chem 1987; 30:1941–1943.

33. Plewig G, Schöpf E. Antiinflammatory effects of antimicrobial agents. Drugs 1976; 11:472–473.

34. Tamargo JB, Demiguel B, Tejerima MT. A comparison of josamycin with macrolides and related antibiotics on isolated rat atria. Eur J Pharmacol 1982; 80:285–293.

35. Tarayre JP, Aliaga M, Barbara M, Villanova G, Ballester R, Tisne-Versailles J, Couzinier JP. Cutaneously applied erythromycin base reduces various types of inflammatory reaction in mouse ear. Int J Tissue React 1987; 9:77–85.

36. Vantrappen G, Janssens J, Peeters TL, Bloom SR, Christofides ND, Hellemans J. Motilin and interdigestive migrating motor complex in man. Dig Dis Sci 1979; 24:497–500.

37. Wilkening RR, Ratcliffe RW, Szymonifka MJ, Shankaran K, May AM, Blizzard TA, Heck JV, Herbert CM, Graham AC, Bartizal K. Synthesis and in vitro activities of 9-deoxo-8a-aza-8a homoerythromycin derivatives, a new series of azalide antibiotics. 33rd Interscience Conference on Antimicrobial Agents and Chemotherapy, New Orleans. 1993: abstr 426.

38. Williams JD, Sefton AM. Comparison of macrolide antibiotics. J Antimicrob Chemother 1993; 31(suppl C):11–26.

39. Zhang ZQ, Antzelevitch C. Erythromycin produces prominent action potential prolongation and early after depolarization-induced triggered activity in M but not epicardial and endocardial regions of the canine ventricle. Circulation 1993; 88(suppl):1753.

40. Jones AB, Herbert CM. J. Antibiotics, 1992; 45:1785–1791.

41. Neu, HC. In: Bryskier AJ, Butzler J-P, Neu HC, Tulkens PM eds., Macrolides, chemistry, pharmacology and clinical uses. Paris: Arnette-Blackwell, 1993, 167–182.

42. Logan MN, et al. J Antimicrob Chemother, 1991; 27:161–170.

43. Hunt E, et al. J. Antibiotics, 1988; 41:1644–1648.

2

Resistance to Macrolides, Azalides, and Streptogramins

Roland Leclercq

Hôpital Henri Mondor
Créteil, France

Patrice Courvalin

Institut Pasteur
Paris, France

INTRODUCTION

Macrolides, which include 14- and 16-membered lactone ring molecules, azalides, lincosamides, and streptogramins (MLS), are chemically distinct, but related by their mechanism of action (inhibition of protein synthesis) and their narrow spectrum of activity. Intrinsic resistance of gram-negative bacilli to macrolides is probably owing to relative impermeability of the cellular outer membrane to these hydrophobic compounds (Table 1). However, azithromycin expands the traditional spectrum of activity of macrolides: this drug contains a nitrogen inserted in the lactone ring, which contributes to improved activity against gram-negative bacteria, in particular *Haemophilus* spp.

BIOCHEMICAL MECHANISM AND GENETIC BASIS OF RESISTANCE

Acquired resistance to MLS antibiotics involves three mechanisms (3,4): modification of the target of the drugs, inactivation, and active efflux of the

Table 1   Intrinsic MLS Resistance

Gram-negative bacilli (except *Campylobacter*, *Legionella*, and *Haemophilus*)
Enterococci (lincosamides and streptogramins A)

antibiotics. In the first type of resistance, a single alteration in 23S ribosomal RNA confers broad cross-resistance to macrolides, azalides, lincosamides, and streptogramin B-type antibiotics (the so-called MLS phenotype), whereas the two other types confer resistance to structurally related antibiotics only. The MLS phenotype emerged in 1956 in staphylococci a few years after the introduction of erythromycin for therapy and, since then, has spread in numerous bacterial genera. This phenotype accounts for nearly all the resistant strains isolated in clinical practice. Modification of the target of the antibiotics by posttranscriptional methylation of 23S rRNA causes cross-resistance to these drugs, probably because their binding sites overlap (6). Streptogramin A-type antibiotics are unaffected, and synergy between the two components of streptogramins against MLS-resistant strains is maintained. Certain modifications of hydroxyl groups on the lactone ring of macrolides can lead to improved activity against erythromycin-resistant organisms. However, these new compounds do not completely overcome resistance.

Ribosomal methylation is due to a minimum of eight classes of erythromycin resistance methylase (*erm*) genes. The determinants representative of these classes have been detected in soil bacteria (*Bacillus*), antibiotic producers (*Streptomyces* and *Arthrobacter*), and human pathogens, *Staphylococcus aureus* (*ermA*), *Streptococcus sanguis* (*ermAM*), *Staph. aureus* (*ermC*), and *Bacteroides fragilis* (*ermF*). Comparison of the amino acid sequences of the methylases encoded by these genes revealed that they are structurally related. These determinants are spread in human pathogens. A particular class of genes can be predominantly associated with a bacterial species, although there are exceptions owing to horizontal gene transfer. In particular, the streptococcal *ermAM* gene is widely spread in streptococci, but is not confined to this genus (Table 2). For example, homologous genes were detected several years ago in *Staph. aureus* borne by transposon Tn*551* and, recently, in *Clostridium perfringens* (*ermP*) and in *Escherichia coli* (*ermBC*). This last finding constitutes evidence for recent in vivo transfer of genetic material from gram-positive cocci to gram-negative bacteria.

In staphylococci, expression of MLS resistance may be constitutive or inducible by 14-membered ring macrolides and azalides, depending on the regulatory region upstream from the structural gene for the methylase. Regulation of expression of the *ermC* determinant from staphylococcal plasmid pE194 has been extensively studied and is explained by a translation attenuation mechanism

Table 2 Distribution of *erm* Determinants in Bacteria

Gene	Bacterial species
ermA	*Staphylococcus* spp.
ermAM	Streptococci (*S. sanguis*, pneumococci: Tn*1545*, streptococci groups A and B)
	Enterococcus faecalis
	Pediococcus acidilactici
	Staphylococcus aureus (*ermB*: Tn*551*)
	Escherichia coli (*ermBC*)
	Klebsiella pneumoniae
	Clostridium perfringens (*ermP*)
	Lactobacillus reuteri
ermC	*Staphylococcus spp.*
	Bacillus subtilis
	Lactobacillus reuteri (*ermGT*)
ermF	*Bacteroides fragilis*, *B. ovatus*

(for reviews see Refs. 1,2,5). Adjacent to the *ermC* structural gene for the methylase is an open-reading frame, encoding a 14-amino acid control peptide (Fig. 1). Both genes are cotranscribed in a single mRNA. The 5′-end of this mRNA presents a set of four inverted repeats that sequester, by base-pairing in the absence of erythromycin, the ribosomal-binding site and the initiation codon for the methylase. When present, erythromycin binds to ribosomes, including those involved in synthesis of the control peptide, and causes them to stall.

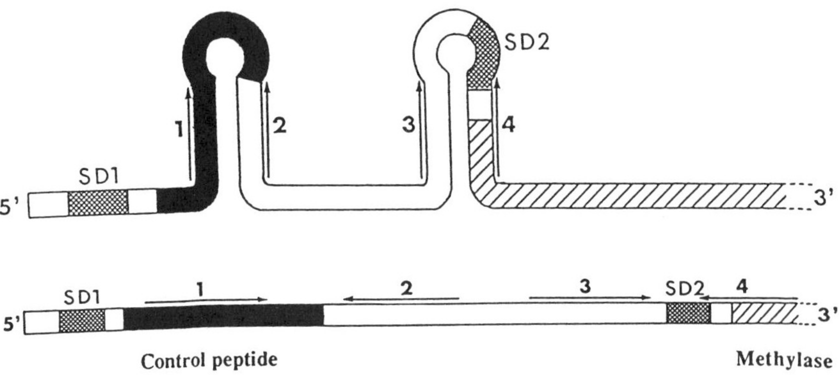

Figure 1 mRNA from *ermC* (pE194) of *S. aureus*. The top drawing is a putative secondary structure. ■ Sequence of the control peptide. ▨ Sequence of the methylase. 1–4, inverted repeats; SD1, SD2, ribosome-binding sites.

Ribosomal stalling probably induces conformational rearrangements in the mRNA and causes displacement of the stem–loop structure (Fig. 2). Because they are free, initiation sequences can then be recognized by ribosomes for translation of the methylase. Activation of mRNA is followed by an increase in its half-life that enhances enzyme synthesis. In this model, regulation is partly due to a methylation-mediated feedback: when all the ribosomes are methylated, stalling does not occur, and mRNA molecules return to the inactive conformation.

Regulation at the level of translation has also been demonstrated: the *ermC*-encoded methylase, when in excess, may bind to the ribosomal-binding site for the methylase, partly blocking its own production (Fig. 3). Specificity of induction is thought to be re, partly blocking its own production (Fig. 3). Specificity of induction is thought to be related to the mode of action of the various macrolides: noninducer macrolides could provoke a premature release or inappropriate stalling of the ribosomes that would not allow mRNA to refold into an active structure. Constitutive expression can be obtained from inducible strains at frequencies of 10^{-7}–10^{-8} by selection on agar plates containing inhibitory concentrations of noninducer macrolide, azalide, lincosamide, or streptogramin B-type antibiotics. Both in these in vitro mutants and in clinical isolates,

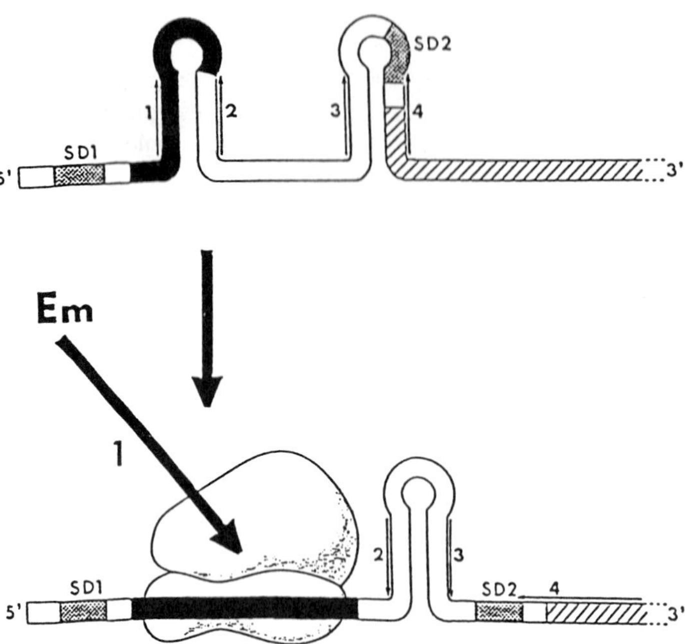

Figure 2 Schematic representation of conformational rearrangements following ribosomal stalling in mRNA from *ermC* (pE194). Em, erythromycin.

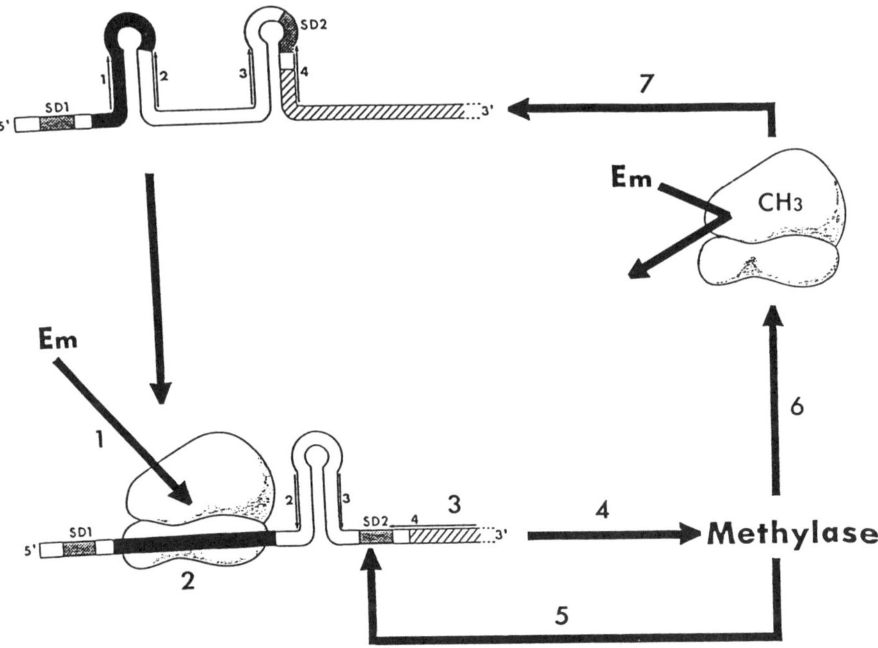

Figure 3 Triple posttranscriptional control of methylase synthesis: 4, increase in the half-life of mRNA; 5, binding of methylase to the ribosome-binding site for the methylase; 6,7, methylation-mediated feedback.

constitutive MLS resistance is also explained by the structure of the regulatory region where deletions, duplications, or direct tandem duplications of repeated segments are observed.

The MLS resistance in streptococci can also be expressed constitutively or inducibly. However, unlike staphylococci, various macrolides or lincosamides may act as inducers. In *Strep. sanguis*, the peculiar features of induction are explained by the complex conformation of the regulatory region upstream from the *ermAM* gene. Constitutive expression of the *erm* determinant of pAMβ1 is explained by deletions in regulatory regions, similar to staphylococci.

The microorganisms can also be resistant to MLS by two other mechanisms: modification of the drugs or active efflux (4,5). Three major MLS-inactivating enzymes have been characterized (Table 3). First, certain enterobacteria inactivate the lactone ring of 14-membered macrolides by production of erythromycin esterases or of a macrolide 2′-phosphotransferase. The 16-membered macrolides are not efficiently utilized as substrates by these enzymes. Two types, I (349 amino acids) and II (419 amino acids), of esterases encoded by *ereA* and *ereB*

Table 3   MLS Resistance by Inactivation

Enzyme	Gene	Host	Ref.
Erythromycin esterase			
Type I	*ereA*	*Escherichia coli*	7
Type II	*ereB*	*E. coli*	8
Macrolide 2′-phosphotransferase		*E. coli*	9
3-Lincomycin, 4-clindamycin	*linA*	*Staphylococcus haemolyticus*	10
O-nucleotidyltransferase	*linA′*	*S. aureus*	
Streptogramin A *O*-acetyltransferase	*vat*	*S. aureus*	11
Streptogramin A *O*-acetyltransferase	*sat*	*Enterococcus faecium*	13
Streptogramin B hydrolase	*vgb*	*S. aureus*	12

(erythromycin resistance esterase) genes, respectively, were found. Second, a plasmid-mediated 3-lincomycin, 4-clindamycin *O*-nucleotidyltransferase (LNT; 3,4) confers resistance to lincosamides in staphylococci. Third, streptogramin A *O*-acetyltransferases in *Enterococcus faecium* and in *Staph. aureus* and a streptogramin B hydrolase in *Staph. aureus*, respectively, are responsible for the inactivation of factors A and B of the streptogramin complex. Active efflux has been reported in *Staph. epidermidis*. The strains harboring the *msrA* (macrolide streptogramin resistance) gene are inducibly resistant to 14-membered ring macrolides, azalides, and streptogramin B-type antibiotics (MS phenotype). Analysis of the sequence of the gene responsible for this resistance suggested that it encodes an ATP-binding protein that functions as a drug efflux pump. The *vga* gene (virginiamycin A), which confers resistance to streptogramin A components, has recently been sequenced (14). The homology of the deduced amino acid sequence with those of proteins acting as ATP-binding efflux pumps suggested that active efflux was responsible for resistance. The overall MLS resistance in staphylococci is shown in Table 4.

EPIDEMIOLOGY OF MLS RESISTANCE DETERMINANTS IN GRAM-POSITIVE COCCI

The Spread of *erm* Genes

Resistance to erythromycin emerged in 1956 in staphylococci, a few years after introduction of the drug in therapy and, since then, has spread in numerous bacterial genera. As developed in the foregoing, the major mechanism of MLS resistance involves modification of the ribosomal target of the antibiotics by methylation and causes cross-resistance to these drugs, the so-called MLS_B

Table 4 Types of MLS Resistance in Staphylococci

Mechanism	Genotype	Ery[a]	16-Mac	Lin	Cli	SgB	SgA	Sg
Target modification	*erm*$_i$[b]	R[c]	S	S	S	S	S	S
	erm$_c$[b]	R	R	R	R	R	S	s
Drug inactivation	*linA*	S	S	R	s	S	S	S
	saa-sbh (*vat-vgb*)	S	S	ND[f]	ND	R	R	R
Active efflux	*msrA*[d]	R	S	S	S	S[e]	S	S
	vga	S	S	ND	ND	S	R	R

Ery, erythromycin; 16-Mac, 16-membered macrolides; Lin, lincomycin; Cli, clindamycin; SgB, streptogramins B-type (pristinamycin factor I, virginiamycin factor S); SgA, streptogramins A-type (pristinamycin factor II, virginiamycin factor M); Sg, streptogramins.
[a]Interpretation for erythromycin is valid for other 14-membered macrolides (clarithromycin) and for azalides (azithromycin).
[b]Subscripts: i, inducible; c, constitutive.
[c]R, resistant; S, susceptible; s, diminished susceptibility to bacteriostatic or bactericidal activity; I, intermediate.
[d]Detected in coagulase-negative staphylococci only.
[e]Resistant after induction by erythromycin.
[f]ND, not determined.

phenotype. This mechanism is due to different classes of *erm* genes. The genes are borne by a variety of elements in staphylococci, enterococci, and streptococci, some of which, such as Tn*1545*, have the remarkable capacity to disseminate horizontally between phylogenetically remote bacterial genera, including transfer from gram-positive to gram-negative hosts (15; Poyart C, et al., unpublished data). In *Staph. aureus*, the incidence of erythromycin resistance ranges from 1 to 50%, depending on local variations. However, resistance is higher in methicillin-resistant strains (>90%). In staphylococci, the presence of *ermA* in the chromosome, borne by the transposon Tn*554*, and of *ermC* on small plasmids appears responsible for erythromycin resistance in most methicillin-resistant and methicillin-susceptible strains, respectively (16). These two determinants are also detected in coagulase-negative strains (16).

So far, in the various species of *Streptococcus*, only genes related to *ermAM* have been detected in macrolide-resistant strains (3). However, lack of hybridization of total DNA of certain of these bacteria with a probe specific for the *ermAM* gene suggests that other determinants, distant from the *ermAM* class, could be involved in resistance. In pneumococci, various frequencies of erythromycin resistance are reported, depending on the country. This type of resistance is currently emerging in the United States, reported with an increasing frequency in Spain, and has reached a minimum of 25–30% of the isolates in France, Israel, and central Europe over the past several years. The *ermAM* gene encoding this resistance is part of the conjugative transposon Tn*1545*. Epidemiological studies have shown that Tn*1545*-like transposons have spread in 50 strains of pneumococci isolated in France (17). The genetic events that lead to the spread of macrolide resistance in pneumococci are probably complex. Horizontal transfer of genes followed by homologous recombination has been reported in pneumococci and this mechanism has been involved in the dissemination of resistance to β-lactams (18). The respective roles of this latter mechanism and of the spread of a conjugative transposon in the evolution of macrolide resistance in pneumococci have not been assessed.

In contrast, erythromycin resistance is usually rare in *Strep. pyogenes*. The resistance determinant is borne, alone or associated with that for chloramphenicol resistance, by large (25- to 30-kb), conjugative plasmids, with a broad host range. In addition, a composite chromosomal transposon, Tn*3701* encoding resistance to erythromycin and tetracycline has been characterized in the genome of plasmid-free *Strep. pyogenes* A454 (19). In Finland, the recent increase of erythromycin resistance to 24% of *Strep. pyogenes* isolated from blood cultures in 1990 was related to the dissemination of several bacterial clones, as suggested by distinct DNA restriction fragment length polymorphism and serotypes of the strains (20). However, the role of plasmids or of transposons in the spread of this type of resistance has not been investigated.

In enterococci, macrolide resistance determinants are borne by various large plasmids that confer resistance to macrolides only or also to chloramphenicol, aminoglycosides, or glycopeptides (for a review, see Ref. 21). On certain of these plasmids, the *ermAM* determinant is part of transposon Tn*917* (22). The presence of this element on large plasmids in the bowels of pigs has been correlated with feeding of tylosin, a 16-membered macrolide, to these animals (23). Similar plasmids are found in the digestive tract of humans. The enterococci could constitute a reservoir of *erm* genes in both humans and animals.

The Efflux Genes

The two genes responsible for antibiotic efflux, *msrA* and *vgA*, have been characterized in staphylococci to which they have so far been confined. The *msrA* gene conferring resistance to 14- and 15-membered macrolides is spread in coagulase-negative staphylococci (7–10% of isolates), but is rarely found in *Staph. aureus* (24). Hybridization experiments have shown that, in the United Kingdom, this gene is borne by large (30- to 32-kb) plasmids (24). In certain strains, the gene is present together with an *ermC* gene. We found a similar location for the *msrA* determinant in coagulase-negative staphylococci isolated in France (Rosato et al., unpublished data). The *vga* gene mediates resistance by active efflux to the streptogramin A-type antibiotics, which is one of the two components of the streptogramin complex. This gene was originally detected on a large plasmid in a strain of *Staph. aureus*, in which it was associated with the *vgb* gene, encoding resistance to the streptogramin B-type antibiotics, and with the *vatA* gene, which specifies an acetyltransferase that inactivates the streptogramin A-type compounds (25). Recently, an increase from 1 to 10% in the incidence of streptogramin resistance among strains of *Strep. epidermidis* in a French hospital was, in large part, related to dissemination of an epidemic strain harboring this determinant on a 7.3-kb plasmid (26).

REFERENCES

1. Bachhofer DH. Triple post-transcriptional control. Mol Microbiol 1990; 4:1419–1423.
2. Dubnau D. Translational attenuation: the regulation of bacterial resistance to the macrolide–lincosamide–streptogramin B antibiotics. Crit Rev Biochem 1984; 16:103–132.
3. Leclercq R, Courvalin P. Bacterial resistance to macrolide, lincosamide, and streptogramin antibiotics by target modification. Antimicrob Agents Chemother 1991; 35:1267–1272.
4. Leclercq R, Courvalin P. Intrinsic and unusual resistance to macrolide, lincosamide, and streptogramin antibiotics in bacteria. Antimicrob Agents Chemother 1991; 35:1273–1276.
5. Weisblum B. Inducible resistance to macrolides, lincosamides and streptogramin type B antibiotics: the resistance phenotype, its biological diversity, and structural element that regulate expression—a review. J Antimicrob Chemother 1985; 16(suppl A):63–90.
6. Fernandez-Munoz R, et al. Substrate- and antibiotic-binding sites at the peptidyl-transferase centre of *Escherichia coli* ribosomes: studies on the chloramphenicol, lincomycin and erythromycin sites. Eur J Biochem 1971; 23:185–193.
7. Ounissi H, Courvalin P. Nucleotide sequence of the gene *ereA* encoding the erythromycin esterase in *Escherichia coli*. Gene 1985; 35:271–278.
8. Arthur M, et al. Analysis of the nucleotide sequence of the *ereB* gene encoding the erythromycin esterase type II. Nucleic Acids Res 1986; 14:4987–4999.
9. O'Hara K, et al. Purification and characterization of macrolide 2′-phosphotransferase from a strain of *Escherichia coli* that is highly resistant to erythromycin. Antimicrob Agents Chemother 1989; 33:1354–1357.
10. Brisson-Noël A, et al. Inactivation of lincosaminide antibiotics in *Staphylococcus*. J Biol Chem 1988; 263:15880–15887.
11. Le Goffic F, et al. Plasmid-mediated pristinamycin resistance: PH1A, a pristinamycin 1A hydrolase. Ann Microbiol (Inst Pasteur) 1977; 128:471–474.
12. Allignet J, et al. Nucleotide sequence of a staphylococcal plasmid gene, *vgb*, encoding a hydrolase inactivating the B components of virginiamycin-like antibiotics. Plasmid 1988; 20:271–275.
13. Rende-Foumier R, et al. Identification of the *satA* gene encoding a

streptogramin A acetyltransferase in *Enterococcus faecium* BM4145. Antimicrob Agents Chemother 1993; 37:2119–2125.

14. Allignet J, et al. Sequence of a staphylococcal plasmid gene, *vga*, encoding a putative ATP-binding protein involved in resistance to virginiamycin A-like antibiotics. Gene 1992; 117:45–51.

15. Courvalin P. Transfer of antibiotic resistance genes between gram positive and gram negative bacteria. Antimicrob Agents Chemother 1994; 38:1447–1451.

16. Thakker-Varia S, et al. Molecular epidemiology of macrolides–lincosamides–streptogramin B resistance in *Staphylococcus aureus* and coagulase-negative staphylococci, Antimicrob Agents Chemother 1987; 31:735–743.

17. Poyart-Salmeron C, et al. Nucleotide sequences specific for Tn*1545*-like conjugative transposons in pneumococci and staphylococci resistant to tetracycline. Antimicrob Agents Chemother 1991; 35:1657–1660.

18. Spratt BG. Resistance to antibiotics mediated by target alterations. Science 1994; 264:388–393.

19. Le Bouguénec C, et al. Molecular analysis of a composite chromosomal conjugative element (Tn*3701*) of *Streptococcus pyogenes*. J Bacteriol 1988; 170:3930–3936.

20. Seppälä H, et al. Resistance to erythromycin in group A streptococci. N Engl J Med 1992; 326:292–297.

21. Horaud T, et al. Molecular genetics of resistance to macrolides, lincosamides and streptogramin B (MLS) in streptococci. J Antimicrob Chemother 1985; 16:111–135.

22. Tomich PK, et al. Properties of erythromycin-inducible transposon Tn*917* in *Streptococcus faecalis*. J Bacteriol 1980; 141:1366–1374.

23. Dunny, et al. Effects of antibiotics in animal feed on the antibiotic resistance of the gram positive bacterial flora of animals and man. In: Levy SB, Clowes RC, Koenig EL, eds. Molecular Biology, Pathogenicity and Ecology of Bacterial Plasmids, 1981.

24. Ross J, et al. Characterisation and molecular cloning of the novel macrolide–streptogramin B resistance determinant from *Staphylococcus epidermidis*. J Antimicrob Chemother 1989; 24:851–862.

25. Dublanchet A, et al. Résistance de *S. aureus* aux streptogramines. Ann Microbiol (Inst Pasteur) 1977; 128A:277–287.

26. Loncle V, et al. Analysis of pristinamycin-resistant *Staphylococcus epidermidis* isolates responsible for an outbreak in a Parisian hospital. Antimicrob Agents Chemother 1993; 37:2159–2165.

3

Clinical Epidemiology of Resistance to Macrolides

Jacques F. Acar and Fred W. Goldstein
Laboratoire de Microbiologie Médicale
Hôpital Saint-Joseph
Paris, France

With the increasing number of antibiotics and the establishment of antibiotic resistance traits in all human pathogens, the clinical epidemiology of antibiotic resistance has become an important problem. The surveillance of antibiotic susceptibility patterns in bacteria is now routine in many hospital laboratories: the prevalence of resistant strains to a particular compound or class, the resistance pattern, the use of such information in a place and at a time to direct the choice of first-line therapy, and to actualize antibiotic policy are well known. However, most information is patchy or missing when one attempts to compare countries, to look at pathogens in community-acquired infections and to understand or predict changes occurring over time (21).

New C_{14} macrolides have overcome many shortcomings of erythromycin, but resistance mechanisms affect them in a way similar to erythromycin. Azalides also share the cross-resistance pattern with erythromycin. Streptogramins have two components that act synergistically, and these may be active against macrolide-resistant strains (4,5,14). The prevalence of resistance in the major bacterial species included in the spectrum of macrolides, azalides, and streptogramins will be reviewed in this report.

Resistance in *Staphylococcus aureus* was recognized in 1953 (28). A clear-cut difference between hospital and community isolates has been shown in several papers. Early on, the prevalence of resistance in hospitals was greater than 25% (up to 70%), contrasting with 3% in the community. In the 1960s, the recognition in hospitals of methicillin-resistant *S. aureus* (MRSA) and their frequent resistance to macrolides confirmed this difference. The prevalence of macrolide resistance in MRSA is greater than 40% (up to 95%). In methicillin-susceptible *S. aureus* (MSSA), 5–14% of strains were macrolide-resistant (4,14,24). In many reports, MRSA and MSSA are not separated and the prevalence of erythromycin-resistant *S. aureus* is then between 20 and 40% (17,26,28). There are also geographic variations in resistance, often reported in relation to the level of macrolide consumption. Trends toward increased or decreased resistance have been observed clearly in parallel with changes in drug consumption (4,24,26).

When comparing staphylococcal resistance phenotypes to C_{14} and C_{16} macrolides, azalides, and streptogramins, three frequent patterns are observed (Table 1) out of a possible six. Interestingly, in 1994, resistance to streptogramins is extremely rare (5). Coagulase- and DNase-negative staphylococci share the same resistance phenotypes as *S. aureus*. Hospital epidemics of coagulase-negative staphylococci resistant to macrolides, azalides, lincosamides, and streptogramins have been recently reported (5,15).

In *Streptococcus pneumoniae*, resistance to erythromycin was recognized in 1967 (1,2); however, the prevalence of resistant strains became a limiting factor in empirical therapy decisions only in the 1980s. France, Hungary, Belgium, Spain, South Africa, and the United States reported resistant strains ranging from 10 to 50% (7,14). From reports that studied the incidence of resistant strains for 5 or more years, the following points can be made:

1. The increase of resistance to macrolides developed unevenly; annual epidemic strains were sometimes susceptible, sometimes resistant.
2. Macrolide-resistance was most frequent in serotypes related to pneumococcal carriage (serotypes 19, 14, 6, 23; Fig. 1). The prevalence of resistant strains was extremely different from country to country: for example, France, with

Table 1 Staphylococcal Resistance Phenotypes

Types	14-Memb.	15-Memb.	16-Memb.	CII (B)	CII (A)	Streptobg[c] (I + II)
1	S	S	S	S	S	S
2[a]	R	R	S	S	S	S
3[b]	R	R	R	R	S	S

[a]Indicuble type.
[b]Constitutive type.
[c]Resistance to streptogramins CI and CII rarely exist alone; in a few strains it is combined with the constitutive type of macrolide resistance.

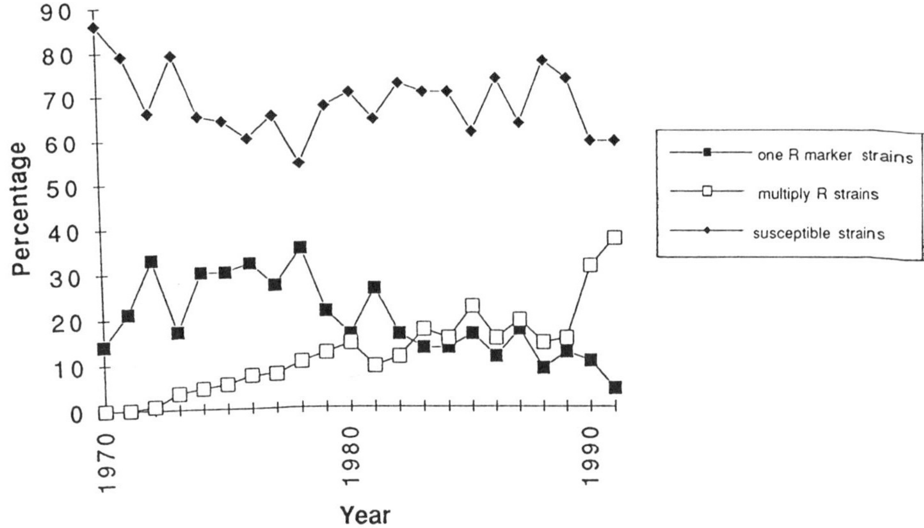

Figure 1 Broussais and Saint-Joseph Hospitals pneumococci resistance patterns 1970–1993.

10–15% compared with United Kingdom and the Netherlands, with 1% erythromycin resistance (14). Resistance to macrolides tends to merge with other resistance traits; it is present in 80% of multiple resistant strains (with penicillin G and tetracycline; personal data; Fig. 2).

Pneumococcal resistance to macrolides is shared equally by C_{14} and C_{16}, macrolides and azalides. These strains remain susceptible to the streptogramins.

Until the Japanese studies (18,20) in the 1970s that reported a large number of group A streptococci resistant to macrolides (15, 23, and 62%), this resistance was considered rare. Of the thousands of strains tested between 1959 and 1970 in the United Kingdom and Canada few strains were resistant (3,23,29). However, since 1980, epidemics have been reported in Australia, United Kingdom, and Finland, with an incidence of 17.6, 22.5, and 13.3% of macrolide-resistant strains, respectively (10,22,27,30). The main difference between the Japanese studies in 1975 and the Finnish multiregional study in 1990 was that primarily one serotype was found in Japan, whereas in Finland, eight serotypes were reported. This phenomenon might represent the horizontal spread of a mobile genetic element.

In non-group A streptococci and nongroupable viridans streptococci, resistance to erythromycin has been reported in only a few studies. Macrolides

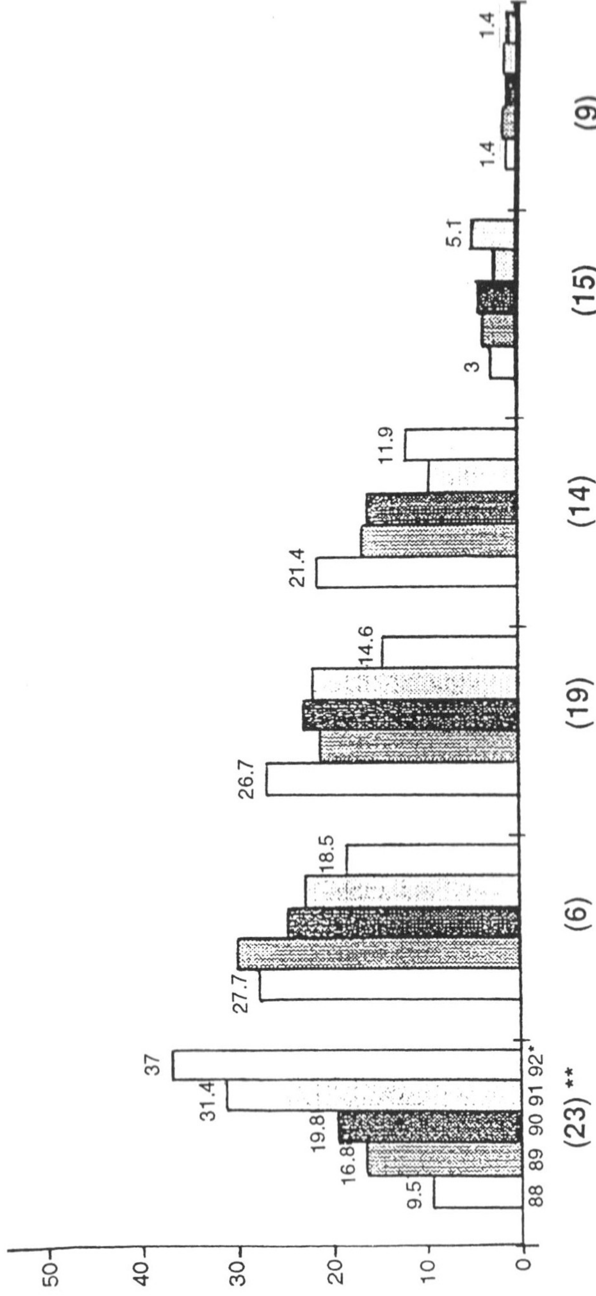

Figure 2 Centre National de Référence des Pneumocoques: Incidence of erythromycin resistance in *S. pneumoniae*: relation with serotype and years (1988–1992) (7608 strains tested). *, years; ** ( ), serotypes.

have been considered of limited importance in the treatment of streptococcal endocarditis or *S. agalactiae* infections. In general, this resistance remains lower than 2% except for one reported study (29). Although the number of studies are limited, macrolide resistance in streptococci is shared with the azalides, but not with the streptogramins.

Enterococci have recently become a major therapeutic concern because of their multiple antibiotic resistance. However, resistance was actually high in the 1970s, as reported by Moellering (19); more than 50% of the strains were resistant. Similar results were found by Duval (4). In recent studies (15,28), all multiple resistant enterococcal strains were resistant to the macrolides.

Susceptibility of anaerobes to macrolides has been interpreted variably. The lack of standardized technical conditions is probably responsible for the noncomparable results among studies. The number of resistant strains may, in fact, be overestimated (25). In the *Bacteroides fragilis* group, studies in the 1980s from the United States, United Kingdom, France, and Spain reported an incidence of resistance ranging from 1 to 8% of the strains. These resistance mechanisms are shared with clindamycin, and C_{15} and C_{16} macrolides. Although streptogramins have rarely been tested, they seem active against most macrolide-resistant strains. Clostridia species, and particularly *Clostridium difficile*, have been repeatedly reported as resistant. Few resistant strains were found among *Fusobacterium*, *Peptococcus*, or *Prevotella* species. Macrolide resistance was not observed in the actinomyces group.

The susceptibility of *Haemophilus influenzae* to macrolides is a controversial subject because the range of minimum inhibitory concentrations (MICs) is broad and overlaps the three zones: susceptible, intermediate, and resistant. Different breakpoints applied in different studies change the percentage of susceptible, intermediate, and resistant strains. The greatest proportion fall in the intermediate zone (Fig. 3). These histograms encompass apparently homogenous populations. Importantly, no strain has been reported with a high MIC (> 8–16 μg/ml for erythromycin) (6,12,13,16). It is obvious that using different breakpoints will generate different frequencies of resistant strains, depending on the cut of the distribution. Such epidemiological results are not comparable. Clinical or experimental studies should preferably define a type of "in vivo" breakpoint. Data on this subject are quite limited and investigators need to improve and standardize methods for testing susceptibility of *Haemophilus* to document tentative breakpoints with experimental and clinical studies, and to assess bacteriological outcome.

Among other species susceptible to macrolides, azalides, and streptogramins, it is of some interest to mention that resistance has been reported in few strains of *Nocardia asteroides* and *Listeria monocytogenes* (8,31). *Corynebacterium* JK and D_2, are mostly resistant to macrolides (11). Further

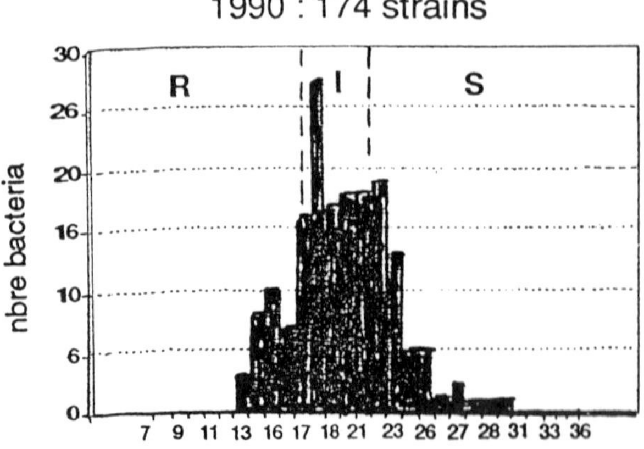

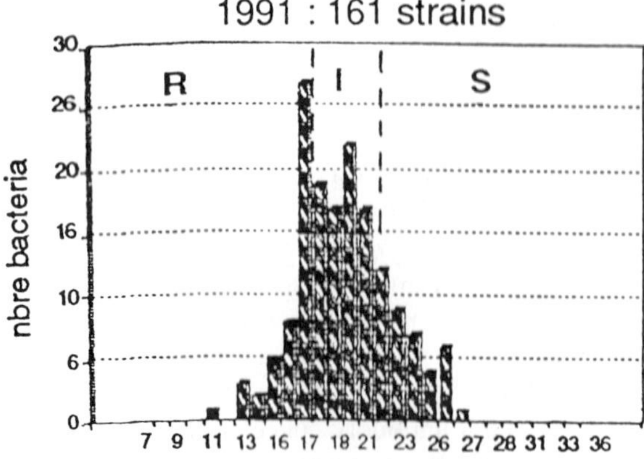

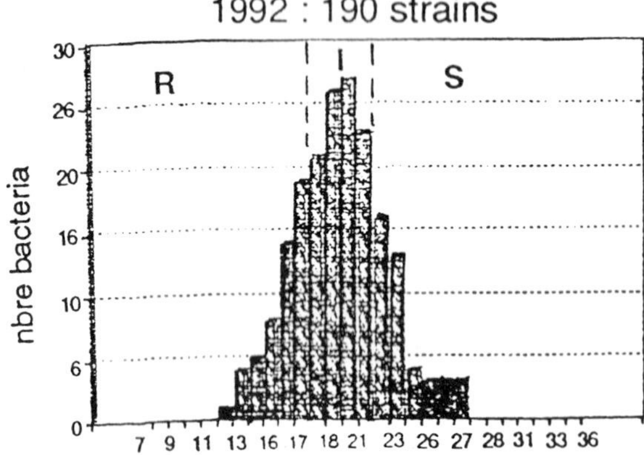

Figure 3 Hôpital Saint-Joseph, Paris, France: Zone size histograms: *Haemophilus influenzae* and erythromycin.

46

studies of macrolide-resistant *C. xerosis*, *C. diphtheriae*, and *Rhodococcus equi* are of interest.

Resistance of *Campylobacter jejuni* varies from 2.4 to 11% in studies collected from 1984 to 1991. *Campylobacter coli* are often reported as more resistant than *Campylobacter jejuni* (28). *Mycobacterium avium* has become an important target for macrolide treatment. Development of acquired resistance under therapy has been demonstrated and this highlights the need for more studies on combined therapy (9).

For many years resistance to macrolides in community-acquired infections was considered to be very infrequent. In fact, susceptibility testing of bacteria, such as *Strep. pneumoniae* or *Strep. pyogenes* were often not performed. The high incidence in some cities or countries of macrolide resistance in these and other bacteria should stimulate better surveys of the occurrence and evolution of antibiotic resistance in general.

REFERENCES

1. Appelbaum PC. World-wide development of antibiotic resistance in pneumococci. Eur J Clin Microbiol 1987; 6:367–377.
2. Cherubin CE, Azabache DB. While nearly no one was watching: the rise of erythromycin and clindamycin resistance in *Streptococcus pneumoniae* and *Streptococcus pyogenes*. Antimicrob Newslett 1992; 8:1–8.
3. Dixon JMS, Lipinski AE. Infections with β-hemolytic *Streptococcus* resistant to lincomycin and erythromycin and observations on zonal-pattern resistance to lincomycin. J Infect Dis 1974; 130:351–356.
4. Duval J. Evolution and epidemiology of MLS resistance. J Antimicrob Chemother 1985; 16(suppl A):137–149.
5. El Solh N, Allignet J, Loncle V, Aubert S, Casetta A, Morvan A. Actualités sur les staphylocoques résistants aux synergistines (pristinamycine). Lett Infectiol 1993; 8:608–615.
6. Geslin P, Buu-Hoi AY, Frémaux A, Acar JF. Antimicrobial resistance in *Streptococcus pneumoniae*: an epidemiological survey in France, 1970–1990. Clin Infect Dis 1992; 15:95–98.
7. Goldstein FW, Emirian MF, Coutrot A, Acar JF. Bacteriostatic and bactericidal activity of azithromycin against *Haemophilus influenzae*. J Antimicrob Chemother 1990; 25:25–28.
8. Hadorn K, Hächler H, Schaffner A, Kayser FH. Genetic characterization of plasmid-encoded multiple antibiotic resistance in strain of *Listeria monocytogenes* causing endocarditis. Eur J Clin Microbiol Infect Dis 1993; 12:928–937.
9. Heifets L, Mor N, Vanderkolk J. *Mycobacterium avium* strains resistant to clarithromycin and azithromycin. Antimicrob Agents Chemother 1993; 37:2364–2370.
10. Holmström L, Nyman B, Rosengren M, Wallander S, Ripa T. Outbreaks

of infections with erythromycin-resistant group A streptococci in child day care centres. Scand J Infect Dis 1990; 22:179–185.

11. Johnson AP, Efstratiou A. *Corynebacterium jeikeium*: a multiresistant nosocomial pathogen. Rev Med Microbiol 1993; 4:242–248.

12. Jones RN, Doern GV, Baker C, Gerlach H, Hindler J. *Haemophilus* test medium (HTM) susceptibility methods: results of evaluations of reproducibility, stability, and medium quality. Antimicrob Newslett 1993; 9:1–8.

13. Jorgensen JH, Doern GV, Maher LA, Howell AW, Redding JS. Antimicrobial resistance among respiratory isolates of *Haemophilus influenzae*, *Moraxella catarrhalis*, and *Streptococcus pneumoniae* in the United States. Antimicrob Agents Chemother 1990; 34:2075–2080.

14. Klugman K. Pneumonococcal resistance in antibiotics. Clin Microbiol Rev 1990; 3:171–196.

15. Leclercq R, Duval J, Courvalin P. Mécanismes et évolution des résistances aux macrolides, lincosamides et streptogramines. In: Pocidalo JJ, Vachon F, Coulaud JP, Vildé JL, eds. Macrolides et Synergistines. Paris: Arnette, 1988:21–40.

16. Machka K, Braveny I, Dabernat H, Dornbusch K, Van Dyck E, Kayser FH, Van Klingeren B, Mittermayer H, Perea E, Powell M. Distribution and resistance patterns of *Haemophilus influenzae*: A European cooperative study. Eur J Clin Microbiol Infect Dis 1988; 7:14–24.

17. Maple PAC, Hamilton-Miller JMT, Brumfitt W. World-wide antibiotic resistance in methicillin-resistant *Staphylococcus aureus*. Lancet 1989; 1:537–540.

18. Mitsuhashi S, Inoue M, Saito K, Nakae M. Drug resistance in *Streptococcus pyogenes* strains isolated in Japan. In: Schlessinger D, ed. Microbiology—1982. Washington, DC: American Society for Microbiology, 1982:151–154.

19. Moellering RC Jr, Krogstad DJ. Antibiotic resistance in enterococci. In: Schlessinger D, ed. Microbiology. Washington, DC: American Society for Microbiology, 1979:293–298.

20. Nakae M, Murai T, Kaneko Y, Mitsuhashi S. Drug resistance in *Streptococcus pyogenes* isolated in Japan (1974–1975). Antimicrob Agents Chemother 1977; 12:427–428.

21. O'Brien TF. Global surveillance of antibiotic resistance. N Engl J Med 1992; 326:339–340.

22. Perez Trallero E, Garcia Arenzana JM, Urbieta Egana M. Erythromycin resistance in streptococci. Lancet 1989; 2:444–445.

23. Phillips G, Parratt D, Orange GV, Harper I, McEwan H, Young N. Erythromycin-resistant *Streptococcus pyogenes*. J Antiomicrob Chemother 1990; 25:723–724.

24. Reverdy ME, Bes M, Brun Y, Fleurette J. Evolution de la résistance aux antibiotiques et aux antiseptiques de souches hospitalières de *Staphylococcus aureus* isolées de 1980 à 1991. Pathol Biol 1993; 41:897–904.

25. Sanchez ML, Jones RN, Croco JL. Use of the E-test to assess macrolide–

lincosamide resistance patterns among *Peptostreptococcus* species. The Antimicrob Newslett 1992; 8:45–49.

26. Schito GC, Varaldo PE. Trends in the epidemiology and antibiotic resistance of clinical *Staphylococcus* strains in Italy—a review. J Antimicrob Chemother 1988; 21(suppl C):67–78.

27. Seppälä H, Nissinen A, Jävinen H, Huovinen S, Henriksson T, Herva E, Holm SE, Jahkola M, Katila M-L, Klaukka T, Kontiainen S, Liimatainen O, Oinonen S, Passi-Metsomaa L, Huovinen P. Resistance to erythromycin in group A streptococci. N Engl J Med 1992; 326:292–297.

28. Shah PM, Bryskier A. Epidemiology of resistance to macrolide antibiotics. In: Bryskier AJ, Butzler JP, Neu HC, Tulkens PM, eds. Macrolides. Paris: Arnette Blackwell, 1993:143–166.

29. Spencer RC, Wheat PF, Magee JT, Brown EH. Erythromycin resistance in streptococci. Lancet 1989; 1:168.

30. Stingemore N, Francis GRJ, Toohey M, McGechie DB. The emergence of erythromycin resistance in *Streptococcus pyogenes* in Fremantle, Western Australia. Med J Aust 1989; 150:626–631.

31. Wallace RJ Jr, Steele LC, Sumter G, Smith JM. Antimicrobial susceptibility patterns of *Nocardia asteroides*. Antimicrob Agents Chemother 1988; 32:1776–1779.

4

Pharmacokinetics of Newer Macrolides

Tom Bergan

Institute of Medical Microbiology
Rikshospitalet
Oslo, Norway

Macrolides have been in clinical use since the 1950s; erythromycin has withstood the challenge from subsequent developments of josamycin, megalomicin, oleandomycin, rokitomycin, and roxithromycin.

Modifications of the erythromycin 14-membered nucleus has rendered derivatives such as clarithromycin, dirithromycin, flurithromycin, lankamycin, megalomicin, and oleandomycin. The first 15-membered nucleus has appeared, azithromycin. Because of its additional methylated nitrogen atom at position 9a within the lactone ring, this is referred to as an azalide. The 16-membered ring structures apply to spiramycin and its subsequent modifications: josamycin, miocamycin, rokitamycin, rosaramicin, turimycin, and tylosin.

Improvements of the biopharmaceutical formulations of erythromycin have resulted in a microencapsulated formulation. Micropellets of the acid-susceptible erythromycin base are individually enteric-coated, to protect the drug from degradation in stomach acid. The microencapsulated formulation is better absorbed than the leading acid-stable salt, the stearate (Josefsson et al., 1982b).

One important aspect of the newer macrolides is the improved pharmacokinetic properties, which will be reviewed in this chapter (the term *macrolide* will also be used to encompass azalide and streptogramins).

SERUM PHARMACOKINETICS

Peak concentrations and total areas under the serum concentration curves of the various macrolides differ. The serum concentrations of most macrolides increase gradually with increasing dose, but by more than would correspond to a multiple of the dose size. This implies a higher bioavailability the higher the dose. Peak concentrations and the time of their occurrence appear in Table 1.

Much interest has centered on serum levels. Thus, for instance, roxithromycin produces much higher serum peaks than the microencapsulated form of the erythromycin base, which results in higher serum concentrations than the erythromycin stearate (Josefsson et al., 1982b). A dose of 150 mg roxithromycin renders maximum serum concentrations of 5.4–7.9 mg/L, compared with peaks of 1.9–3.8 mg/L after 500 mg of the microencapsulated erythromycin base (Kees et al., 1988; Nilsen, 1987). Lower serum levels compared with dose are achieved by azithromycin; although there is no direct comparison of the pharmacokinetics of azithromycin and erythromycin within the same volunteer cohort, they appear to be achieving comparable serum concentrations—at least as far as the least absorbable erythromycin formulations are concerned. Clarithromycin produces serum levels that are intermediate between the higher levels of roxithromycin, on the one hand, and those of azithromycin and erythromycin, on the other.

One aspect of macrolide pharmacokinetics that is often overlooked is the frequent occurrence of double serum peaks after one single dose of the drug. This has been clearly described for both erythromycin and azithromycin (Bergan et al., 1992; Josefsson et al., 1982a,b), but it should also apply to other macrolides. For erythromycin, the second peak may even be considerably larger than the primary serum concentration peak (Josefsson et al., 1982a,b). For azithromycin, the second serum peak is accompanied by a second, and parallel, rise in the concentration in peripheral fluids (human lymph; Bergan et al., 1993). This is because the macrolide is concentrated in bile which is stored within the gallbladder during fasting; the bile is then discharged quantitatively and suddenly when food is consumed. The healthy volunteers included in our studies received the oral dose while fasting and were allowed to eat only after 2–3 h. This stimulates the discharge of bile containing high concentrations of macrolide, leading to subsequent reabsorption from the gut and, consequently, a second serum peak.

This serum concentration pattern has important consequences for pharmacokinetic studies. One consequence of erratic serum concentration courses is that the number of individuals who should be included in studies determining the pharmacokinetics of a macrolide (e.g., healthy, young individuals) should be considerably higher than has been customary. An appropriate number of volunteers would be at least 25, if the statistical predictive force is to be meaningful.

Protein binding of macrolides involves α-$_1$-acid-glycoproteins (Table 2).

Table 1 Concentrations and Time of Occurrence of Serum Peaks of Macrolides

Antibiotic	Dose (mg)	Time to peak (h)	Peak conc. (mg/L)	AUC (mg · h/L)	Ref.
Azithromycin	500	2–3	0.4	6.7	Foulds et al., 1990
Clarithromycin	500	2–3	0.4	18.9	Pechere, 1993
14-OH clarithromycin			0.7	6.0	Pechere, 1993
Dirithromycin	500	4 – 4.5	0.1–0.5		Sides et al., 1993
Erythromycin base	500	1–5	1.9–3.8	5.8–11.2	Nilsen, 1987; Josefsson et al., 1982a
Flurithromycin	500	1–2	1–2	16.0	Pechere, 1993
Josamycin				12	Wildfeuer and Lemme, 1985
Roxithromycin	150	1–3	5.4–7.9	53.0–81.0	Nilsen et al., 1988
	300	1.6	10.8	81.0	Pechere, 1993
Spiramycin	1000			54	Osono et al., 1985

Table 2   Serum Protein Binding of Macrolides

Antibiotic	Concentration (mg/L)	Serum protein binding (%)	Ref.
Azithromycin	0.02–0.05	50	[a]
	0.1	23	[a]
	1.0	7	[a]
Clarithromycin	0.45–4.5	70	[b]
	45	20–40	[b]
Dirithromycin		15–30	Sides, 1993[c]
Erythromycin	1.0	74	Dette and Knothe, 1986
	8.5	65	Dette and Knothe, 1986
Roxithromycin	3.3	96	Nilsen et al., 1988
	8.4	92	Nilsen et al., 1988
Spiramycin		18	Frydman et al., 1988

[a]Azithromycin Clinical Investigator Brochure, 1990.
[b]Data on file, Abbott, Chicago.
[c]Data on file, Eli Lilly, Indianapolis.

Less of the drug is non–protein-bound at higher concentrations with both erythromycin and roxithromycin.

Food does not influence the absorption of the microencapsulated form of erythromycin base (Josefsson et al., 1982a,b), dirithromycin (Sides et al., 1993), or roxithromycin (Segre et al., 1988), but enhances the absorption of erythromycin stearate. Food reduces the absorption of azithromycin and roxithromycin, but has reportedly little consequence for clarithromycin (Puri and Lassman, 1987; Sörgel et al., 1993).

DERIVED PHARMACOKINETIC CHARACTERISTICS

By *derived pharmacokinetic properties* we mean, in particular, serum half-life ($t_{1/2}$) and serum clearance (Table 3).

Considerable interest is appropriately focused on the bioavailability of the macrolides, and this is usually low. The term *bioavailability* is designed to express the amount of drug absorbed. The accepted approach to determining bioavailability is by comparing the total area under the serum concentration vs. time curve (AUC) after the same single dose is given intravenously and orally to a group of healthy volunteers (assuming that oral absorption is in focus). This approach presumes that rapid introduction of the drug intravenously is, indeed, comparable with what occurs when the serum levels increase more gradually after an orally administered dose. Cellular and tissue uptake of some macrolides is both rapid and high; if a major portion of a dose disappears rapidly and almost quantitatively from the serum compartment to the tissue compartment, I suspect

Table 3 Derived Pharmacokinetic Properties of Macrolides

Antibiotic	Dose (mg)	Serum half-life (h)	AUC/ 1 g	Ref.
Azithromycin	1000	44	7.9	Bergan et al., 1992
	500	35–40	6.7	Foulds et al., 1990
	500	54	9.8	Mazzei et al., 1993
Clarithromycin	500	4.9	19	Pechere, 1993
14-OH clarithromycin		7.2	6	Pechere, 1993
Dirithromycin	500	44(16–65)		Sides et al., 1993
Erythromycin base	250	2.0	18	Nilsen, 1987
	500	2.5	22	Nilsen, 1987
	1000	3.0	27	Nilsen, 1987
Flurithromycin	500	8.0	16	Pechere, 1993
Josamycin		1.5–2.5		Wildfeuer and Lemme, 1985
Roxithromycin	150	10.5	54	Nilsen, 1987
	300	11.3	44	Nilsen, 1987
	450	13.8	37	Nilsen, 1987
Spiramycin	1000	3.5–7.0	54	Osono and Umezawa, 1985

[a]Data on file, Eli Lilly, Indianapolis.

that the AUC after an oral dose may appear relatively lower than after an intravenous dose. This would ensue simply because a more gradual appearance in serum after an oral dose enables more of the drug to be transferred to tissues, from the very beginning of the dosage interval, than occurs with an intravenous bolus. This will, undoubtedly, lead to bioavailability underestimates that are proportionate to the degree of macrolide tissue affinity.

Another problem that reduces the precision level of bioavailability assessments of oral doses of macrolides is their erratically occurring, bimodal serum concentration peak profiles. The double peaks are not consistent; they do not appear after every dose, and they differ in size, even in the same individual. Since a second peak increases the total AUC and the recognized method of bioavailability determination consists of computing the ratio of the total AUCs of oral and intravenous doses (in the same subject, after doses of the same sizes), it follows that the outcome involves uncertainties and constraints. Consequently, the published figures for bioavailabilities, which are usually relatively low for macrolides, appear to be rather imprecise estimates.

Bioavailability figures must be viewed in this context. The published value of 37% (Foulds et al., 1990) for azithromycin may very well be a gross underestimate, although the figure was perfectly generated by the method that is currently accepted as appropriate. The algorithm accepted internationally for the determination of bioavailability is more appropriate for drugs that are primarily lodged extracellularly, and thus entails sources of error when a major proportion of the dose is transferred rapidly to cells and tissues, and when an irreproducible and unpredictable double peak occurs in serum, as occurs with drugs that have a sizable enterohepatic circulation, such as the macrolides.

A bioavailability figure of 54% for roxithromycin (Nilsen, 1987) may reflect the lower tissue affinity of roxithromycin compared with the very much higher tissue and cell concentrations of azithromycin. The bioavailability of clarithromycin is 55%, and of erythromycin is 50–70%; these figures correlate well with the intermediate serum levels afforded by these drugs. Published values for spiramycin are rather disparate; consequently, they are difficult to assess.

Notably though, the bioavailability of many macrolides is dose-dependent. Such a pattern has been described for erythromycin (Josefsson et al., 1982a,b; Nilsen, 1987) and roxithromycin (Nilsen, 1987; Puri and Lassmann, 1987; see Table 3). For erythromycin, higher doses are afforded by relatively higher bioavailabilities (AUC per dose unit; see Table 3). Roxithromycin exhibits the opposite pattern, relatively lower serum levels—and bioavailabilities—for higher doses (see Table 3). The pattern points to nonlinear pharmacokinetics for the macrolides.

The nonlinearity is underscored by relatively longer serum half-life values for higher doses of erythromycin and roxithromycin. Why erythromycin and roxithromycin show completely opposite patterns is difficult to say. We may be dealing with saturated mechanisms of absorption, or with inhibition of enzymes involved in metabolic transformation, but also with transfer to cells and with cellular and tissue accumulation. A concentration-dependent serum protein binding may also play a role. The lower the non–protein-bound moiety, the greater will be the effect of changes in serum protein binding; for roxithromycin, the binding is more than 90%, and the free portion is increased by a factor of 3, as the serum level is raised from 3.3 to 8.4 mg/L.

After multiple dosing, increases in both serum half-life and AUC have been described for azithromycin (Foulds et al., 1990; Wildfeuer et al., 1993) and roxithromycin (Puri and Lassman, 1987).

PHARMACOKINETICS IN CHILDREN

The pharmacokinetics of roxithromycin in children resembles the properties described in adults (Bégue et al., 1987; Kafetzis et al., 1988).

PHARMACOKINETICS IN ELDERLY

Roxithromycin exhibits a much longer serum half-life and higher serum concentrations in elderly patients than in young subjects. In the former, the values are two to three times longer than in young subjects (Nilsen et al., 1988; Puri and Lassman, 1987). Whereas steady-state serum concentrations of roxithromycin in the elderly are higher than after the first dose, the serum half-life remains the same (Nilsen et al., 1988). This pattern has been explained by the rather high serum protein binding of roxithromycin for which increased serum levels (in the steady state) are accompanied by a several times higher free drug concentrations and, consequently, result in a higher renal elimination by simple glomerular filtration (Nilsen, 1987).

MODES OF ELIMINATION

Macrolides are metabolized in the liver to a series of biotransformation products (Table 4). These are eliminated in the bile and, thereafter, discharged into the gut. Metabolites also appear in the urine. Renal elimination of the unchanged parent compound accounts for but a minor portion (5–10%) of the dose (see Table 4).

A reduced renal function has a minor effect on the serum half-life of macrolides such as erythromycin (Disse et al., 1986) and azithromycin (Höffler et al., 1992). Roxithromycin elimination, in contrast, is significantly slower in patients with severely reduced renal function. Thus, one study reported a serum half-life in healthy subjects of 10.5 h and in patients with renal failure of 17.9 h, with respective AUCs of 81 mg·h/L and 211 mg·h/L (Periti and Mazzei, 1987).

Renal clearances of azithromycin, clarithromycin, and spiramycin have been described as 150, 180, and 144 ml/min, respectively (Sörgel et al., 1993). Given these observations that the total renal clearance exceeds the glomerular filtration rate, it has been proposed that active tubular secretion of the relevant metabolites may occur, possibly by the proximal tubular base transport system (Sörgel et al., 1993). If that is true, then the considerably lower renal clearances of 35 ml/min for erythromycin and 6 ml/min for roxithromycin (Sörgel et al., 1993) may, at least partly, be due to renal tubular reabsorption.

Alcoholic liver cirrhosis increases the serum half-life of erythromycin (Hall et al., 1982). Roxithromycin serum half-life is not increased in either subjects with severely reduced renal function (Tremblay et al., 1988b) or in those with impaired hepatic capacity (Lebrec et al., 1988). Azithromycin elimination

Table 4 Metabolites of Macrolides

Dirithromycin: erythromycylamine (Sides et al., 1993)
Roxithromycin: decladinose roxithromycin, *N*-monodemethylated
  roxithromycin, *N*-didemethylated roxithromycin (Puri and
  Lassmann, 1987)

---

half-life is unaffected by hepatic cirrhosis (Mazzei et al., 1993). The same has been described for dirithromycin (LaBreque et al., 1993).

TISSUE PENETRATION

One of the distinctive properties of the macrolides generally is that they tend to accumulate in granulocytes, macrophages, and tissue cells. Levels in tissues and leukocytes, including macrophages, exceed those in serum or the extracellular concentrations. The presence of high concentrations in phagocytosing cells is an advantage, because this enhances the ability of the cells to eliminate the infecting organisms.

High cellular levels apply to both the newer and the older macrolides (e.g., erythromycin). The phenomenon gave impetus to successful relaunching of spiramycin. The ability to reach high tissue levels differs for different compounds, but for lack of broad encompassing comparative studies, it is deemed impossible to describe in detail how the different compounds compare.

Still, it appears that azithromycin is the compound that reaches the highest tissue levels, compared with serum concentrations and those outside the cells (lymph in tissues and extracellular levels in vitro studies of leukocytes and macrophages; Bergan et al., 1992).

Azithromycin achieves low serum concentrations and higher tissue levels than other macrolides. Roxithromycin, which shows the inverse pattern, lies at the other end of the spectrum; namely, the highest serum levels of any macrolide, but also relatively low tissue and cellular levels. The extremely high serum protein binding may account for this.

The tonsillar tissue levels of clarithromycin, erythromycin, and roxithromycin are higher than in serum (Bergogne-Bérezin, 1987, 1993; Sörgel et al., 1993), but only by a factor of approximately 10%. These macrolides thus enhibit only a minor organotropy compared with azithromycin (Sörgel et al., 1993; Gerard et al., 1990).

Comparisons of drug levels in other tissues are confusing. Although it is generally accepted as an axiom that tissue penetration is a function of the lipid solubility of the drug, correlation with tissue penetration and lipophilicity is as yet difficult to make because valid comparisons of the various macrolides is missing. A further reason for reserved judgment is that evaluable studies have presented mostly tissue homogenate data (e.g., for azithromycin; Shepard and Falkner, 1990; Girard et al., 1990; Foulds et al., 1990, 1993), erythromycin and dirithromycin (Bergogne-Bérezin, 1993), and roxithromycin (Bergogne-Bérezin, 1987). The sampling of extracellular fluid, such as peripheral human lymph or skin blister fluid, would render more appropriate and conclusive data.

Levels of macrolides are very low to undetectable in cerebrospinal fluid, as exemplified by roxithromycin (Puri and Lassman, 1987).

Concentrations in human milk are extremely low for roxithromycin (Puri and Lassman, 1987) and probably for other macrolides as well. Concentrations in sputum and tear fluid are comparable with serum concentrations (Sörgel et al., 1993).

REFERENCES

Bégue P, Kefetzis DA, Albin H, Safran C. Pharmacokinetics of roxithromycin in paediatrics. J Antimicrob Chemother 1987; 20(suppl B):101–106.

Bergan T, Engeset A, Olszewski W, Josefsson K, Larsen N. Penetration of erythromycin into human peripheral lymph. J Antimicrob Chemother 1982; 10:319–324.

Bergan T, Jørgensen NP, Olszewski W, Zhang Y. Azithromycin pharmacokinetics and penetration to lymph. Scand J Infect Dis [Suppl] 1992; 83:15–21.

Bergogne-Bérezin E. Tissue penetration of roxithromycin. J Antimicrob Chemother 1987; 20(suppl B):113–120.

Bergogne-Bérezin E. Tissue distribution of dirithromycin: comparison with erythromycin. J Antimicrob Chemother 1993; 31(suppl C):77–87.

Carlier M-B, Zenebergh A, Tulkens PM. Cellular uptake and subcellular distribution of roxithromycin and erythromycin in phagocytic cells. J Antimicrob Chemother 1987; 20(suppl B):47–56.

Dette GA, Knothe M. The binding of erythromycin to human serum. Biochem Pharmacol 1986; 35:959–966.

Disse B, Gundert-Remy U, Weber E, Andrassy K, Sietzen W, Lang A. Pharmacokinetics of erythromycin in patients with different degrees of renal impairment. Int J Clin Pharmacol Ther Toxicol 1986; 24:460–464.

Foulds G, Shepard RM, Johnson RB. The pharmacokinetics of azithromycin in human serum and tissues. J Antimicrob Chemother 1990; 25(suppl A):73

Foulds G, Johnson RB. Selection of dose regimens of azithromycin. J Antimicrob Chemother 1993; 31(suppl E):39–50.

Frydman AM, LeRoux Y, Desnottes JF, Kaplan P, Djebhar F, Coumot A, Dachier J, Gaillot J. Pharmacokinetics of spiramycin in man. J Antimicrob Chemother 1988; 22(suppl B):93–103.

Girard D, Bergeron JM, Milisen WB, Retsema JA. Comparison of azithromycin, roxithromycin, and cephalexin penetration kinetics in early and mature abscesses. J Antimicrob Chemother 1993; 31(suppl E):17–28.

Hall KW, Nightingale CM, Gibaldi M, Nelson E, Bates TR, DiSanto AR. Pharmacokinetics of erythromycin in normal and alcoholic liver disease subjects. J Clin Pharmacol 1982; 22:321–325.

Höffler D, Paeske B, Koeppe P, Kinzig M, Sörgel F. Plasma levels of azithromycin in patients with renal failure and healthy volunteers. 1st International Conference on the Macrolides, Azalides and Streptogramins. Santa Fe, NM, January 1992: abstr 213.

Josefsson K, Bergan T, Magni L. Dose-related pharmacokinetics after oral administration of a new formulation of erythromycin base. Br J Clin Pharmacol 1982a; 13:685–691.

Josefsson K, Steinbakk M, Bergan T, Midtvedt T, Magni L. Pharmacokinetics of a new, microencapsulated erythromycin base after repeated oral doses. Chemotherapy 1982b; 28:176–184.

Kafetzis DA, Krotsi-Laskari X, Tremblay D, Saint-Salvi B. Multiple dose pharmacokinetics in infants and children treated with roxithromycin. Br J Clin Pract 1988; 42(suppl 55):58.

Kees F, Grobecker H, Fourtillan JB, Tremblay D, Saint-Salvi B. Comparative pharmacokinetics of single dose roxithromycin (150 mg) versus erythromycin stearate (500 mg) in healthy volunteers. Br J Clin Pract 1988; 42(suppl 55):51.

Lebrec D, Benhamou JP, Fourtillan JB, Tremblay D, Saint-Salvi B, Manuel C. Roxithromycin: pharmacokinetics in patients suffering from alcoholic cirrhosis. Br J Clin Pract 1988; 42(suppl 55):63.

Mazzei T, Surrenti C, Novelli A, Crispo A, Fallani S, Carla V, Surrenti E, Periti P. Pharmacokinetics of azithromycin in patients with impaired hepatic function. J Antimicrob Chemother 1993; 31(suppl E):57–63.

Nilsen O, Saint-Salvi B, Lenfant B, Tremblay D, Manuel C. Pharmacokinetics of roxithromycin in the elderly—linearity and repeat dose studies. Br J Clin Pract 1988; 42(suppl 55):59–60.

Nilsen O. Comparative pharmacokinetics of macrolides. J Antimicrob Chemother 1987; 20(suppl B):81–88.

Osono T, Umezawa H. Pharmacokinetics of macrolides, lincosamides and streptogramins. J Antimicrob Chemother 1985; 16(suppl A):151–166.

Pechere, J-C. The use of macrolides in respiratory tract infections. Int J Antimicrob Agents 1993; 3:S53–S61.

Periti P, Mazzei T. Pharmacokinetics of roxithromycin in renal and hepatic failure and drug interaction. J Antimicrob Chemother 1987; 20(suppl B):107–112.

Puri SK, Lassman HB. Roxithromycin: a pharmacokinetic review of a macrolide. J Antimicrob Chemother 1987; 20(suppl B):89–100.

Segre G, Bianchi E, Zanolo G, Bartucci F, Sassella D. Influence of food on the bioavailability of roxithromycin versus erythromycin stearate. Br J Clin Pract 1988; 42(suppl 55):55–57.

Shepard RM, Falkner FC. Pharmacokinetics of azithromycin in rats and dogs. J Antimicrob Chemother 1990; 25(suppl A):49–60.

Sides GD, Cerimele BJ, Black HR, Busch U, DeSante KA. Pharmacokinetics of dirithromycin. J Antimicrob Chemother 1993; 31(suppl C):65–75.

Sörgel F, Kinzig M, Naber KG. Physiological disposition of macrolides. In: Bryskier AJ, Butzler J-P, Neu H, Tulkens PM. Macrolides. Chemistry, Pharmacology and Clinical Use. Paris: Arnette Blackwell, 1993:421–435.

Wildfeuer A, Lemme JD. Zur Pharmacokinetik von Josamycin. Arzneimittelforschung 1985; 35:3–9.

Wildfeuer A, Leufen H, Leitold M, Zimmermann T. Comparison of the pharmacokinetics of three-day and five-day regimens of azithromycin in plasma and urine. J Antimicrob Chemother 1993; 31(suppl E):51–56.

5

Safety and Drug–Drug Interactions of Macrolides, Azalides, and Streptogramins

S. Ragnar Norrby

Chinese University of Hong Kong
Prince of Wales Hospital
Sha Tin, Hong Kong

INTRODUCTION

Macrolides cause few serious adverse reactions. The most common adverse effects of erythromycin, the best-documented macrolide, are gastrointestinal, especially nausea or vomiting. Such reactions are usually dose-dependent and have limited the possibilities to increase erythromycin doses to cover less susceptible pathogens, or to achieve sufficient drug concentrations in difficult-to-treat infections. It is important to realize that altered indications for use of macrolides, azalides, and streptogramins (the two latter referred to in this article as macrolides) have increased the importance of drug–drug interactions. For example, clarithromycin is now often used in patients with acquired immunodeficiency syndrome (AIDS) to treat infections with atypical mycobacteria, and such patients regularly receive a multitude of other drugs.

This overview will concentrate on erythromycin, clarithromycin, roxithromycin, dirithromycin, and azithromycin, drugs for which there is now abundant information. Other derivatives (e.g., josamycin and streptogramins) will be less well covered owing to limited availability of published information.

In the evaluation of the safety profile of these antibiotics, it is important to realize that, with time, the methods used for assessments of safety have changed. Until the mid-1980s, emphasis was put on adverse effects, and often only reactions considered related to the drug given were reported. Lately, adverse events (i.e., any unwanted experience occurring during or shortly after treatment) have been reported. The consequence of this is a marked increase in the frequencies of adverse experiences reported in clinical trials. Although adverse event registration may give falsely high frequencies, it is more likely that unexpected events and events that are rare will be detected in the clinical evaluation of a new compound. Another factor to consider in this context is that there has been, and still is, a tendency to report lower rates of adverse events in some geographic areas than in others. Thus, studies performed in Japan or southern Europe tend to show fewer adverse experiences than trials in Scandinavia, the United Kingdom or, particularly, the United States.

SAFETY PROFILES

Gastrointestinal Reactions

Table 1 summarizes some relatively recent trials comparing various new macrolides in different types of infections. Four trials (1,2,9,10) showed significant differences, favoring roxithromycin, clarithromycin, and dirithromycin over erythromycin. The latter was given at a high dosage (2 g/day) in one of these trials (2). In the other studies, no significant differences were demonstrated among the various macrolides. Table 1 also demonstrates the difficulties in comparing adverse event reports from different countries. For example, two trials of dirithromycin were performed using similar protocols and identical regimens. The United States studies generated more than 20% adverse events, whereas the European ones reported rates of only 5–6% (12,13).

A possible explanation for the relatively high frequency of upper gastrointestinal side effects seen with erythromycin is that it increases the rate of gastric emptying by functioning as a motilin agonist (14). However, this does not explain the differences in adverse event profiles between erythromycin and roxithromycin, since, at least in vitro, both antibiotics have the same effects on motilin activity (15).

Lower-gastrointestinal tract adverse events are relatively rare with macrolides, although diarrhea is reported with all of them. Brismar et al. (16) studied the effects on the fecal microflora of a 7-day treatment with either 250 mg bid of roxithromycin or 1 g bid of erythromycin ethyl succinate. The gram-positive and anaerobic gram-negative stool floras were markedly altered by both antibiotics, and the changes were more pronounced with erythromycin, which

Table 1 Comparative Frequencies of Gastrointestinal (GI) Adverse Events in Controlled Trials

Comparison (dose in mg)	Study design[a]	GI events (patients)[b]	Ref.
Roxithromycin, 150 bid, vs. erythromycin stearate, 500 bid	DB	6/40(15%) 14/39(36%)*	1
Clarithromycin, 250 bid, vs. erythromycin stearate, 500 qid	DB	7/96(7%) 30/112(27%)*	2
Clarithromycin, 250 bid, vs. erythromycin stearate, 500 bid	OR	7/120(6%) 12/202(10%)	3
Clarithromycin, 500 bid, vs. josamycin 500, tid	OR	3/52(7%) 4/51(8%)	4
Clarithromycin, 500 bid, vs. josamycin, 1000 bid	OR	2/48(4%) 3/24(13%)	5
Azithromycin, 10/kg qd, vs. erthyromycin ethyl succinate, 10–15/kg tid	OR	4/46(9%) 6/47(13%)	6
Azithromycin, 500 qd, vs. clarithromycin, 250 bid	OR	14/191(7%) 10/189(5%)	7
Azithromycin, 500 qd, vs. clarithromycin, 250 bid	OR	15/252(6%) 10/258(4%)	8
Dirithromycin, 500 qd, vs. erythromycin base, 250 qid	DB	70/265(26%) 97/288(34%)*	9
Dirithromycin, 500 qd, vs. erythromycin base, 250 qid	DB	20/193(10%) 33/196(17%)*	10
Dirithromycin, 500 qd, vs. erythromycin base, 250 qid	DB	73/260(28%) 54/257(21%)*	11
Dirithromycin, 500 qd, vs. erythromycin base, 250 qid	DB	90/393(23%) 102/409(25%)	12
Dirithromycin, 500 qd, vs. erythromycin base, 250 QID	DB	29/640(5%) 34/608(6%)	13

[a]DB, double-blind; OR, open, randomized.
[b]In five trials (9–13) only events were reported; several patients had more than one event.
*Significant difference ($p < 0.05$).

may have been due to the considerably larger amounts of this drug excreted in the stools. These changes are probably more important from an ecological point of view (i.e., selection of macrolide-resistant organisms) than from safety aspects (16).

Dose dependence has been suggested for erythromycin-induced gastrointestinal adverse events. This does not seem to be so for clarithromycin (Table 2). With the other new compounds such analyses cannot be made, since they have been studied at fixed doses.

Table 2 Gastrointestinal Adverse Events with Clarithromycin Given 250 mg bid or 500 mg bid

Type of event	Clarithromycin dosage	
	250 mg bid (*n* = 2664)	500 mg bid (*n* = 773)
Any gastrointestinal	248 (9.3%)	60 (7.8%)
Nausea	98 (3.7)%	20 (2.6%)
Diarrhea	78 (2.9%)	14 (1.8%)
Dyspepsia	44 (1.7%)	12 (1.6%)
Abdominal pain	47 (1.8%)	8 (1.0%)
Vomiting	23 (0.9%)	11 (1.4%)

Source: Abbott, data on file.

Other Adverse Events

The new macrolides have been evaluated in extensive clinical trials. Events other than gastrointestinal, including liver transaminase increases, have occurred at frequencies similar to, or lower than, those observed with comparators (other macrolides, β-lactams, doxycycline, fluoroquinolones, and trimethoprim–sulfamethoxazole; 17,18; Eli Lilly, data on file; Abbott, data on file). Ototoxic reactions have been extremely rare or nonexistent.

Drug–Drug Interactions

The subject of drug interactions has been previously reviewed by Polk (19). As he pointed out, macrolides are metabolized in the liver by the cytochrome P-450 system. It is now well known that this system consists of many isoenzymes that can be classified in three main groups—cytochrome P-450 I, II, and III—each of which contains several subgroups. By identifying the isoenzyme group responsible for metabolism, possible candidates among other drugs for metabolic interactions may be identified. Most macrolides seem to be metabolized by cytochrome P-450 IIIA. A systematic mapping of metabolic pathways would markedly facilitate the selection of candidates for drug–drug interaction studies. In this context, it is also important to realize that drug interactions may be two-sided (i.e., drug A can affect the metabolism of drug B or vice versa). Thus, the demonstration of lack of effects of a macrolide on the hepatic metabolism of another drug does not exclude the possibility that the other drug might affect the metabolism of the macrolide.

There are various ways to study the possible interactions between two drugs: in vitro and in vivo studies on inductions of cytochrome P-450; Phase I trials in healthy volunteers or patients; and clinical observations. The last of these is likely to be very insensitive, since only interactions leading to adverse clinical symptoms will be detected. Phase I trials are cumbersome, and it cannot reasonably be mandatory for a drug manufacturer to actively study more than a limited number of possible interactions. The in vitro and in vivo studies of cytochrome P-450 induction, on the other hand, offer means to identify possible interactions and to warn against them.

Table 3 lists documented interactions between macrolides and other drugs. There is a clear predominance of erythromycin, whereas other macrolides are less represented. This is partly because erythromycin seems more prone to induce cytochrome P-450 metabolism than the newer macrolides (e.g., roxithromycin and azithromycin, and probably also clarithromycin and dirithromycin). It may also reflect that the new macrolides have been in clinical use for a limited time (47–49). Virtually no systematic documentation is available on interaction between nucleoside analogues and macrolides, although such combinations are becoming increasingly common (e.g., for the treatment of atypical mycobacterial infections in AIDS patients). Moreover, zidovudine and didanosine are metabolized by the cytochrome P-450 system.

Table 3 Interactions Between Macrolides and Other Drugs

Drug	Interacts with[a]	Interaction	Refs.
Alfentanile	ERY	Reduced alfentanile metab.	20
Bromocriptine	ERY	Reduced bromocriptine metab.	21
Carbamazepine	ERY > CLA > ROX > AZI	Reduced carbamazepine metab.	17,22–24
Cyclosporine	ERY > ROX	Reduced cyclosporine metab.	25–27
Digoxin	ERY	Increased digoxin conc.	28
Disopyramide	ERY	Reduced dispyramide metab.	29
Ergotamine	ERY	Increased ergotamine bioav.?	30
Felodipine	ERY	Reduced felodipine metab.	31
Midazolam	ERY, ROX	Increased midazolam conc.	32
Prednisolone	ERY	Reduced prenisolone metab.?	33
Theophylline	ERY = CLA = ROX = DIR > AZI	Reduced theophylline metab.	24,34–40
Terfenadine	ERY > AZI	Reduced terfenidine metab.	41–42
Triazolam.	ERY	Reduced triazolam metab.	43
Warfarin	ERY >> ROX	Reduced warfarin metab.?	44–46

[a]AZI, azithromycin; CLA, clarithromycin; DIR, dirithromycin; ERY, erythromycin; ROX, roxithromycin.
Note: Lack of indication of an interaction does not exclude the possibility, but reflects that no documentation has been found.
Source: Modified from Ref. 19.

SUMMARY

In general, the new macrolides are drugs with a high degree of safety. Importantly, the frequencies of upper gastrointestinal tract events caused by these antibiotics have been reduced in comparison with erythromycin, and the risk of drug–drug interactions appears to be lower. However, systematic evaluations of the risks for drug–drug interactions with this group of new antibiotics are needed.

REFERENCES

1. Paulsen O, Christensson BA, Hebelka M, Ljungberg B, Nilsson-Ehle I, Nyman L, Svensson R, Tüll P, Varga Z. Efficacy and tolerance of roxithromycin in comparison with erythromycin stearate in patients with lower respiratory tract infections. Scand J Infect Dis 1992; 24:219–225.

2. Anderson G, Esmonde TS, Coles S, Macklin J, Carnegie C. A comparative safety and efficacy study of clarithromycin and erythromycin stearate in community-acquired pneumonia. J Antimicrob Chemother 1991; 27(suppl A):117–124.

3. Scaglione F. Comparison of the clinical and bacteriological efficacy of clarithromycin and erythromycin in the treatment of streptococcal pharyngitis. Curr Med Res Opinion 1990; 12:25–33.

4. Frachini F. Clinical efficacy and tolerance of two new macrolides, clarithromycin and josamycin, in the treatment of patients with acute exacerbations of chronic bronchitis. J Int Med Res 1990; 18:171–176.

5. Straneo G, Scarpazza G. Efficacy and safety of clarithromycin versus josamycin, in the treatment of hospitalized patients with bacterial pneumonia. J Int Med Res 1990; 18:164–170.

6. Weippi G. Multicentre comparison of azithromycin versus erythromycin in the treatment of paediatric pharyngitis or tonsillitis caused by group A streptococci. J Antimicrob Chemother 1993; 31(suppl E):95–101.

7. Müller O. Comparison of azithromycin versus clarithromycin in the treatment of patients with upper respiratory tract infections. J Antimicrob Chemother 1993; 31(suppl E):137–146.

8. Bradbury F. Comparison of azithromycin versus clarithromycin in the treatment of patients with lower respiratory tract infections. J Antimicrob Chemother 1993; 31(suppl E):153–162.

9. Derrienic M, Conforti PM, Sides GD. Dirithromycin in the treatment of streptococcal pharyngitis. J Antimicrob Chemother 1993; 31(suppl C):89–95.

10. Müller O, Wettisch K. Clinical efficacy of dirithromycin in pharyngitis and tonsillitis. J Antimicrob Chemother 1993; 31(suppl C):97–102.

11. Jacobson K. Clinical efficacy of dirithromycin in pneumonia. J Antimicrob Chemother 1993; 31(suppl C):121–129.

12. Sides GD. Clinical efficacy of dirithromycin in acute exacerbations of chronic bronchitis. J Antimicrob Chemother 1993; 31(suppl C):131–138.

13. Gaillat J. Multicentre study comparing the safety and efficacy of dirithromycin with erythromycin in the treatment of bronchitis.

14. Peeters TL, Matthys G, Depootere I, Cachet T, Hoogmartens J, Vantrappen G. Erythromycin is a motilin receptor agonist. Am J Physiol 1989; 257:G470–474.

15. Depootere I, Peeters TL, Matthys G, Cachet T, Hoogmartens J, Vantrappen G. Structure activity relation of erythromycin-related macrolides in inducing contractions and in displacing bound motilin in rabbit duodenum. J Gastrointest Motil 1989; 1:150–159.

16. Brismar B, Edlund C, Nord CE. Comparative effects of clarithromycin and erythromycin on the normal intestinal microflora. Scand J Infect Dis 1991; 23:635–642.

17. Hopkins S. Clinical toleration and safety of azithromycin. Am J Med 1991; 91(suppl 3A):40–45S.

18. Blanc F, D'Enfert J, Fiessinger S, Lenoir A, Renault M, Rezvani Y. An evaluation of tolerance of roxithromycin in adults. J Antimicrob Chemother 1987; 20(suppl B):170–183.

19. Polk RE. Drug interactions with macrolide antibiotics. In: Neu HC, Young LS, Zinner SH, eds. The New Macrolides, Azalides, and Streptogramins. Pharmacology and Clinical Applications. New York: Marcel Dekker, 1993:73–81.

20. Bartkowski RR, Goldberg ME, Larijani GE, Boerner Y. Inhibition of alfentanil metabolism by erythromycin. Clin Pharmacol Ther 1989; 46:99–102.

21. Nelson MV, Berchou RC, Kateri D, LeWitt PA. Pharmacokinetic evaluation of erythromycin and caffeine administered with bromocriptine. Clin Pharmacol Ther 1990; 47:694–697.

22. Wong YY, Ludden TM, Bell RD. Effect of erythromycin on carbamazepine kinetics. Clin Pharmacol Ther 1983; 33:460–464.

23. Albani F, Riva R, Baruzzi A. Clarithromycin–carbamazepine interaction; a case report. Epilepsia 1993; 34:161–162.

24. Saint-Salvi B, Tremblay D, Surjus A, Lefebvre MA. A study of the interaction of roxithromycin with theophylline and carbamazepine. J Antimicrob Chemother 1987; 20(suppl B):121–129.

25. Lysz K, Rosenberg JC, Kaplan MP, Migdal S, Sillix D. Interaction of erythromycin with cyclosporin. Transplant Proc 1988; 20:543–548.

26. Gupta SK, Bakran A, Johnson RWG, Rowland M. Cyclosporin–erythromycin interaction in renal transplant patients. Br J Clin Pharmacol 1989; 27:475–481.

27. Billaud E, Guillemain R, Kitzis M, Fortineau N, Dreyfus G, Amrein C, Kreft-Jais C, Chétien P, Husson JM. Roxithromycin and cyclosporin interaction: heart transplant recipient study [abtr]. 16th International Congress on Chemotherapy, Jerusalem, 1989.

28. Lindenbaum J, Rund DG, Butler VP, Tse-Eng D, Aaha JJ. Inactivation of digoxin by the gut flora; reversal by antibiotic therapy. N Engl Med J 1981; 305:789–794.

29. Echisen H, Kawasaki H, Ohiba K, Tani M, Tshizaki T. A potent inhibitory effect of erythromycin and other macrolide antibiotics on the monodealkylation metabolism of disopyramide with human liver microsomes. Am J Med 1989; 86:465–466.

30. Larcan A. Lérgotism thérapeutique. J Pharmacol (Paris) 1979; 10:413–430.

31. Liedholm H, Nordin G. Erythromycin–felodipine interaction. Drug Intel Clin Pharm 1991; 25:1007–1008.

32. Backman J, Aranko K, Himberg JJ, Olkkola KT. Effect of roxithromycin on pharmacokinetics of midozalam. 18th International Congress on Chemotherapy, Stockholm, 1993:abstr 397.

33. LaForce CF, Szefler SJ, Miller MF, Ebling W, Brenner M. Inhibition of methylprednisolone elimination in the presence of erythromycin therapy. J Allergy Clin Immunol 1983; 72:34–39.

34. Jenne JW. Theophylline. A remarkable window to the hepatic microsomal oxidase. Chest 1982; 81:529–530.

35. Maddux MS, Leeds NH, Organek HW, Hasegawa GR, Bauman JL. The effect of erythromycin on theophylline pharmacokinetics at steady state. Chest 1982; 81:563–565.

36. May DC, Jarboe CH, Ellenburg DT, Roe EJ, Karibo J. The effects of erythromycin on theophylline elimination in normal males. J Clin Pharmacol 1982; 22:125–130.

37. Niki Y, Nakajima M, Tsukiyama K, Nakagawa Y, Umeki S, Moriya O, Watanabe M, Yagi S, Kawane H, Soejima R. Effect of TE-031 (A-56283), a new oral macrolide antibiotic on serum theophylline concentrations. Chemotherapy (Tokyo) 1985; 36(suppl 3):515–519.

38. Ruff F, Chu SY, Sonders RC, Sennello LT. Effect of multiple dose clarithromycin on the pharmacokinetics of theophylline. 30th Interscience Conference on Antimicrobial Agents and Chemotherapy, Atlanta, GA, 1990:abstr 761.

39. Polk RE, Gillum JG, Israel DS, Scott RB, Climo MW. Effect of ciprofloxacin and clarithromycin on the metabolism of theophylline in healthy volunteers. 33rd Interscience Conference on Antimicrobial Agents and Chemotherapy, New Orleans, 1993:abstr 596.

40. Bachman K, Nunlee M, Martin M, et al. Changes in steady-state pharmacokinetics of theophylline during treatment with dirithromycin. J Clin Pharmacol 1990; 30:1001–1005.

41. Konig PK, Woosley RL, Zamani K, Conner DP, Cantilena LR Jr. Changes in the pharmacokinetics and electrocardiographic pharmacodynamics of terfenadine with concomitant administration of erythromycin. Clin Pharmacol Ther 1992; 52:231–238.

42. Harris S, Morse I, Hilligoss DM, Colangelo PM, Eller M, Okerholm R. Azithromycin and terfenadine. 33rd Interscience Conference on Antimicrobial Agents and Chemotherapy, New Orleans, 1993:abstr 597.

43. Phillips JP, Antal EJ, Smith RB. A pharmacokinetic drug interaction between erythromycin and triazolam. J Clin Psychopharmacol 1986; 6:297–299.

44. Bachmann KA, Schwartz JI, Forney R, Frogameni A, Janregui LE. The effect or erythromycin on the disposition kinetics of warfarin. Pharmacology 1984; 28:171–176.

45. Weibert RT, Lorentz SM, Townsend RJ, Cook CE, Klauber MR, Jagger PI. Effects of erythromycin on patients receiving long-term warfarin therapy. Clin Pharmacol 1989; 8:210–214.

46. Paulsen O, Nilsson LG, Saint-Salvi B, Manuel C, Lunell E. No effect of roxithromycin on pharmacokinetic or pharmacodynamic properties of warfarin and its enantiomers. Pharmacol Toxicol 1988; 63:215–220.

47. Delaforge M, Sartori E, Mansuy D. In vivo and in vitro effects of a new macrolide antibiotic roxithromycin on rat liver cytochrome P-450, comparison with troleandomycin and erythromycin. Chem Biol Interact 1988; 68:179–188.

48. Villa P, Sassella D, Corada M, Bartosek I. Effects of roxithromycin, a new semisynthetic macrolide, and two erythromycins on drug metabolizing enzymes in rat liver. J Antibiot 1988; 41:563–569.

49. Amacher DE, Schomaker SJ, Retsema JA. Comparison of the effects of the new azalide antibiotic, azithromycin, and erythromycin estolate on rat liver cytochrome P-450. Antimicrob Agents Chemother 1991; 35:1186–1190.

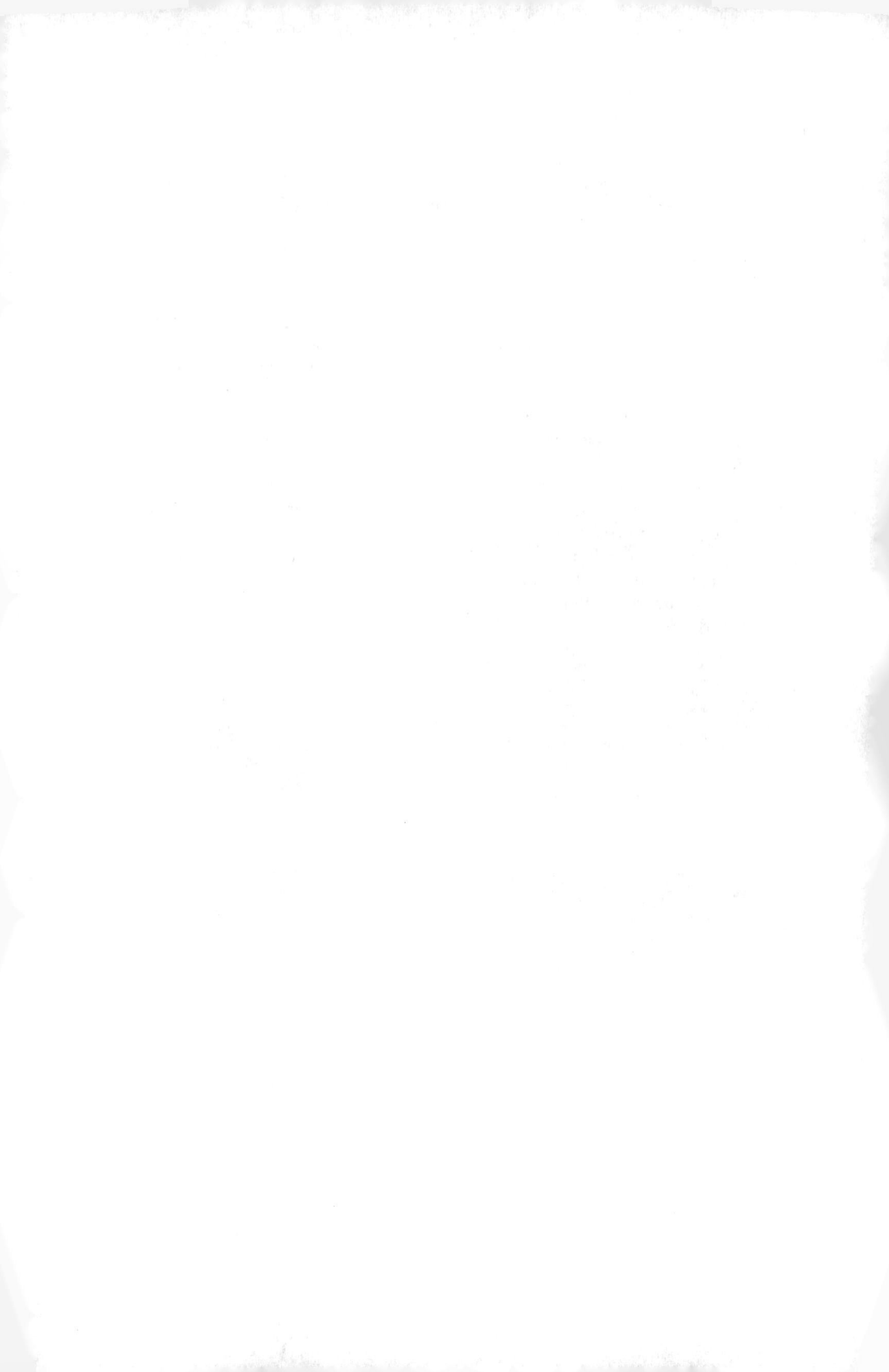

Biology and Pharmacology: Discussion

MORNING SESSION

Young: Dr. Labro, do you find in your studies much difference between antimicrobial uptake by neutrophils, which are short-lived cells in the circulation and probably in the tissues, and macrophages? Does neutrophil uptake parallel what is happening in macrophages, which remain viable and persist for weeks or months?

Labro: The differences in uptake between macrophages, monocytes, and neutrophils have been reported for macrolides, tetracyclines, and other antimicrobial agents. Differences relate to experimental conditions. For in vitro experiments, there are different results, depending on the medium used. Much work is still necessary to standardize test conditions.

Neu: What is the uptake of macrolides by M cells in the gut? The translocation of a lot of bacteria through the gut is thought to be across the M cell. I wonder whether yersinia would respond to macrolides in the same manner as *M. avium*, which is probably acquired orally.

Bryskier: Cellular transport of macrolides is different from quinolones. Work has been published about the transefflux of quinolones between the blood and the interstitial cells. With macrolides, to my knowledge, there is only one work—presented 2 years ago at ICMAS I—using clarithromycin. The work suggested that after uptake there is efflux from the cells. Probably high concentrations in one part of the cells could be very useful for treating infections such as shigella or *M. avium*.

Young: Professor Scaglione has several posters here on tissue penetration, and intracellular and extracellular concentrations.

Scaglione: Perhaps it is most important to understand if the drug inside the cell is active: not only the absolute quantity, but how much active antibiotic is located inside the cell. Another point is whether bacteria and antibiotics are located in the same site intracellularly.

Wise: We have some information that sheds a certain amount of light on what is happening both in vitro and in vivo. Certainly, all the macrolides are rapidly taken up by the phagocytic cells we have looked at—the alveolar macrophages, both in vitro and in vivo—but there are differences in their rate of efflux. Professor Bergan alluded to this, inasmuch as azithromycin elutes in vitro, or is released in vivo, far, far more slowly. He showed that with azithromycin you do not see the peak concentration in alveolar macrophages until 2 days after a single oral dose. But with the other macrolides, using our inflammatory fluid model, looking at the polymorphs, all the drugs enter rapidly and also are eluted rapidly from those cells.

Young: You have also shown that macrophages from smokers actually take up more antimicrobic than those of nonsmokers. Is that because they are "activated" by various cytokines liberated during their response to infection?

Wise: I don't know if that is the answer to the question. It could be, but one thing is for sure, and that is you have to be very careful of the models you're using. It's so much easier, of course, to obtain macrophages from smokers, because their lungs are loaded with them. It's very difficult actually to wash out macrophages from nonsmokers. So I'm not sure whether it's that or whether it's a methodological problem.

Young: Dr. Retsema, what do you see from your perspective, as far as the targets for the next 5–10 years?

Retsema: I think, as usual in industry, we all identify the same targets, most of the time very rapidly. I agree with what Dr. Bryskier said about the targets. I personally feel, and I think a lot of people agree with me in industry, that probably the major target that we would like to achieve within, I'll say, a decade, is activity against the macrolide-resistant strains that exist and appear to be increasing and spreading throughout the world. Concerning the target of increased spectrum, I think, to a certain degree, something is attainable there. However, from a discovery standpoint, part of the problem is that these are macrocyclic structures, and they are probably too big already to hope for a tremendous increase in spectrum. I think that the same thing that would make it difficult to have an increase in spectrum, their size, could possibly be used to an advantage to help achieve activity against the MLSB-resistant ribosomes and possibly the efflux mechanisms. So I look at resistance again as the major objective.

Young: Let's just look at one group of organisms, enterococci. Is there any hope for new macrolides? We really may not have an effective agent to treat vancomycin and penicillin-resistant enterococci. Can you manipulate the molecule to get 'cidality against the enterococcus? You don't need a broad spectrum.

Retsema: I think there is hope at overcoming the resistance that's in enterococci as far as MIC is concerned. As far as the bactericidal activity, that is a problem with enterococcus with many drugs. It appears to me that bactericidal activity is innate in the structure or innate in the class of an antibiotic. It has to do with the whole physiology of the organism and the antibiotic that's acting on it. I don't know of anybody yet who has taken a bacteriostatic antibiotic and turned it into a bactericidal antibiotic. That may relate more to the physiology of the bacterial cell, and you're asking to really change the pathogen at the same time as the drug. That may be impossible.

Neu: Endocarditis obviously has to have a bactericidal antibiotic. We treated a lot of patients in the early 1960s with erythromycin, and even Synercid isn't bactericidal for organisms like *Enterococcus faecium*. The other comment I should make is that these compounds show a postantibiotic effect. I think this is a very important thing, in the sense that, for example, Synercid shows a most potent postantibiotic effect with pneumococci and streptococci. Even though it has a very short half-life, it will kill for about 8 h and thereafter. The other problem that is very important is that, all macrolides and Synercid itself, can be combined with β-lactams, aminoglycosides, fluoroquinolones, chloramphenicol, and other similar drugs. They do not show an antagonistic effect. You can use these drugs to cover the gram-positive cocci, or the legionella, or the mycoplasma, at the same time you use other antibiotics.

Young: Dr. Bryskier, do you want to respond to Dr. Retsema?

Bryskier: I think, for the moment, we do not have any macrolide with a 'cidal activity against enterococci. I agree with my colleague that due to the physiology of the cells, because the macrolides act on the ribosomes, for the moment they are bacteriostatic drugs and not bactericidal drugs. Even if we can find, let's say, a new structure within the macrolides, it is a great challenge. But for enterococci there are also other approaches, and probably the lipopeptides are promising against the enterococci. Some compounds have been withdrawn because of high-level serum binding. We hope that in this peptide field, we will find a new drug against enterococci.

Young: Professor Acar and Professor Leclercq, we are impressed by the interest that French scientists have had in resistance to macrolides. Is it because these compounds have been so traditionally popular in France that you seem to be experiencing more resistance than, say, the United States, where it has only been in the last 2 or 3 years that this group of agents has become so popular. Is it just duration of popularity, or does it have to do with what Dr. Neu implied: persons are given macrolides, such as erythromycin; these are poorly tolerated, the persons stop treatment, and that is the setting in which resistance develops—partially treated infection.

Acar: From what has been published, I think that the macrolides are among the few antibiotics for which there is a little evidence that when using more of the compound, you have greater prevalence of resistance in the place where the compound has been used. Compared with other antibiotics, there is, perhaps, a clearer relation when you look at what's published. In my opinion, using a compound at a given time triggers the beginning of resistance. Then the phenomenon has its own dynamic, which is becoming more complex and more multifactorial, so ultimately changing the habits of use does not change anything. I would like to mention that there are two countries where erythromycin resistance in pneumococci was monitored a number of times by the same groups: South Africa and France. The resistance to erythromycin appeared in both countries, first linked to use of tetracycline. Subsequently, a number of strains with erythromycin resistance alone belonged to different serotypes. Then it was felt that the more resistant serotype was becoming more prevalent. This is happening now in France and also in South Africa, where serotype 23 is increasing, but with multiresistance, not just erythromycin resistance. In this case, I wonder if when you change prescribing habits, you will impinge on the problem of resistance. If there is no selection pressure by one antibiotic, there will be a selection pressure by another.

Leclercq: I agree with Professor Acar on this point. The characteristic of erythromycin resistance is that it's very often borne of plasmids with other associated resistance genes, in particular, tetracycline and aminoglycoside resistance. You can select erythromycin resistance by the use of other antibiotics. It is a very complex issue.

Neu: How do you account for *The New England Journal of Medicine* paper in which the resistance in Finland went from 0% in respiratory isolates to about 13% in respiratory isolates that cause disease and in skin isolates, over the period that the use of erythromycin increased?

Bryskier: This paper is a very good one, but the same author published exactly the same profile of resistance in *Lancet* precisely 1 year earlier. One interpretation of the two papers is that there is probably an outbreak of one strain that is very resistant. I am not sure there is really an increase only because of an increased level of drug use.

Acar: I would like to add about the paper published from Finland that there was no publication about the genetic basis of the type of resistance observed. In the Japanese strains, the resistance was against the whole group of macrolides. In the Finnish publications, the lincosamides and maybe 16-membered macrolides were still active. Is it a completely different mechanism, is it a plasmid, or is it another system? I think maybe the molecular epidemiology might explain what happened in Finland.

Young: Professor Norrby, can you comment on the differences in antibiotic usage and control practices in Europe for some specific countries.

Norrby: Finland has a very high usage rate of antibiotics. Because of the paper published in *The New England Journal of Medicine*, the sales of erythromycin dropped by 50%. I think if you were to go out and revisit the problem, you might get your answer. We have seen similar tendencies, not to the same extent, but we have increasing frequencies of streptococcal A resistance, which seem to parallel the increased consumption of macrolides.

Young: Professor Bergan, those of us who treat AIDS are now starting patients on clarithromycin and azithromycin. They are taking these pills for the rest of their lives, up to 2-plus years now, because of the desire to suppress not only the mycobacterial infections, but also some of the others. Has anybody looked at what happens in terms of long-term pharmacokinetics? I have been impressed by the incredible safety, and I wouldn't have anticipated that, knowing that traditionally macrolides may have some hepatotoxicity. Have you or anyone else looked at pharmacokinetics after 2 months of clarithromycin or azithromycin?

Bergan: I don't know that anybody has done that. The type of studies that have been done have been carried on for maybe a week or so. Just from a pharmacokinetic theory point of view, I think there are going to be very few of my colleagues who are going to be intrigued by looking at the pharmacokinetics in AIDS patients.

Young: But you should. Where are the drugs going? Are they staying in the gut, or coming out of tissues at more rapid rates?

Bergan: My guess is they are staying in the tissues. You get an accumulation of course.

Young: More of it is being added every day. Look at the doses that are being used. One of the concerns we had is that macrolides would crystallize out in our patients, but it doesn't seem to be happening.

Bergan: I'm sure there's going to be an equilibrium, so that you have so much in the tissues and so much is going out in the urine and in feces everyday. The study that Dr. Bryskier referred to that has not been published was the rat intestine study of Sorgel and his group. They postulated a transintestinal elimination of the macrolides. They have used the same model and demonstrated transintestinal elimination in an in vitro model of fluoroquinolone turnover. For the fluoroquinolones, this has been studied and demonstrated in humans as well, but I am not aware of any study that has examined the transintestinal elimination of macrolides. I would suspect that because we have high concentrations of all the macrolides in feces, including after intravenous administration, you get some transintestinal elimination. In the case of the macrolides, it is probably going to be impossible to do a good study in humans, because you have copious amounts eliminated in the bile, which is not the case for the quinolones.

Norrby: I think you have a very good point, Dr. Young, because there are several issues that should be directed in these patients, not only the pharmacokinetics of the macrolides, but the possibility of induction of enzymes of various kinds. We do remember the old azoles, which committed a sort of metabolic suicide after 3 weeks. You couldn't find any azoles at all in the patients after 3 weeks.

Young: So you're suggesting that these studies which Professor Bergan doesn't want to do should be done.

Norrby: I think they have to put on the gloves and do them.

Scaglione: Tissue concentration depends mainly on the intracellular concentration. If you compare macrolides with β-lactams, you find that the concentration of macrolide is higher than that of the β-lactam, because β-lactams are mainly in the extracellular compartment, not the intracellular. Among macrolides there are very different pharmacokinetic differences between roxithromycin and azithromycin. What are the clinical implications of these differences?

Bergan: I don't think that there is necessarily a clinical implication. All of the newer macrolides have, by and large, the same spectrum of activity. It is always a question of dose–tissue concentrations in relation to the susceptibility of the organism. With roxithromycin, you have doses of 150 mg, and you reach very high concentrations. It is an active compound in vitro. Extracellular versus intracellular levels pose a very difficult issue in interpretation. That is one of the reasons why I avoided commenting about the tissue concentrations of the various compounds. You have in investigators' brochures and publications what amounts to huge menus of concentrations in different tissues, which is actually in the tissue homogenates. I'm not sure that this means anything.

Wise: Can I pursue that matter a little bit further with Professor Bergan, that is, to return to the thorny problem of what tissue levels are important. Because we have, on the one hand, a drug, such as erythromycin, which gets into relevant tissues, such as the respiratory tract—because that's where these drugs are used—moderately well, and its serum levels are quite high. You have a drug, such as azithromycin, on the other hand, that has vanishingly small serum levels after a moderate period, but exists in tissue concentrations, again in relevant cells, maybe a thousandfold greater than the serum. Then you have a disease, such as a pneumococcal infection, that can be both a tissue infection and a bacteremic condition—this is a problem that has been rehearsed many times—but maybe you could give us your thoughts on it.

Bergan: I think the point of having high tissue concentrations means that you have at least a reservoir from which the drug is released over time, for instance, to expose the bacteria to be taken up by new macrophages that enter the area. I think tissue concentration must be important.

Neu: Professor Norrby, you did not say anything about the deafness that occurs with erythromycin at high doses. What occurs with other macrolide drugs? The other problem is that sometimes the patient is so ill that he or she requires intravenous therapy. And phlebitis has been a problem with all of these compounds. Additionally, with Synercid the concentration that one can use is limited.

Norrby: One of the reasons that I briefly touched on is that we are lacking dose-finding studies, also in terms of adverse events, with the new macrolides, azalides, and streptogramins. Most of the studies that you see test a very narrow range of doses and conclude that there are no differences either in terms of toxicity or in terms of safety. But that only tells you that the ranges have been wrong. Many studies should be redone. I think one of the explanations for the fact that there are no deafness reports with the new agents is that only low doses have been used. I think we must have that in mind when we go into higher doses, such as used in AIDS patients. As to phlebitis, there is still very little data available, but my understanding is that phlebitis is a common problem with all macrolides.

AFTERNOON SESSION

Zinner: A question about RP 59500, which is also known as Synercid. This drug kills most pneumococci. Do we know if anything increases the bactericidal rate associated with the use of this drug in vitro, something that increases the rate of killing of pneumococci in the presence of Synercid?

Baquero: In general it is not appreciated that macrolides and streptogramins are bactericidal agents. In the case of *Streptococcus pneumoniae* they are bactericidal, but we can't predictably increase the rate.

Neu: As you indicated RP 59500 binds to two different sites and, therefore, is bactericidal for susceptible strains. None of our penicillin-resistant pneumococci, which are type 23, were also macrolide- or streptogramin-resistant.

Mayer: I agree. I think the question would be how the drug performs in more complex situations, in other words, bacteremia—one would expect it to be highly effective. If you're dealing with an empyema or more complex infection with a lower pH, you might be a little bit more concerned.

Neu: But you can probably achieve a blood level of 10, and the MIC would probably be 0.12. So you would obviously be many times over the minimum bactericidal concentration, and even at 10 in the lung, even though the pH might be 6, it probably would exceed the minimal therapeutic level. I think that in animal models RP 59500 has been active.

Zinner: We don't really know what the intracellular pH is within a phagosome or within certain compartments of the cell. Yet these drugs are active intracellularly when the pH might be lower than 7 in certain compartments within that cell. I just wonder if there's any comment on that phenomena. Does anyone either on our panel or in the audience know of any data on macrolide or streptogramin activity in bacterial endocarditis models? I didn't see any of those presented today. We have to wait for further studies.

Tulkens: I want to comment about the pH effect. It is clear that the activity of the macrolides will be decreased by acidic pH. At the same time, acidic pH would drive the macrolide into that compartment. Interestingly enough, the lysosomes tend to be fairly acidic, which concentrates much of the macrolide, but the drug would be mostly inactive in these compartments. Those phagosomes that do contain a legionella, for instance, would not fuse any longer with the lysosomes, and their pH would tend to be more alkaline, or let's say less acidic than the lysosomes. So in the same phagosome with legionella you would anticipate the macrolide to show better activity, but because the pH is not as low, the concentration would be less. I'm not certain that the concentration within the most acidic compartment would eventually make the compound globally less active. There would be more compound and the compound would be less active per se. So the two actually may balance out.

Neu: What's the concentration, for example, of magnesium and calcium in the lysosome? That is a problem for the quinolones.

Tulkens: I don't know, and I think very few people have addressed this question. It's very difficult for us to isolate the lysosomes or the phagosomes and make a determination of cations or anions within the intact organisms. That has not been done very clearly.

Unidentified (France):   I have two comments. One about intracellular concentration of streptogramin and about RP 59500. We studied the accumulation of this streptogramin inside macrophages, and we obtained a ratio of intracellular to extracellular concentration of about 30 for the p1 component and between 40 and 50 for the p2 component. We observed bactericidal activity of the two compounds inside the macrophages.

Zinner: For which organisms?

Unidentified (France):   For *Staphylococcus aureus*. The second comment is about endocarditis and the streptogramins. Several studies have been done for RP 59500 in a model of experimental endocarditis in rabbits. This compound displayed activity equal to vancomycin in a model of endocarditis caused by methicillin-resistant *S. aureus*.

Neu: The problem with that is that vancomycin is an overrated drug for *S. aureus*. It's not bactericidal, and you will have a prolonged bacteremia. I wonder whether with these drugs that stay in the tissues for a long period, you have to keep the animals for a much longer time to see whether they might have some sort of relapse.

Bergan: I would like to carry on the discussion with Dr. Tulkens. A low pH and lower activity in noninfected lysosomes and the higher pH in infected lysosomes I think would lead to another conclusion than the one that is lingering around: that the active pH and the low pH more or less inactivate the high concentrations. Because once you get the bacteria there, then the pH is going up.

Zinner: Is that true?

Bergan: That was going to be my question to Tulkens. So that you actually do have an advantage. Because of the high concentrations once the bacteria get there, you will have higher pH.

Tulkens: I think one should distinguish two things. I was referring to the fact the phagosomes that are infected with the legionella do not fuse with the lysosomes. Those phagosomes always remain less acidic, so there would be less tendency for the macrolide to accumulate into those infected phagosomes. If you now take a lysosome that is infected by *S. aureus* or by *Salmonella typhi*, we don't know, but it is possible indeed that the pH rises a little bit. At that time, the macrolide that has accumulated in those lysosomes would also leak out. The point might be that, indeed, they may have bound to the bacteria before, so that might indeed help in the activity. But it has not been demonstrated; it is pure speculation.

Mellis (USA):   A point concerning the intracellular activity, I think that whatever the considerations are regarding flux between different compartments, we always need to go back to fundamental biological activity. Clearly, we know that lysosomes are the primary site of concentration. Yet a single dose of azithromycin eradicates chlamydial infection, which typically requires 7 days of treatment. Likewise, in animal models of legionella, at least in Dr. Fitz-George's work, the PD_{100} was far lower for either erythromycin or clarithromycin when azithromycin was administered just once daily, even at lower doses. I think with regard to concentrations in nonlysosomal compartments, we need to remember there is still a vast reservoir of drug present in serum, as well as that which is present in the lysosome. There will be a tendency to concentrate in any compartment that has a lower pH than the surrounding compartment. The fact that there is still a lot of drug present in serum or interstitial space will still drive large quantities of drug into compartments that have a pH of even 6, even though the concentration in the lysosome might be even lower at pH 4.

LeBel (Canada): Relative to the important pharmacodynamic parameters for macrolides, time above at MIC was reported by Dr. William Craig at ICAAC (1993). Additionally, we observed with aminoglycosides that the magnitude of that concentration was important. In other words, as with β-lactams, it might be more complex than just the time above MIC. We may have to consider the size of the dose, and with once-a-day administration of some of the macrolides using a large dose, rather than a small dose.

Mayer: In studying genital tract secretions we are dealing with two- and three-compartment situations. In many patients we have examined for risk of HIV and with HIV, we find huge numbers of white cells, even when they do not have other STDs, so that the activity of these antibiotics in white cells is a very important part of the treatment of STDs.

Tulkens: But I am not saying that the macrolides are not active intracellularly. We have published many data concluding quite the opposite. However, we do not know whether macrolides fully express their activity within the cell. My bias today is that they express about a 10th to a 40th of the activity they could show if they were totally free, depending on the organism we use. Interestingly enough, you get almost the same value whether you use a cytosolic organism, such as listeria, a phagosomal organism, such as chlamydia, or a lysosomal one, such as *S. aureus*. Hence, the idea that whatever the situation of the organism, the concentration is undermined by the pH. One exception is *Mycobacterium avium*, for which you get more activity than you would anticipate. That might be due to the long incubation period and also because the macrolide is given in combination with other antimicrobials.

CLINICAL APPLICATIONS

6

Macrolides, Azalides, and Streptogramins in Staphylococcal and Other Gram-Positive Infections

Stephen H. Zinner

Brown University
Rhode Island Hospital
and Roger Williams Medical Center
Providence, Rhode Island

INTRODUCTION

Most of the currently available antibiotics in the macrolide, azalide, and streptogramin (MAS) class are known to be effective in over 90% of patients with acute bronchitis, acute exacerbations of chronic bronchitis, acute otitis media, acute bacterial sinusitis, pharyngitis, tonsillitis, odontogenic infections, and in 80–90% of patients with community-acquired pneumonias. Also, these agents are effective in about 80–85% of cases of infections involving the skin and soft tissues.

This review will concentrate on recent clinical studies of the newer MAS antibiotics in infections caused by *Staphylococcus aureus* and other gram-positive organisms.

STAPHYLOCOCCUS AUREUS

Several studies report in vitro susceptibilities to the MAS drugs. Against 62 erythromycin-sensitive strains of *S. aureus*, Bauernfiend reported that azithromycin, dirithromycin, and roxithromycin had 90% minimum inhibitory concentrations (MIC_{90}) of 4 $\mu g/ml$ (respective ranges, 0.25–8, 0.25–8, and 0.13–16 $\mu g/ml$). Clarithromycin was somewhat more active, with an MIC_{90} of 1 $\mu g/ml$ (range, 0.13–4 $\mu g/ml$). However, against 24 erythromycin-resistant strains of *S. aureus* with erythromycin MIC of 8 $\mu g/ml$ or higher, the MIC_{90}s for all of the new MAS drugs were >64 $\mu g/ml$ (1). In vitro studies with the new pristinamycin combination, RP 59500 (Synercid) reported at the Second International Conference on Macrolides, Azalides, and Streptogramins (ICMAS II) revealed this drug to be at least as active, if not more active, than vancomycin against strains of methicillin-sensitive and methicillin-resistant *S. aureus* and against methicillin-sensitive strains of coagulase-negative staphylococci (Table 1) (2).

In clinical studies (Table 2), results with the new MAS compounds have been comparable with, or somewhat better than, those obtained with erythromycin. For example, in a double-blind, double-dummy study of skin infections from 30 centers in North America and 31 in Europe, Derriennic and Escande reported favorable clinical responses to dirithromycin, 500 mg qd for 7 days, in 162 of 188 (86%) patients with *S. aureus* infections, compared with 137 of 156 (88%) such patients treated with erythromycin, 250 qid (3). One hundred percent of 29 and 30 infections caused by coagulase-negative staphylococci responded favorably in each group, respectively. In this trial, the infecting organism was eradicated in 223 of 256 (86%) patients in the dirithromycin group and from 198 of 226 (88%) in the erythromycin-treated patients. Similar results were obtained in an Italian trial comparing dirithromycin with miocamycin (4).

In a study of 60 patients with cellulitis, abscesses, and other skin infections in Mexico, azithromycin at 500 mg/day for 3 days compared favorably with 7

Table 1 In Vitro Susceptibilities to RP 59500 and Vancomycin

	RP 59500	Vancomycin
MSSA ($n = 48$)		
MIC_{90}	0.25	0.5
MBC_{90}	0.50	1.0
MRSA ($n = 22$)		
MIC_{90}	0.5	1.0
MBC_{90}	1.0	1.0
MRSE ($n = 30$)		
MIC_{90}	0.25	1.0
MBC_{90}	0.50	2.0

MSSA, methicillin-sensitive *Staphylococcus aureus*; MRSA, methicillin-resistant *S. aureus*; MRSE, methicillin-resistant coagulase-negative staphylococci.
Source: From Ref. 2.

Table 2 Selected Clinical Results with New Macrolides and Azalides in Infections Caused by *Staphylococcus aureus* and *Streptococcus pneumoniae*

Organism/site	Cured or improved		Ref.
	New macrolide	Comparator	
S. aureus			
Skin	162/188(86%)[b]	137/156(88%)[g]	3
Skin	25/30(83%)[a]	26/30(87%)[h]	5
Skin (children)	57/59(97%)[d]	57/58(98%)[i]	
Skin	242/256(95%)[b]	217/226(96%)[g]	7
Skin	297/321(93%)[e]	32/39(82%)[j]	8
S. pneumoniae			
Pneumonia[a]	12/13(92%)[b]	14/15(93%)[g]	17
Pneumonia[a]	4/5(80%)[c]	4/5(80%)[f]	18
Bronchitis[a]	53/53(100)[k]	52/55(95%)[j]	16

[a]Bacterial eradication rates.
[b]Dirithromycin, 500 mg pd × 7d
[c]Azithromycin, 500 mg pd × 3d
[d]Azithromycin, 10 mg/kg × 3d
[e]Roxithromycin, qd or bid
[f]Amoxicillin–clavulanate, × 7–10d
[g]Erythromycin, 250 mg qid × 7d
[h]Dicloxacillin, 250 mg qid × 7d
[i]Cloxacillin, 5 mg/kg qid × 7d
[j]Various nonmacrolides
[k]Clarithromycin, 500 mg bid

days of dicloxacillin at 250 mg qid (5). In this study, clinical resolution occurred in 25 of 30 (83%) patients receiving azithromycin and in 26 of 30 (87%) dicloxacillin-treated patients. *Staphylococcus aureus* was eradicated from all 15 patients in the azithromycin group and from 18 of 19 patients (95%) treated with dicloxacillin. Both drugs were well tolerated.

In a study of children with skin infections in South and Central America, azithromycin at 10 mg/kg for 3 days was compared with cloxacillin at 5 mg/kg qid for 7 days. These children with impetigo, furunculosis, folliculitis, paronychias, and other skin infections, were cured or improved in 97% (57 of 59) of patients receiving azithromycin and in 98% (57 of 58) patients treated with cloxacillin (6). Eradication of *S. aureus* occurred in 31 of 34 (91%) azithromycin-treated patients and in 34 of 35 (97%) cloxacillin recipients.

In several studies reported at the ICMAS II meeting, the new macrolide drugs responded favorably when compared with erythromycin or nonmacrolide comparators. For example, once daily dirithromycin for 7 days was successful clinically and microbiologically in 242 of 256 (95%) and 223 of 256 (87%) cases, respectively, with similar results for 7 days of erythromycin qid at 96% (217/226) and 88% (196/226), respectively (7). Similar results were reported by Schupbach (8). In another nonblinded study, roxithromycin once or twice daily administered to 321 patients was slightly more effective clinically (297 of 321; 93%) and microbiologically (184 of 197; 93%) than various nonmacrolide comparators given more frequently (32 of 39; 82% and 9 of 11; 82%, respectively) (8).

In large multihospital studies involving over 750 patients with various skin and soft-tissue infections, clarithromycin was as effective clinically and microbiologically and as well tolerated as cefadroxil and erythromycin (9).

Staphylococcal infections are certainly amenable to treatment with the new macrolide–azalide–streptogramin antibiotics. In general, staphylococcal strains that are susceptible to erythromycin will be susceptible to these drugs, but erythromycin-resistant strains are less likely to be sensitive to the new MAS drugs. Similarly, methicillin-resistant strains of *S. aureus* may be resistant to the new macrolides, but many such strains might be susceptible to RP 59500 (Synercid). There is good experience with staphylococcal skin infections, as reviewed in the foregoing, but there is little published experience with the new MAS drugs in the treatment of osteomyelitis. Also, these drugs should not yet be recommended in the treatment of bacteremia or endocarditis. However, as new intravenous formulations are under development, future studies might alter this opinion.

STREPTOCOCCUS PNEUMONIAE

Erythromycin has long been a standard alternative to penicillin in the therapy of pneumococcal infections. Against 20 penicillin-susceptible strains of *S. pneumoniae*, Bauernfeind reported the MIC_{90} for azithromycin, dirithromycin, and roxithromycin at 0.25 μg/ml and for clarithromycin at 0.06 μg/ml (1). For 17 penicillin-resistant pneumococci the MIC_{90} was 8 μg/ml for azithromycin and dirithromycin, 4 μg/ml for roxithromycin, and 1 μg/ml for clarithromycin (1). Scriver et al., reported MIC_{90} of 0.5 for RP 59500 (Synercid) against 451 penicillin-susceptible strains and 1.0 μg/ml for 51 penicillin-resistant strains of *S. pneumoniae* (10). At this meeting, Berthaud reported that the RP compound is rapidly bactericidal for penicillin-susceptible and penicillin-resistant pneumococci and also for erythromycin-resistant strains, as tested in a dynamic in vitro model and in mouse septicemia (11). Similar results were found in serum of human volunteers following intravenous administration of RP 59500 (12).

Clarithromycin is bactericidal for susceptible pneumococci in vitro (13) and, in another in vitro study, Perri et al. reported clarithromycin to have better in vitro activity than ciprofloxacin and penicillin when tested against 47 clinically isolated bacteremic strains of *S. pneumoniae* (14). Clarithromycin MICs for four penicillin- and ciprofloxacin-resistant pneumococci ranged from 0.007 to 2.0 μg/ml (14).

Consistent with these in vitro results, bacteriological cures were reported for clarithromycin in 4 of 4 patients with pneumonia, 66 of 70 (94%) with sinusitis, and 22 of 23 patients (96%) with bronchitis, compared, respectively, with β-lactam comparators at 6 of 7 (86%), 52 of 59 (88%), and 17 of 22 (77%) (15). In another published report, pneumococci were eradicated in 53 of 53 patients with bronchitis treated with clarithromycin, 500 mg bid, as compared with 52 of 55 (95%) bronchitis patients treated with a reference β-lactam (16).

Clinically, the new macrolide or azalide drugs have performed well in pneumococcal infections. In a multicentered study of 173 patients with community-acquired pneumonia, dirithromycin at 500 mg qd was compared with erythromycin at 250 mg qid. Pneumococci were eradicated from 12 of 13 patients (92%) in the dirithromycin group and from 14 of 15 (93%) of the erythromycin-treated patients (17). Both drugs were tolerated similarly. In a Dutch study, Hoepelman reported that azithromycin, at 500 mg/day for 3 days, was comparable with amoxicillin–clavulanic acid for 7–10 days; each drug eradicated the infecting pneumococcus in four of five patients (18). Similarly, Myburgh reported that this dose of azithromycin eradicated sputum pneumococci in 27 of 27 pneumonia patients and that four of six patients with pneumococcal bacteremia had sterile blood at 48 h (19). Three days of azithromycin were comparable with 10 days of clarithromycin in lower respiratory tract infections caused by various organisms (20). In a large survey of 14,038 patients with respiratory tract infections, roxithromycin produced excellent or good results in 1654 (93%) patients with pneumonia caused by various organisms (21).

In a study reported at this meeting, 12 bacteremic pneumococcal infections treated with dirithromycin, at 500 mg qd for 10–14 days, were compared with 9 episodes treated with erythromycin, 250 mg qid. Overall, clinical responses were similar (83 and 89%, respectively) and blood isolates were ultimately eradicated in 100% of both groups (22).

OTHER STREPTOCOCCAL SPECIES

The susceptibilities of other *Streptococcus* species to the new macrolide or azalide drugs are quite respectable, with MIC_{90} values against *S. pyogenes* (22 strains) reported as 0.13 μg/ml for azithromycin, 0.03 μg/ml for clarithromycin, 0.25 μg/ml for dirithromycin, and 0.06 μg/ml for roxithromycin (1). Similarly, for 38 strains of group B streptococci (*S. agalactiae*) Bauernfeind reported MIC_{90}s of 0.13 μg/ml for azithromycin, 0.06 μg/ml for clarithromycin, and 0.25 μg/ml for dirithromycin and roxithromycin (1).

Several clinical trials have studied the role of the new macrolide and azalide drugs in the treatment of upper respiratory bacterial infections, presumably caused by *S. pyogenes* and other gram-positive cocci. For example, Müller and O'Doherty reported at the ICMAS II meeting results from multicenter open comparative trials in adult patients with pharyngitis, tonsillitis, otitis, and sinusitis (23,24). Similar clinical "cure or improved" rates were reported for 3 days of 500 mg azithromycin (224 of 242; 93%) and 10 days of cefaclor, at 250 mg qid (214 of 224; 96%) (23). Azithromycin, at 500 mg qd for 3 days, compared favorably with roxithromycin, 150 mg bid for 10 days, in patients with upper respiratory infections (99 and 98%, respectively; 24). In another study, 3 days of azithromycin were comparable with 10 days of bid clarithromycin in upper respiratory tract infections (25).

Several studies of the new macrolide–azalide drugs in streptococcal pharyngitis have been reported. In a randomized double-blind trial in 257 patients with streptococcal pharyngitis and tonsillitis, McCarty et al. reported equivalent clinical and bacteriological responses with dirithromycin, 500 mg qd (97 and 90%, respectively), and phenoxymethyl-penicillin, 250 mg qid (94 and 90%, respectively), both given for 10–14 days (26). In another study of 444 adults and 367 children with streptococcal pharyngitis, diagnosed with a streptococcal antigen test, clarithromycin, at 250 mg bid (or 7.5 mg/kg) for 10 days, was similar to phenoxymethyl-penicillin, at 250 mg tid or qid (or 13.3 mg/kg), in clinical successes (27). However, group A β-hemolytic streptococci were eradicated from 208 of 222 adults (94%) who received clarithromycin compared with 197 of 224 (88%) penicillin recipients ($p = 0.048$). Bacterial eradication rates for the children were 168 of 183 (92%) clarithromycin recipients and 162 of 199 (81%) penicillin-treated patients ($p = 0.004$). Azithromycin suspension, 10 mg/kg for 3 days, compared favorably with penicillin V suspension, 125–250 mg qid for 10 days; in 96 children treated for streptococcal pharyngitis or tonsillitis (93% clinical cure, 95% bacterial eradication in each group; 28).

Other studies report similar results (29), and azithromycin for 3 days was as effective as erythromycin qid for 10 days in an Austrian pharyngitis study (30). In an open study of 638 patients with pharyngitis or tonsillitis, 181 of whom had *S. pyogenes* isolated on culture, roxithromycin, at 150 mg bid for 7 days, was clinically effective in 94% of patients (31).

Erysipelas is classically caused by group A β-hemolytic streptococci. One multicenter study randomized hospitalized patients with erysipelas to receive roxithromycin, 150 mg orally bid, or intravenous penicillin (switched to oral penicillin with defervescence; 32). Roxithromycin (without any additional antibiotics) cured 26 of 31 (84%) patients compared with 29 of 38 (75%) treated with penicillin. Side effects were similar, but two penicillin-treated patients developed a rash.

OTHER INFECTIONS

Although penicillins are usually preferred for oral infections, erythromycin has been used. The new azalide–macrolide drugs have had limited trials in odontogenic infections and, in one open study, roxithromycin, at 150 mg bid, cured 94% of these infections and compared favorably with erythromycin, at 1 g bid (33). Similar side effect profiles were found in each group (20%). In another report, azithromycin for 3 days was more effective in 30 patients with acute odontogenic infections (29/30; 97%) than spiramycin, 3 million units tid for 7 days (22/30; 73%; 34).

A few reports suggest that the azalide–macrolide drugs might be useful in preventing bacteremia following dental procedures. Rahn and colleagues reported that roxithromycin, at 150 mg, was as effective as 1 g of erythromycin in the prevention of viridans streptococcal bacteremia following dental procedures (35). However, there are no studies documenting the efficacy of MAS drugs in the prevention of endocarditis.

In another context, Kern and colleagues were able to show that a combination of roxithromycin plus ofloxacin was statistically significantly more effective in preventing streptococcal bacteremia in neutropenic patients than ofloxacin alone (0/64 vs. 6/67; $p = 0.03$) (36).

Several unanswered questions remain for future research concerning the use of the new macrolide, azalide, and streptogramin drugs. As the parenteral product Synercid (RP 59500) is developed, its role in the treatment of enterococcal infections and in bacteremia caused by *Corynebacterium jeikeium* and other gram-positive organisms will be evaluated. Also, the role of these new drugs in the treatment of infections caused by *Listeria monocytogenes* needs to be determined. In addition, the role of these oral drugs in the long-term treatment of osteomyelitis caused by susceptible gram-positive organisms needs evaluation, as does the use of these agents in the prophylaxis against endocarditis following oral and dental procedures. More studies are needed to determine the clinical efficacy of these agents against anaerobic gram-positive bacteria.

As new intravenous preparations of the macrolide, azalide, and streptogramin antibiotics are developed their indications for use against gram-positive infections will need specification.

SUMMARY

The new oral azalide–macrolide antibiotics are clearly effective against gram-positive bacterial infections, such as pharyngitis, tonsillitis, sinusitis, otitis, bronchitis, pneumonia, as well as skin and soft tissue infections. The new parenteral pristinamycin derivative RP 59500 has genuine potential in the treatment of methicillin-resistant staphylococcal infections as well as in the treatment of enterococcal infections caused by resistant organisms. These and other applications need continued evaluation, but it is likely that these new agents will prove to be worthy additions to our anti-infective armamentarium.

REFERENCES

1. Bauernfeind A. In-vitro activity of dirithromycin in comparison with other new and established macrolides. J Antimicrob Chemother 1993; 31(suppl C):39–49.

2. Raad I, Sacilowski M, Hachem R, Bodey G. The activity of streptogramin RP 59500 (RP) against methicillin sensitive and resistant staphylococci. Second International Conference on the Macrolides, Azalides and Streptogramins Program and Abstracts, Venice, Italy, January 19–22, 1994:abstr 130.

3. Derriennic M, Escande JP. Dirithromycin in the treatment of skin and skin structure infections. J Antimicrob Chemother 1993; 31(suppl C):159–168.

4. Ruggiero G, Utili R, Adionolfi LE, et al. Clinical efficacy of dirithromycin versus miocamycin in tonsillopharyngitis. J Antimicrob Chemother 1993; 31(suppl C):103–109.

5. Amaya-Tapia G, Aguirre-Avalos G, Andrade-Villanueva J, et al. Once-daily azithromycin in the treatment of adult skin and skin-structure infections. J Antimicrob Chemother 1993; 31(suppl E):129–135.

6. Rodriguez-Solares A, Pérez-Gutiérrez F, Prosperi J, Milgram E, Martin A. A comparative study of the efficacy, safety and tolerance of azithromycin, dicloxacillin and flucloxacillin in the treatment of children with acute skin and skin-structure infections. J Antimicrob Chemother 1993; 31(suppl E):103–109.

7. Varanese L, Sides G. Dirithromycin efficacy in skin and skin structure infections. Second International Conference on the Macrolides, Azalides and Streptogramins Program and Abstracts, Venice, Italy, January 19–22, 1994:abstr 308.

8. Portier H. Overview of the efficacy and safety of roxithromycin (ROX) vs control antibiotics in the treatment of infections in adults. Second International Conference on the Macrolides, Azalides and Streptogramins Program and Abstracts, Venice, Italy, January 19–22, 1994:abstr 223.

9. Parish LC. Clarithromycin in the treatment of skin and skin structure infections: two multicenter clinical studies. Int J Dermatol 1993; 32:528–532.

10. Scriver SR, Lai STF, Chong LY, Gonsales A, Levi M, Low DE. In vitro activity of RP 59500 against *Streptococcus pneumoniae* including isolates moderately susceptible and resistant to penicillin. Second International Conference on the Macrolides, Azalides and Streptogramins Program and Abstracts, Venice, Italy, January 19–22, 1994:abstr 120.

11. Berthaud N, Desnottes JF. RP 59500: in vitro and in vivo bactericidal activity against *Streptococcus pneumoniae*. Second International Confer-

ence on the Macrolides, Azalides and Streptogramins Program and Abstracts, Venice, Italy, January 19–22, 1994:abstr 117.

12. Pangon B, Bray P, Couzon B, et al. Serum bactericidal activity of RP 57669/RP 54476:RP 59500 (RP) against *S. pneumoniae*. Second International Conference on the Macrolides, Azalides and Streptogramins Program and Abstracts, Venice, Italy, January 19–22, 1994:abstr 118.

13. Lemmen SW, Anding K, Engels I, Daschner FD. Bactericidal activity of clarithromycin vs cefaclor against *Streptococcus pneumoniae* and *Moraxella catarrhalis*. Second International Conference on the Macrolides, Azalides and Streptogramins Program and Abstracts, Venice, Italy, January 19–22, 1994:abstr 119.

14. Perri MB, Zervos MJ. Comparative in-vitro activity of ciprofloxacin, clarithromycin and penicillin versus blood isolates of *Streptococcus pneumoniae*. Second International Conference on Macrolides, Azalides and Streptogramins Program and Abstracts, Venice, Italy, January 19–22, 1994:abstr 116.

15. Siepman N, Pixton G, Notario G. Clarithromycin in the treatment of *S. pneumoniae* infections. Second International Conference on Macrolides, Azalides and Streptogramins Program and Abstracts, Venice, Italy, January 19–22, 1994:abstr 260.

16. Wettengel R, Vetter N, Waardenburg FA. Clarithromycin versus cefaclor for the treatment of mild-to-moderate acute bacterial bronchitis. J Antimicrob Chemother 1993; 31:963–972.

17. Jacobson K. Clinical efficacy of dirithromycin in pneumonia. J Antimicrob Chemother 1993; 31(suppl C):121–129.

18. Hoepelman AIM, Sips AP, van Helmond JLM, et al. A single-blind comparison of three-day azithromycin and ten-day co-amoxiclav treatment of acute lower respiratory tract infections. J Antimicrob Chemother 1993; 31(suppl E):147–152.

19. Myburgh J, Nagel GJ, Petschel E. The efficacy and tolerance of a three-day course of azithromycin in the treatment of community-acquired pneumonia. J Antimicrob Chemother 1993; 31 (suppl E):163–169.

20. Bradbury F. Comparison of azithromycin versus clarithromycin in the treatment of patients with lower respiratory tract infection. J Antimicrob Chemother 1993; 31(suppl E):153–162.

21. Marsac JH. An international clinical trial on the efficacy and safety of roxithromycin in 40,000 patients with acute community-acquired respiratory tract infections. Diagn Microbiol Infect Dis 1993; 15(suppl 4):81S–84S.

22. Smietana M, Conforti PM, Smits P, Sides GD. Intent-to-treat analysis of outcome of pneumonia patients with bacteremia enrolled in two dirithromycin clinical trials. Second International Conference on Macrolides, Azalides and Streptogramins Program and Abstracts, Venice, Italy, January 19–22, 1994:abstr 272.

23. Müller O. A multicenter trial comparing azithromycin and roxithromycin in the treatment of adults with acute upper respiratory tract infections.

Second International Conference on Macrolides, Azalides and Streptogramins Program and Abstracts, Venice, Italy, January 19–22, 1994:abstr 230.

24. O'Doherty B (on behalf of the Azithromycin Study Group). An open comparative study of azithromycin versus cefaclor in the treatment of patients with upper respiratory tract infections. Second International Conference on Macrolides, Azalides and Streptogramins Program and Abstracts, Venice, Italy, January 19–22, 1994:abstr 229.

25. Müller O. Comparison of azithromycin versus clarithromycin in the treatment of patients with upper respiratory tract infections. J Antimicrob Chemother 1993; 31(suppl E):137–146.

26. McCarty J, Good C, Renteria A, Siepman N, Craft J. Comparative safety and efficacy of clarithromycin (C) vs amoxicillin/clavulanate (A/C) or cefaclor (Cf) in the treatment of acute otitis media (AOM) in children. Second International Conference on Macrolides, Azalides and Streptogramins Program and Abstracts, Venice, Italy, January 19–22, 1994:abstr 234.

27. Still JG, Palmer R. An evaluation of clarithromycin and penicillin in patients with streptococcal pharyngitis. Second International Conference on Macrolides, Azalides and Streptogramins Program and Abstracts, Venice, Italy, January 19–22, 1994:abstr 240.

28. Hamill J. Multicentre evaluation of azithromycin and penicillin V in the treatment of acute streptococcal pharyngitis and tonsillitis in children. J Antimicrob Chemother 1993; 31(suppl E):89–94.

29. Principi N, Ambrosioni G, Bianco R, et al. Randomized multicenter study of azithromycin vs erythromycin in pediatric patients with acute pharyngotonsillitis due to group A beta-haemolytic streptococci. Second International Conference on Macrolides, Azalides and Streptogramins Program and Abstracts, Venice, Italy, January 19–22, 1994:abstr 239.

30. Weippl G. Multicenter comparison of azithromycin versus erythromycin in the treatment of paediatric pharyngitis or tonsillitis caused by group A streptococci. J Antimicrob Chemother 1993; 31(suppl E):95–101.

31. Sanchez L. Roxithromycin in the treatment of pharyngotonsillitis. Second International Conference on Macrolides, Azalides and Streptogramins Program and Abstracts, Venice, Italy, January 19–22, 1994:abstr 244.

32. Bernard P, Plantin P, Roger H, et al. Roxithromycin versus penicillin in the treatment of erysipelas in adults: a comparative study. Br J Dermatol 1992; 127:155–159.

33. Deffez JP, Scheimberg A, Rezvani Y. Multicenter double-blind study of the efficacy and tolerance of roxithromycin versus erythromycin ethylsuccinate in acute orodental infection in adults. Diagn Microbiol Infect Dis 1992; 15(suppl 4):133S–137S.

34. Lo Bue AM, Sammartino R, Chisari G, Gismondo MR, Nicoletti G. Efficacy of azithromycin compared with spiramycin in the treatment of odontogenic infections. J Antimicrob Chemother 1993; 31(suppl E):119–127.

35. Rahn R, Linde JH, Riffel C, Dornauf C, Shah PM. Macrolides in prophylaxis for endocarditis. Second International Conference on Macrolides, Azalides and Streptogramins Program and Abstracts, Venice, Italy, January 19–22, 1994:abstr 312.

36. Kern WV, Hay B, Kern P, Marre R, Arnold R. Efficacy of roxithromycin to prevent viridans streptococcal bacteremia following cytotoxic chemotherapy. A randomised trial in patients with acute leukemia and bone marrow transplant patients receiving ofloxacin prophylaxis. Second International Conference on Macrolides, Azalides and Streptogramins Program and Abstracts, Venice, Italy, January 19–22, 1994:abstr 314.

7

Clinical Application of Macrolides and Azalides in *Legionella, Mycoplasma,* and *Chlamydia* Respiratory Infections

Giuliana Gialdroni Grassi and Carlo Grassi

Pavia University
Pavia, Italy

INTRODUCTION

The broad use of antibiotics and the increasing number of patients with special characteristics (elderly, immunocompromised and transplant patients, drug addicts, or others) have effected remarkable changes in the etiology of respiratory infections, not only in hospital settings, where the selective pressure of antibiotics is higher, but also in community-acquired pneumonia (CAP) and in exacerbations of chronic bronchitis (COPD) (Pennington 1989a,b; Sachs, 1989; Meyer and Finch, 1992; Kayser, 1992; Fass, 1993; MacFarlane et al., 1993). In the growing number of possible respiratory pathogens, a special place has to be reserved for agents responsible for "atypical pneumonia." In the past, this entity was attributed to viruses, lacking the possibility to demonstrate an etiological agent. However, when new, better diagnostic techniques became available, the group of atypical pneumonia was shown to include forms caused by different, previously unrecognized microorganisms belonging to the genera *Mycoplasma, Legionella, Chlamydia,* and possibly to others (Berntsson et al., 1986; Atmar and Greenberg, 1989; Tuazon and Murray, 1989; Glynn and Jones, 1990; Fang et al., 1990).

The incidences of viral and *Mycoplasma pneumoniae* infections are not clearly known (Sachs, 1988). The incidence of the latter is quite variable in different studies of CAP, ranging from 0.5 to 18% of cases (MacFarlane, 1993). Differences can be ascribed, at least in part, to the difficulties in microbiological and serological diagnosis and to unequal application in the search for this pathogen among different laboratories.

Comparison between the most important series of studies performed before and after the discovery of legionellosis and the adoption of reliable laboratory methods to diagnose *Legionella pneumophila* indicated that the frequency of this species as a cause of CAP was of some relevance (Pennington, 1989a). The percentage of CAP attributed to *Legionella* is extremely variable, ranging from zero to 30% (Bertsson et al., 1985; Woodhead et al., 1985; MacFarlane et al., 1985; Research Committee British Thoracic Society, 1987). Epidemiological differences among countries likely exist, but lack of diagnostic facilities may also lead to an underestimation of the presence of the disease.

Chlamydia pneumoniae (TWAR), the most recently discovered species of the *Chlamydia* genus, is a frequent etiologic agent of lower respiratory tract infections (LRTI), both bronchitis and pneumonia (Grayston et al., 1986). Studies carried out in different countries have indicated that *C. pneumoniae* is associated with CAP in 6–15% of cases (Fang et al., 1990; Kirby et al., 1991; Blasi et al., 1993; Torres and El-Ebiary, 1993), but in some studies, even higher percentages have been found (Almirall et al., 1993). Some cases also could be of nosocomial origin (Grayston et al., 1989). An incidence of 4–5% has been found in exacerbations of COPD in two studies (Beaty et al., 1991; Blasi et al., 1993b).

Considering the importance of *M. pneumoniae*, *L. pneumophila*, and *C. pneumoniae* in the etiology of LRTI, it is of paramount importance to know their susceptibility to antimicrobial agents and to adopt the most adequate treatment schedules to obtain satisfactory clinical results.

ACTIVITY OF ANTIMICROBIAL AGENTS AGAINST *LEGIONELLA*, *MYCOPLASMA*, AND *CHLAMYDIA* SPECIES

Legionella

For different reasons the genera causing so-called atypical pneumonia (*Legionella*, *Mycoplasma*, *Chlamydia*) are not susceptible to β-lactams: in fact, on the one hand *Mycoplasma*, which lacks the cell wall that is the target of β-lactam activity, cannot be influenced by the action of these agents, and on the other hand, *Legionella* and *Chlamydia*, which are intracellular pathogens, are susceptible only to antibiotics that can penetrate the infected cell.

Therefore, the determination of in vitro antibiotic activity does not always reflect the real activity in vivo and in human disease. In fact, some β-lactams and aminoglycosides that exert antibacterial activity at low minimum inhibitory concentrations (MICs) in vitro do not show any efficacy clinically. In vitro assays in cell lines should be more predictive of in vivo activity. A recent study carried out in a human macrophagelike cell line (U-937) infected with *L. pneumophilla* showed that the ampicillin or sulbactam had no significant activity on the intracellular organism, whereas the combination of ampicillin plus sulbactam showed greater bactericidal activity than erythromycin (Ramirez et al., 1993). This finding should be considered cautiously, in light of the limited clinical activity in legionella infections. A report of clinical failure in a patient treated with amoxicillin–clavulanic acid also confirmed that this in vitro model does not transfer well to clinical settings (Hohl et al., 1992).

The most active antibiotics that show in vitro and in vivo activity are the macrolides, followed by quinolones and rifampin (Table 1; Liebers et al., 1989; Gump, 1991; Roig et al., 1993; Edelstein and Edelstein, 1991; Barker and Farrel, 1990). Experimental legionellosis in guinea pigs has been the most useful animal model. Intratracheal or aerosol delivery of legionella into the lungs causes

Table 1 In Vitro Activity of Some Antibiotics Against *Legionella*, *Mycoplasma*, and *Chlamydia* MIC (mg/L)

Antibiotic	*L. pneumophila*[a]	*M. pneumoniae*[a]	*C. pneumoniae*[b]	*C. psittaci*[b]
Erythromycin	0.25–2	$\leq$0.01	0.06	0.1
Roxithromycin	0.25–0.5	$\leq$0.01–0.03	0.05–0.125	0.025–2
Dirithromycin	4–16	0.01–0.02	0.5	2.5
Clarithromycin	0.12–0.25	$\leq$0.01–0.05	0.5	0.05
Azithromycin	0.12–2	$\leq$0.01	0.06	0.02
Josamycin	0.5–1	$\leq$0.01–0.02	0.25	0.25
Miokamycin	0.12	$\leq$0.01	0.5	2
Rokitamycin	0.12–0.25	0.03		
Rifampin	0.002–0.125			
Ofloxacin	0.03–0.06	0.39–1.56		
Ciprofloxacin	0.03–0.12	2.5–8		
Pefloxacin	0.008–1	0.78–12.5		
Tetracycline	>16	0.06–0.4	0.05–0.1	
Chlortetracycline		0.8–25		
Demethylchlor- 　tetracycline		0.05–0.4		
Minocycline	2–4	0.1–3.1		
Sulfisoxazole			>400	
Penicillin	8–16		>100	
Ampicillin	2–4		>100	
Ceftazidime	0.05			
Gentamicin	0.25			

[a]In some cases, MICs represent MIC_{90} and, in other cases, scattered data on a few strains.
[b]MICs of a few strains.

pneumonia that closely resembles human legionellosis. Peritoneal infection of guinea pigs with *L. pneumophila* results in peritonitis, bacteremia, and spreads to different organs, including the lungs. Pneumonia produced in this manner does not resemble human disease, but the inhalation model does (Edelstein et al., 1984; Edelstein, 1993b). In these models, erythromycin was more active than β-lactam antibiotics and gentamicin, whereas clarithromycin and azithromycin were more active than erythromycin (Kohno et al., 1989; Fitzgeorge et al., 1990).

Quinolones appear to have higher bactericidal activity against legionella. Pefloxacin resulted in more activity than erythromycin in animal infection, but comparisons with clinical results were inconclusive (Pocidalo, 1989; Rajagopalan et al., 1990). In vitro and in vivo data testify to the excellent activity of rifampin against legionella. However, there is evidence that rifampin used alone induces rapid appearance of resistance in legionella. Therefore, it is preferably combined with erythromycin in severe cases of legionellosis to prevent emergence of resistance (Roig et al., 1993).

Tetracyclines, the activity of which has been demonstrated in in vitro and in animal models, are very rarely employed to treat legionellosis in clinical practice. However, in a few clinical cases of erythromycin failure, they have shown satisfactory efficacy (Ruiz-Santana et al., 1986). Co-trimoxazole was active in the guinea pig model of legionellosis, but very few clinical cases have been treated (Edelstein et al., 1984).

Mycoplasma

Methods to test the in vitro susceptibility of *Mycoplasma pneumoniae* are not satisfactory. Assays are usually carried out using an agar dilution method, which needs better standardization. Macrolides are very active, with MICs $\leq$ 0.01 mg/L. Quinolones are less active. The MICs of ofloxacin range from 0.39 to 1.50 mg/L, whereas those of ciprofloxacin are higher, varying from 2.5 to 8 mg/L. Tetracyclines are endowed with good activity, although they are less active than macrolides (Kenny, 1991) (Table 1). Experimental pneumonia, caused by *Mycoplasma pneumoniae*, in young golden hamsters was cured by administration of roxithromycin and erythromycin (Hara et al., 1987).

Chlamydia

Because of the obligate intracellular nature of the organism, the determination of susceptibility of *Chlamydia* species to antibiotics is carried out in tissue culture. Various cell lines may be used. The MIC and minimum bactericidal concentration (MBC) can be determined. However, the methods need to be standardized to obtain more homogeneous results. The MICs of macrolides are quite low. The most active derivatives are erythromycin, roxithromycin, and azithromycin.

Chlamydia psittaci shows good susceptibility to macrolides and tetracycline (Orfila, 1993a) (Table 1).

PHARMACOKINETIC CONSIDERATIONS

To exert their therapeutic activity, antibiotics must reach the infectious focus. When infection is localized to the respiratory tract, it is necessary that an antibiotic reach the lung parenchyma, bronchial tissue, bronchial secretions, and the interior of cells if the infection is intracellular. The determination of antibiotic concentration in lung parenchyma is usually carried out on surgical specimens. Aminoglycosides and β-lactams reach lung concentrations that, respectively, are equal to or somewhat lower than blood levels, whereas macrolides and quinolones reach tissue concentrations that are much higher than those of serum, with some variability between compounds (Table 2). Approximately the same behavior can be demonstrated in bronchial mucosa.

Table 2 Concentration of Some Antibiotics in Lung Parenchyma After Administration of Therapeutic Dosages

Antibiotic	Lung/serum ratio (at serum peak)	
β-Lactams		
Amoxycillin	0.6–0.8	(s.d.)[a]
Cefotaxime	0.1–0.3	(s.d.)
Aminoglycosides		
Gentamicin	~1.0	(m.d.)[a]
Macrolides		
Erythromycin	2–5	(m.d.)
Roxithromycin	0.6–0.9	(m.d.)
Clarithromycin	6–8	(m.d.)
Azithromycin	~20–100	(s.d.)
Dirithromycin	19–40	(m.d.)
Quinolones		
Ciprofloxacin	~3.5	(s.d.)
Ofloxacin	~4	(m.d.)

[a]s.d., single dose; m.d., multiple dose.
Sources: Baldwin et al., 1992; Bergogne-Berezin, 1981, 1993; Foulds et al., 1990; Fraschini et al., 1991; Gialdroni Grassi, 1980; Smith and Le Frock, 1983; Valcke et al., 1990.

Profound differences among derivatives belonging to the same or to different antibiotic classes are observed for the concentrations in bronchial secretion and sputum. In fact penetration into these secretions implies the passage through what has been called the "hematobronchial barrier" made up of cellular membranes, mucus, bacterial debris, and proteinaceous material. This passage is influenced by the physicochemical properties of the drug, its lipophylicity, degree of ionization, and the degree of inflammation and tissue injury. Inflammation and tissue damage favor the passage of antibiotics. When inflammation subsides, an antibiotic's concentration in tissue and secretions falls.

Inflammation has a different influence on the degree of antibiotic passage: for example, tetracyclines are indifferent, whereas β-lactam penetration is correlated to inflammation. β-lactams usually penetrate very poorly in bronchial secretions, in which their concentrations represent only 10–20% or less of serum levels. Aminoglycoside concentrations can reach values equal to 30–40% of peak serum levels and can persist for some time after the serum level falls. Better penetration in bronchial secretions is achieved with the quinolones, the levels of which usually approximate those of serum. Macrolides reach high concentrations in bronchial secretions, up to five- to sixfold (and even 16-fold for roxithromycin) higher than in serum (Table 3; Gialdroni Grassi, 1980; Bergogne-Berezin, 1981; Baldwin et al., 1992).

A recently developed "microlavage technique" performed by fiberoptic bronchoscopy allows investigators to obtain specimens of epithelial lining fluid of alveoli and macrophages, in addition to bronchial secretions and bronchial tissue in which antibiotic concentrations can be measured. Therefore, antibiotic concentrations at the different sites of respiratory tract can be determined (Baldwin et al., 1992). In bronchitis, it remains a matter of discussion whether the major importance should be attributed to mucosal levels of antibiotics, where infection takes place, rather than sputum levels (Gialdroni Grassi, 1980; Valcke et al., 1990; Baldwin et al., 1992). Although the higher mucosal levels are the major determinant of infection eradication, sputum levels are also important in hastening the clearance of bacteria.

Several studies have been devoted to determination of antibiotic concentration in phagocytic cells, with the aim of determining predictions of antibiotic clinical activity in intracellular infection. β-Lactams do not accumulate in cells. Conflicting opinions exist on the behavior of aminoglycosides. According to many authors, aminoglycosides do not penetrate mammalian cells, whereas according to others, they do, albeit at a very low rate, localizing almost exclusively within lysosomes. The short-term experiments usually performed with phagocytic cells do not allow the detection of possible intracellular concentrations of these antibiotics (Tulkens, 1991a).

Clindamycin, macrolides, rifampin, and fluoroquinolones accumulate in phagocytes. Rifampin accumulation is low, reaching an extracellular/intracellular

Table 3 Bronchial Mucosa and Secretion/Serum Concentration Ratio of Some Oral Antimicrobial Agents After Administration of a Standard Dosage

	Ratio	
Antibiotic	Mucosa/serum	Bronchial secretions/serum
β-Lactams		
Amoxicillin	0.7	0.10–0.20
Cefixime	0.5–0.7	0.10–0.20
Macrolides		
Erythromycin		0.3–0.5
Josamycin		0.3–0.6
Miokamycin		3–6
Spiramycin		0.8–2
Roxithromycin		1–16
Clarithromycin	~4	
Azithromycin	30	2.5–5
Dirithromycin	26–24	5–6
Quinolones		
Ciprofloxacin	1.5–2.3	~0.4
Ofloxacin	1.2–1.9	~ 0.8–1
Lomefloxacin	~2	~0.9
Sparfloxacin	~2	~0.5

Sources: Baldwin et al., 1992; Bergogne-Berezin, 1987, 1988, 1993; Foulds et al., 1990; Gialdroni Grassi, 1980; Peters and Clissold, 1992; Smith and Le Frock, 1983; Valcke et al., 1990.

(C/E) ratio of 2–3. In spite of a higher C/E ratio (C/E = 11; Prokesh and Hand, 1982), clindamycin shows sparse activity against intracellular *Staphylococcus aureus*, possibly because of the slow growth rate of the microorganism and the rapid efflux of the antibiotic from cells (Tulkens, 1991b). Fluoroquinolones accumulate in phagocytes at C/E ratios of 2–8: both uptake and release are rapid, but the antimicrobial activity is excellent. Macrolides show great capacities to accumulate in phagocytes and other cells, with remarkable differences existing among various derivatives. According to different authors, C/E ratios in polymorphonuclear (PMN) cells may vary from 2 to 14 for erythromycin, from 14 to 21 for roxithromycin, from 4 to 10 for flurithromycin, and from 40 to >200 for azithromycin. This ratio approximates 10 for clarithromycin and 80 for dirithromycin. Even higher concentrations can be found in alveolar macrophages (Table 4). They are further increased in alveolar macrophages of smokers, probably because these cells are in an activated state or show some alterations in membrane functions (Hand et al., 1985). A peculiar behavior is shown by azithromycin, which has a very long half-life, about 50 h. Whereas serum levels

Table 4 Intracellular/Extracellular Concentration Ratio of Some Macrolide Derivatives in Human PMN, AM, and Fibroblasts[a]

Derivative	PMN	AM	Fibroblast
Erythromycin	2–14	15–40	35
Roxithromycin	14–22	~60	
Flurithromycin	4–10	ND	
Clarithromycin	~12	ND	
Dirithromycin	83	ND	
Azithromycin	40–> 200	200–> 500	> 1000
Josamycin	~13	ND	
Rokitamycin	~25		

[a]PMN, polymorphonuclear granulocytes; AM, alveolar macrophages; ND, not determined.
Sources: Anderson et al., 1988; Andrews et al., 1992; Baldwin et al., 1990; Carlier et al., 1987; Fietta et al., 1992; Hand et al., 1985; McDonald and Pruul, 1991; Tulkens, 1991a,b.

are low, extremely high tissue and intracellular levels are reached, particularly in phagocytic cells. Azithromycin is released very slowly from phagocytes. This behavior allows antibiotic laden PMN to deliver the drug to the site of infection, where these cells accumulate (Gladue et al., 1989).

The correlation between intracellular accumulation and antimicrobial activity has been submitted to careful analysis. Large quantities of drug in the cell do not always assure higher antibacterial activity. Cell penetration of macrolides correlates with extracellular concentrations, and antimicrobial activity correlates with intracellular accumulation in experimental models (Tulkens, 1991a).

The main question that arises from these experimental observations is their effect on clinical activity. Animal models, such as legionella infection in guinea pigs and in immunocompromised mice and *M. pneumoniae* infection in golden hamster, demonstrate the in vivo activity of macrolides (Edelstein et al., 1984; Blander et al., 1990; Orfila, 1993b; Hara et al., 1987). On the other hand, ex vivo experiences in patients undergoing fiberoptic bronchoscopy and treated with clarithromycin or azithromycin showed that alveolar macrophages in bronchoalveolar lavage (BAL) fluid accumulated macrolides approximately to the same extent as in vitro (Baldwin et al., 1992, 1990; Andrews et al., 1992).

Again, because of methodological difficulties in assessing intracellular antibiotic concentrations in this setting and the discrepancies that might exist between concentrations and intracellular activity, it is arbitrary to infer that intracellular concentrations are predictive of clinical efficacy against intracellular pathogens. Only clinical trials can offer answers to this question.

CLINICAL ACTIVITY OF MACROLIDES IN RESPIRATORY INFECTIONS

The antimicrobial activity and the spectrum of action of macrolides include most respiratory pathogens, such as *Steptococcus pneumoniae*, *Moraxella catarrhalis*, and *Haemophilus influenzae* (against which recent derivatives, clarithromycin, azithromycin, and dirithromycin are most active) and *Legionella*, *Mycoplasma*, *Chlamydia*, and *Coxiella* spp. Moreover, their pharmacokinetic behavior predicts satisfactory results from their use in respiratory infections. In addition to the classic respiratory pathogen, recent data show that *Legionella pneumophila*, *Mycoplasma pneumoniae*, and *Chlamydia pneumoniae* have a relevant role in the etiology of community-acquired pneumonia (CAP). Most often, the precise bacteriological diagnosis of CAP is not possible. Therefore, it is of interest to determine the clinical results obtained with the use of macrolides for the empirical treatment of CAP. Very few comparative, controlled studies on this subject have been carried out with older macrolides.

Recently, some clinical studies that compare newer macrolides with older ones, or with other antibiotics, for the empirical treatment of CAP have given us better insights into the activity of these derivatives in respiratory infections (Gialdroni Grassi and Grassi, 1993). Tables 5, 6, and 7 summarize recent clinical studies comparing roxithromycin, clarithromycin, and azithromycin with other macrolide derivatives or with β-lactams in CAP. Clinical bacteriological results are reported in these tables. Bacteriological results are available from fewer patients (about 40–50%) than are clinical results.

In only a few studies have serological data been examined as evidence for causation by *Legionella*, *Mycoplasma*, or *Chlamydia* species. However, in several cases, clinical symptoms and signs support the possibility of atypical pneumonia. Roxithromycin, at a dose of 150 mg bid, was as active as erythromycin, midecamycin, ampicillin, amoxicillin, amoxicillin–clavulanic acid, cephradine, cefixime, doxycycline, and ciprofloxacin, employed at standard dosages, for periods of treatment ranging from 5 to 15 days. A large study of 344 patients demonstrated that treatment with roxithromycin, at 150 mg bid, was equivalent to 300 mg od (see Table 5). Clarithromycin, at 250 or 500 mg bid, was compared with erythromycin, josamycin, and roxithromycin at standard dosage, and excellent results were obtained. Clinical and bacteriological results were similar to those obtained with comparative drugs (see Table 6).

Clinical trials with azithromycin deserve particular attention, since the drug has been administered according to its unique pharmacokinetic properties. Treatment for 5 days (500 mg in single dose on day 1, followed by 250 mg od on days 2–5) achieved the same results as those obtained with cefaclor, amoxicillin, and amoxicillin–clavulanic acid prescribed at standard dosage for 10 days. Moreover, a 3-day course of treatment (500 mg od), based on pharmacokinetic

Table 5 Clinical Efficacy of Roxithromycin in Community-Acquired Pneumonia: Comparative Studies

Drugs	Daily dosage[a]	No. pts. with satisfactory clinical results (cure + improvement)/ no. evaluable pts. (%)	Bacteriological eradication[b] % strains eradicated	Refs.
Roxithromycin	150 mg bid	39/42 (93)	76	Bertrand et al., 1988
vs.				
erythromycin	1 g bid	32/39 (82)	80	
Roxithromycin	150 mg bid	43/46 (93)	83	Zeluff et al., 1988
vs.				
cephradine	1 g bid	44/44 (100)	76	
Roxithromycin	150 mg bid	14/18 (80)	73	Rahlews et al., 1987
vs.				
amoxicillin	750 mg bid	11/15 (73)	73	
Roxithromycin	150 mg bid	14/15 (93)	ND	Dautzenberg et al., 1991
vs.				
amoxicillin + clavulanic acid	500 + 125 mg tid	10/16 (63)	ND	
Roxithromycin	150 mg bid	7/7 (100)	96[c]	Bhasin, 1991
vs.				
ampicillin	250 mg qid	7/8 (88)	63[c]	

Roxithromycin	150 mg bid	55/61 (90)	72	Marsac et al., 1988
vs.			80	
doxycycline	200 mg od	55/65 (85)		
Roxithromycin	150 mg bid	18/20 (90)	ND	Brückner et al., 1989
vs.				
cefixime	200 mg bid	24/28 (86)	ND	
vs.				
Ciprofloxacin	250 mg bid	15/19 (79)	ND	
Roxithromycin	150 mg bid	166/178 (93.3)	53/56 (94.6)	Perianu and Grassi, 1991
vs.				
roxithromycin	300 mg od	149/166 (89.8)	58/59 (98.3)	
Roxithromycin	150 mg bid	57/70 (81.4)	75	Soejima and Hara, 1989
vs.				
midecamycin	200 mg tid	56/80 (70)	70	

[a]The common duration of treatment ranged between 5 and 15 days.
[b]Bacteriological data concern fewer patients than for those on clinical efficacy.
[c]Results obtained in LRTI other than pneumonia are included (mostly exacerbations of chronic bronchitis).
ND, not determined.

Table 6 Clinical Efficacy of Clarithromycin in Community-Acquired Pneumonia: Comparative Studies

Drugs	Daily dosage[a]	No. pts. with satisfactory clinical results (cure + improvement)/ no. evaluable pts. (%)		Bacteriological eradication[b] % strains eradicated	Refs.
Clarithromycin	500 mg bid	84/93	(90)	87	Periti et al., 1990
vs.					
josamycin	1000 mg bid	58/65	(89)	94	
Clarithromycin	500 mg bid	43/47	(91)	86	Straneo and
vs.					Scarpazza, 1990
josamycin	1000 mg bid	20/23	(87)	90	
Clarithromycin	250 mg bid	33/34	(97)	ND	Dubois et al.,
vs.					1990
erythromycin	500 mg q6h	32/32	(100)	ND	
Clarithromycin	250 mg bid	21/23	(91)	100	Futterman and
vs.					Drnec, 1990
erythromycin	250 mg qid	24/24	(100)	89	
Clarithromycin	250 mg bid	57/64	(89)	ND	Anderson et al.,
vs.					1991
erythromycin	500 mg q6h	43/44	(98)	ND	
Clarithromycin	250 mg bid	137/142	(96)	92	Nicotra et al, 1991
vs.					
erythromycin (250)	250 mg q6h	48/48	(100)	92	
vs.					
erythromycin (500)	500 mg q6h	78/81	(96)	100	
Clarithromycin	250 mg bid	26/34	(76)	57	Poirier, 1991
vs.					
roxithromycin	150 mg bid	26/31	(84)	83	
Clarithromycin	250–500 mg bid	26/30	(87)	ND	Cassell et al.,
vs.					1991a
erythromycin	250–500 mg qid	30/30	(100)	ND	

[a]The common duration of treatment ranged between 7 and 15 days.
[b]Data on bacteriological eradication concern fewer patients than for those on clinical effects.
ND, not determined.

Table 7 Clinical Efficacy of Azithromycin in Lower Respiratory Tract Infections (LRTI)

Drugs	Daily dosage and duration of treatment	No. pts. with satisfactory clinical results (cure + improvement)/ no. evaluable pts. (%)	Bacteriological eradication[a] % strains eradicated	Refs.
Azithromycin vs.	500 mg single dose on day 1 + 250 mg od (on days 2–5)	184/191 (96.3)	88.2	Dark, 1991
cefaclor	500 mg tid (10 days)	77/81 (95.1)	87.8	
Azithromycin	500 mg single dose	30/32 (93.8)	80.4	Kinasewitz and Wood, 1991
vs.	on day 1 + 250 mg od (on days 2–5)			
cefaclor	500 mg tid (10 days)	39/39 (100)	92.6	

(continued)

Table 7 Continued

Drugs	Daily dosage and duration of treatment	No. pts. with satisfactory clinical results (cure + improvement)/ no. evaluable pts. (%)	Bacteriological eradication[a] % strains eradicated	Refs.
Azithromycin	500 mg single dose	48/52 (92) (10 days)	91	Balmes et al., 1991
vs.	on day 1 + 250 mg od (on days 2–5)			
amoxicillin + clavulanic acid	500 mg + 125 mg tid (10 days)	47/54 (87)	89	
Azithromycin (open study in CAP—3 days treatment)	500 mg od (3 days)	39/40 (98)	97	Myburgh et al., 1993
Azithromycin	500 mg od (3 days)	61/62 (98)	90.4	Bisetti et al., 1992[b]
vs. erythromycin	500 mg qid (7 days)	55/59 (93)	96.5	
Azithromycin	500 mg od (3 days)	230/241 (95.4)	100	Bradbury 1993
vs. clarithromycin	250 mg bid (5–10 days)	240/247 (97.1)	95	
Azithromycin	500 mg od (3 days)	43/48 (90)	31	Hoepelman et al., 1993
vs. amoxicillin + clavulanic acid	500 mg + 125 mg (10 days)	45/81 (88)	25	

[a]Bacteriological data concern fewer patients than for those on clinical efficacy.
[b]In this study 35 patients were affected with URTI (42.3%), 34 with pneumonia (28%), and the other with acute bronchitis and exacerbations of chronic bronchitis.

considerations (prolonged half-life and long-lasting accumulation of azithromycin in tissues and cells), was as effective as a 5-day course, and compared favorably with treatment with erythromycin and clarithromycin for 7–10 days (see Table 7). The study of Myburgh et al. (1993), carried out exclusively in patients with CAP, is of particular relevance: 66 patients, 40 of whom were evaluable, were treated with a 3-day course of azithromycin at 500 mg/day in a single dose. Clinical and bacteriological outcomes were very satisfactory, with positive results in 98% of cases, similar to those obtained with a 5-day course (500 mg as single dose on day 1, followed by 250 mg/day for 4 days).

A few studies are now available on the clinical efficacy of dirithromycin in CAP. Because of its long half-life, dirithromycin is administered in a single daily dose of 500 mg. In a double-blind, double-dummy, multicenter study (Jacobson, 1993), dirithromycin was compared with erythromycin at a daily dose of 1 g (250 mg qid) in the treatment of pneumonia. The duration of treatment with both drugs ranged from 10 to 14 days. At 3–5 days posttherapy and also later posttherapy, favorable responses in 90 dirithromycin-treated patients were 94.5 and 98.7%, respectively, and in 83 erythromycin-treated patients, 100 and 94.8%, respectively. Bacterial eradication was achieved in 91.4% of patients in the dirithromycin-treated group and in 87.8% of patients in the erythromycin-treated group. *Mycoplasma pneumoniae* and *L. pneumophila* pneumonia could be serologically ascertained in 41 and 14 patients, respectively, in the dirithromycin-treated group, and in 31 and 8 patients in the erythromycin-treated group. Satisfactory clinical responses were obtained with dirithromycin in 38 of 41 patients with mycoplasmal pneumonia and in all patients (14) with legionellosis. All patients with mycoplasmal and Legionella pneumonia treated with erythromycin recovered (Table 8).

A special use for macrolides exists in the treatment of atypical pneumonia; however, data are still scanty. Several isolated cases of pneumonia, caused by *Legionella*, *Mycoplasma*, or *Chlamydia* species, who were successfully treated with macrolides have been reported, but very few prospective studies are available.

Erythromycin is considered the first-choice drug in legionellosis, and it is initially administered intravenously at high doses (up to 4 g daily), and then subsequently by the oral route. Quite often in severe cases, it has been combined with rifampin or other drugs; hence, the evaluation of its role is not always clear-cut (Edelstein, 1993). Spiramycin, josamycin, and miokamycin have been used with success in a limited number of patients (Mayaud et al., 1988; Stahl, 1987; Croce et al., 1987). Also recent derivatives, such as roxithromycin, clarithromycin, azithromycin, and dirithromycin, which reach higher tissue and intracellular concentrations, have satisfactory activity, although major experience is still lacking (see Table 8). Because of their favorable pharmacokinetic characteristics the new macrolides and azalides can be administered once or twice

Table 8 Clinical Efficacy of Macrolides in Atypical Pneumonia

Drugs	Daily dosage and duration of treatment	No. pts. with satisfactory clinical results (cure + improvement)/no. evaluable pts. (%) in					Refs.
		Atypical pneumonia (pathogen not identified)	*Legionella pneumophila*	*Mycoplasma pneumoniae*	*C. pneumoniae* *C. psittaci*	*Coxiella burnetii*	
Roxithromycin	150 mg bid (9–14 days)				13/13		Astarloa et al., 1988
Roxithromycin	300 mg od or 150 mg bid (10 days)	17/18	4/4	17/19	21/21	1/1	Perianu and Stamboulian, 1991
Clarithromycin	500–1000 mg bid (14–35 days)		43/44				Hamedani et al., 1991
Clarithromycin vs.	250 mg bid				4/6		Martin et al., 1990
erythromycin	250–500 mg qid (14 days)				4/6		
Clarithromycin vs.	250 mg bid			18/18	9/11		Cassell et al., 1991b
erythromycin	250–500 mg qid (up to 14 days)			11/12	11/11		
Clarithromycin vs.	250 mg bid (7–14 days)			10/11	2/2		Chien et al., 1993
erythromycin	500 mg qid (7–14 days)			7/8	2/2		

Azithromycin vs.	250 mg bid on day 1 and 250 mg od (on days 2−5)		31/31	8/8		Schönwald et al., 1990
erythromycin	500 mg qid (10 days)		24/24	8/8		
Azithromycin	500 mg od (3 days)	8/8				Myburgh et al., 1993
Azithromycin vs.	500 mg od (3 days)		19/19	4/4	3/3	Schönwald et al., 1991
azithromycin	250 mg bid on day 1 and 250 mg od on days 2−5		24/24	4/4	3/3	
Azithromycin vs.	500 mg od (3 days)	2/2	3/3	2/2		Rizzato et al., 1993
clarithromycin	250 mg bid (8 days)		3/3	0/1		
Dirithromycin vs.	50 mg od (10−14 days)	14/14	38/41			Jacobson, 1993
erythromycin	250 mg qid (10−14 days)	10/10	32/32			

daily, an advantage for tolerability and compliance. Clarithromycin is available also in an intravenous formulation. The duration of therapy with most of these derivatives is 2–3 weeks, with the exception of azithromycin, which has been employed successfully in 3-day courses (Myburg et al., 1993). Future trials should assess if additional 3-day courses could help ensure persistence of cure or improvement.

Alternative choices in legionellosis, when macrolides or macrolides plus rifampin fail, are quinolones (ciprofloxacin or ofloxacin) or doxycycline. Co-trimoxazole has occasionally been effective, mostly in combination with erythromycin or rifampin, but clear evidence of its efficacy is lacking (Edelstein, 1993).

Macrolides and tetracyclines are also effective in *Mycoplasma pneumoniae* pneumonias. Erythromycin still remains the most widely used macrolide, but the new macrolides have been tested in this pneumonia with excellent results (see Table 8; Orfila, 1993b).

In the treatment of respiratory infection caused by the recently described new chlamydial species *Chlamydia pneumoniae* TWAR, it has been noted that erythromycin or tetracycline for 10–14 days may fail. New macrolides, particularly clarithromycin and azithromycin, are highly active in vitro against *C. pneumoniae*. The limited available clinical data indicate good efficacy for these derivatives in human disease. Again, a 3-day course of azithromycin is equivalent to the longer treatment necessary with the other antimicrobial agents effective in this infection (Grayston, 1992). The most recent data on the activity of the new macrolides in pneumonia caused by *Chlamydia psittaci* and *Coxiella burnetii*, suggest their efficacy in these clinical settings (see Table 8), although only a small number of patients have been studied.

In conclusion, new reliable diagnostic methods and extensive epidemiological surveys have led to a better understanding of the microbial etiology of atypical pneumonia and to a more rational classification of the different clinical entities previously grouped under this heading. Macrolides show good activity against *L. pneumophila*, *M. pneumoniae*, and *C. pneumoniae*, but several aspects of treatment need to be clarified.

The clinical use of erythromycin in legionellosis has been largely based on empirical observations and its activity in experimental *L. pneumophila* infections. In clinical settings, newer derivatives should be better accepted by patients, owing to their favorable pharmacokinetics that allow one or two daily doses and to their good toleration by patients. However, clinical data are available in only a limited number of patients. Larger clinical experience is needed to assess their value in this infection.

Satisfactory results have been obtained with old and new macrolide derivatives in the treatment of *M. pneumoniae* infection. Comparative studies have been performed, although the number of patients is limited.

Preliminary clinical data on the treatment of *C. pneumoniae* infection is disappointing. Treatment failures with erythromycin were more frequent than with tetracycline. Recent clinical data, however, indicate good activity with erythromycin as well as with the newer derivatives in *C. pneumoniae* pneumonia.

One hopes that more prospective, randomized, comparative clinical studies on the efficacy of different macrolide derivatives will be performed to develop more specific indications for their use in atypical pneumonia. To achieve this target, there is a need for more reliable, simple, and rapid methods of microbiological or serological diagnosis. Moreover, it will be of paramount importance to assess and monitor the existence and the emergence of resistant strains among different populations of pathogens.

REFERENCES

Almirall J, Morató I, Riera F, et al. Incidence of community-acquired pneumonia and *Chlamydia pneumoniae* infection: a prospective multicentre study. Eur Respir J 1993; 6:14–18.

Anderson R, Joone G, van Rensburg CEJ. An in vitro evaluation of the cellular uptake and intraphagocytic bioactivity of clarithromycin (A-56268, TE-031), a new macrolide antimicrobial agent. J Antimicrob Chemother 1988; 22:923–933.

Anderson G, Esmonde TS, Coles S, et al. A comparative safety and efficacy study of clarithromycin stearate in community-acquired pneumonia. J Antimicrob Chemother 1991; 27(suppl A):117–124.

Andrews JM, Honeybourne D, Greaves I, et al. Clarithromycin levels in human bronchial mucosa, alveolar macrophages and serum. Eighth Mediterranean Congress of Chemotherapy, Athens, Greece, May 24–27, 1992:abstr 714.

Astarloa L, Maglio F, Congelosi D, Garcia-Messina O. Roxithromycin in the treatment of atypical pneumonia in adult patient. Br J Clin Pract 1988; 42:94–95.

Atmar RL, Greenberg SB. Pneumonia caused by *Mycoplasma pneumoniae* and the TWAR agent. Semin Respir Infect 1989; 4:19–31.

Baldwin DR, Honeybourne D, Wise R. Pulmonary disposition of antimicrobial agents: "in vivo" observations and clinical relevance. Antimicrob Agents Chemother 1992; 36:1176–1180.

Baldwin DR, Wise R, Andrews JM, et al. Azithromycin concentrations at the sites of pulmonary infection. Eur Respir J 1990; 3:886–890.

Balmes P, Clerc G, Dupont B, et al. Comparative study of azithromycin and amoxicillin/clavulanic acid in the treatment of lower respiratory infections. Eur J Clin Microbiol Infect Dis 1991; 10:437–439.

Barker JE, Farrel ID. The effects of single and combined antibiotics on the growth of *Legionella pneumophila* using time-kill studies. J Antimicrob Chemother 1990; 26:45–53.

Bartlett JG. Atypical and *Legionella* infections. Curr Opin Infect Dis 1989; 2:526–530.

Beaty CD, Grayston JY, Wang SP, et al. *Chlamydia pneumoniae*, strain TWAR, infection in patients with chronic obstructive pulmonary disease. Am Rev Respir Dis 1991; 144:1408–1410.

Bergogne-Bérézin E. Penetration of antibiotics into the respiratory tree. J Antimicrob Chemother 1981; 8:171–174.

Bergogne-Bérézin E. Tissue distribution of roxithromycin. J Antimicrob Chemother 1987; 20(suppl B):113–20.

Bergogne-Bérézin E. Spiramycin concentrations in the human respiratory tract: a review. J Antimicrob Chemother 1988; 22(suppl B):117–22.

Bergogne-Bérézin E. Tissue distribution of dirithromycin: comparison with erythromycin. J Antimicrob Chemother 1993; 31(suppl C):77–87.

Berntsson E, Lagergard T, Strannegard O, Trollfors B. Etiology of community-acquired pneumonia. Eur J Microbiol Infect Dis 1986; 5:446–447.

Bertrand A, Caubarrere I, Chapman A, et al. Multicentre comparative study of the efficacy and safety of roxithromycin and erythromycin ethylsuccinate in the treatment of lower respiratory infections. Br J Clin Pract 1988; 42(suppl 55):98–99.

Bhasin RC. An open comparative clinical study of roxithromycin versus ampicillin in acute respiratory tract infections. 17th International Congress of Chemotherapy, Berlin, June 23–28, 1991:abstr 152.

Bisetti A, Grassi L, Marelli G, et al. Confronto tra azitromicina ed eritromicina nel trattamento delle infezioni acute delle vie respiratorie superiori ed inferiori in pazienti adulti. Farm Ter 1992; 9(2–3):135–142.

Blander SJ, Szeto L, Shuman HA, Horwitz MA. An immunoprotective molecule, the major secretory protein of *Legionella pneumophila*, is not a virulence factor in a guinea pig model of legionnaires disease. J Clin Invest 1990; 86:817–824.

Blasi F, Cosentini R, Legnani F, Denti F, Allegra L. Incidence of community-acquired pneumonia caused by *Chlamydia pneumoniae* in Italian patients. Eur J Clin Microbiol Infect Dis 1993a; 12:696–699.

Blasi F, Legnani D, Lombardo VM, et al. *Chlamydia pneumoniae* infection in acute exacerbations of COPD. Eur Respir J 1993b; 6:19–22.

Bradbury F. Comparison of azithromycin versus clarithromycin in the treatment of patients with lower respiratory tract infections. J Antimicrob Chemother 1993; 31(suppl E):153–162.

Brueckner O, Trautmann M, Kemmerich B. Roxithromycin (ROX) compared to a new cephalosporin cefixime (CEF) and ciprofloxacin (CIP) in purulent chest disease and pneumonia. In: Rubinstein E, Adam D, eds. Recent Advances in Chemotherapy. 16th Int. Congr. Chemother., Jerusalem, June 11–16, 1989. Jerusalem: E Lewin-Epstein, 1989:436–441.

Carlier MB, Zenebergh A, Tulkens PM. Cellular uptake and subcellular distribution of roxithromycin and erythromycin in phagocytic cells. J Antimicrob Chemother 1987; 20(suppl B):47–56.

Cassell G, Bates J, Drnec J. Clarithromycin vs erythromycin in the treatment of atypical community acquired pneumonia. 17th International Congress of Chemotherapy, Berlin, June 23–28, 1991b:abstr 1810.

Cassell GH, Drnce J, Waites KB, et al. Efficacy of clarithromycin against *Mycoplasma pneumoniae*. J Antimicrob Chemother 1991a; 27(suppl A):47–59.

Chien SM, Pichotta P, Siepman, Chan CK. Treatment of community-acquired pneumonia—a multicenter, double-blind, randomized study comparing clarithromycin with erythromycin. The Canada–Sweden clarithromycin–pneumonia study group. Chest 1993; 103:697–701.

Croce GF, Mazzei L, Zechini F, et al. Terapia con miocamicina della polmonite da *Legionella pneumophila*: tre casi clinici. Ann Inst Forlanini 1987; 7:201–212.

Dark D. Multicenter evaluation of azithromycin and cefaclor in acute lower respiratory tract infections. Am J Med 1991; 91(suppl 3A):31S–35S.

Dautzenberg B, Scheimberg A, Brambilla C, et al. Comparison of 2 oral antibiotics, roxithromycin and amoxicillin plus clavulanic acid, in lower respiratory tract infections. 17th International Congress of Chemotherapy, Berlin, June 23–28, 1991:abstr 755.

Dubois J, St Pierre C, Prokocimer P. Treatment of community-acquired pneumonia: a comparison of clarithromycin and erythromycin. 30th Interscience Conference on Antimicrobial Agents and Chemotherapy (ICAAC), Atlanta, October 21–24, 1990:abstr 1336.

Edelstein PH. Legionnaires' disease. Clin Infect Dis 1993; 16:741–749.

Edelstein PH, Edelstein MAC. In vitro activity of azithromycin against clinical isolates of *Legionella* species. Antimicrob Agents Chemother 1991; 35:180–181.

Edelstein PH, Calarco K, Yasui VK. Antimicrobial therapy of experimentally induced legionnaires' disease in guinea pigs. Am Rev Respir Dis 1984; 130:849–856.

Fang GD, Fine M, Orloff J, et al. New and emerging etiologies for community-acquired pneumonia with implications for therapy. Medicine 1990; 69:307–316.

Fass RJ. Aetiology and treatment of community-acquired pneumonia in adults: an historical perspective. J Antimicrob Chemother 1993; 32(suppl A):17–27.

Fietta A, Boeri P, Colombo ML, Merlini C, Gialdroni Grassi G. Uptake of flurithromycin by human polymorphonuclear phagocytes: partial characterization of the entry mechanism. Chemotherapy 1992; 38:433–440.

Fitzgeorge RB, Featherstone ASR, Baskerville A. Efficacy of azithromycin in the treatment of guinea pigs infected with *Legionella pneumophila* by aerosol. J Antimicrob Chemother 1990; 25(suppl A):101–108.

Foulds G, Shepard RM, Johnson RB. The pharmacokinetics of azithromycin in human serum and tissues. J Antimicrob Chemother 1990; 25(suppl A):73–82.

Fraschini F, Scaglione F, Pintucci G, et al. The diffusion of clarithromycin and roxithromycin into nasal mucosa, tonsil and lung in humans. J Antimicrob Chemother 1991; 27(suppl A):61–65.

Futterman M, Drnec J. Safety and efficacy of clarithromycin compared with erythromycin in the treatment of community acquired pneumonia. 30th Interscience Conference on Antimicrobial Agents and Chemotherapy, Atlanta, GA, 1990: abstr 1337.

Gialdroni Grassi G. Passaggio degli antibiotici nelle secrezioni bronchiali. In: Gialdroni Grassi G, Grassi C, eds. Aggiornamenti di Chemioterapia. Pavia: La Goliardica Pavese, 1980:68–88.

Gialdroni Grassi G, Grassi C. Lower respiratory tract infections: (II) parenchymal infections. In: Bryskier AJ, Butzler JP, Neu HC, Tulkens PM, eds. Macrolides. Paris: Arnette Blackwell, 1993:535–550.

Gladue RP, Bright GM, Isaacson RE, New Borg MF. In vitro and in vivo uptake of azithromycin (CP-62, 993) by phagocytic cells: possible mechanism of delivery and release at sites of infection. Antimicrob Agents Chemother 1989; 33:277–282.

Glynn JR, Jones AC. Atypical respiratory infections, including *Chlamydia* TWAR infection and *Legionella* infection. Curr Opinion Infect Dis 1990; 3:169–175.

Grayston JT. Infections caused by *Chlamydia pneumoniae* strain TWAR. Clin Infect Dis 1992; 15:757–763.

Grayston JT, Kuo CC, Wang SP, Alman J. A new *Chlamydia psittaci* strain, TWAR, isolated in acute respiratory tract infections. N Engl J Med 1986; 315:161–168.

Grayston JT, Diwan VK, Cooney M, Wang SP. Community and hospital acquired pneumonia associated with *Chlamydia* TWAR infection demonstrated serologically. Arch Intern Med 1989; 149:169–173.

Gump DW. Antimicrobial susceptibility testing for some atypical microorganism: chlamydiae, mycoplasmas, rickettsia and spirochetes. In: Lorian V, ed. Antibiotics in Laboratory Medicine, 3rd ed. Baltimore: Williams & Wilkins, 1991:279–294.

Hamedani P, Hafeez S, Bachand R Jr, et al. The safety and efficacy of clarithromycin in patients with *Legionella* pneumonia. Chest 1991; 100:1503–1506.

Hand WL, Boozer RM, King-Thompson NL. Antibiotic uptake by alveolar macrophages of smokers. Antimicrob Agents Chemother 1985; 27:42–45.

Hara K, Suyama N, Yamaguchi K, Kohno S, Saito A. Activity of macrolides against organism responsible for respiratory infection with emphasis on *Mycoplasma* and *Legionella*. J Antimicrob Chemother 1987; 20(suppl B):75–80.

Hoepelman AIM, Sips AP, van Helmond JLM, et al. A single-blind comparison of a three-day azithromycin and ten-day co-amoxicillin treatment of acute and lower respiratory tract infections. J Antimicrob Chemother 1993; 31(suppl E):147–152.

Hohl P, Buser V, Frei R. Fatal *Legionella pneumophila* pneumonia: treatment failure despite early sequential oral–parenteral amoxicillin–clavulanic acid therapy. Infection 1992; 20:99–100.

Jacobson K. Clinical efficacy of dirithromycin in pneumonia. J Antimicrob Chemother 1993; 31(suppl C):121–129.

Kayser FH. Changes in the spectrum of organism causing respiratory tract infections: a review. Postgrad Med J 1992; 68(suppl 3):S17–S23.

Kenny GE. Mycoplasmas. In: Balows A, Hausler WJ, Herrmann L, Jenberg HD, Shadomy HJ, eds. Manual of Clinical Microbiology, 5th ed. Washington DC: American Society for Microbiology, 1991:478–482.

Kinasewitz G, Wood RG. Azithromycin versus cefaclor treatment for acute bacterial pneumonia. Eur J Clin Microbiol Infect Dis 1991; 10:872–877.

Kirby BD, Snyder KM, Meyer RD, Finegold SM. Legionnaires' disease: report of sixty-five nosocomially acquired cases and review of the literature. Medicine 1980; 59:188–205.

Kohno S, Koga H, Yamaguchi K, et al. A new macrolide, TE 031 (A-56268) in treatment of experimental legionnaires' disease. J Antimicrob Chemother 1989; 24:397–405.

Liebers DM, Baltch AL, Smith RP, et al. Susceptibility of *Legionella pneumophila* to eight antimicrobial agents including four macrolides under different assay conditions. J Antimicrob Chemother 1989; 23:37–41.

MacDonald PJ, Pruul H. Phagocyte uptake and transport of azithromycin. Eur J Clin Microbiol Infect Dis 1991; 10:828–833.

MacFarlane JT, Finch RG, Ward MJ, Macrae AD. Hospital study of adult community-acquired pneumonia. Lancet 1982; 2:255–258.

MacFarlane JT, Calville A, Guian A, et al. Prospective study of aetiology and outcome of adult lower-respiratory-tract infections in the community. Lancet 1993; 341: 511–514.

Mansel JK, Rosenow EC, Smith TF, Martin JW. *Mycoplasma pneumoniae* pneumonia. Chest 1989; 95:3.

Marsac JH, Akoun G, Balmes P, et al. Multicentre comparative study of the efficacy and safety of roxithromycin and doxycycline in the treatment of lower respiratory infections. Br J Clin Pract 1988; 42(suppl 55):100–101.

Martin R, Rank R, Person K, et al. *Chlamydia pneumoniae* (TWAR): comparative-efficacy of clarithromycin and erythromycin. 30th International Conference on Antimicrobial Agents and Chemotherapy, Atlanta, October 1990:abstr 1334.

Mayaud C, Dournon E, Montagne V, et al. Efficacy of intravenous spiramycin in the treatment of severe legionnaire disease. J Antimicrob Chemother 1988; 22(suppl B):179–182.

Meyer RD, Finch RG. Community-acquired pneumonia. J Hosp Infect 1992; 22(suppl A):51–59.

Myburgh J, Nagel GJ, Petschel E. The efficacy and tolerance of a three day course of azithromycin in the treatment of community-acquired pneumonia. J Antimicrob Chemother 1993; 31(suppl E):163–169.

Nicotra MB, Northcutt VJ. Results of comparative trials of clarithromycin and erythromycin in the treatment of community acquired pneumonia. 17th International Congress of Chemotherapy, Berlin, June 23–28, 1991:abstr 1809.

Orfila J. Chlamydial infections. In: Bryskier AJ, Butzler JP, Neu HC, Tulkens PM, eds. Macrolides. Paris: Arnette Blackwell, 1993a:241–252.

Orfila J. Antimycoplasmal activity of macrolides. In: Bryskier AJ, Butzler JP, Neu HC, Tulkens PM, eds. Macrolides. Paris: Arnette Blackwell, 1993:253–260.

Pennington JE. Hospital acquired pneumonia. In: Pennington JE, ed. Respiratory Infections: Diagnosis and Management, 2nd ed. New York: Raven Press, 1989a: 171–186.

Pennington JE. Community-acquired pneumonia and acute bronchitis. In: Pennington JE, ed. Respiratory Infections: Diagnosis and Management, 2nd ed. New York: Raven Press, 1989b:159–170.

Perianu M, Grassi C. The clinical and bacteriological efficacy of roxithromycin (300 mg once-daily or 150 mg bid) in acute lower respiratory tract infection in a double-blind multicentre international study. 17th International Congress of Chemotherapy, Berlin, June 23–28, 1991:abstr 762.

Perianu M, Stamboulian D. The efficacy of roxithromycin (300 mg once-daily or 150 mg bid) in the treatment of "atypical" pneumonia in an international multicentre study. 17th International Congress of Chemotherapy, Berlin, June 23–28, 1991: abstr 785.

Periti P. Recenti progressi nella chemioterapia antimicrobica orale: la claritromicina. Farm Ter 1990; 7(suppl 1):37–63.

Peters DH, Clissold SP. Clarithromycin. A review of its antimicrobial activity, pharmacokinetic properties and therapeutical potential. Drugs 1992; 44:117–164.

Pocidalo JJ. Use of fluoroquinolones for intracellular pathogens. Rev Infect Dis 1989; 11(suppl 5):S979–S984.

Poirier R. Comparative study of clarithromycin and roxithromycin in the treatment of community-acquired pneumonia. J Antimicrob Chemother 1991; 27(suppl A):109–116.

Prokesh RC, Hand WL. Antibiotic entry into human polymorphonuclear leukocytes. Antimicrob Agents Chemother 1982; 21:373–378.

Rahlwes M, Wagner J, Schuster L, et al. Prospective of community-acquired pneumonia and comparison of amoxicillin versus roxithromycin therapy. In: Berkarda B, Kuemmerle HP, eds. Progress in Antimicrobial and Anticancer Chemotherapy, vol 2. Proc 15th Intern Congr Chemother, Istanbul, July 19–24, 1987. Landberg/Lech, Germany: Ecomed, 1987:1376–1378.

Rajagopalan-Levasseur P, Dournon E, Dameron G, Vilde JL, Pocidalo JJ. Comparative postantibacterial activities of pefloxacin, ciprofloxacin and ofloxacin against intracellular multiplication of *Legionella pneumophila* serogroup 1. Antimicrob Agents Chemother 1990; 34:1733–1738.

Ramirez JA, Summersgill JT, Miller D, Meyers TL, Raff MJ. Comparative study of the bactericidal activity of ampicillin–sulbactam and erythromycin against intracellular *Legionella pneumophila*. J Antimicrob Chemother 1993; 32:93–99.

Research committee of the British Thoracic Society and the Public Health Laboratory Service. Community-acquired pneumonia in adults in British hospitals in 1982–1983: a survey of aetiology, mortality, prognostic factors and outcome. Q J Med 1987; 239:195–220.

Rizzato G, Montemurro L, Fraioli P, et al. Studio pilota con azitromicina per tre giorni versus claritromicina per otto giorni nelle polmoniti comunitarie: i nostri primi venti casi. L'Internista 1993; 1:115–122.

Roig J, Carreres A, Domingo C. Treatment of legionnaires' disease. Drugs 1993; 46(suppl 1):63–79.

Ruiz-Santana, Agauado-Bourrey JM, Narvaez-Bermejo JM, Gonzalez-Mediere G. *Legionella bozemanii* pneumonia and tetracyclines. Ann Intern Med 1986; 105:969–970.

Sachs FL. Chronic bronchitis. In: Pennington JE, ed. Respiratory Infections: Diagnosis and Management, 2nd ed. New York: Raven Press, 1989:142–158.

Schonwald S, Gunjaca M, Kolacny-Babic L, et al. Comparison of azithromycin and erythromycin in the treatment of atypical pneumonias. J Antimicrob Chemother 1990; 25(suppl A):123–126.

Schonwald S, Skerk V, Petricevic I, et al. Comparison of three-day and five-day courses of azithromycin in the treatment of atypical pneumonia. Eur J Clin Microbiol Infect Dis 1991; 10:877–880.

Smith BR, LeFrock JL. Bronchial tree penetration of antibiotic. Chest 1983; 83:904–908.

Soejima R, Hara K. Double blind comparison of roxithromycin and midecamycin acetate in the treatment of pneumonia. In: Rubinstein E, Adam D, eds. Recent Advances in Chemotherapy. 16th Intern Congr Chemother, Jerusalem, June 11–16, 1989. Jerusalem: E. Lewin-Epstein, 1989:435.1–435.2.

Stahl JP, Leclenq P, Bru JP, et al. Empiric therapy of 246 acute pneumonias of adults. 15th International Congress of Chemotherapy, Istambul, July 19–24, 1987:abstr 91.

Straneo G, Scarpazza G. Efficacy and safety of clarithromycin versus josamycin in the treatment of hospitalized patients with bacterial pneumonia. J Int Med Res 1990; 18:164–170.

Torres A, El-Ebiary M. Relevance of *Chlamydia pneumoniae* in community-acquired respiratory infections. Eur Respir J 1993; 6:7–8.

Tuazon CU, Murray HW. Atypical pneumonias. In: Pennington JE, ed. Respiratory Infections: Diagnosis and Management, 2nd ed. New York: Raven Press, 1989: 341–363.

Tulkens PM. Intracellular pharmacokinetics and localization of antibiotics as predictors of their efficacy against intraphagocytic infections. Scand J Infect Dis [Suppl] 1991a; 74:209–217.

Tulkens PM. Intracellular distribution and activity of antibiotics. Eur J Clin Microbiol Infect Dis 1991b; 10:100–106.

Valcke Y, Pauwels R, Van Den Straeten M. Pharmacokinetics of antibiotics in the lungs. Eur Respir J 1990; 3:715–722.

Woodhead MA, MacFarlane JT, Rodgers FG, et al. Aetiology and outcome of severe community-acquired pneumonia. J Infect 1985; 10:204–210.

Woodhead MA, MacFarlane JT, McCracken JS, et al. Prospective study of the aetiology and outcome of pneumonia in the community. Lancet 1987; 1:671–674.

Zeluff BJ, Lowe P, Koornhof HJ, Gentry LO. Evaluation of roxithromycin (RU-965) versus cephradine in pneumococcal pneumonia. Eur J Clin Microbiol Infect Dis 1988; 7:69–71.

8

Macrolides as Antimycobacterial Agents

Lowell S. Young

Kuzell Institute for Arthritis and Infectious Diseases
California Pacific Medical Center
San Francisco, California

INTRODUCTION

We live in a time when mycobacterial diseases are important concerns in the minds of every infectious disease clinician. Tuberculosis remains the most lethal of all infectious diseases (malaria may be more common, but tuberculosis is associated with greater mortality; 1). Worldwide, leprosy afflicts approximately some 20 million individuals. With the advent of the acquired immunodeficiency syndrome (AIDS) the atypical mycobacteria, and *Mycobacterium avium-intracellulare* complex (MAC), in particular, have assumed a major clinical role as opportunistic pathogens (2). Organisms of the MAC now represent the most common cause of disseminated bacterial infection in patients in the advanced stages of AIDS (3). The profound immune deficiency observed in AIDS patients appears to set the stage not only for systemic MAC disease, but other mycobacterial pathogens have become increasingly appreciated (2). These include *M. haemophilum*, *M. genovense*, and *M. malmoense*. Other mycobacteria appear to be even more fastidious, and their existence has been identified by molecular techniques. To further compound the problem, the atypical mycobacteria are often resistant to conventional antituberculous chemotherapy. A widely appreciated upsurge in MAC disease seems to have paralleled the advent of the AIDS pandemic (4). Serious MAC infections are now being seen with increased frequency in patients *without* underlying human immunodeficiency virus (HIV) disease.

IN VITRO TESTING OF MACROLIDES AGAINST MYCOBACTERIA

In vitro test conditions are likely to influence considerably the outcome of laboratory studies. Many investigators have noted that the activity of macrolides is pH-dependent (5,6). Macrolides are most active at neutral or alkaline pHs and are relatively inactive at acid pHs. The pH of media, such as is present in standard mycobacterial culture systems using Middlebrook broth, are buffered in the acid range to facilitate the growth of organisms (i.e., provide optimal growth conditions). Although the pH within phagocytes is normally acid during the process of phagolysosomal fusion (which follows bacterial ingestion), it has been noted that several important pathogens, such as mycobacteria and legionella, inhibit acidification of phagosomes. Rather than testing organisms in pH-altered media, we believe that it may be useful to proceed with any promising compound using phagocytic (macrophage) cell lines, which are buffered at physiological pH. One factor that also needs to be borne in mind is that the in vivo situation is likely to be influenced by host factors or components of the host cellular response. Thus, cytokines may actually have a beneficial effect in enhancing intracellular penetration of drugs such as macrolides (7). Figure 1 is an attempt to depict the in vitro activity of four of the new macrolides or azalides in Middlebrook 7H11 broth medium. The minimum inhibitory concentrations

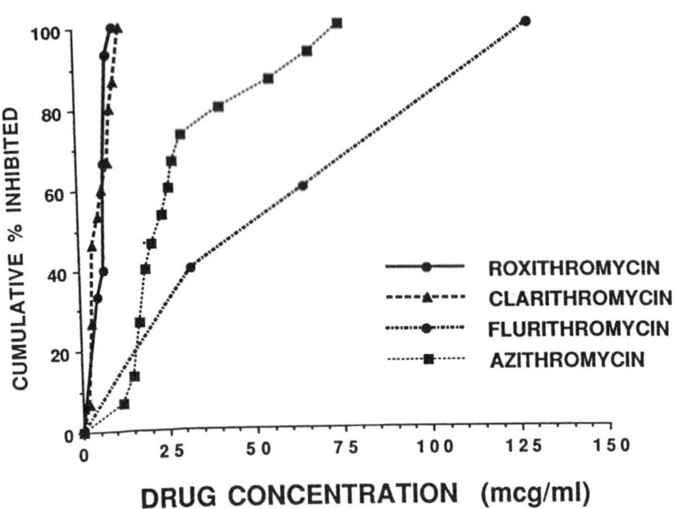

Figure 1   Comparative activity of the four new macrolides (azalides) against 15 isolates of *M. avium* from AIDS patients with disseminated disease. (Method of Inderlied, Ref. 6.)

(MICs) of 15 isolates of MAC from AIDS patients, as determined by the method of Inderlied, are shown (6).

MYCOBACTERIUM AVIUM COMPLEX

Historical Perspective

The first suggestion that the new macrolides might be effective for atypical mycobacterial organisms, and *M. avium* complex in particular, was a publication by Casal in 1987 (Table 1; 8). This report focused on the activity of roxithromycin in vitro. The work received little attention until we and others investigated the effect of roxithromycin alone and in combination with immunomodulators, such as tumor necrosis factor (9). In 1989, Fernandes et al. (10) and Inderlied et al. (11) reported on the in vitro and in vivo activity of clarithromycin and azithromycin, respectively. The in vivo test system employed was the beige mouse model of systemic disease, which has reliably identified every compound that has been used successfully either to treat or to prevent *M. avium* disease in humans. Even though agents such as azithromycin achieve relatively low serum levels ($<$ 1 μg/ml peak serum level), the extremely high tissue concentrations and the long serum half-life suggested that this compound might be effective against intracellular organisms with long replication times.

Encouraged by the initial in vitro studies, Dautzenberg and colleagues in France (12) and ourselves in the United States initiated the first human clinical trials with clarithromycin and azithromycin, respectively (13). The design of these studies, although involving relatively few patients, used quantitative blood culture methodology for assessing the microbiological effect of the compound in vivo. As a result of these pilot studies much larger clinical trials of macrolide monotherapy have been organized in the United States. These have included trials of treatment and prophylaxis organized by several multicenter groups including the AIDS Clinical Trial Groups and the California Collaborative Treatment Group.

Table 1 New Macrolides/Azalides vs. *M. avium*

Date	Author/agent/ref.
1987	Casal on roxithromycin [RU-28965] *Chemotherapy* 33:255
1989	Fernandes on clarithromycin (in vitro/in vivo) *Antimicrob Agents Chemother* 33:1531
1989	Inderlied on azithromycin (in vitro/in vivo) *J Infect Dis* 159:994
1991	Dautzenberg on clarithromycin in AIDS *Am Rev Respir Dis* 144:564
1991	Young on azithromycin in MAC bacteremia *Lancet* 338:1107

Studies with Clarithromycin, Azithromycin, and Roxithromycin

Clarithromycin has an approved indication for the treatment of *M. avium* bacteremia in AIDS patients. Clinical trials in the United States demonstrated, in a dose-ranging manner, that doses of 0.5–2 g twice a day led to a convincing reduction in bacteremia by 4–8 weeks (14). The approved dose of clarithromycin in the United States is at the lower level because of concern about side effects and survival. It has been noted that the microbiological response to clarithromycin is maintained for approximately 4 months before significant numbers of organisms are isolated from blood cultures that show a fourfold or greater increase in MIC. The significance of this finding is ominous. Nonetheless, in vitro testing of the atypical mycobacteria is a controversial field, and it is unclear whether organisms with MICs of 32 or greater still might be effectively treated by larger doses of clarithromycin. More extended clinical trials are now in progress in which clarithromycin is being combined with other agents. A paramount issue is whether or not the combination of clarithromycin with agents, such as ethambutol, clofazimine, rifabutin, and possibly other agents, might accelerate the rate of clinical response and yet limit the emergence of "resistant strains."

Azithromycin, the first 15-membered macrolide, or azalide, was used at a dose of 500 mg/day in our pilot study, in which the duration of treatment was progressively increased from 5, to 20, to 30 days (13). A convincing microbiological response was observed that was paralleled by an improvement in symptoms (mainly fever and chills) and an objective reduction in organomegaly (splenomegaly in patients presenting with this finding). After an initial induction phase with 500 mg/day, a maintenance dose of 250 mg was then employed; a few patients who had follow-up isolates of MAC had organisms that had increased significantly from an initial MIC of 16 to levels that were eightfold or greater than pretreatment levels. At this meeting, we have data presented by Koletar, Williams, and Berry indicating that doses of 600 and 1200 mg of azithromycin as monotherapy are successful in bringing about an approximate 2-log reduction in bacteremia by 6–8 weeks of treatment (abstr 292, this conference). In fact, no significant difference in microbiological response was seen with these two doses of azithromycin, leading some to speculate that an even lower initial dose might be equally effective, or that a loading dose followed by a smaller maintenance dose might be the optimal way to treat systemic disease with azithromycin. As with clarithromycin the eventual selection of strains with increased MICs relative to pretreatment values is a major medical concern.

Roxithromycin has MICs that roughly parallel those of clarithromycin. Figure 1 is representative of 15 strains from our collection that were tested by the method of Inderlied (6). Roxithromycin is active in in vitro test systems employing cultured macrophages, a favored method for evaluating intracellular activity against an intracellular pathogen such as MAC. Furthermore, roxithromycin achieves the highest serum levels of any of the newer macrolides or azalides and might be an attractive candidate for either therapy or prophylaxis. However, no human data have yet been published and studies in experimental murine systems, while anticipated, have not been presented or published.

Present and Future Problems

A major trend in the management of patients with AIDS is an increasing emphasis on the prevention of opportunistic infections, given their serious morbidity. Rifabutin has been studied in two well-controlled clinical trials and was moderately active in the prevention of MAC bacteremia (3). A clear-cut objective has been to compare the efficacy of the newer macrolides with rifabutin (which is FDA approved for this indication) and to determine whether these newer macrolides are as effective or more effective and whether combinations with rifabutin could offer the potential of reducing drug resistance by providing greater prophylactic efficacy. These trials are currently underway, but have encountered some problems. For instance, there now appear to be interactions between rifabutin and fluconazole, but equally of concern are interactions between clarithromycin and rifabutin (15). It is not known whether such interactions also relate to roxithromycin and azithromycin.

EFFECT OF MACROLIDES AGAINST RAPIDLY GROWING MYCOBACTERIA

The so-called rapidly growing mycobacteria include more than a dozen species: organisms tend to form colonies on solid media within less than a week. Clinically important infections before the AIDS pandemic were limited to *M. fortuitum* and *M. chelonae*. Rapidly growing organisms are susceptible to erythromycin, which was successfully used to treat infections with *M. fortuitum* and *M. chelonae*. More recent studies include a beneficial effect from the use of agents such as clarithromycin to treat *M. chelonae* complex disease when coupled with appropriate surgery (debridement and excision; 2).

MACROLIDES FOR *MYCOBACTERIUM LEPRAE*

Effective medications exist for the treatment of leprosy, but the persistence of this ancient disease in the world is probably related more to socioeconomic factors and limited access of its victims to appropriate modern drug treatment. Macrolides have been active in vitro, and there are promising reports of the effect of various drug regimens both in animal models and in human clinical trials. Ji and colleagues compared clarithromycin, minocycline (an established agent for leprosy), and the combination of the two agents in a trial in West Africa: both single agents and the combinations appeared to be potently bactericidal when evaluated in humans (16). Similarly, Franzblau and colleagues assessed the activity of clarithromycin monotherapy in a clinical setting and found clinical and microbiological evidence for efficacy (17).

OTHER ATYPICAL MYCOBACTERIA ASSOCIATED WITH AIDS

The limited data available on *M. genovense* and *M. malmoense* suggest that these organisms are susceptible to macrolides. Combination regimens aimed primarily at MAC may well prove to be effective in reducing organism burden due to these fastidious atypical agents.

MYCOBACTERIUM TUBERCULOSIS

One of the tantalizing issues is whether any of the new macrolides or azalides might be effective against the most virulent of the "typical" mycobacteria, *M. tuberculosis*. Although the new macrolides have been more potent than erythromycin against *M. tuberculosis* in vitro, the activity is probably marginal, at best (18). More recently, Luna-Herrera and colleagues have reported the synergistic effect of clarithromycin when used with isoniazid and rifampin against tubercle bacilli (19). These investigators used a liquid broth solution method for in vitro studies and found that clarithromycin caused a significant enhancement of susceptibility of a "virulent" strain of *M. tuberculosis* to subinhibitory concentrations of rifampin. A similar potentially beneficial interaction was also observed when clarithromycin was tested in the presence of isoniazid.

Realistically, the treatment of tuberculosis, whether susceptible to conventional agents or so-called multiple drug-resistant (MDR) isolates, will require combination chemotherapy. Thus, a potential role for the new macrolides or azalides against tuberculosis should not be overlooked. At least in vitro and in animal test systems, combination studies containing a macrolide are justified. What seems reasonable to infer from the limited number of experimental data available is that macrolides, by themselves, (at least those compounds presently available) do not promise even transiently effective monotherapy for tuberculosis, and combination therapy requires rather complicated assessment.

CONCLUDING PERSPECTIVE

Table 2 summarizes what is currently accepted about the role of the new macrolides, or azalides, in the treatment of mycobacterial diseases. The best-established indication for the use of macrolides is in the treatment of disseminated *M. avium* infection in AIDS patients. Although treatment results

Table 2 Mycobacteria and the New Macrolides/Azalides

Organism	Treatment	Prophylaxis
M. avium[a]	established[b]	Investigational
M. tuberculosis	?	?
M. leprae	Some	NA
M. chelonae	Established	NA

[a]AIDS associated.
[b]Combinations advisable.

in patients with localized pulmonary disease and non–HIV-underlying disorders is limited, the anecdotal clinical observations of the author suggest that regimens similar to those used in AIDS patients could benefit non-AIDS patients who have pulmonary *M. avium* disease. The results of large-scale prophylaxis studies have yet to be reported, but the same animal models that predicted the efficacy of macrolides for treatment of established *M. avium* infection now suggest that prophylaxis with macrolides is likely to be effective (20). Concern has been expressed that single-agent prophylaxis may select for macrolide-resistant mycobacteria.

Tuberculosis remains an open question. A desperate search for new agents with activity against *M. tuberculosis* is underway, and one of the tantalizing questions is whether a new macrolide, or azalide, when added to three or four other antituberculous agents might result in some enhancement of overall activity.

Mycobacterium leprae has been treated in a series of pilot studies in African and Filipino patients, and the results are encouraging. For the rapidly growing mycobacteria, *M. chelonae* infections have been adequately treated in combination with surgical debridement.

Overall, the new macrolide or azalides represent an important advance in the treatment of some mycobacterial diseases, particularly those opportunistic pathogens that complicate AIDS. Given the well-established experience, the treatment of an established mycobacterial infection should probably involve combination therapy. Current investigative efforts are aimed at defining optimal combination regimens. Prophylaxis is another important issue, with a major emphasis now being placed on developing versatile preventative regimens that will obviate the development of multiple opportunistic infections complicating AIDS, including those caused by mycobacteria (20).

REFERENCES

1. Young LS. The Garrod lecture: mycobacterial diseases in the 1990s. J Antimicrob Chemother 1993; 32:179–194.
2. Young LS. Atypical mycobacteria. In: Broder S, Merigan TC Jr, Bolognesi

D, eds. Textbook of AIDS Medicine. Baltimore: Williams & Wilkins, 1993: 283–294.

3. Nightingale SD, Cameron DW, Gordin FM, Sullam PM, Cohn DL, Chaisson R, Eron LJ, Sparti PD, Bihari B, Kaufman DL, Stern JJ, Pearce DD, Winberg WG, LaMarca A, Siegal FP. Two placebo controlled trials of rifabutin prophylaxis against *Mycobacterium avium* complex infection in AIDS. N Engl J Med 1993; 329:828–833.

4. Prince DS, Peterson DD, Steiner RM, Gottlieb JE, Scott R, Israel HL, Figueroa WG, Fish JE. Infection with *Mycobacterium avium* complex in patients without predisposing conditions. N Engl J Med 1989; 130:863–868.

5. Truffot PC, Ji B, Grosset J. Effect of pH on the in vitro potency of clarithromycin against *Mycobacterium avium* complex. Antimicrob Agents Chemother 1991; 35:1677–1678.

6. Young LS, Bermudez LE, Wu M, Inderlied CB. Potential role of roxithromycin against the *Mycobacterium avium* complex. Infection 1994; (in press).

7. Bermudez LE, Inderlied C, Young LS. Stimulation with cytokines enhances penetration of azithromycin into human macrophages. Antimicrob Agents Chemother 1991; 12:2625–2629.

8. Casal M, Rodriguez F, Villalba R. In vitro susceptibility of *Mycobacterium avium* to a new macrolide (RU 28564). Chemotherapy (Basel) 1987; 33:255–258.

9. Bermudez LE, Young LS. Activities of amikacin, roxithromycin and azithromycin alone or in combination with tumor necrosis factor against *Mycobacterium avium* complex. Antimicrob Agents Chemother 1988; 32:1149–1153.

10. Fernandes PB, Hardy DJ, McDaniel D, Hanson CW, Swanson RN. In vitro and in vivo activities of clarithromycin against *Mycobacterium avium*. Antimicrob Agents Chemother 1989; 33:1531–1536.

11. Inderlied CB, Kolonoski PT, Wu M, Young LS. In vitro and in vivo activity of azithromycin (CP 62,993) against the *Mycobacterium avium* complex. J Infect Dis 1989; 159:994–997.

12. Dautzenberg B, Truffot C, Legris S, Meyohas MC, Berlie HC, Mercat A, Chevret S, Grosset J. Activity of clarithromycin against *Mycobacterium avium* infection in patients with the acquired immune deficiency syndrome. Am Rev Respir Dis 1991; 144:564–569.

13. Young LS, Wiviott L, Wu M, Kolonoski PT, Bolan R, Inderlied CB. Azithromycin reduces *Mycobacterium avium* complex bacteremia and relieves the symptoms of disseminated disease in patients with AIDS. Lancet 1991; 338:1107–1109.

14. Chaisson RE, Benson C, Dube M, Korvick A, Wu S, Licheter M, Dellerson M, Smith T, Sattler F. Clarithromycin therapy for *Mycobacterium avium* complex (MAC) in AIDS. 32nd Interscience Conference on Antimicrobial Agents and Chemotherapy (ICAAC), Anaheim, CA, 1992: abstr 891.

15. The DATRI 001 Study Group Albany Medical College, Albany NY, University of Maryland, Baltimore MD, Westat, Inc., Rockville, MD,

Division of AIDS/NIADS Baltimore MD. Coadministration of clarithromycin alters the concentration-time profile of rifabutin. 34th Interscience Conference on Antimicrobial Agents and Chemotherapy (ICAAC), Orlando, FL, 1994: abstr A2.

16. Ji B, Jamet P, Perani EG, Bobin P, Grosset JH. Powerful bactericidal activity of clarithromycin and minocycline against *Mycobacterium leprae* in the treatment of lepromatous leprosy. J Infect Dis 1993; 168:188–190.

17. Chan GP, Garcia-Ignacio BY, Chavez VE, Livelo JB, Jimenez CL, Parrilla MLR, Franzblau SG. Clinical trial of clarithromycin for lepromatous leprosy. Antimicrob Agents Chemother 1994; 38:515–517.

18. Gorzynski EA, Gutman SI, Allen W. Comparative antimycobacterial activities of difloxacin, temafloxacin, enoxacin, pefloxacin, reference fluoroquinolones, and a new macrolide, clarithromycin. Antimicrob Agents Chemother 1989; 33:591–592.

19. Luna-Herrera J, Reddy VM, Gangadharam PRJ. Synergistic effect of clarithromycin and isoniazid and rifampin against tubercle bacilli. 34th Interscience Conference on Antimicrobial Agents and Chemotherapy (ICAAC), Orlando, FL, 1994: abstr E134.

20. Bermudez LE, Inderlied CB, Kolonoski P, Petrofsky M, Young LS. Clarithromycin, dapsone and their combination to treat or prevent disseminated *Mycobacterium avium* infection in beige mice. Antimicrob Agents Chemother 1994; (in press).

9

Macrolides in Toxoplasmosis

Hernan R. Chang

*National University of Singapore
Lower Kent Ridge, Singapore*

Jean-Claude Pechère

*University of Geneva School of Medicine
Geneva, Switzerland*

INTRODUCTION

Toxoplasma gondii is a pandemic, obligate, intracellular protozoan parasite of humans and various animal species. Toxoplasma infection can occur in a variety of ways, including ingestion of tissue cysts present in raw or undercooked meat, consumption of water or food contaminated with oocysts from cat feces (Jacobs et al., 1960; Frenkel et al., 1981), transplacental contamination, blood transfusion, and organ transplantation. The infection has an initial acute phase in which the parasite multiplies rapidly within host cells and causes tissue destruction. With the onset of the immune response, which appears to be mainly cell-mediated, the infection enters a chronic phase in which the parasite forms tissue cysts, mainly in the central nervous system and muscle (Remington et al., 1965). The cysts persist for long periods, possibly for life.

In humans, most *T. gondii* infections remain asymptomatic. When symptomatic toxoplasmosis occurs, four categories of disease can be distinguished. Acute acquired toxoplasmosis in immunocompetent individuals often induces cervical lymphadenopathy, sometimes with fever, myalgia, sore throat, rash, splenomegaly, and a mononucleosislike syndrome. Acquired or reactivated toxoplasmosis can develop in patients with the acquired immunodeficiency syndrome (AIDS) or other immunodeficiencies, and this usually involves the central nervous system. Congenital toxoplasmosis results from an acute infection contracted by the mother during pregnancy and can produce various sequelae or progressive infection in the fetus. Chorioretinitis typically occurs in congenital toxoplasmosis, but often becomes clinically apparent later in life in immunocompetent subjects (Koppe et al., 1986).

The current treatment of choice for toxoplasmosis is the synergistic combination of pyrimethamine, a dihydrofolate reductase inhibitor, and sulfadiazine or trisulfapyrimidines [sulfamethazine (sulfadimidine or sulfadimerazine), sulfamerazine, or sulfapyrazine], which are competitive inhibitors of dihydropteroate synthetase (Eyles et al., 1955; Wettingfeld et al., 1956; Kayhoe et al., 1957; Frenkel et al., 1960). Such treatment, however, is active only against the replicating (intracellular) form of the parasite, not extracellular parasites and tissue cysts. Pyrimethamine is considered potentially teratogenic, and its use is not recommended during the first trimester of pregnancy (Kutscher et al., 1954; Kaufman et al., 1960).

The mortality rate among AIDS patients with toxoplasmic encephalitis treated with the combination of pyrimethamine and sulfadiazine is 70–92% (Levy et al., 1985; Haverkos, 1987; Wanke et al., 1987; Leport et al., 1988). This high mortality rate is mainly related to relapse because of the toxicity (mainly bone marrow suppression and skin rash) of the sulfonamide component of the combination (Levy et al., 1985; Haverkos, 1987). In addition, the bone marrow toxicity of the pyrimethamine–sulfonamide combination may interfere with the prescription of antiviral agents, such as zidovudine, particularly since it has been suggested that AIDS patients with toxoplasmic encephalitis should receive maintenance treatment to avoid relapse (Glatt et al., 1988). Safer compounds are thus urgently needed to treat this disease.

Since the report by Bogacz (1954) on the activity of spiramycin against *T. gondii* in animals (confirmed by Garin et al., 1958; Bonaduce, 1960; Milovanovic et al., 1965; Mas Bakal et al., 1965), this antibiotic has been used in many countries for the treatment of human toxoplasmosis, with no evidence of toxicity. More recently, a number of new macrolide molecules with improved pharmacokinetics have been synthesized, and their activities against *T. gondii* have been assessed. Here, we review the results of the in vitro, experimental and clinical investigations performed with these compounds. Clindamycin also has a major role in the treatment and prophylaxis of toxoplasmosis, especially in patients with AIDS. This lincosamide is not considered in this review.

IN VITRO STUDIES

Toxoplasma gondii readily invades most mammalian cells and multiplies. Extracellular forms do not multiply, they show relatively little metabolic activity, and they are commonly resistant to antiparasitic compounds. As a result, in vitro systems using mammalian cell monolayers have been developed to test compounds for antitoxoplasmic activity. The in vitro activity of macrolides against intracellular *T. gondii* has been evaluated with several methods. These include light microscopy (number of infected cells and toxoplasma bodies per infected vacuole), specific uptake of [^{3}H]uracil by intracellular parasites, and an enzyme immunoassay on fixed cell monolayers (Kieng Truong et al., 1970; Chang et al., 1988; Derouin et al., 1988; Derouin et al., 1990; Chamberland et al., 1991). The IC_{50} (50% inhibitory concentrations) in terms of [^{3}H]uracil uptake in infected mouse peritoneal macrophages, together with the 95% confidence limits, have been estimated at 54 (38–73), 140 (98–201), 147 (101–204), and 246 (187–325) for roxithromycin, azithromycin, clarithromycin, and spiramycin, respectively, following intramuscular injection (Chang et al., 1988). The respective IC_{50} values using MRC5 human fibroblasts and an enzyme immunoassay were 3 (erythromycin), 12 (midecamycin), 12 (spiramycin), 2 (roxithromycin), 1.7 (josamycin), 6.5 (oleandomycin), 1.2 (azithromycin), and 0.8 mg/L (clarithromycin) (Derouin et al., 1988, 1990). None of the macrolides tested seemed to exert a complete killing effect on the intracellular parasites.

Azithromycin has exhibited a killing effect against cysts in vitro (Huskinson-Mark et al., 1991).

ANIMAL MODELS

Several groups have tested macrolides in the treatment of experimental toxoplasmosis in mice, rabbits, and monkeys.

Murine Models

Acute Toxoplasmosis

Intraperitoneal injection of a virulent strain of *T. gondii* and a large inoculum of a relatively virulent strain, both produce a lethal infection in mice. The activity of a given drug is assessed in terms of its ability to protect mice for a given observation time. Spiramycin has protected, respectively, 80 and 75% of mice at doses of 400 mg/kg per day and 250–320 mg/kg per day s.c. (Garin et al., 1958; Milovanovic et al., 1965); the SD_{50} (50% survival dose) of oral spiramycin has been calculated at 300 mg/kg per day (Chang et al., 1987). Full protection has been achieved, respectively, with 540 mg/kg per day for 5 days, 200 mg/kg per day for 10 days and 300 mg/kg per day for 9 days, of roxithromycin (Chang et al., 1987), azithromycin (Araujo et al., 1988), and clarithromycin (Chang et al., 1988). Midecamycin and josamycin are inactive in this model (Garin et al., 1984).

Toxoplasmic Encephalitis

Toxoplasmic encephalitis is induced by intraperitoneal injection of a low-virulence (acute-phase) strain into mice rendered immunodeficient with cortisone acetate, and by intracerebral inoculation of a similar strain (Luft et al., 1986; Hofflin et al., 1987). Roxithromycin gave significant protection in both models (Luft et al., 1986; Hofflin and Remington, 1987) and, in the intracerebral inoculation model, acted synergistically with interferon gamma (Hofflin and Remington, 1987).

Congenital Toxoplasma *Infection*

Experiments with congenitally toxoplasma-infected mice treated with the combination of pyrimethamine and sulfadimidine or spiramycin from the age of 4–8 weeks showed that both treatments were effective in preventing the histopathological changes observed during the early weeks of life (Beverley et al., 1973). Given the similar efficacy of the two treatments, it was suggested that spiramycin was preferable for the treatment of congenital toxoplasmosis because of the potential toxicity of pyrimethamine–sulfadimidine.

Rabbit Model

Spiramycin is effective and nontoxic in the treatment of inflammation in induced toxoplasmic anterior uveitis (Giles et al., 1964).

Monkey Model

A fatal systemic disease has been induced in squirrel monkeys by oral challenge with a relatively virulent strain of *T. gondii*. Spiramycin had no effect on survival (Harper et al., 1985), whereas sulfonamides, alone or in combination with trimethoprim or pyrimethamine, had a significant effect.

Although spiramycin is readily available in most countries, in the United States it can only be obtained directly from the Food and Drug Administration.

CLINICAL STUDIES

Toxoplasmosis in Pregnancy and Congenital Toxoplasmosis

Acute toxoplasmosis acquired during pregnancy is associated with a significant incidence of congenital infections. Moreover, the risk of congenital toxoplasmosis may be increased when the mother has AIDS (Cohen-Addad et al., 1988). Rare cases of congenital toxoplasmosis in infants born to mothers with a history of toxoplasmic infection before pregnancy have been reported (Desmonts et al., 1990). The risk and severity of infection in the fetus is related to the time at which the mother acquires the infection. Severity is greatest when the maternal infection is acquired during the first trimester, whereas the risk of fetal infection is highest when the maternal infection is acquired during the third trimester. Because there seems to be a lag period between the maternal and fetal infection, antitoxoplasmic therapy can be started in the hope of preventing transmission to the fetus when the diagnosis is made sufficiently early.

Three-week courses of spiramycin, alternating with 2-week periods without treatment, until term have been reported to reduce the incidence of congenital infection from 17 to 5% (Desmonts et al., 1974) and from 61 to 23% (Desmonts et al., 1984). Correlations between negative results in mouse inoculation tests of placental tissues and spiramycin treatment have suggested that spiramycin might reduce the risk of maternal–fetal transmission of *T. gondii* by decreasing the severity and duration of placentitis (Couvreur et al., 1988). When spiramycin was used with combined courses of pyrimethamine and sulfadiazine in the early treatment of pregnant women acutely infected with *T. gondii*, there was a marked reduction in the incidence of congenital infection and a correspondingly low incidence of sequelae (Daffos et al., 1988). Congenital toxoplasmosis has been treated with spiramycin and the combination of pyrimethamine and sulfadiazine, with encouraging results (Couvreur et al., 1980). Similarly, treatment of fetal toxoplasmic infection (followed by postnatal treatment) with pyrimethamine and sulfonamides alternating with spiramycin significantly reduced severe congenital toxoplasmosis and decreased the ratio of benign to subclinical forms (Hohlfeld et al., 1989). The authors of this study recommended that spiramycin be started as soon as possible when maternal toxoplasmic infection is proved or strongly suspected during pregnancy, because a delay between the onset of infection and therapy may be associated with severe fetal lesions (Hohlfeld et al., 1989).

Toxoplasmic Chorioretinitis

Patients with active chorioretinitis must be treated with specific agents without delay. The use of corticosteroids should be considered when there are optic nerve or macular lesions. Unfortunately, controlled trials of systemic therapy in toxoplasmic chorioretinitis are lacking. Some authors have found that spiramycin is effective in the treatment of posterior uveitis (Chodos et al., 1961), whereas others have reported a lack of efficacy (Canamucio et al., 1963; Cassidy et al., 1964). The combination of pyrimethamine and sulfadiazine appears to be more active than systemic steroids alone or in combination with spiramycin (Fajardo et al., 1962; Timsit et al., 1987).

Toxoplasmic Encephalitis in Immunocompromised Hosts

Many conditions, such as cancer, autoimmune diseases, and organ transplantation, require immunosuppression and, therefore, are associated with a greater risk of severe primary or reactivated toxoplasmosis. In patients with AIDS, toxoplasmosis is one of the leading central nervous system infections, causing abscess, encephalitis, and other encephalopathies. Few authors have studied the efficacy of macrolides in this setting. Failures with spiramycin and roxithromycin as single-drug therapy in sporadic cases of AIDS-associated toxoplasmic encephalitis (Leport et al., 1986; Decazes et al., 1988) may have been due to poor diffusion of the drugs across the blood–brain barrier. Roxithromycin, however, has been reported to achieve measurable concentrations in human brain tissue (Manuel et al., 1988), suggesting that failures with this antibiotic result from inadequate dosing or from the intrinsic pharmacological properties of the drug. Indeed, in vitro and animal studies have shown that macrolides inhibit rather than kill the parasite. A pilot study has indicated that clarithromycin in combination with pyrimethamine, which kills the parasite in vitro, is as effective in the treatment of *T. gondii* encephalitis in AIDS patients as the combination of pyrimethamine with clindamycin (Leport et al., 1990). However, several adverse effects were observed, suggesting that careful selection of eligible patients is needed in further evaluations. The increasing number of AIDS patients with toxoplasmic encephalitis makes prophylactic treatment an urgent necessity. Hygiene measures must be recommended to toxoplasma-seronegative AIDS patients (primary prevention), whereas seropositive AIDS patients can require prophylaxis to avoid reactivation (secondary prevention). The use of macrolides as prophylactic agents alone or in combination with other drugs in these clinical settings must await the results of carefully designed clinical trials.

In addition to the inhibitory activity on intracellular tachyzoite replication, several other observations support the concept of using the newer macrolide compounds, those with improved pharmacokinetics, as agents of primary or secondary prevention of toxoplasmosis in the severely immunocompromised patients at risk. Compounds such as roxithromycin, clarithromycin, or azithromycin show high tissue specificity, including in the brain (Araujo et al., 1991); impressive accumulation into macrophages; prolonged half-life, allowing simplified dosing schedules; good tolerability; lack of effects on zidovudine disposition in patients with AIDS receiving azithromycin (Chave et al., 1992); and possible activity against cryptosporidiosis and *Mycobacterium avium–intracellulare* (Vargas et al., 1993; Brown et al., 1993). Given these advantageous properties, several trials are on the way for determining the potential of these drugs in the prevention of toxoplasmosis in patients with AIDS.

CONCLUDING REMARKS

Many members of the macrolide family of antibiotics, including roxithromycin, azithromycin, and clarithromycin, exert an antitoxoplasmic effect, although it is more static than cidal. Macrolides should not be recommended alone in the most severe forms of the disease, particularly toxoplasmic encephalitis in AIDS patients. On the other hand, macrolides have no harmful side effects, and might

Table 1 Potential Indications for Macrolides in the Treatment of Toxoplasmosis

---

Macrolide alone
  Acute acquired toxoplasmosis
    Nonpregnant, nonimmunocompromised host
    No damage to vital organs
    Lymphadenopathy and/or high, persistent fever
  Toxoplasmosis acquired during pregnancy
    Before documentation of fetal infection
  Healthy newborn of a mother with high levels of anti-toxoplasma IgG
    Before diagnosis ascertained
  Secondary prevention of toxoplasmic encephalitis in immunocompromised host?
Combined with pyrimethamine and sulfadiazine
  Confirmed fetal toxoplasmosis
  Confirmed congenital toxoplasmosis
Combined with pyrimethamine
  When sulfonamides are toxic or produce adverse effects?
  Prophylaxis in the immunocompromised host?

---

be used safely under certain circumstances, such as in the prevention of congenital toxoplasmosis. The new macrolide compounds, with improved intracellular pharmacokinetics, merit further investigations in this setting. Potential indications for macrolides in the prevention and treatment of toxoplasmosis are proposed in Table 1.

REFERENCES

Araujo FG, Guptill DR, Remington JS. Azithromycin, a macrolide antibiotic with potent activity against *Toxoplasma gondii*. Antimicrob Agents Chemother 1988; 32:755–757.

Araujo FG, Shepard RM, Remington JS. In vivo activity of the macrolide antibiotics azithromycin, roxithromycin and spiramycin against *Toxoplasma gondii*. Eur J Clin Microbiol Infect Dis 1991; 10:519–524.

Beverly JKA, Freeman AP, Henry L, Whelan JPF. Prevention of pathological changes in experimental congenital toxoplasma infections. Lyon Med 1973; 230:491–498.

Bogacz J. Action comparée sur les toxoplasmes des diverses substances synthétiques et de quelques antibiotiques dont la spiramycine. Bull Soc Pathol Exot 1954; 47:903–915.

Bonaduce A. Ricerche sull'azione della spiramicina nella toxoplasmosi sperimentale del topino bianco. Boll Soc Ital Biol Speriment 1960; 36:57–59.

Brown ST, Edwards FF, Bernard EM, Tong W, Armstrong D. Azithromycin, rifabutin and rifapentine for treatment and prophylaxis of *Mycobacterium avium* complex in rats treated with cyclosporine. Antimicrob Agents Chemother 1993; 37:398–402.

Canamucio CJ, Hallet JW, Leopold JM. Recurrence of treated toxoplasmic uveitis. Am J Ophtalmol 1963; 55:1035–1039.

Cassidy HR, Bahler JW, Minken MV. Spiramycin for toxoplasmosis. Am J Ophtalmol 1964; 57:227–255.

Chamberland S, Kirst HA, Current WL. Comparative activity of macrolides against *Toxoplasma gondii* demonstrating utility of an in vitro assay. Antimicrob Agents Chemother 1991; 35:903–909.

Chang HR, Pechère JC. Effect of roxithromycin on acute toxoplasmosis in mice. Antimicrob Agents Chemother 1987; 31:1147–1149.

Chang HR, Pechère JC. In vitro effect of four macrolides (roxithromycin, spiramycin, azithromycin [CP-62, 993], and A-56268) on *Toxoplasma gondii*. Antimicrob Agents Chemother 1988; 32:524–529.

Chang HR, Rudareanu FC, Pechère JC. Activity of A-56268 (TE-031), a new macrolide, against *Toxoplasma gondii* in mice. J Antimicrob Chemother 1988; 22:359–361.

Chave JP, Mufano A, Chatton JY, Daye P, Glauser MP, Biollaz J. Once a week azithromycin in AIDS patients: tolerability, kinetics and effects on zidovudine disposition. Antimicrob Agents Chemother 1992; 36:1010–1026.

Chodos JB, Habegger-Chodos HE. The treatment of ocular toxoplasmosis with spiramycin. Arch Ophtalmol 1961; 65:401–409.

Cohen-Addad NE, Joshi VV, Sharer IR, Epstein LG, Gubitosi TA, Oleske JM. Congenital acquired immuno-deficiency syndrome and congenital toxoplasmosis: pathologic support for a chronology of events. J Perinatol 1988; 8:328–331.

Couvreur J, Nottin N, Desmonts G. La toxoplasmose traitée. Résultats cliniques et biologiques. Ann Pediatr 1980; 27:647–652.

Couvreur J, Desmonts G, Thulliez P. Prophylaxis of congenital toxoplasmosis. Effects of spiramycin on placental infection. J Antimicrob Chemother 1988; 22(suppl B):193–200.

Daffos F, Forestier F, Capella-Pavlovsky M, Thulliez P, Aufrant C, Valenti D, Cox WL. Prenatal management of 746 pregnancies at risk for congenital toxoplasmosis. N Engl J Med 1988; 318:271–275.

Decazes JM, Doco-Lecompte T, Modai J. Échec de fortes doses de roxithromycine dans le traitement de la toxoplasmose cérébrale des patients atteints de SIDA. Réunion Interdisciplinaire de Chimiothérapie Antiinfectieuse, Société Française de Microbiologie et Société de Pathologie Infectieuse de Langue Française, Paris, France, 1988: abstr 202/C12.

Derouin F, Nalpas J, Chastang C. Mesure in vitro de l'effet inhibiteur des macrolides, lincosamides et synergistines sur la croissance de *Toxoplasma gondii*. Pathol Biol 1988; 36:1204–1210.

Derouin F, Chastang C. Activity in vitro against *Toxoplasma gondii* of azithromycin and clarithromycin alone and in combination with pyrimethamine. J Antimicrob Chemother 1990; 26:708–711.

Desmonts G, Couveur J. Congenital toxoplasmosis. A prospective study of 378 pregnancies. N Engl J Med 1974; 290:1110–1116.

Desmonts G, Couvreur J. Toxoplasmose congénitale. Étude prospective de l'issue de la grossesse chez 542 femmes atteintes de toxoplasmose acquise en cours de gestation. Ann Pediatr 1984; 31:805–809.

Desmonts G, Couvreur J, Thulliez P. Toxoplasmose congénitale. Cinq cas de transmission à l'enfant d'une infection maternelle antérieure à la grossesse. Presse Med 1990; 19:1445–1449.

Eyles DE, Coleman N. An evaluation of the curative effects of pyrimethamine and sulfadiazine, alone and in combination, on experimental mouse toxoplasmosis. Antibiot Chemother 1955; 5:529–539.

Fajardo RV, Furgiule FP, Leopold JM. Treatment of toxoplasmic uveitis. Arch Ophtalmol 1962; 67:712–720.

Frenkel JK, Weber RW, Lunde MN. Acute toxoplasmosis. Effective treatment with pyrimethamine, sulfadiazine, leucovorin calcium, and yeast. JAMA 1960; 173: 1471–1476.

Frenkel JK, Ruiz A. Endemicity of toxoplasmosis in Costa Rica: transmission between cats, soil, intermediate hosts and humans. Am J Epidemiol 1981; 113:254–269.

Garin JP, Eyles DE. Le traitement de la toxoplasmose expérimentale de la souris par la spiramycine. Presse Med 1958; 66:957–958.

Garin JP, Paillard B. Toxoplasmose expérimentale de la souris. Activité comparée de: clindamycine, midécamycine, josamycine, spiramycine, pyriméthamine–sulfadoxine, et triméthoprime–sulfaméthoxazole. Ann Pediatr 1984; 31:841–845.

Giles CL, Jacobs L, Melton M. Chemotherapy of experimental toxoplasmosis. Evaluation of spiramycin alone and in combination. Arch Ophtalmol 1964; 71:119–127.

Glatt AE, Chirgwin K, Landesman SH. Treatment of infections associated with human immunodeficiency virus. N Engl J Med 1988; 318:1439–1448.

Harper JS, London WT, Sever JL. Five drug regimens for treatment of acute toxoplasmosis in squirrel monkeys. Am J Trop Med Hyg 1985; 34:50–57.

Haverkos H. Assessment of therapy for toxoplasma encephalitis. The TE study group. Am J Med 1987; 82:907–914.

Hofflin JM, Remington JS. In vivo synergism of roxithromycin (RU 965) and interferon against *Toxoplasma gondii*. Antimicrob Agents Chemother 1987; 31:346–348.

Hofflin JM, Conley FK, Remington JS. Murine model of intracerebral toxoplasmosis. J Infect Dis 1987; 155:550–557.

Hohlfeld P, Daffos F, Thulliez P, Aufrant C, Couvreur C, MacAleese J, Descombey D, Forestier F. Fetal toxoplasmosis: outcome of pregnancy and infant follow-up after in utero treatment. J Pediatr 1989; 115:765–769.

Huskinson-Mark J, Araujo FG, Remington JS. Evaluation of the effect of drugs on the cyst form of *Toxoplasma gondii*. J Infect Dis 1991; 164:170–177.

Jacobs L, Remington JS, Melton MN. A survey of meat samples from swine, cattle, and sheep for the presence of encysted *Toxoplasma*. J Parasitol 1960; 46:23–8.

Kauffman HE, Geisler PH. The hematologic toxicity of pyrimethamine (Daraprim) in man. Arch Ophtalmol 1960; 64:140–146.

Kayhoe DE, Jacobs L, Beye HK, McCullough NB. Acquired toxoplasmosis. Observations of two parasitologically proved cases treated with pyrimethamine and triple sulfonamides. N Engl J Med 1957; 257:1247–1254.

Kieng Truong T, Garin JP, Ambroise-Thomas P, Despeignes J, Maillard MA. Concentration minimale inhibitrice de spiramycine sur deux souches de toxoplasme (RH Sabin et DC Lyon) entretenues sur système cellulaire BK. Rev Inst Pasteur Lyon 1970; 3:127–134.

Koppe JG. Loewer-Sieger DH, de Roever-Bonnet H. Results of 20-year follow-up of congenital toxoplasmosis. Lancet 1986; 1:254–256.

Kutscher AH, Lane SL, Segael R. The clinical toxicity of antibiotics and sulfonamides. A comparative review of the literature based on 104,672 cases treated systemically. J Allergy 1954; 25:135–150.

Leport C, Vildé JL, Katlama C, Regnier B, Matheron S, Saimot AG. Failure of spiramycin to prevent neurotoxoplasmosis in immunosuppressed patients [letter]. JAMA 1986; 255:2290.

Leport C, Raffi F, Matheron S, Katlama C, Regnier B, Saimot AG, Marche C, Vedrenne C, Vildé JL. Treatment of central nervous system toxoplasmosis with pyrimethamine/sulfadiazine combination in 35 patients with the acquired immunodeficiency syndrome. Efficacy of long-term continuous therapy. Am J Med 1988; 84:94–100.

Leport C, Fernández-Martín J, Morlat P, Meyohas MC, Chauvin JP, Vildé JL. Combination of pyrimethamine–clarithromycin for acute therapy of toxoplasmic encephalitis. A pilot study in 13 AIDS patients. 30th Interscience Conference on Antimicrobial Agents and Chemotherapy, Atlanta, 1990: abstr 1158.

Levy RM, Bredesen DE, Rosemblum ML. Neurological manifestations of the acquired immunodeficiency syndrome (AIDS): experience at UCSF and review of the literature. J Neurosurg 1985; 62:475–485.

Luft BJ, Hofflin J, Chan J, Remington JS. The activity of RU 28965, a macrolide, in the treatment of toxoplasmic encephalitis. 26th Interscience Conference on Antimicrobial Agents and Cheomtherapy. Washington, DC: American Society for Microbiology, 1986:abstr 1105.

Manuel C, Dellamonica P, Rosset MJ, Safran C, Pirot D, Audegond L, Pechère JC. Penetration of roxithromycin into brain tissue. 28th Interscience Conference on Antimicrobial Agents and Chemotherapy. Washington, DC, American Society for Microbiology, 1988:abstr 1224.

Mas Bakal P, Int'Veld N. Postponed spiramycin treatment of acute toxoplasmosis in white mice. Trop Geogr Med 1965; 17:254–260.

Milovanovic M, Stretenovic M. L'action de la spiramycine sur la toxoplasmose expérimentale chez la souris. Ann Parasitol 1965; 40:639–642.

Remington JS, Cavanaugh EN. Isolation of the encysted form of *Toxoplasma gondii* from human skeletal muscle and brain. N Engl J Med 1965; 273:1308–1310.

Timsit JC, Bloch-Michel E. Efficacité de la chimiothérapie spécifique dans la prévention des récidives des choriorétinites toxoplasmiques dans les quatre années qui suivent le traitement. J Fr Ophtalmol 1987; 10:15–23.

Vargas SL, Shenep JL, Flynn PM, Pui CH, Santana VM, Huges WT. Azithromycin for the treatment of severe cryptosporidium diarrhea in two children with cancer. J Pediatr 1993; 123:154–156.

Wanke C, Tuzaon CU, Kovacs J, Dina T, Davis DO, Barton N, Katz D, Lunde M, Levy C, Conley FK, Lane HC, Fauci AS, Masur H. Toxoplasma encephalitis in patients with acquired immune deficiency syndrome: diagnosis and response to therapy. Am J Trop Med Hyg 1987; 36:509–516.

Wettingfeld RF, Rose J, Eyles DF. Treatment of toxoplasmosis with pyrimethamine (Daraprim) and triple sulfonamide. Ann Intern Med 1956; 44:557–564.

10

Treatment of Early Lyme Borreliosis with Macrolide Antibiotics

Benjamin J. Luft and Elizabeth M. Bosler

State University of New York at Stony Brook
Stony Brook, New York

Lyme borreliosis is a progressive infectious disease, commonly found in North America, Europe, and Northern Asia. Infection begins locally after the spirochete, *Borrelia burgdorferi*, is inoculated into the skin by a feeding tick, usually *Ixodes* species. In most individuals, the initial sign of infection is the development of erythema migrans, an annular erythematous skin lesion that is characteristic for this illness (1). Erythema migrans usually develops 3–14 days after the tick bite. Hematogenous dissemination, with seeding of multiple organs, occurs early and can produce a wide array of clinical manifestations, including multiple erythema migrans lesions, fever, arthralgias, myalgias, conjunctivitis, and meningismus (2–5). However, some persons are relatively asymptomatic at the time of dissemination. Acute meningitis, myocarditis with or without conduction block abnormalities, hepatitis, myositis, and less commonly, frank arthritis are the most dramatic manifestations of the chronic phase of infection (6). Unfortunately, there is no objective sign or laboratory abnormality that can universally identify patients with disseminated infection. Between the time of acute dissemination and the onset of the manifestations of chronic disease, there is usually a disease-free interval in which the infection remains latent.

Although erythema migrans is virtually diagnostic, it is recognized in only three-quarters of the patients with this spirochetosis and, then, only early in the course of infection. In the absence of erythema migrans, a definitive diagnosis of Lyme borreliosis can be difficult. *Borrelia burgdorferi* is difficult to culture and, in the chronic phase of the disease, it is rarely observed in clinical samples. Therefore, unlike most bacterial diseases that can be defined microbiologically by direct observation or culture of the pathogen, Lyme borreliosis is defined indirectly. The basis for diagnosis is the demonstration of an immune response against *B. burgdorferi* in an appropriate clinical setting.

In the previous ICMAS symposium, the in vitro, in vivo, and clinical data for the macrolides, erythromycin and roxithromycin, were discussed. Neither proved to be valuable as first- or second-line therapeutic agents for this disease. Therefore, we will focus this report on recent laboratory and clinical studies involving the more promising new macrolides, azithromycin and clarithromycin.

Two problems must be considered in any discussion of the treatment of *B. burgdorferi* infection. First, although a number of in vitro sensitivity studies have been performed, they have not been conducted in a standardized manner, and their relation to in vivo efficacy has not been established. Second, the diagnosis and the assessment of response to treatment are based solely on clinical grounds, not on microbiological criteria. Macrolides appear to be among the most active class of antimicrobial agents when tested against *B. burgdorferi* in vitro (7–9; Table 1). Azithromycin is well-absorbed and able to maintain tissue concentrations above the minimal inhibitory and bactericidal concentrations for prolonged periods. Similarly, Levin et al. (9) tested clarithromycin [^{14}OH]clarithromycin, and dirithromycin against 11 strains of *B. burgdorferi* and reported excellent in vitro activity. The pharmacokinetic data further enhanced their potential as therapeutic agents because of their ability to maintain

Table 1 In Vitro Sensitivity of *Borrelia burgdorferi* to Macrolides

Antibiotic	MIC/MBC (ug/ml)	No. strains	Ref.
Azithromycin	0.04	1	7
Erythromycin	0.16	1	7
Tetracycline	1.6	1	7
Azithromycin	0.015–0.03	10	8
Clarithromycin	0.015–0.06	10	8
Erythromycin	0.03–0.12	10	8
Roxithromycin	0.015–0.012	10	8
Clarithromycin	0.03–0.125	11	9
[^{14}OH]Clarithromycin	0.03–0.5	11	9
Dirithromycin	0.03–0.125	11	9
Erythromycin	0.03–0.5	11	9

high tissue concentrations. This conclusion is further supported by Alder et al. (10). The pharmacokinetic data for clarithromycin and [^{14}OH]clarithromycin suggest that these drugs are capable of maintaining high concentrations in blood and tissues throughout the long exposure period necessary to kill *B. burgdorferi*. In the hamster model, clarithromycin (bid) was effective for the treatment of *B. burgdorferi* infection.

We conducted a large, multicenter (12 sites in the United States), double-blind, randomized, prospective trial to compare the efficacy of azithromycin and amoxicillin for the treatment of erythema migrans (11). We used a standardized weighted examination for recording objective clinical manifestations and a self-reported symptom score that used an analog scale to measure initial manifestations and response to therapy. This approach was necessary because of the lack of accurate, reproducible, microbiological and immunological markers of persistent infection. Furthermore, the long-term sequelae of partially treated erythema migrans is unknown. Therefore, relatively "minor" signs of continued or recrudescent infection may be important indicators of the failure of a given therapeutic regimen to eradicate the infection and may portend more serious long-term sequelae. It remains unclear whether persistent signs and symptoms are due to continued infection, permanent tissue damage, or some undefined immune mechanism.

In this trial comparing azithromycin, 500 mg daily for 7 days, with amoxicillin, 1500 mg daily in three divided doses for 20 days, amoxicillin was significantly more effective than azithromycin in completely preventing relapse within 6 months after infection. Of the 217 evaluable patients, only 4% (4 of 106) of patients treated with amoxicillin relapsed compared with 16% (17 of 108) treated with azithromycin (Table 2). Patients who did not have a complete response to therapy at the end of treatment were significantly ($p < 0.002$) more likely to relapse. This study was designed with stringent entry criteria and

Table 2 Late (Major and Minor) Manifestations of Patients Treated with Azithromycin

Dose	Patients (no.)	Relapsed (%)	Ref.
250 mg bid for 2 d, then 250 mg qod for 8 d	20	15	13
500 mg on day 1, then 250 mg for 5 d	16	6	12
500 mg bid day 1, then 500 mg qod for 4 d	55	18	14
500 mg daily for 7 d	108	16	11

standardized assessments of key signs and symptoms that were used at the time of entry and throughout the 6-month study period. As a result, important information was obtained, not only about the comparative efficacy of these two treatment regimens, but even more importantly, about the clinical and laboratory presentation of acute Lyme disease and its relapse. For instance, there was a significant association ($p < 0.04$) between the development of an antibody response to *B. burgdorferi* and a complete response to treatment with azithromycin, and approximately 40% of patients who developed objective signs of relapse of their Lyme borreliosis were seronegative for *B. burgdorferi* at the time of relapse. Our findings are in contrast with the recently published small, open-trial study (12) that showed comparability between amoxicillin plus probenecid, doxycycline, and azithromycin. Fifty-five patients were randomized to receive oral azithromycin, 500 mg on the first day and 250 mg for the following 4 days; oral amoxicillin, 500 mg, and probenecid, 500 mg, three times a day for 10 days; or doxycycline, 100 mg twice a day for 10 days. If symptoms persisted at the end of treatment for the latter groups, patients received 10 more days of amoxicillin plus probenecid or doxycycline. The differences in size and design (open versus double-blind) of these studies, including objective entry criteria specific for *B. burgdorferi* infection and objective measurement of clinical endpoints, irrespective of serology, may account for the differences between these findings.

In a study from Europe (13), 64 patients with erythema migrans were randomized to treatment with either azithromycin, 250 mg bid for 2 days followed by 250 mg qod for 8 days; phenoxymethylpenicillin 1 million units tds for 14 days; or doxycycline, 100 mg bid for 14 days. Patients were followed for 24 months. None of the patients treated with azithromycin developed later (major) manifestations of disease, whereas four patients (two each) receiving the other drug regimens developed major manifestations of Lyme borreliosis, including meningopolyradiculitis, arthritis, facial palsy (with positive CSF findings), and severe intermittent arthralgia (see Table 2). A larger follow-up study comparing azithromycin, 500 mg bid the first day and 500 mg qod for 4 days, and doxycycline, 100 mg bid for 14 days, conducted by the same research team demonstrated a significantly shorter duration of erythema migrans for the azithromycin group (14). No patients treated with azithromycin developed major manifestations of disease during the 12-month follow-up period, whereas three relapsed in the doxycycline treatment group (see Table 2). The major late manifestations of Lyme borreliosis were meningoradiculitis, arthritis, and meningitis, with peripheral facial palsy.

Recently, 41 patients were entered into an open-labeled, pilot study of clarithromycin, conducted on Long Island, New York, for the treatment of early Lyme disease. In this study it appeared that clarithromycin, at a dose of 500 mg twice daily, was effective in preventing the late manifestations of infection within a 6-month follow-up period. Further, randomized comparative trials are needed to fully assess the usefulness of this agent for the treatment of Lyme borreliosis.

REFERENCES

1. Luft BJ, Dattwyler RJ. Lyme borreliosis: problems in diagnosis and treatment. Curr Clin Top Infect Dis 1989; 11:56–81.
2. Stiernstedt G, Ericksson G, Enfors W, et al. Erythema chronicum migrans in Sweden: clinical manifestations and antibodies to *Ixodes ricinus* spirochete measured by indirect immunofluorescence and enzyme-linked immunosorbent assay. Scand J Infect Dis 1986; 18:217.
3. Steere AC, Hutchinson GJ, Rahn DW, et al. Treatment of the early manifestations of Lyme disease. Ann Intern Med 1983; 99:22–26.
4. Steere AC, Hutchinson GJ, Craft JE, et al. The early clinical manifestations of Lyme disease. Ann Intern Med 1983; 99:76–82.
5. Luft BJ, Steinman CR, Schubach WH, Muralidhar B, Neimark HC, Polin D, Ruch T, Finkel MF, Kunkel M, Gorevic PD, Dattwyler RJ. Invasion of the central nervous system by *Borrelia burgdorferi* in acute disseminated infection. JAMA 1992; 267:1364–1367.
6. Asbrink E, Hovmark A. Early and late cutaneous manifestations in *Ixodes*-borne borreliosis (erytherma migrans, borreliosis, Lyme borreliosis). Ann NY Acad Sci 1988; 539:4–15.
7. Johnson RC, Kodner C, Russell M, and Girard D. In vitro and in vivo susceptibility of *Borrelia burgdorferi* to azithromycin. J Antimicrob Chemother 1990; (suppl 25A):33–38.
8. Preac-Mursic V, Wilske B, Schierz G, Suss E, Gross B. Comparative antimicrobial activity of the new macrolides against *Borrelia burgdorferi*. Eur J Clin Microbiolol 1989; 8:651–653.
9. Levin JM, Nelson JA, Segreti J, Harrison B, Benson CA, Strle F. In vitro susceptibility of *Borrelia burgdorferi* to 11 antimicrobial agents. Antimicrob Agents Chemother 1993; 37:1444–1446.
10. Alder J, et al. Antiborrelial activity of clarithromycin. Antimicrob Agents Chemother 1993; 37:1331–1333.
11. Luft BJ, Dattwyler RJ, Johnson RC, Luger S, Bosler EM, Rahn D, Nadelman R, Masters E, Melski J, Grunwaldt E, Gadgil SD. A randomized, double-blind prospective study in the treatment of erythema migrans. (manuscript submitted)
12. Massarotti EM, Luger SW, Rahn DW, Messner RP, Wong J, Johnson RC, Steere AC. Treatment of Lyme disease. Am J Med 1992; 92:396–403.
13. Strle F, Ruzic E, Cimperman J. Erythema migrans comparison of treatment with azithromycin, doxycycline and phenoxymethylpenicillin. J Antimicrob Chemother 1992; 30:543–550.
14. Strle F, Preac-Mursic V, Cimperman J, Ruzic E, Maraspin V, Jereb M. Azithromycin versus doxycycline for treatment of erythema migrans: clinical and microbiological findings. Infection 1993; 21:83–88.

11

Chlamydia and Other Sexually Transmitted Diseases

Geoffrey L. Ridgway

*University College London Hospitals
London, England*

INTRODUCTION

The antimicrobial spectrum of the macrolides is ideally suited for the chemotherapy of sexually transmitted bacterial infections. Tables 1–3 give an indication of the activity of the more widely used members of this group against *Chlamydia trachomatis*, the genital mycoplasmas, and *Neisseria gonorrhoeae*.

Erythromycin continues to be widely used for nongonococcal genital infections, including syphilis, albeit often as a second-choice agent. Failure of erythromycin to be effective against *N. gonorrhoeae* in a single dose, problems of resistant gonococci, and the gastrointestinal side effects are important factors restricting the use of this agent. Handsfield (1993) reviewing this topic at the First International Congress on Macrolides, Azalides, and Streptogramins (ICMAS-I) noted that the in vitro activity, unique pharmacokinetics of some of the new agents (acid stability, gastrointestinal tolerance, extended plasma half-life, tissue affinity, and intracellular penetration) should lead to their gaining a prominent role in sexually transmitted diseases (STD) management. Furthermore, he noted that few clinical studies had been reported. Two years after that conference, there has been surprisingly little advance. Several small studies have been reported at workshops and international conferences, but they are frequently difficult to evaluate owing to different protocols, lack of suitable control

Table 1 Activity of Various Macrolides and Azalides Against *Chlamydia trachomatis*

Antimicrobial	MIC (mg/L)
Clarithromycin	0.007
Josamycin	0.03
Rosithromycin	0.03
Midecamycin acetate	0.06
Erythromycin	0.06
Azithromycin	0.125
Spiramycin	0.5

Source: From Ridgway (1992).

treatments, small numbers, and short follow-up. Major studies have been restricted to one particular agent, azithromycin, extending the preliminary studies reported at the first ICMAS. Published studies with other new macrolides are lacking in this area.

GONORRHEA

Handsfield (1993) reported that a preliminary multicentre study, in the United States, of the treatment of gonorrhea with a single 1-g oral dose of azithromycin was abandoned when a cure rate of only 85–90% was documented. Further studies reported that 2 g of azithromycin cured 370 of 374 patients with culture-confirmed gonorrhea (99%). However, of 431 patients receiving the 2-g dose, 152 (37%) complained of gastrointestinal effects, reported as severe in 56 (17%). In light of these findings, the United Kingdom single-center study reported by Waugh (1993) was most interesting. Men and women with gonorrhea

Table 2 Activity of Various Macrolides and Azalides Against *Mycoplasma hominis*, and *Ureaplasma urealyticum*

Antimicrobial	*M. hominis* MIC (mg/L)	*U. urealyticum* MIC (mg/L)
Clarithromycin	8–64	0.025–1.0
Josamycin	Not available	0.02–0.5
Roxithromycin	8–>64	0.06–1.0
Midecamycin acetate	0.008–0.12	0.03–0.25
Erythromycin	>32	0.12–2.0
Azithromycin	2–16	0.12–1.0

Source: After Ridgway (1993).

Table 3 Activity of Macrolides and Azalides Against
Neisseria gonorrhoeae

Antimicrobial	MIC$_{50}$ (mg/L)	MIC$_{90}$ (mg/L)
Clarithromycin	1.0	2.0
Josamycin	0.25	1.0
Roxithromycin	0.25	1.0
Midecamycin acetate	1.0	1.0
Erythromycin	0.06	2.0
Azithromycin	0.12	0.25

Source: From Ridgway (unpublished data).

received a single 1-g oral dose of azithromycin. Bacteriological cure was achieved in 78 of 82 (95%) men (including 4 rectal and 2 pharyngeal infections), and all of 9 women with cervical infection. Clinical cure was reported in 72 (90%), and improvement in 5 of the remaining 8 men initially symptomatic. All women with symptoms were cured. The minimum inhibitory concentration (MIC) of azithromycin for the strains isolated from the treatment failures was 0.25 mg/L; that is at the high end of the expected range of MIC reported as clinically effective (0.003–0.25 mg/L). It would appear that 1 g of azithromycin should be effective against *N. gonorrhoeae* infection; however, the CDC did not include this regimen in its 1993 recommendations (Centers for Disease Control, 1993b). Side effects were low, one patient vomited the tablets.

SYPHILIS

Erythromycin continues to be recommended as an alternative to penicillin or tetracyclines for the treatment of primary and secondary syphilis (Centers for Disease Control, 1993a). It is not as effective as the other regimens, and patients need careful monitoring. The efficacy of azithromycin in a rabbit model for active syphilis was previously reported by Lukehart and colleagues (1990). In view of the difficulty usually encountered with clinical trials for syphilis therapy, there was considerable interest in the poster presentation at the first ICMAS by Mashkilleyson and co-workers on the successful treatment of syphilis with azithromycin (Mashkilleyson and Gomberg, 1992). This study was extended and, at the 18th International Congress on Chemotherapy (ICC) in Stockholm in 1993, they reported on an open study of 40 patients with primary or secondary disease (Mashkilleyson et al., 1993). Thirty-two patients received 500 mg of azithromycin daily by mouth for 10 days, and 8 patients received 500 mg on alternate days for a total oral dose of 3 g. Treponemes became undetectable within a mean of 26 h (range 24–30 h), compared with 37 h for erythromycin (1.5 g daily for total dose of 30 g), and 10.5 for penicillin (300,000 units IM q3h for 16–30 days). The resolution of clinical signs was subjectively quicker with azithromycin compared with benzyl penicillin G, and particularly, compared with erythromycin. Six patients had concurrent chlamydial infection, and received a daily dose of 1 g of azithromycin. The authors recommend azithromycin for penicillin-allergic patients with early syphilis. Controlled studies from this and other centers are necessary to confirm these findings.

CHLAMYDIAL AND NONGONOCOCCAL INFECTIONS

Table 4 summarizes successful treatment regimens described in Handsfield's 1993 review. The clarithromycin study of Stein et al. was extended with further reports at the Eighth Mediterranean Congress of Chemotherapy in Athens (1992) and at the 18th ICC. At the latter meeting they reported on the treatment of 40 adult patients (sex not stated) with nongonococcal genital infection (NGI). Twenty received oral clarithromycin, 250 mg bid for 7 days, and 20 received oral doxycycline, 100 mg bid for 7 days. All cases of proved chlamydial infection (14 of 20 and 13 of 20, respectively) were microbiologically cured. Thirteen of 20 patients (65%) in the azithromycin group and 12 of 20 patients (60%) in the doxycycline group were clinically cured or improved at follow-up 3 weeks after completion of therapy (Stein and Mummaw, 1993). Fedele (1992) at a meeting entitled "Josamycin: New Clinical Perspectives," reported an open study on the treatment of chlamydial cervicitis with 1 g of josamycin bid for 10 days. Microbiological cure was achieved in 227 of 259 cases (87.6%). Of 20 patients retreated, 15 were reported as culture-negative at follow-up.

Table 4 Treatment of Nongonococcal Genital Infection with Macrolides and Azalides

Drug/dose	Comments	Refs.
Roxithromycin 150 mg q12h, 300 mg daily, or 450 mg daily, for 7 to 10 days	Chlamydial and nonchlamydial genital infection in men and women	Lassus et al., 1987; Worm et al., 1989
Josamycin, 500 mg q12h or q8h	Chlamydial infection in pregnancy	Söltz-Szöts et al., 1989
Clarithromycin, 250 mg q12h for 7 days	Chlamydial and nonchlamydial genital infection in men and women	Stein et al., 1992

Source: From Handsfield (1993).

Preliminary studies reported at ICMAS-I (Handsfield, 1993) indicated that single-dose therapy of chlamydial infection was possible with azithromycin. Clearly, this finding could revolutionize the treatment of nongonococcal urethritis (NGU) and mucopurulent cervicitis (MPC). Over the last 2 years, azithromycin studies have dominated the few peer reviewed English language reports on macrolides and the treatment of STDs.

Nilsen et al. (1992) compared a single 1-g oral dose of azithromycin with standard doxycycline therapy (100 mg bid for 7 days), for the treatment of chlamydial urethritis in men. This study is of particular interest because placebos were used to blind the study, such that all patients took the same number of capsules. Follow-up was at 6–12 days and 13–21 days after start of therapy. *Chlamydia trachomatis* was eradicated from 100% of patients in both groups at first follow-up (44/44 azithromycin; 42/42 doxycycline) and 100% (35/35) and 97% (34/35), respectively, at second follow-up. There was no significant difference between clinical cure rates in either group at either follow-up (64 vs. 69% and 89 vs. 94%, respectively, at first and second follow-up). Side effects (mild gastrointestinal) were reported by 30% of the azithromycin group and 22% of the doxycycline group. Efficacy in cervical infection was demonstrated by Ossewarde et al. (1992), who treated 14 women with cervical chlamydial infection with standard doxycycline therapy and 17 with a single 1-g oral dose of azithromycin. At follow-up at 1 and 4 weeks after start of therapy, all culture samples were negative.

Martin et al. (1992) reported on the U.S. multicenter trial of oral azithromycin, 1 g (single dose), versus oral doxycycline, 100 mg bid for 7 days, for treatment of chlamydial urethritis or cervicitis. Azithromycin was again found to be as effective as 7 days of doxycycline therapy. Cumulative results for eradication of *C. trachomatis* (i.e., attendance at one or more follow-up clinics) were 41/43 (95%) men and 95/98 (97%) women with azithromycin and 37/38 (97%) men and 185/187 (99%) women in the doxycycline group. Assessment of clinical cure was subjective and nonstandardized, varying between 91 and 98% between sexes and therapies. There was no significant difference between clinical cure rates.

Unfortunately, patients with chlamydial lower genital infection do not have specific signs. *Chlamydia trachomatis* is present in less than half of patients with NGU or MPC. Therefore, it is important to evaluate clinical response in both *C. trachomatis*-positive and -negative patients. Two recently published studies looked at chlamydial and nonchlamydial urethritis in men. Both studies compared a single 1-g oral dose of azithromycin with 100 mg of doxycycline bid for 7 days.

Lauharanta et al. (1993) followed patients for up to 35 days after the start of treatment. They had 60 patients in each treatment arm, and half of the patients in each group were chlamydia-positive. The results are shown in Table 5. Lister

Table 5 Treatment of Nongonococcal Genital Infection with Macrolides and Azalides

Follow-up (days)	Antibiotic	*C. trachomatis*-positive		*C. trachomatis*-negative
		Clinically resolved or improved (%)	Eradication of *C. trachomatis* (%)	Clinically resolved or improved (%)
8	Azithromycin	28/28 (100)	27/28 (96)	26/27 (96)
	Doxycycline	28/29 (96)	29/29 (100)	23/24 (96)
35	Azithromycin	19/21 (91)	20/21 (95)	15/19 (79)
	Doxycycline	23/24 (96)	22/24 (92)	8/17 (47)
Overall	Azithromycin		26/30 (87)	
	Doxycycline		28/30 (93)	

Source: From Lauharanta et al. (1993).

Table 6 Treatment of Nongonococcal Genital Infection with Macrolides and Azalides

Follow-up (days)	Antibiotic	*C. trachomatis*-positive		*C. trachomatis*-negative
		Clinically resolved or improved (%)	Eradication of *C. trachomatis* (%)	Clinically resolved or improved (%)
7–10	Azithromycin	24/29 (83)	27/29 (93)	27/32 (84)
	Doxycycline	17/22 (77)	21/22 (95)	40/45 (89)
14–21	Azithromycin	12/16 (75)	13/16 (81)[a]	21/23 (91)
	Doxycycline	11/12 (92)	12/12 (100)	30/30 (100)

[a]Two patients reinfected.
Source: From Lister et al. (1993).

et al. (1993) treated 143 men (72 with azithromycin and 71 with doxycycline). Of 128 evaluable men with NGU, 51 (39.8%) were positive for *C. trachomatis*. The results are shown in Table 6. Neither study revealed any significant differences between antibiotics, nor with chlamydial eradication, or clinical response in either *C. trachomatis*-positive or -negative NGU. Side effects, again mainly mild gastrointestinal, were reported in Lauharanta's studies as 18% for azithromycin and 16% for doxycycline, and in Lister's study as 8 and 14%, respectively. Both studies concluded that azithromycin was an effective and convenient alternative to doxycycline for the treatment of chlamydial and nonchlamydial NGU. This conclusion is reflected in the "Recommendations for prevention and management of *Chlamydia trachomatis* infections, 1993" (Centers for Disease Control, 1993b), and the recently published CDC *1993 Sexually Transmitted Diseases Treatment Guidelines* (Centers for Disease Control, 1993a).

Preliminary results on the treatment of chancroid with azithromycin were previously reported (Handsfield, 1993). Definitive reports are still awaited. Other areas of potential therapeutic use for azithromycin include bacterial vaginosis and pelvic inflammatory disease. Studies are under way in these areas, but results are not yet available.

There continues to be a number of important gaps in our knowledge on the use of macrolides in STDs. Properly controlled studies are still required for syphilis, gonorrhea, female chlamydial infection, chancroid, bacterial vaginosis, and pelvic inflammatory disease. Preliminary results of open studies presented in international conferences may fire enthusiasm, but it is the controlled clinical trial published after peer review that will convince the sceptic.

REFERENCES

Centers for Disease Control (CDC) Report. Recommendations for the prevention and management of *Chlamydia trachomatis* infections, 1993. MMWR 1993a; 42(RR-12):27–28.

Centers for Disease Control (CDC) Report. 1993 sexually transmitted diseases treatment guidelines. MMWR 1993b; 42(RR-14):47–52.

Fedele L. Multicentre epidemiological study in gynaecology and treatment of *Chlamydia trachomatis* infections with josamycin. Symposium: Josamycin: New Clinical Perspectives, Paris, 1992.

Handsfield HH. Sexually transmitted chlamydial infections, gonorrhoea and syphilis. In: Neu HC, Young LS, Zinner S, eds. The New Macrolides, Azalides and Streptogramins, New York: Marcel Dekker, 1993:167–172.

Lassus A, Seppala A. Roxithromycin in nongonococcal urethritis. J Antimicrob Chemother 1987; 20(suppl B):157–165.

Lauharanta J, Saarinen K, Mustonen M-T, Happonen H-P. Single oral azithromycin versus seven day doxycycline in the treatment of nongonococcal urethritis in males. J Antimicrob Chemother 1993; 31(suppl E):177–183.

Lister PJ, Balechandran T, Ridgway GL, Robinson AJ. Comparison of azithromycin and doxycycline in the treatment of non-gonococcal urethritis in men. J Antimicrob Chemother 1993; 31(suppl E):185–192.

Lukehart SA, Fohn MJ, Baker-Zander SA. Efficacy of azithromycin for therapy of active syphilis in the rabbit model. J Antimicrob Chemother 1990; 25(suppl A):91–99.

Martin DH, Mroczdowski TF, Dalu ZA, et al. A controlled trial of a single dose of azithromycin for the treatment of chlamydial urethritis and cervicitis. N Engl J Med 1992; 327:921–925.

Mashkilleyson AL, Gomberg MA. Azithromycin in patients with syphilis. First International Conference on the Macrolides, Azalides and Streptogramins, Santa Fe, 1992:abstr 260.

Mashkilleyson AL, Gomberg MA, Mashkilleyson N, Katin SA. New azalide azithromycin in the treatment of clinical syphilis. 18th International Congress of Chemotherapy, Stockholm 1993:abstr 866.

Nilsen A, Halsos A, Johansen A, Hansen E, Tørud E, Moseng D, Ånestad, Størvold G. A double blind study of single dose azithromycin and doxycycline in the treatment of chlamydial urethritis in males. Genitourin Med 1992; 68:325–327.

Ossewarde JM, Plantema FHF, Rieffe M, Nawrocki RP, de Vries A, van Loon AM. Efficacy of single-dose azithromycin versus doxycycline in the treatment of cervical infections caused by *Chlamydia trachomatis*. Eur J Clin Microbiol Infect Dis 1992; 11:693–697.

Ridgway GL. Advances in the antimicrobial therapy of chlamydial genital infections. J Infect 1992; 25(suppl 1):51–59.

Ridgway GL. In vitro activity against *Mycoplasma* spp. and intracellular organisms. In: Neu HC, Young LS, Zinner S, eds. The New Macrolides, Azalides and Streptogramins. New York: Marcel Dekker, 1993:25–30.

Söltz-Szöts J, Schneider S, Niebauer B, Knobler RM, Lindmaier A. Significance of the dose of josamycin in the treatment of chlamydia infected pregnant patients. Z Hautkr 1989; 64:129–131.

Stein GE, Mummaw N, Christensen S. Randomised trial of clarithromycin and doxycycline in the treatment of nongonococcal urethritis/cervicitis (NGU). First International Conference on the Macrolides, Azalides and Streptogramins, Santa Fe, 1992:abstr 257.

Stein GE, Mummaw NL. Randomised, double blind, clinical trial of clarithromycin and doxycycline in the treatment of nongonococcal urethritis/cervicitis. 18th International Congress of Chemotherapy, Stockholm, 1993:abstr 867.

Waugh MA. Open study of the safety and efficacy of a single oral dose of azithromycin for the treatment of uncomplicated gonorrhoea in men and women. J Antimicrob Chemother 1993; 31(suppl E):193–198.

Worm AM, Hoff G, Kroon S, Petersen CS, Christensen JJ. Roxithromycin compared with erythromycin against genitourinary chlamydial infections. Genitourin Med 1989; 65:35–38.

Clinical Applications: Discussion

MORNING SESSION

Young: Dr. Cassell, I'd like to have your thoughts about atypical pneumonia and its causes.

Cassell: I was pleased to hear Professor Grassi from Italy say that perhaps we should no longer consider *Mycoplasma pneumoniae* as a cause of atypical pneumonia. Clearly, I think that what we are beginning to appreciate is that this organism can cause pneumonias that are classic lobar pneumonias. The other thing that I would just share with this group is that over the past 5 years we've been fortunate in being able to serve as a reference center for several large multicenter studies in various AIDS populations. One consistent finding is that *M. pneumoniae* does cause atypical pneumonias or community-acquired pneumonias in anywhere from 12 to 20% of the cases that we've seen, regardless of the AIDS group. Certainly, diagnosis is a major problem and continues to be with *M. pneumoniae*. These studies that I mentioned are documented not only by culture, but serology, immunoblot, and also now polymerase chain reaction (PCR), so I feel relatively confident in talking about the percentage caused by *M. pneumoniae*. Dr. Neu alluded to *M. pneumoniae* and its effect on cilia in the respiratory tract. Although early animal studies had suggested that *M. pneumoniae* could be a cause of coinfections, this is certainly something that we see now with increasing frequency. We recently investigated two disease outbreaks in closed populations, along with CDC, in which both *Bordetella pertussis* and *M. pneumoniae* were documented in these populations. In a number of studies where we've been looking for *Chlamydia pneumoniae* and *M. pneumoniae*, again by culture, we have, in fact, documented coinfection, so indeed they do occur. This is something that should be taken into consideration both for diagnosis and treatment. Relative to hospitalized patients and the role of *M. pneumoniae* in causing pneumonia in these patients—this is an area that has not been previously much appreciated.

Neu: I think that *B. pertussis* is a particularly important organism. With advancing age antibody levels against this organism decline. The symptomatic patient has cough for a long period, and this feature makes macrolides the drugs of choice. There are techniques today to make a rapid diagnosis of *B. pertussis*. In Japan it was surprising to me how common *C. pneumoniae* was in that population. The antibody levels declined with advancing age so one could develop *C. pneumoniae* again.

Hammerschlag: I think there are a lot of myths about *C. pneumoniae*. Actually, culture really is not that difficult, any laboratory that is relatively competent in culturing *C. trachomatis* can culture *C. pneumoniae*, if the right cell lines are used, and the methods have been well established. Hep2 cells are very sensitive. We have also been able to serve as a central laboratory for several drug studies. Unfortunately, the data are basically in abstract form or unpublished. We presented at ICAAC in 1993 a multicenter pneumonia study in children 3 through 12 years of age inclusive, who had to have radiographically proved pneumonia, who were seen at 30 sites in 20 states. We isolated *C. pneumoniae* from 42, or 16%, of these children, and it was pretty equal in the children under 6 and over 6. Over 20% had *M. pneumoniae* infection, as documented by culture or serology, and seven children were coinfected. The only child in this group who had pneumococcal bacteremia also had *C. pneumoniae*, so I think that it may set you up for other things to come in, probably also by interfering with local clearance mechanisms. What was really interesting is that the serology is correlating poorly with actual culture isolation. We're finding this in adults, we're finding this in children, and the positives are going in opposite directions. We've seen this now in several populations, with different laboratories with the microimmunofluorescence (MIF) test: maybe only 20%, especially younger children, will have detectable antibody by MIF or even seroconvert. The majority remain seronegative, so the serosurveys actually greatly underestimate the burden of disease in children. Conversely, with a population of asymptomatic adults—not only ourself, but a study in Rhode Island firefighters—we found that in a group of over 100 adults, over 80% of them had antibody, and these were individuals who were asymptomatic and both culture- and PCR-negative. Twenty percent would have met Grayston's serological criteria for infection based on a single sample, but they were asymptomatic. There are clearly serological cross-reactions between *C. trachomatis*. A number of subjects had antibody to both organisms in similar titers. Because of this I rely primarily on cultures. The problem there is the organism is beginning to behave more and more like *C. trachomatis*, in that there are a large number of asymptomatic subclinical infections that can persist for protracted periods.

Young: Could you comment, Professor Dautzenberg, on your experience with the new macrolides for *Mycobacterium avium* lung disease.

Dautzenberg: We have treated some patients with *M. avium* lung disease and also *M. xenopi* lung disease in non-AIDS patients. We have the same results as in AIDS patients. We have an improvement of more of the patients, decrease of fever, decrease of symptoms, but we have relapse after 3 years in approximately 30% of patients. With *M. xenopi* we now have two patients with relapse, we do not know what the MIC is now.

Young: What would you combine the macrolide with?

Dautzenberg: For *M. avium* disease, we combine ethambutol with all patients, and we give clofazimine. We don't know why. And for *M. xenopi* we give a quinolone and ethambutol.

Neu: What is the basis of the resistance?

Young: Decreased cell wall permeability is one of the mechanisms, but some of these other mechanisms that were discussed yesterday are being looked at actively. I think there are lots of these strains now, so if anybody wants them, we and Professor Dautzenberg can provide them.

Unidentified (Italy): I need to know the opinion of Dr. Young about the use of azithromycin as a wide prophylactic agent in HIV-positive patients, and the practical use and dosage of azithromycin that may be useful in the prophylaxis of mycobacteriosis, toxoplasmosis, and mycoplasmosis. I think that there are very few works about this type of infection.

Young: The reason that these trials are being undertaken is to come up with an appropriate dose and dosing interval. I don't think we should assume that these trials have shown efficacy. What I've tried to give this audience is the thinking of the various collaborative groups in the United States. Let me give you an example, however, from the CCTG trial. The dose of azithromycin is 1200 mg once a week, because of the long half-life. For clarithromycin the prophylaxis trials are using 1 g/day. Does that work for *M. avium*? We don't know, because the studies are in progress. Does it work for toxoplasmosis? I'm going to defer to Professor Pechére. He is going to talk about this during the next session. For pneumocystis, the preliminary work of Dr. Walter Hughes, is that a macrolide, whether it is erythromycin, azithromycin, or clarithromycin— and maybe roxithromycin from the Dellamonica data—should be combined with a sulfonamide or a sulfone. A common dose of dapsone currently being used in the United States is 100 mg every other day. Dapsone may also have some effect, or the sulfa may also have some effect on toxoplasmosis. Your question reminds me to emphasize that these trials have been designed with great planning and deliberation, but we shouldn't assume that they've automatically proved efficacy.

Neu: Dr. Young, you said that rifabutin in the United States was available for prophylaxis. I think that's fine in San Francisco, but in New York City, where we have 22% resistance to isoniazid plus rifampin, we have to start with the five-drug regimen. What do you think about that?

Young: For concern about tuberculosis?

Neu: We're concerned about tuberculosis, because this is not a pulmonary infection.

Young: No, I certainly don't disagree with that. Professor Dautzenberg had some comments.

Dautzenberg: We have treated some patients with multidrug-resistant tuberculosis with clarithromycin, but we have had no successes. When we compare the MIC before and after 6 months of treatment, we have no change of MIC. So probably the drug, macrolide, was not effective in tuberculosis. I can comment also about the question before about the toxoplasmosis. We have four patients in the treatment study in France with toxoplasmosis after receiving 2 g/day of clarithromycin for *M. avium* disease. Thus clarithromycin was not totally effective in the prevention of toxoplasmosis in these patients.

Fong (Canada):   Dr. Young, as you reported, in the States you've seen nine cases of uveitus to the rifabutin-containing combination.

Young: The uveitis is attributed to rifabutin.

Fong: In the Canadian prophylaxis trial employing rifabutin and clarithromycin, there are 25 uveitis cases in the arm receiving 600-mg rifabutin daily, and we've now cut the dose to 300 mg. It is not clear to me whether this is in fact directly due to rifabutin or whether it is an interaction with ethambutol, because ethambutol is in both arms.

Young: In the ongoing ACTG trial that I referred to the nine cases of uveitis are attributed to rifabutin. In the large prophylaxis trials, published in the *New England Journal of Medicine* last year, the prophylactic dose of rifabutin was 300 mg; in the ACTG trial it is 450 mg. Both fluconazole and clarithromycin raise the serum levels of rifabutin, and above 300 mg of rifabutin you start to get the complication of uveitis. Again, this emphasizes the need to conduct very careful prospective trials, because sometimes the initial aim is to make prophylaxis or treatment better, when in fact, unanticipated complications arise.

Dautzenberg: We used 5 years ago a combination of ethambutol and rifabutin in 180 patients, and we never observed uveitis and so on. We used 600 mg/day. It was a high dose of rifabutin.

Young: This is why there is a suspicion that it's due to the interaction with fluconazole.

Gialdroni Grassi: Do you think this is an interaction with fluconazole?

Dautzenberg: I don't know, but in these patients we observed no uveitis, and the Canadian clinicians observed 50% interactions.

G. Grassi: Was this in AIDS patients?

Dautzenberg: Yes, AIDS patients. But at this time, it was 5 years ago, we didn't use fluconazole in France.

Neu: What I don't understand is why fluconazole? It doesn't affect any one of the three ribosome components, the P-450 components in the cell, does it? Do you understand the mechanism?

Young: Not at this time.

Mayer: A question for Dr. Grassi and the panel members. I'm impressed that legionellosis, particularly nosocomial infection, is quite a severe disease. Your review showed how common it is. Are you comfortable with starting with oral agents, since these agents have variable bioavailability. Do you have parameters for when you would be concerned about starting the newer macrolide or azalide orally for patients with severe respiratory distress caused by legionellosis or other severe pulmonary disease?

Grassi: Of course this is a cause for concern. With legionellosis, erythromycin is more often given by IV. But what we can see from the data is that these new agents seem to be active by the oral route. A problem in some studies is that the severity of the disease is not clearly assessable. So I would say that we need some well-planned studies with well-defined severity of legionellosis, to see how far we can go with an oral antibiotic in the treatment of this disease.

Young: I'd like to get a feeling from Dr. Luft about treatment of toxoplasmosis with macrolides.

Luft: At this time in the immunocompromised host, macrolides have no role when used as a single agent. Perhaps as an alternative in patients who are not able to tolerate pyrimethamine/sulfa, clindamycin, and probably atovaquone, there may be a role for macrolides when used in combination with pyrimethamine. In the ACTG trial that I was involved in, which used azithromycin with pyrimethamine, the dose of azithromycin that had to be given was between 1200 and 1500 mg daily along with 50–75 mg of pyrimethamine. Any reduction in the dose of azithromycin led to a prompt recrudescence of the disease. Furthermore, this would be a lifelong type of therapy.

Young: Dr. Raffi has a poster here on clarithromycin and toxoplasmosis, so I invite him to comment on his experiences and any other experiences that he is aware of.

Raffi: Our study was of patients treated for MAC infection with clarithromycin. We observed a breakthrough of cerebral toxoplasmosis. As Professor Dautzenberg said, in the French cohort of patients treated with clarithromycin in France, we also observed a breakthrough cerebral toxoplasmosis. We are concerned about that because we have no clearly effective drug for primary prophylaxis of toxoplasmosis. What we found in these four patients with cerebral toxoplasmosis on clarithromycin is as suggestion of possible interaction with companion drugs given for MAC infection, such as rifampin. Others have suggested that there is a clarithromycin interaction with rifabutin, and that could be one explanation. It will be interesting to look in the clarithromycin prophylaxis studies for MAC infection for the incidence of toxoplasmosis in this population, especially in the French, German, and Italian studies, where the prevalence of toxoplasmosis is high.

Young: I believe that's part of the intention of all of the prophylaxis studies. Let me ask if Professor Gasser would like to comment on the controversies in the treatment of Lyme disease. I know that there has been considerable interest in central Europe with this problem. What insights can you provide us about new chemotherapeutic approaches?

Gasser: I think that the controversy is primarily, as Professor Luft has already stated, based on the dose and duration of treatment. We are currently investigating the right dose and the right duration of treatment. There is a major difference between early and late Lyme disease, which has also been brought up by Professor Luft. Macrolides have been shown to be effective in early disease.

Unidentified: What advice would you give a woman with a positive toxoplasma antibody titer who wants to be pregnant?

Pechère: To my knowledge, there are three cases where toxoplasmosis has been acquired by the woman before fertilization who later had offspring with congenital toxoplasmosis. It has been assumed in these three cases that the primary infection in the pregnant woman was very soon before conception. It is a very rare event to have congenital toxoplasmosis when the disease has been acquired by the woman before fertilization. More importantly, just tell this woman, wait 1 or 2 months and you will be more secure in not having a child with toxoplasmosis.

Young: Dr. Luft, some additional comments?

Luft: I'd tell her to get pregnant.

Young: Professor Adam, there are now a series of papers claiming that clindamycin is more effective than penicillin for the treatment of streptococcal pharyngitis. At this meeting, we have heard the same evidence for the new macrolides. Some people believe that the failures with penicillin are due to the presence of β-lactamase-producing staphylococci in the pharynx and that the clindamycin or, let's say, one of the new macrolides, would target both of those gram-positive cocci.

Adam: Yes, I have had the discussion very often with microbiologists. They say it is impossible that such small amounts of β-lactamases in the mouth of the patient can destroy the penicillin. But, as a clinician, I would say if there is poor compliance, a very low drug concentration in the tonsils, and perhaps some β-lactamase-producing anaerobes in the oral flora, then several factors could be responsible for relapses with penicillin V. Perhaps β-lactamase plays a role.

Ridgway: I'm a microbiologist, so perhaps I can defend our side of the fence. Penicillin has always had a pretty poor track record when it comes to eliminating the carrier state. It doesn't matter whether you're talking about diphtheria carriage, group A streptococcal carriage, or gonococcal carriage in the pharynx. None of those diseases are reliably treated with oral penicillin V. I don't think it is anything to do with β-lactamase. I think it's simply that you get poor tissue levels at the site where you need it.

Young: Dr. Andriole, this reminds me of some of the early studies done with a rabbit model of endocarditis. Isn't it true that erythromycin in some of those studies was not effective in the prophylaxis of endocarditis? Yet you cited this study in which they did the blood cultures. So the recommendations for erythromycin as dental prophylaxis in patients who were penicillin-allergic have always been hedged. What do you think now in view of these animal studies?

Andriole: The rabbit model is like all animal models: we use it as a bridge to clinical studies. The rabbit model that was designed in New Haven with Larry Friedman is a very traumatic model. The aortic valve is practically destroyed with a Silastic catheter, so the model is applicable to a very small percentage of patients who have underlying heart disease and risk for endocarditis. To produce the animal model, you have to inject the organism shortly after you disrupt the valve, and the valve is traumatized and bleeding. You're quite right, erythromycin did not prevent endocarditis in the animal model. The number of patients who have been treated with erythromycin as a prophylactic agent and who have penicillin allergy are relatively small, first. Moreover, there's never been a good prospective, double-blind, trial demonstrating that erythromycin is effective in clearing that bacteremia. In the studies presented here, I don't know how many of these patients were given erythromycin or the macrolide as prophylaxis, or how many of them had underlying heart disease. It might have just been the first 150 patients who had a dental extraction.

Young: Sometimes underlying cardiac abnormalities are hard to tell, such as mitral valve prolapse.

Andriole: I wouldn't discount a role for macrolides. I think they are a reasonable alternative, but I certainly would not bring them up to first-line prophylactic therapy.

Young: Professor Adam, you raised the issue about the shorter courses of treatment of streptococcal A disease, looking for sequellae, such as rheumatic fever or glomerulonephritis. How often do you, as a pediatrician, see this?

Adam: We had about three or four cases in 2 or 3 years. But we are a big university hospital, and cases will be brought to our hospital. Overall these complications are very rare. Some physicians do not use penicillin treatment, and some doctors, in our country, do not prescribe treatment of pharyngitis. You must be aware of rheumatic fever. I don't know what the rate is at the moment, for example, in Germany.

Young: There have been major geographic differences in the United States. The Rocky Mountain area, Salt Lake City and Denver, have had a higher attack rate than the low-lying areas.

Young: I didn't have a chance to really look at the helicobacter papers, which as a group were quite fascinating. Was there anything mentioned about emergence of resistance?

Andriole: No.

Young: That's a big issue with metronidazole and helicobacter. I'm wondering if anybody here has any data about helicobacter.

Logan: I'm the author of the three papers on *Helicobacter pylori* and would like to make a plea, before answering a question about microbial resistance by *H. pylori*, that in your next ICMAS meeting you devote an entire session to *H. pylori*. This is an infection that at least half of this audience are probably harboring, which, if they have had it long enough, will cause them to die of gastric cancer. It is an incredibly important infection with which we need as much help as possible. As a gastroenterologist, I make this plea to you who are mainly microbiologists that we need help in trying to treat this infection and treat it in the same way we would treat any other infectious condition. We have just finished a study of United Kingdom gastroenterologists and how they manage *H. pylori* infection. Although only a few gastroenterologists treated duodenal ulcers that presented for the first time in men younger than 30 with anti-*H. pylori* therapy, over 80% treated chronic recurrent duodenal ulcer disease with anti-*H. pylori* therapy. Only 10% took cultures before starting treatment. Otherwise, they chose to ignore their microbiologists. So, although we ignore our microbiologists, I would hope that the microbiologists do not ignore their *H. pylori*.

Your question about microbial resistance, is an extremely important issue. For metronidazole and the other imidazoles, if we know that patients harbor resistant strains, they are very likely to fail with standard triple therapy with bismuth, amoxycillin, and an imidazole. You mentioned, in your introduction the problem of the fluoroquinolones, how ciprofloxacin was hailed as possibly a very exciting treatment, but was rapidly dismissed. The reason for that was because people used it as monotherapy and did not use it in combination with other antibiotics. There is a paper from our group that was published in January of this year in *Alimentary Pharmacology and Therapeutics*, in which we discuss the use of ciprofloxacin, but in combination with two other antibiotics, and have shown it to be quite an effective treatment for *H. pylori*. The more important point is the resistance to macrolides. The posters presented at this meeting employed clarithromycin. A recent multicenter study in the United Kingdom found that none of the strains were resistant to clarithromycin at the start of treatment. This no doubt accounts for one of the reasons why it is such an effective treatment. At the same time, it must be said that there are countries where macrolide resistance is a problem. This almost certainly relates to the way the macrolides are used to treat other infections. As I view the posters at this meeting describing the use of macrolides to treat lower respiratory tract infections, upper respiratory tract infections, or sexually transmitted diseases, I wonder how many of these patients whose *H. pylori* is being exposed to low doses of clarithromycin will subsequently develop resistant strains. I think it is something we have to bear in mind, not only when we're treating an *H. pylori* infection, but also when we're treating other infections.

Andriole: The quinolones were used as single agents against *H. pylori*. Nobody knew enough to use an H2 blocker in those very early studies. My question when I read your abstract was why did you use a single macrolide with an H2 blocker without using metronidazole or a third agent with it? Share with us the design of your study.

Logan: I would like to make it clear that omeprazole is not an H2 blocker. Omeprazole is a proton-pump inhibitor.

Andriole: Right. Sorry for that slight oversight.

Logan: Omeprazole is a far more effective agent for suppressing acid secretion.

Our rationale for using a proton-pump inhibitor is based on the in vitro data, which shows that the MIC of many of these antibiotics, as reflected against *H. pylori*, is critically dependent on the pH. This is one of the challenges that we're faced with in treating *H. pylori* in infections. It's getting your antimicrobial to work not only in the antrum and the fundus of the stomach, where there can be a fourfold difference in concentration, but also across the mucous layer. *Helicobacter pylori* has this very specific habitat. You have to get the antibiotics to penetrate the mucus, where the pH gradient will go from 7.5 on the mucosal side to 2.1 on the luminal side. This is why we wanted to use it with the proton-pump inhibitor, so that you decrease that gradient and increase the efficacy of your antibiotic. Although ranitidine is a very effective drug for healing duodenal ulcers, it has a very small effect on pH. It actually inhibits only nocturnal acid secretion, but not acid secretion during the rest of the day.

Young: I think the issue is that everyone agrees that a three-drug regimen works for helicobacter, but the goal will be to get down from three to two and maybe even one. However, that one will have to be a pretty unusual agent, and a macrolide that works in a very acid pH is not on the immediate horizon.

POSTER RAPPORTEURS'
SUMMARIES

Biology and Pharmacology

Kenneth H. Mayer

Brown University AIDS Program
Providence, Rhode Island
Memorial Hospital of Rhode Island
Pawtucket, Rhode Island

Fernando Baquero

Ramon E. Cajal Hospital
Madrid, Spain

MICROBIOLOGICAL CONSIDERATIONS

Since this International Macrolide Symposium is taking place in the historic city of Venice, we should reflect on the lessons of the past. One famous ancient Venetian site of medical interest is the Ospedale Degli Incurabili, which is the hospital for incurable diseases, a 16-century edifice that was mainly used to treat syphilis patients. Medicine now does much better with the treatment of syphilis in this part of the 20th century, but the historical perspective is important because medicine is often one step behind the evolution of the microbes. I shall review the posters that provide key insights to the spectrum of activity of some of the newer agents, the macrolides, azalides, and streptogramins (MAS). Dr. Baquero will discuss the posters that deal with pharmacokinetics and specific issues concerning mechanism of actions of these exciting agents.

The emergence of multiresistant pneumococci in different parts of the world presents complex management problems for the clinician. Certainly, the good

Dr. Mayer contributed the discussion on Microbiological Considerations, while Dr. Baquero contriubuted the discussion on Pharmacokinetics of Macrolides.

news is that the newer macrolides and streptogramins tend to be very active against multiresistant pneumococci, but there are some potential clouds on the horizon. Fremaux and the French National Pneumococcal Reference Center found that between 1984 and 1992, erythromycin resistance increased from 18.9 to 27.6% in the 10,000 isolates they looked at. Penicillin resistance was at 20%. All but two of these isolates were pristinamycin-susceptible, which is certainly good news, especially since many of the penicillin-resistant pneumococci (almost two-thirds) were erythromycin-resistant, and over 40% of these were blood isolates. Fleites and colleagues found that 13% of Spanish isolates were erythromycin-resistant, and almost half of these were multiresistant, including penicillin resistance. Thus, a role is evolving for the use of streptogramins against these pneumococci in certain parts of the world.

However, in the United States, pneumococcal susceptibility to macrolides still tends to be very good. Barry and colleagues in the United States found that only 4% of the *Streptococcus pneumoniae* isolates were resistant to macrolides: High levels of penicillin resistance were found in some of these. Casellas and colleagues found that minimum inhibitory concentrations (MICs) were also satisfactory for the newer macrolides against Argentinian isolates. Other agents that were highly effective against the resistant pneumococci included virginiamycin (Freumaux and colleagues). Perri and Zervos in Michigan found that among their pneumococcal blood isolates, clarithromycin was ten times as effective as penicillin, and the susceptibility of isolates to clarithromycin was 5 logs greater than to ciprofloxacin, as assesed with time–kill curves. RP 59500 was effective against pneumococci, including those that were multiresistant to β-lactams, erythromycin, and aminoglycosides. Scriver and colleagues globally collected erythromycin-resistant pneumococci, and serum bactericidal activity was demonstrated against 99.9% at a 1:16 dilution 5 h following a dose of RP 59500.

As Professor Courvalin discussed earlier in the symposium, there are multiple ways in which macrolide and streptogramin resistance can evolve. Lonks in Providence described pneumococci that did not possess either of the previously described mechanisms among pneumococci (i.e., efflux and methylation). This may represent some of the first isolates of pneumococci that could modify the erythromycin substrate itself, but, as yet, no plasmid or other determinant has been found. This raises the specter of alternative mechanisms of pneumococcal resistance, as Courvalin and colleagues have shown in other species. Bidirectional gram-positive and gram-negative transfer of resistance determinants has been described in vitro and is a phenomenon that can be anticipated.

The enterococci certainly have been clinically problematic, particularly with the increasing emergence of vancomycin-resistant strains. Scriver, with Canadian and U.S. colleagues, tested RP 59500 against sensitive and resistant *Enterococcus faecalis*, *E. faecium*, *E. mundtii* and *E. gallinarum*, and found an

MIC_{90} for all species at about 4 μg/ml. But there were three isolates (one *E. faecalis* that had the VanA-resistant determinant, one *E. faecium* with VanA, and one *E. faecium* with a VanB) that had MICs of 16 μg/ml. Five other enterococci in this series had MICs of 8 μg/ml. This is a worrisome finding. Perri and colleagues found that the MIC_{90}s for RP 59500 versus enterococci from around the globe were quite satisfactory (0.5 μg/ml), even though the MIC_{90} for teicoplanin and that for vancomycin were greater than 16 μg/ml. Coignard and French colleagues found that virginiamycin was effective against 27 of 31 isolates of enterococci. Hence, there are "Achilles heels" with enterococci that are resistant to these antibiotics. The question for future clinical studies will be to look at the addition of second agents to some of these newer compounds, such as combinations of macrolides and aminoglycosides or rifamyacins.

With *Staphylococcus aureus* there are also increasing problems in global macrolide resistance. Reverdy and colleagues in France looked at 925 nonepidemic isolates, and they found great increases in methicillin-resistant *S. aureus* (MRSA), doubling to 20%, erythromycin resistance up to 28%, lincomycin resistance going from 11 to 17%, and aminoglycoside (gentamicin) resistance doubling to 18%. Most of these isolates were sensitive to vancomycin and completely susceptible to pristinamycin. However, Bismuth and French colleagues found some examples of pristinamycin resistance among 89 isolates. They found two different mechanisms of resistance in their collection: acetylation and efflux. They also found some resistance among coagulase-negative staphylococci. Accordingly, the clinical significance of the potential problems with the staphylococci will have to await further epidemiological studies.

RP 59500 may be useful for these multiresistant *S. aureus* strains. The MIC_{90} against MRSA from Texas was 1 μg/ml, and against *S. epidermidis* was 0.5 μg/ml. This was compared with much higher MIC_{50} and MIC_{90} for vancomycin, teicoplanin, and as high as 32 and 64 for ciprofloxacin (Raad and colleagues). Hamilton-Miller and Brumfitt, in the United Kingdom found RP 59500 to be equally effective in a biofilm model (which simulates catheter related infection) as in conventional broth, with 99.9% killing in 17–36 h. Slime production among strains did not alter the efficacy of RP 59500 in this model. Thus, even virulent strains seem to be readily inhibited by RP 59500. Turcotte and colleagues in Montreal found that RP 59500 decreased colony-forming units in a fibrin clot model colonized with MRSA, but this did not result in sterilization, as there was some level of strain persistence in this model. Although these compounds were not completely bactericidal, the model used three drug doses, and resistance did not develop during therapy. Clinical relevance awaits future trials.

The new MAS compounds appear to be extremely effective against respiratory tract pathogens. Torun and colleagues, in Turkey, found that all respiratory isolates of *Streptococcus pneumoniae, S. pyogenes, Moraxella catarrhalis*, *Haemophilus influenzae*, and *H. parainfluenzae* were inhibited by clarithromycin; but, interestingly, 3 of 20 β-hemolytic streptococci strains were not inhibited. Chin and Neu looked at the activity of clarithromycin and its 14-hydroxy derivative and found the compounds to be synergistic against most respiratory pathogens. One worrisome finding was that 10% of group B streptococci were resistant to the combination and did not show synergism. Whether group B streptococci will present an increasing problem once these drugs are more widely used remains to be seen.

Lamen, in a German series, found that the MIC$_{90}$ of clarithromycin, was 0.5 μg/ml for *M. catarrhalis* and 0.03 μg/ml for penicillin-resistant pneumococci, indicating excellent activity. In an Argentinian study by Tome, roxithromycin inhibited 88% of *H. influenzae* at concentrations achievable using a dose of 150 mg bid. It appears that the achievable levels are adequate to inhibit most, but not all, *H. influenzae*. Dabernat and French colleagues found that virginiamycin was highly effective with these organisms, as well as other respiratory pathogens. With *Pseudomonas aeruginosa*, Kita and Japanese colleagues found, in a biofilm production model, that very low concentrations of roxithromycin (0.2 μg/ml) decreased the activity of the pseudomonads, but there were no changes in exotoxin production until a dose of 2 μg/ml was reached. Whether this will have any significance relative to pulmonary virulence in patients chronically colonized with *P. aeruginosa* remains to be seen.

Another important pulmonary pathogen that the newer macrolides, azalides, and streptogramins inhibit is *Legionella* spp., and there were a number of important posters in this area. Jones and colleagues found that roxithromycin was twice as effective as erythromycin, but less active than rifampin against *Legionella* spp. Dubois and colleagues in Quebec found similar findings against 190 legionella isolates. Edelstein in the United States, using a guinea pig model, found that azithromycin was very active and highly concentrated in *Legionella pneumophila*-infected pulmonary alveolar macrophages; thus, the increased intracellular activity was very useful. Martin and colleagues, in the United States, found that roxithromycin appeared to be the best of the newer agents against legionella in vitro.

Roblin and Hammerschlag in New York studied *Chlamydia pneumoniae* and found that clarithromycin was two to ten times more active than erythromycin. They also found that the organism could persist in some patients, without increases in the MICs of the isolates. However, infected patients improved clinically, indicating that use of the newer macrolides could result in partial clearing, without necessarily resulting in the complete eradication of the organisms. Segreti and U.S. colleagues performed time–kill curves with *C. pneumoniae* and *C. trachomatis* and found a great deal of activity with the newer macrolides. Minimum bactericidal concentrations (MBCs) were as low as 0.008 μg/ml with clarithromycin.

Mentis and Greek colleagues examined *C. trachomatis* isolates taken from patients with nongonococcal urethritis and found roxithromycin to be quite effective. Kowalski-Foray and French colleagues found virginiamycin to be effective, as well, with MICs lower or similar to pristinamycin. The findings were very similar when these compounds were tested against gonococci. Sednaoui, in Paris, also found virginiamycin to be effective. Martens, in Texas, found that azithromycin was effective against penicillinase-producing *N. gonorrhoeae*, with 100% activity, which was better than the in vitro efficacy of third-generation cephalosporins. Ureaplasmas and mycoplasmas tend to exhibit significant resistance to erythromycin, but very good levels of activity have been noted for josamycin, pristinamycin, and virginiamycin. In a study from Israel, Samra and colleagues found roxithromycin to be the most active in vitro compound against ureaplasma isolates when compared with erythromycin and doxycycline. Dr. Neu discussed *Haemophilus ducreyi* and its very important role in sub-Saharan Africa in potentiating the spread of human immunodeficiency virus (HIV). However, it is increasingly resistant to trimethoprim–sulfameth-oxazole, but isolates tested from Rwanda revealed exquisite sensitivity to azithromycin with MIC_{90} of 0.008 μg/ml.

Keren and colleagues in Israel looked at them as agents against *Rickettsia conorii*, *R. typhi*, and *Coxiella burnetti* in Vero cell systems and found MIC_{90}s in the 0.01–1.0 μg/ml range. The clinical role of the new macrolides deserves further investigation. Rubinstein and colleagues in Israel looked at brucellar infection in animal models and found a great deal of in vitro synergism of roxithromycin with gentamicin and with streptomycin. Further clinical studies of these combinations are warranted.

Steele-Moore and colleagues from the United States found that RP59500 was the most active compound against *Corynebacterium jeikeium*. All of these new MAS agents were somewhat weak against *Listeria* strains, except clar-ithromycin, which had an MIC_{90} of 8 μg/ml. Clarithromycin could be considered for serious listerial infections, but one might have to use combination therapy.

Other presentations investigated the potential use of MAS agents in *Plasmodium falciparum* malarial infection (Anderson and Berman). Because of the increased hepatic concentrations of azithromycin, it might be more useful than doxycycline for both malarial prophylaxis and treatment. Early human trials suggest an excellent role of azithromycin for prophylaxis. Because the drugs are schizonticidal and are very effective for the interhepatic phase of malaria, they could be used in combination with an agent, such as quinine, that would cause initial rapid killing. Combinations of newer macrolides, such as azithromycin with quinine or mefloquin, need to be studied.

Dr. Young's remarks reviewed the current management of mycobacterial infection, but several excellent posters contained very new data and are worth highlighting. Klemens reported that azithromycin was found in higher concentrations in splenic cells of mice that were infected with *Mycobacterium avium* complex than in spleens treated with clarithromycin. Scorneaux and Tulkens looked at intracellular and extracellular concentrations of the different macrolides and found that intracellular concentrations were higher than extracellular concentrations in their studies of *M. avium* infection. The highest concentrations were noted when sparfloxacin–isepamicin were given with azithromycin, so that this combination of an aminoglycoside, a quinolone, and a macrolide might prove to be effective combination therapy. Casal and colleagues, in Spain, looked at the postantibiotic effect in *M. avium* infection and in *M. tuberculosis*. They found that this effect with azithromycin persisted up to 2 days in a *M. tuberculosis* model and up to 3 days in their MAI model. These very favorable pharmacological characteristics may result in the macrolides being a key component in the treatment of serious mycobacterial diseases, such as *M. avium* infection.

Lastly, several posters described the susceptibility of *Helicobacter pylori* to clarithromycin and amoxicillin. Flamm's studies showed that clarithromycin exhibited early bactericidal activity with MIC_{90} from 0.015 to 0.03. The reason it is appropriate to end these remarks by mentioning *Helicobacter* is that the organism has only recently become recognized as a pathogen in human gastrointestinal infection, and by the same token, that the clinical roles of the newer macrolides are also being newly appreciated. By the next meeting, one can hope for even more insights on how the clinical usefulness of these agents achieves some of the potential efficacy suggested by the presentations at this meeting, which are based primarily on in vitro and animal model activities of the new macrolides, azalide, and streptogramins against the emerging pathogens of the 1990s.

PHARMACOKINETICS OF MACROLIDES

The first group of posters is related to an important subject, the intracellular activity of macrolides and, particularly, their activity at the subcellular level. One of the most relevant posters is from P. Tulkens, which shows that macrolides accumulated both in the cytosol and in lysosomes of most cells. The position is about 50% in the lysosomes and 50% in the cytosol. This study used a very interesting approach with noninvasive and invasive *Listeria monocytogenes*, bacteria that are able to enter the vesicles in the lysosomes, but are not able to get outside in the cytoplasma. Obviously, the problem is that macrolides inside the lysosomes are doing something; the same author stated that there is an increase in the lipid phosphate content of lysosomes related to the presence of macrolides inside. The clinical significance of this is still to be investigated. It is interesting that probably part of the macrolides are collected in some of these acidic compartments inside the cell, either the lysosomes or the azurophilic granules, as H. J. Labro also presented. We do not really know what the antibacterial effect of macrolides in these organelles is. We can infer that because of the low pH of some of these compartments, the local effect of macrolides will be relatively lower. This morning it was discussed that macrolides act preferentially at alkaline pHs. The presence of macrolides in subcellular compartments and also in the cytosol is a major factor that explains the effects of macrolides on intracellular bacteria.

Another group of posters encompassing this subject of intracellular activity concern differences between when a cell is infected or noninfected. Edelstein and Tulkens performed some experiments looking at the intracellular concentration of different macrolides in infected or noninfected cells. There is a certain amount of controversy between two posters, because Tulkens says that infected and noninfected cells have exactly the same intracellular concentration, as assessed in models with *Legionella pneumophila*, *Staphylococcus aureus*, and *Listeria monocytogens*. Conversely, Edelstein says that, at least azithromycin is slightly more concentrated, 20–40%, in *L. pneumophila*-infected macrophages.

Another question is, why are there differences in antibiotic concentrations in different cells. This was commented on this morning, and we really do not have a good answer. Several posters presented by Kees, Wise, Tulkens, and others have data on the concentrations of macrolides in polymorphonuclear neutrophils (PMNs) or in mononuclear cells. In general, all agree that mononuclear cells are able to concentrate more macrolides than PMNs, and in macrophages the concentration is 20–40 times that outside the cell.

I would also like to mention the theory from Tulkens that we can quantitatively compare intracellular antibiotics as a reflection of what will happen if the same concentrations are in the extracellular compartment. That means a quantitative comparison of intracellular activity with extracellular activity. For instance, if 8 μg is captured intracellularly by cells and produces an effect equivalent to 24 μg extracellularly, can we assume that 8 μg intracellular is equivalent to 24 μg extracellular? This is an important question.

The second group of papers is related to drug delivery at the sites of extracellular infections. Macrolides accumulate in cells, but what happens outside the cells? In general, the concentrations of macrolides outside of the cells or in tissue fluids are very low, as with azithromycin. Hence, what is the role of drug retention by cells and the microbial effect of macrolides? Drug retention is more common for one macrolide in comparison with others; azithromycin has a higher drug retention power in the cells than other macrolides. This results in a certain continuity for the presence of the antibiotic in a fluid, particularly if this fluid contains cells. Probably the cells are destroyed, and the antibiotic is released from them. There are two or three papers, related to this process that compare the macrolide concentrations in blisters, with simultaneous determination in inflammatory blisters with cells and in noninflammatory blisters without cells. Obviously, if cells are present, the concentration is much higher. So we understand that the concentration of a macrolide in a given tissue or fluid is dependent on the quantity of inflammatory or other cells present in this site.

Azithromycin is very well retained in cells and is probably released very slowly when cells die, or is released by other mechanisms. Other macrolides, such as clarithromycin or roxithromycin, are probably balanced in such a way that the extracellular and intracellular concentrations are more equalized. Is the antibacterial effect of high drug concentrations inside a cell positive or negative? It appears negative if the concentration of antibiotic in periplasmic lymph or in interstitial fluid is considered, because if the antibiotic is trapped in a cell, it is released in small amounts. However, inside the cell, even a low concentration, over a long time, serves to increase the bactericidal activity of these macrolides. Craig has presented satisfactory results in animal models in which time above the MIC relates very well to the antibacterial efficacy of macrolides. Time above the MIC is a good pharmacological consideration for those bacteria that are trapped in the cell, as there is a period of contact with any drug that is present, and this results in a bactericidal effect. This factor is probably not as clearly related to the extracellular effect of macrolides.

If we consider drug levels in different tissues, a great deal of data has been presented. Blood levels of macrolides are consistent. Dunn, Worm, and Stratchunsky presented a range of 0.02–0.2 mg/L in blood after a 1-g dose of azithromycin. Clarithromycin, at doses of 700 mg or 1 g, results in levels of 1–7 mg/L, according to data from Gustavson, Giamarellou, Craft, Kees, and others. Dirithromycin achieves serum levels of about 0.5 mg/ml. Tissue levels depend on the cellular content of a particular sample. In prostate, clarithromycin reaches a level twice that of serum; namely, approximately 2–3 μg/ml after a dose of 750 mg. In semenal fluid, about 1 μg/ml of azithromycin is found following a 1-g dose. This same result was obtained by LeBel, in Canada, and Stratchunsky, from Russia. This level is slightly higher than the MIC of *Neisseria gonorrhoeae*, *Chlamydia trachomatis*, and *Ureaplasma* spp.

Some other posters dealt with the concentrations of different antibiotics in cervical mucosa: 2–3 μg/ml could be achieved with a 1-g dose of azithromycin.

The macrolides have direct effects on some cells. Erythromycin induces small-bowel contraction. Matera and collaborators report that smooth muscles in guinea pig trachea also contract in the presence of erythromycin, but we do not know the physiological or pathological consequences of this fact. All macrolides are immunosuppressive to a certain degree: roxithromycin inhibits neutrophil recruitment, as presented by Tamaoki and others, for example. Also, the inhibition of oxidant production in polymorphonuclear neutrophils by different macrolides has been presented by Labro. Macrolides probably compensate for this, as suggested by the synergistic effect of macrolides with some non–oxygen-related antibacterial effects in cells.

Some puzzling data have been presented by Sorgel on biliary secretion of macrolides. For instance, according to the data of Foulds, LeBrecque, and Sorgel, dirithromycin peaks in bile at 0.7–500 μg/ml in different patients. We do not know what accounts for the differences among patients. It is likely that the low trough levels of clarithromycin at 24 h after dosing can be compensated by the postantibiotic effect, which depends, according to some papers presented here by Capobianco, Goldman, and Scaglione, on the slow dissociation rate constant of clarithromycin in the ribosomes of gram-negative bacteria. Thus, the binding of the drug to the ribosome is dissociated. If this dissociation takes a long time, protein synthesis is blocked for all of that period, which might explain part of the postantibiotic effect.

Some other posters presented data on pharmacology in special clinical situations. For example, the kinetics of macrolides are not modified in patients with AIDS, except if cryptosporidiosis is present. The associated diarrhea results in a lower absorption of macrolides.

In hepatic failure, no pharmacological effects were reported in two consistent papers by Mazzei and LaBrecque. In renal failure, data from Sorgel and Shiba suggest that a dose adjustment is not needed for azithromycin. In dialysis patients, roxithromycin is not dialyzed; therefore, its dosage does not need to be adjusted. In a paper from Kisicki on dirithromycin in elderly populations, no need for a dose adjustment was reported.

The increase of erythromycin resistance in France is well known. However, the potential appearance of a novel mechanism of resistance in *Streptococcus pneumoniae* and *S. mitis* was reported in a paper by Lonks and Medeiros. There are some pneumococci that present resistance to erythromycin and 14-membered macrolides, but are susceptible to the 16-member macrolides, clindamycin, lincomycin, and streptogramin B. This is like an MLS-inducible phenotype, but it is not inducible, and is similar to that mentioned by Leclercq and Courvalin. Lonks and Medeiros looked with probes of *ermB* and *msrA*, at the genes involved in efflux-mediated resistance, and the result was negative. So there must be another efflux-mediated mechanism.

Clinical Applications

Dieter Adam

Children's Hospital of the University of Munich
Munich, Germany

Vincent T. Andriole

Yale University School of Medicine
New Haven, Connecticut

NEW MACROLIDES IN RESPIRATORY TRACT INFECTIONS

Professor Vincent Andriole and I reviewed 98 clinical posters, but we will report on only 41 of them that describe randomized studies.

Azithromycin, at 500 mg/day for 3 days, was compared with 10 days of roxithromycin or cefaclor in the treatment of patients with upper respiratory tract infections in two open, comparative, randomized studies. In the cefaclor comparative study, 519 patients with acute pharyngitis, acute otitis media, and sinusitis were included. At the end of therapy, the overall satisfactory response rates were 93% with azithromycin and 96% with cefaclor. The eradication rate in tonsillitis was 99% with azithromycin and 96% with cefaclor. The 3-day azithromycin regimen was as good as 10 days of the comparator. It is possible to treat those infections for only 3 days with azithromycin with good clinical results.

In another comparative, randomized, open study done in Italy, azithromycin versus amoxicillin–clavulanic acid was compared in pediatric patients with acute otitis media. Azithromycin was administered in a 10 mg/kg per day dosage

Dr. Adam contributed the discussion on New Macrolides in Respiratory Tract Infections, while Dr. Andriole contributed the discussion on Newer Macrolides in MAI, *Helicobacter pylori*, SBE, and STD.

for 3 days in children (97 patients), or amoxicillin–clavulanic acid, 50 mg/day bid was administered for 10 days (99 patients). In both groups a 97.9 and 96.7%, respectively, cure rate was observed. After 10 or 13 days, no significant differences appeared. Azithromycin therapy was better tolerated: gastrointestinal side effects were reported in 1% of the azithromycin group and in 9% of the amoxicillin–clavulanic acid group. Three days of treatment with azithromycin was equally as effective as 10 days of amoxicillin–clavulanic acid in children with acute otitis media.

There were two very good studies on sinusitis. In one, with 739 patients, clarithromycin resulted in high efficacy rates in the treatment of acute maxillary sinusitis. Clarithromycin was compared with amoxicillin–clavulanic acid in another study with 284 adult patients with symptoms of acute maxillary sinusitis: 86 versus 85% success rate. The incidence of adverse events was similar in both groups, and the most common was nausea in the clarithromycin group and diarrhea in the amoxicillin–clavulanic acid group. The success rate was 84% when *Haemophilus influenzae* was isolated, which means that clarithromycin is very effective in infection caused by *H. influenzae*. Yesterday, Dr. Harold Neu questioned the clinical antimicrobial activity of the metabolite. As can be seen from these studies, the metabolite must be active, because the success rates in *H. influenzae* infections are excellent.

In the next group, five posters on tonsillitis and pharyngitis were presented. In a randomized, multicenter study of azithromycin versus erythromycin in pediatric patients with acute tonsillopharyngitis caused by group A β-hemolytic streptococci, 3 days of azithromycin, 10 mg/kg versus 5 days azithromycin, 10 mg/kg on day 1 and 5 mg/kg on days 2–5, versus erythromycin, 50 mg three times daily for 10 days—a three-arm study—showed the clinical response rate at day 3 was better in group 1 (azithromycin 3 days—10 mg/kg), with 36% cured patients, than in group 2, with 19.6% (day 3) cured patients, or in group three with 17% cured patients. At day 10 in group 1, success rates were 94%, in group 2, 91%, and in group 3, 74%. The eradication rates of group A β-hemolytic streptococci at days 3 and 10 were 96, 95.7, and 95.8%, respectively. Hence, 3-day treatment of acute tonsillopharyngitis with azithromycin is possible. This study indicates that a 3-day regimen can treat patients successfully, but there were no data on acute rheumatic fever following the infection. Studies must be done comparing outcome relative to acute rheumatic fever, comparing 3-day, 5-day, and 10-day regimens: The recommendation now is still to use penicillin V, but if we can shorten the time, better compliance is likely.

In other studies, clarithromycin versus penicillin V for 10 days in adults and children were both highly effective, with an eradication rate of 94% in clarithromycin and 88% in the penicillin V group. In adults, the rate was 92 versus 81% in children. This difference was statistically significant. Also dirithromycin was successfully used in acute tonsillopharyngitis versus penicillin

V in a multicenter, randomized, double-blind, double-dummy study. Dirithromycin was given in a single daily dose of 500 mg in adults versus four daily doses of penicillin V for 10–14 days. The outcomes were 96.7% success rate with the macrolide versus 94% with penicillin. Sixty-four percent of dirithromycin-treated and 67% of penicillin-treated patients reported at least one adverse event. Notably, there are big differences in reported side effects from country to country and on how patients are questioned. One must be very careful with reported side effect rates of 64 or 65%. I think there may be differences between the study situation and what happens in general practice. In another study, dirithromycin versus erythromycin base were both comparable in safety and efficacy in the treatment of acute tonsillopharyngitis.

Let us turn to chronic bronchitis. In a pooled analysis of five double-blinded, multicenter, randomized studies comparing clarithromycin, 500 mg bid, with amoxicillin, amoxicillin-clavulanate (Augmentin), cefaclor, cefixime, and others in the treatment of patients with bronchitis or sinusitis caused by *H. influenzae*, an overall success rate of 91% was shown for clarithromycin, compared with 95% with all the reference agents. Adverse events were 32% in both groups: gastrointestinal 15% with clarithromycin and 20% with the reference agents. Clarithromycin was also highly effective in the treatment of *H. influenzae* infections in these multicenter, randomized studies.

Azithromycin was studied versus clarithromycin in acute purulent tracheobronchitis. Azithromycin was administered for 3 days, 500 mg orally once daily, or for 5 days in measured dose. Clarithromycin was given orally for 7–10 days. Clinical efficacy was the same in both groups, but time to improvement was significantly shorter for azithromycin-treated patients (3.1 days) than for clarithromycin-treated patients (4.2 days). Duration of work incapacity was shorter for the azithromycin patients (4 days) than for clarithromycin (5 days). This may be a very important finding. If one can shorten treatment days, it can save money on lost work.

In a pooled analysis of six double-blinded, randomized studies comparing clarithromycin with ampicillin or cephalosporins in the treatment of acute bacterial exacerbations of chronic bronchitis, no difference could be shown in clinical success rate. Therapy with clarithromycin, 250 mg or 500 mg bid, led to high pathogen eradication rates, and both dosages were well tolerated. Also erythromycin versus dirithromycin in acute bacterial exacerbations of chronic bronchitis comparing 5 days with 7 days was effective, and the advantage of once-daily dosage for dirithromycin may improve patients' compliance. Similar results also could be shown with roxithromycin—5 days dirithromycin versus 7 days roxithromycin—in acute bacterial exacerbations of chronic bronchitis.

Also lower respiratory tract infections were treated. Azithromycin was compared in one study with clarithromycin and in another study with amoxicillin–clavulanate (Augmentin). It was concluded that the 3-day course of azithromycin is as effective and well-tolerated as 10 days of clarithromycin or 10 days Augmentin in patients with lower respiratory tract infections. Clarithromycin showed a high success rate of 98% also in children compared with amoxicillin (95%) or cefaclor (96%). Twice-daily clarithromycin resulted in high rates of clinical success, comparable with that of tid amoxicillin or cefaclor in pediatric lower respiratory tract infections.

Also chlamydial studies were reviewed. There were three contributions on lower respiratory tract infections caused by *Chlamydia pneumoniae*. In one study, chlamydia was identified by bronchial secretions, by using fluorescent species-specific monoclonal antibodies; also cultures were positive. All patients were clinically cured, 100%, with no relapses at 2-week and 4-week follow-ups. After treatment with clarithromycin, all patients with positive cultures were bacteriologically cured. This was a study from Scaglione from Milano. I think the macrolides are absolutely, 100% active in *C. pneumoniae*. This study was done with clarithromycin; perhaps there is no difference between azithromycin and roxithromycin, and erythromycin as well. In another study, azithromycin was also used for *C. pneumoniae*; eradication from the respiratory tract was 75% of the culture-positive patients. In another study, azithromycin was successfully used against *Mycoplasma pneumoniae* and *C. pneumoniae*; 1229 patients from the United States were enrolled in the study. Results indicate that *Mycoplasma* and *Chlamydia pneumoniae* together may constitute a substantial proportion of community-acquired infections. A five-dose 1.5-g total-dose regimen of azithromycin showed high rates of efficacy in all infections studied. In pediatric community-acquired pneumonia, a 3-day azithromycin course compared with erythromycin 10 days bid, indicated a faster cure rate, with better gastrointestinal tract tolerance with the new azalide.

Dirithromycin was successfully compared with erythromycin in mycoplasma, and in another study with legionella. Also clarithromycin was successful for treatment of community-acquired pneumonia caused by legionella. In upper respiratory tract infections all the substances used in the studies were active. Also in otitis media and pharyngitis caused by usual microorganisms, including mycoplasma and chlamydia, the new azalide–macrolide drugs were highly active.

NEWER MACROLIDES IN MAI, *HELICOBACTER PYLORI*, SBE, AND STD

For two days I have listened and I have thoroughly enjoyed all of the presentations, I want to thank my colleagues, Harold Neu, Steve Zinner, and Lowell Young, for putting together a very fine program. When Professor Adam and I reviewed the abstracts, we were very pleased with the numbers that we had and the work that was presented in the abstracts. Out of necessity we decided that we should pick the comparative studies.

There were 14 posters on *Mycobacterium avium intracellulare* infections. I have selected two of these abstracts, one in which azithromycin was used and one in which clarithromycin was used, because they each make important points that need to be resolved in the future.

The first is Koletar, Williams, and Berry's study from Texas and from Pfizer Research in Groton, Connecticut. The title is "Serum Level and Minimum Inhibitory Concentrations Do Not Correlate with Efficacy of Azithromycin for Disseminated MAC Infection in Patients with AIDS." There were 65 HIV-positive patients who were treated. One group received 600 mg of azithromycin a day, a second group received 1200 mg monotherapy. They were then monitored with quantitative cultures. The results were really quite good. These patients were followed for a period of 6 weeks. What is the important point in this study? For me it was the following: This morning Dr. Young showed that patients with *Mycobacterium avium* complex (MAC) bacteremia who receive therapy do well for a period and then, after a while, their bacteremia becomes worse. These authors showed that this is not caused by resistance of the organism to azithromycin. The MICs did not change, so the question is why do they get worse? This is an area for future research. The second point is that the patients who received the high dose of 1200 mg did not do any better than the patients who received 600 mg/day. This is in contrast to the clarithromycin study, by Craft and Henry from Abbott Laboratories. They report on the efficacy of clarithromycin in disseminated MAC. They had 469 HIV-positive patients in two groups. One group received 500 mg and one received 1000 mg, for 12 weeks, and they were followed. The clearance rate in the clarithromycin-treated patients is almost identical with the clearance rate in the azithromycin-treated patients. Although the higher dose of azithromycin did not do any better, the higher dose of clarithromycin had a more favorable bacteriological and clinical response. I do not understand this difference. Maybe it is not so important, but we need to follow these patients further to see if there is truly any difference. I was impressed by the fact that the results of clearing the bacteremia, whether you used azithromycin or clarithromycin, were much the same.

Also, in the area of MAI infection, there are two papers in which a macrolide was investigated in terms of increased toxicity when it was used with other antimycobacterial agents. Notario and Henry from Abbott have an abstract on the safety of clarithromycin in combination with other antimycobacterial drugs. They used clofazimine, ethambutol, and ciprofloxacin, each one with clarithromycin, and also a three-drug combination of clarithromycin, ethambutol, and clofazimine. They looked at the adverse events in this large number of patients (866). The adverse event rate when clarithromycin was added to ciprofloxacin was only 4.1%, that was the lowest. The highest was when clarithromycin was added to clofazimine, and it was 9.7%. When clarithromycin was combined with ethambutol, it was 5.9%, and when the three-drug combination was used the adverse event rate was only 7.4%. The message was that combination therapy that includes a macrolide in this seriously ill group of patients, is well tolerated.

To carry on that concept, one abstract by Rastogi and Bryskier from France looked at combinations of drugs in vitro (this was not done in patients), in which roxithromycin was looked at in combination with ethambutol, rifampin, amikacin, ofloxacin, and clofazimine. The intent here is to see which of the combinations might have better antimycobacterial activity. They had ten clinical isolates of *Mycobacterium avium–intracellulare* (MAI) in which they studied the combination. They showed that the antibacterial activity of roxithromycin was enhanced in all ten strains by ethambutol, but it was not enhanced in all of those strains by other combinations. For example, only three strains responded in an enhanced way when roxithromycin was added to rifampin, and the same number when roxithromycin was added to clofazimine; only two strains responded when roxithromycin was added to amikacin, and only one strain when it was added to ofloxacin. They also showed that a three-drug combination—roxithromycin (and I assume it would be good for any of the other macrolides) plus ethambutol with a third antimycobacterial agent—achieved the most significant antimycobacterial activity in vitro.

Continuing again with *Mycobacterium avium–intracellulare*, there were three papers that dealt with very early studies on prophylaxis with clarithromycin in these patients. The total number in the three abstracts is only about 30 patients. When 500 mg bid of clarithromycin was used as a prophylactic agent, it appears as though there is some future for the macrolides in prophylaxis. The ATCG studies are underway and there are numerous patients involved in these.

The remaining abstracts that I want to emphasize are isolated issues that I found of great interest. The first of these was reported by Raffi and his colleagues from France on the use of clarithromycin for MAI in AIDS patients, who then went on to develop cerebral toxoplasmosis. There were 21 AIDS patients with disseminated MAI who were treated with clarithromycin with a variety of different combination agents. Four of these patients developed very strong evidence of cerebral toxoplasmosis; the first patient after 1 month of treatment. There were two patients who developed it at 3 months, and one case at 6 months into treatment. The clarithromycin was continued throughout that time. I am not singling out clarithromycin in this circumstance. What I am singling out is that we have to be worried about this development.

Yesterday, Dr. Neu raised the issue that he had not seen any studies on prophylaxis for bacterial endocarditis with the macrolides and azalides. We have so many effective agents to treat bacterial endocarditis, but the issue of using macrolides for prophylaxis in penicillin-allergic patients is different. The numbers of patients for whom we might have to revert to using a macrolide or an azalide because of allergies and who have endocarditis is so small, yet the prophylactic issue is much, much greater. There is a paper by Rahn and his colleagues from Germany, in which they report treatment of 150 patients who received either erythromycin 1 g, roxithromycin 150 mg, or no treatment at all, and who underwent dental procedures. They did blood cultures at 3, 6, and 9 min after the dental procedure, and found bacteremia in 29 of the 50 control patients, in 4 of the 50 erythromycin-treated patients, and in 4 of the 50 roxithromycin-treated patients. *Streptococcus viridans* was isolated from 21 of the 29 control patients, but from none of the erythromycin- or roxithromycin-treated patients. This is early evidence to support our clinical view that the macrolides and the azalides might be alternative prophylactic agents for patients who are allergic to β-lactams, who have underlying valvular disease and are subjected to the potential for bacterial endocarditis, and who require prophylaxis during different procedures.

Helicobacter pylori was touched on. In one abstract, Logan and his colleagues from Central Middlesex and St. Mary's Hospitals in London, studied patients who had biopsy, culture-proved, and urea–test-positive *H. pylori* gastritis. This study had four arms. The first arm was the use of clarithromycin, 500 mg, with omeprazole 20 mg. The second arm was the same dose of clarithromycin, but with double the dose of omeprazole, 40 mg. The last two arms were amoxicillin plus the two different doses of omeprazole, 20 mg in one arm and 40 mg in the other arm. The results with clarithromycin plus omeprazole at the high dose, 40 mg, cured 30 of 37 patients (81%). That was substantially different from the results with the lower dose of omeprazole and clarithromycin, during which only 56% of the patients were cured. When the higher dose of omeprazole with amoxicillin was used the cure rate was only 30%. This gives some evidence that the macrolides and azalides might have activity here. I remember many years ago when we thought we were going to cure *H. pylori* with the quinolones. Many studies and many gastric biopsies were done, only to prove that, even though improvement occurred during treatment, patients relapsed after treatment.

There was an abstract by Lilue and colleagues from Caracas, Venezuela, in which they studied roxithromycin compared with doxycycline in both mycoplasmal and chlamydial gynecological infections. Patients were randomly assigned to receive either roxithromycin, 150 mg twice daily, or doxycycline, 100 mg twice daily, and both groups were treated for 10 days. At the end of treatment, the bacteriological cure seen with roxithromycin was 93%, and with doxycycline it was 92%. Only small numbers of patients were studied, but it provides preliminary clinical data to support the use of macrolides as reasonable alternative agents to doxycycline for the treatment of lower gynecological infections caused by chlamydiae or by mycoplasmas.

Early studies have shown that azithromycin, as a 1 g single dose, cured chlamydial urethritis. There is no question about that. But in studies for single-dose treatment of gonorrhea, a failure rate was observed in two areas of the world. At this meeting, however, a paper by Lijnen and his colleagues from the Netherlands unequivocally shows that 1 g of azithromycin cures uncomplicated gonorrhea. There were four conclusions: One, a single-dose treatment of 1 g cures uncomplicated gonorrhea. The second was that patients who received the tablet form, rather than the capsule, seemed to do better. The third was that a single of 1-g azithromycin dose was also effective with concomitant infections, such as chlamydia; we suspected that would happen. The fourth was that in contrast with the 2-g dose, which we had studied years ago, the single, 1-g dose of azithromycin had few and very mild adverse effects.

The last abstract, again in the area of sexually transmitted diseases, is so unique that I wanted to mention it. It is the study by Mashkilleyson and his colleagues from Moscow, in which azithromycin was used to treat early syphilis. The numbers accrued in this study are 100 patients with early clinical syphilis. The patients received azithromycin, 500 mg once daily for 10 days, and the comparative arm was penicillin. Lesions disappeared in both groups, but serological tests reverted faster with azithromycin. Adverse reactions were very mild and did not require cessation of treatment.

POSTERS

Determination of the Inherent Antimicrobial Activity of Dirithromycin by Measuring Cell-Free Inhibition of Protein Synthesis

H. A. Kirst and L. C. Creemer

Lilly Research Laboratories, Eli Lilly and Company
Greenfield, Indiana

W. E. Alborn, Jr. and D. A. Preston

Lilly Research Laboratories, Eli Lilly and Company
Indianapolis, Indiana

The macrolide class of antibiotics has witnessed a remarkable renaissance during the last decade, culminating in the commercial development of several new semisynthetic 14- and 16-membered macrolide derivatives. Dirithromycin is a member of the new group of second-generation semisynthetic 14-membered macrolides derived from erythromycin (1). The structure of dirithromycin features a 9-N-11-O-oxazine moiety that is formed by condensation of 2-methoxyethoxyacetaldehyde and 9(S)-erythromycylamine [Fig. 1; (2–4)]. The latter is a well-known and very potent antibiotic previously synthesized from erythromycin.

The substituent of the oxazine ring system that is present in dirithromycin possesses the absolute configuration denoted as the R-configuration, as depicted in Figure 1. The isomer that possesses the alternative S-configuration of the oxazine substituent, named epidirithromycin (see Fig. 1), has also been prepared and characterized (5,6). Although epidirithromycin is the kinetically formed product of the synthetic reaction, it rapidly epimerizes under the reaction conditions to dirithromycin, the thermodynamically more stable compound (5–7). These two epimeric compounds readily interconvert with each other, and under a variety of solvent conditions, they reach an equilibrium mixture containing approximately 85–88% dirithromycin.

Both dirithromycin and epidirithromycin readily hydrolyze back to erythromycylamine, as do structurally related oxazine derivatives (5,8). This

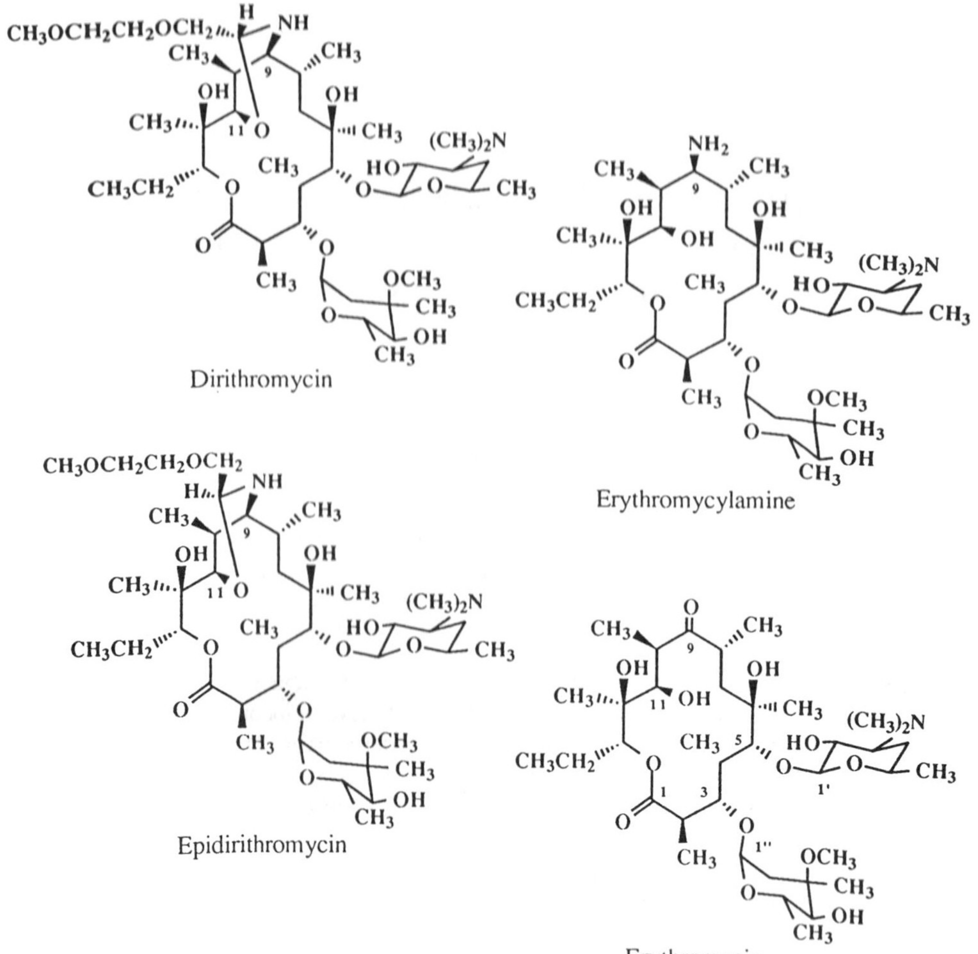

Figure 1   Structures of dirithromycin and related macrolides.

facile hydrolysis, which occurs both in vitro and in vivo, is responsible for the complex pharmacokinetic features of dirithromycin (9). Because hydrolysis also occurs under the prolonged conditions normally employed for determining minimum inhibitory concentration (MIC) values, and because dirithromycin and erythromycylamine generally yield the same MIC values when tested under standard conditions, it is not possible under the usual methods for in vitro evaluation to ascertain whether dirithromycin itself possesses inherent antibacterial activity or whether it must first hydrolyze to erythromycylamine to exert its antibiotic effects.

Inhibition of ribosomal protein synthesis is presumed to be the mechanism of action of all macrolide antibiotics (10). Measurement of protein synthesis inhibition is a well-precedented technique for 2′-esters of erythromycin, a well-known group of compounds that are also subject to facile hydrolysis (11). Consequently, we undertook to measure the inhibition of protein synthesis of dirithromycin while concomitantly using analytical high-performance liquid chromatography (HPLC) to measure its rate of hydrolysis and epimerization in the same test medium. Dirithromycin was rapidly hydrolyzed in Tris buffer at 37°C, such that >50% erythromycylamine was produced within 1 h. Furthermore, epidirithromycin also rapidly hydrolyzed to erythromycylamine under these same conditions; thus, the small proportion (<10%) of epidirithromycin in the sample did not increase. As a result of these pilot studies, procedures were subsequently developed to measure inhibition of protein synthesis in which the time period was reduced to only 5 min, during which an acceptable level of only 10% hydrolysis to erythromycylamine occurred. The rate of hydrolysis was relatively constant from 0.102 mM to 6 mM dirithromycin.

An Amersham kit number N.380 was used to measure the inhibition of cell-free protein synthesis on ribosomes from *Escherichia coli*. The progression of protein synthesis from a DNA template was followed by measuring the incorporation of tritiated leucine into protein. The effects of drug on protein synthesis were then compared with results from drug-free controls. From the HPLC analysis of the hydrolysis of dirithromycin in the same buffer solution, a protocol was adopted in which components were assembled and mixed in the following order: 1 μl DNA (pBluescript II SK-) + 1.5 μl supplement solution + 0.6 μl leucine + 0.4 μl [^{3}H]leucine + 1.0 μl S30 ribosome extract. The mixture was incubated at 37°C for 15 min to initiate protein synthesis, which was linear over this time period. The test antibiotics were dissolved as quickly as possible in dilution buffer (1 mM Tris acetate buffer at pH 7.5 plus one crystal of tartaric acid to facilitate dissolution) at a concentration of 3.7 mg in 925 μl; 1:10 serial dilutions were rapidly prepared, and 1.5 μl of the antibiotic solution was added immediately to the protein synthesis mixture. After incubation for 5 min, protein synthesis was quenched by submersion of the reaction tubes into an ice bath; 500 μl of 1N sodium hydroxide was added and the mixture was incubated for 15 min at 37°C. After adding 1 ml of 25% trichloroacetic acid (TCA) containing 1 mg/ml casein hydrolysate, the mixture was incubated at 0°C for 30 min to precipitate protein, which was then collected on Whatman glass-fiber filters, washed with 5% TCA and ethanol, and counted for radioactivity in a liquid scintillation counter. Each experiment was conducted in triplicate.

Erythromycyclamine inhibited protein synthesis to the extent of 63, 70,

63, and 0% at 100, 10, 1, and 0.1 μg/ml, respectively, whereas dirithromycin inhibited protein synthesis at 61, 72, 62, and 0% at 1000, 100, 10, and 1 μg/ml, respectively. Thus, an approximately tenfold higher concentration of dirithromycin was required to produce the same degree of inhibition of protein synthesis compared with erythromycylamine. Since analytical HPLC measurements had indicated that approximately 10% of dirithromycin was hydrolyzed to erythromycylamine under these buffer conditions, erythromycylamine accounted for >90% of the protein synthesis inhibition that had been observed in this experiment. Thus, under these particular test conditions, dirithromycin exhibited no greater than 10% of the inhibitory effect of erythromycylamine on ribosomal protein synthesis.

Consequently, the advantages of dirithromycin lie in its unique pharmacokinetic features, in which the oxazine ring system appears to facilitate the penetration and uptake of the antibiotic into cells and tissues. Intracellular hydrolysis of dirithromycin to erythromycylamine may then account for its extended in vivo half-life and its high and prolonged tissue and intracellular concentrations of antibiotic, thereby permitting once-a-day administration for the eradication of susceptible pathogens.

REFERENCES

1. Kirst HA. Prog Med Chem 1993; 30:57–88.
2. Counter FT, Ensminger PW, Preston DA, Wu C-YE, Greene JM, Felty-Duckworth AM, Paschal JW, Kirst HA. Antimicrob Agents Chemother 1991; 35:1116–1126.
3. Luger P, Maier R. J Cryst Mol Struct 1979; 9:329–338.
4. McGill JM. Synthesis 1993; 1089–1091.
5. Kirst HA, Greene JM, Amos JG, Clemens RL, Sullivan KA, Creemer LC, Paschal JW, Counter FT. 32nd Interscience Conference Antimicrobial Agents Chemotherapy, Anaheim, CA, October 11–14, 1992:abstr 1365.
6. Firl J, Prox A, Luger P, Maier R, Woitun E, Daneck K. J Antibiot 1990; 43:1271–1277.
7. McGill JM, Johnson R. Tetrahedron 1994; 50:3857–3868.
8. Massey EH, Kitchell BS, Martin LD, Gerzon K. J Med Chem 1974; 17:105–107.
9. Sides GD, Cerimele BJ, Black HR, Busch U, DeSante KA. J Antimicrob Chemother 1993; 31(suppl C):65–75.
10. Aumercier M, Le Goffic F. In: Bryskier AJ, Butzler J-P, Neu HC, Tulkens PM, eds. Macrolides: Chemistry, Pharmacology and Clinical Use. Paris: Arnette Blackwell, 1993:115–123.
11. Tardrew PL, Mao JCH, Kenny D. Appl Microbiol 1969; 18:159–165.

Characterization of the Bacterial Ribosomal-Binding Site for Lankacidin C

J. A. Retsema, M. Norcia, J. M. Bergeron, and W. U. Schelkly

Pfizer Inc.
Groton, Connecticut

INTRODUCTION

The recent increase in multiple antibiotic resistance among community-acquired pathogens has prompted a review of fermentation-derived antibiotics that might be useful against these new resistant strains. The 17-membered ring neutral macrolide antibiotic, lankacidin C, is such an antibiotic (1).

METHODS

Lankacidin C and streptogramins were isolated at Central Research, Pfizer Inc., all other antibiotics were from commercial sources. The minimum inhibitory concentration (MIC) values were determined, as previously described (2); all strains were clinical isolates. Natural mRNA-directed cell-free peptide synthesis assays were carried out with *Escherichia coli* subcellular fractions, as described (1), using three times 0.5 M NH$_4$Cl-washed ribosomes and 4.0 mM Mg^{2+} in the assays. The *E. coli* macrolide–lincosamide–streptogramin B (MLS$_B$) ribosomes were obtained from a strain carrying a plasmid Erm C construct (3). Assay component preparation and peptide synthesis assay procedures for *Staphylococcus aureus*-susceptible and MLS$_B$ ribosomes were exactly as described (2). Rat liver extracts were prepared, and polyphenylalanine synthesis was assayed, as described (4). The competitive ribosomal-binding assays, using washed ribosomes and [^{14}C]erythromycin or [^{3}H]chlorampenicol, were as described (2,5).

RESULTS

Lankacidin C had equivalent activity against macrolide-susceptible and macrolide-resistant gram-positive and fastidious gram-negative organisms. Its MIC_{90} versus macrolide-resistant isolates of *Streptococcus pyogenes, Staphylococcus* and *Haemophilus influenzae* strains was ≤ 1.6 $\mu g/ml$, compared to ≥ 50 $\mu g/ml$ for the 16-membered ring macrolide josamycin (Table 1).

To better understand the mechanism of action for lankacidin C against resistant isolates, ribosomes from susceptible and constitutive MLS_B-resistant gram-positive and gram-negative strains were prepared and used in biochemical assays to compare the activities of lankacidin C and MLS_B antibiotics. Lankacidin C was more potent than the representative macrolides, clindamycin and streptogramin B, for inhibiting peptide synthesis on susceptible gram-positive and gram-negative ribosomes. As expected, the macrolides (both 14- and 16-membered ring), clindamycin, and streptogramin B, all failed to inhibit peptide synthesis on MLS_B gram-positive- and gram-negative-resistant ribosomes (Table 2). Tetracycline, chloramphenicol, and streptogramin A are not affected by MLS_B resistance and showed equal potency (IC_{50} values) on both the susceptible and MLS_B ribosomes. In agreement with the MIC values in Table 1, lankacidin C demonstrated equal peptide synthesis inhibition on macrolide-susceptible and macrolide-resistant ribosomes (see Table 2).

Both competitive-binding data (5) and ribosomal protection studies (6) have shown that the 50S ribosomal subunit-binding sites for the 14- and 16-membered macrolides, lincosamides (clindamycin), streptogramin B, and chloramphenicol overlap. Thus, it was of interest to see what effect lankacidin C had on the binding of erythromycin and chloramphenicol to the ribosome. Nonradioactive erythromycin and chloramphenicol displaced [^{14}C]erythromycin and [^{3}H]chloramphenicol at the expected concentrations, that is the IC_{50} for the nonradioactive isomer was similar to the concentration of the isotope used in the assay (1.5 and 15 μM, respectively; see Table 2). The negative control tetracycline, which binds to the 30S ribosomal subunit, was inactive. The 16-membered macrolides (tylosin, josamycin), clindamycin, and the streptogramins, all displaced erythromycin and chloramphenicol from the susceptible ribosomes, as predicted (5,6). However, lankacidin C demonstrated no activity for displacing erythromycin from either *S. aureus* or *E. coli* ribosomes (see Table 2). Lankacidin C did compete for the chloramphenicol-binding site, although its IC_{50} values were slightly higher than those of the other MLS antibiotics.

The data in Table 2 clearly show that lankacidin C binds to ribosomes differently from the 14- and 16-membered ring macrolides. This raises the question: Does lankacidin retain the prokaryotic specificity of the macrolide class? To answer this, its ability to inhibit eukaryotic peptide synthesis was

Table 1 In Vitro Activity of Lankacidin C Against Resistant Pathogens

Organism	No. of strains	MIC_{90} (μg/ml)			
		Lankacidin C	Erythromycin	Josamycin	Clindamycin
Streptococcus pyogenes					
Susceptible	2	0.4	0.05	0.4	0.1
Resistant	8	0.4	>50	>50	>50
Staphylococcus[a]					
Susceptible	17	1.6	0.2	0.8	ND[b]
Resistant	27	1.6	>50	>50	
Haemophilus influenzae	46	1.6	6.3	50	>50[c]

[a] *S. aureus* (28), *S. epidermidis* (16) strains.
[b] ND, not done.
[c] Ampicillin, not clindamycin.

Table 2 Activity of Lankacidin C in Ribosomal Function Tests as Compared with Other Protein Synthesis Inhibitors Concentration Giving 50% Inhibition: IC$_{50}$ Values (μM)

Antibiotic	Ribosomes[a]	Peptide synthesis inhibition		Competitive binding	
		Susceptible[b]	MLSB[b]	Erythromycin[c]	Chloramphenicol[d]
Erythromycin	G$^-$	0.3	>200	1.9	0.4
	G$^+$	2.4	1000	1.7	0.8
Tylosin	G$^-$	0.11	>74	2.5	0.4
Josamycin	G$^+$	3.2	>1000	3.9	0.6
Clindamycin	G$^-$	8	>50	ND[e]	ND
	G$^+$	ND	ND	4.1	0.8
Streptogramin					
Mixture	G$^-$	0.04	0.045	0.31	0.36
A component	G$^-$	0.05	0.07	0.8	ND
B component	G$^-$	7	>50	55	ND
Lankacidin C	G$^-$	0.021	0.02	>150	1.1
	G$^+$	0.4	0.5	>>50	5.3
Chloramphenicol	G$^-$	2.9	2.9	>150	15
	G$^+$	40	30	>50	13.4
Tetracycline	G$^-$	4	4	>150	>250

[a]Source ribosomes, G$^-$ *Escherichia coli*, G$^+$ *Staphylococcus aureus*
[b]Ribosomes from erythromycin-susceptible or MLS$_B$-resistant strain.
[c]Displacement of 1.5 μM[^{14}C]erythromycin from susceptible ribosomes.
[d]Displacement of 1.5 μM[^{3}H]chloramphenicol from susceptible ribosomes.
[e]ND, not done.

Table 3 Comparison of the Activity of Lankacidin C to Inhibit Cell-Free Peptide Synthesis[a] in an *E. coli* and a Rat Liver System

	$IC_{50}(\mu M)$	
Agent	*E. coli*	Rat liver
Cycloheximide	ND[b]	22
Tylosin	0.085	>>800
Lankacidin C	0.28	>>800

[a]Poly-U–directed polyphenylalanine synthesis.
[b]ND, not done.

determined. Lankacidin inhibited poly-U–directed polyphenylalanine synthesis in an *E. coli* system in a manner similar to the 16-membered macrolides (tylosin; Table 3), but demonstrated no activity for inhibiting polyphenylalanine synthesis in a rat liver system. The positive control cycloheximide was active in the rat liver system (see Table 3).

In conclusion, the lankacidin class of macrolides should be reviewed for their potential to meet the challenge of increasing multidrug-resistant community pathogens.

REFERENCES

1. McFarland JW, Perie DK, Retsema JA, English AR. Side chain modifications in lankacidin group antibiotics. Antimicrob Agents Chemother 1984; 25:226–233.
2. Retsema J, Girard A, Schelkly W, Manousos M, Bright G, Borovoy R, Brennan L, Mason R. Spectrum and mode of action of azithromycin (CP-62,993), a new 15-membered-ring macrolide with improved potency against gram-negative organisms. Antimicrob Agents Chemother 1987; 31:1939–1947.
3. Macrina FL, Tobian JA, Jones KR, Evans RP, Clewell DB. A cloning vector able to replicate in *Escherichia coli* and *Streptococcus sanguis*. Gene 1982; 19:345–353.
4. Weinstein IB, Ochoa M Jr, Friedman SM. Fidelity in the translation of messenger ribonucleic acids in mammalian subcellular systems. Biochemistry 1966; 5:3332–3339.
5. Pestka S. Antibotics as probes of ribosome structure: binding of chloramphenicol and erythromycin to polyribosomes; effect of other antibiotics. Antimicrob Agents Chemother 1974; 5:255–267.
6. Moazed D, Noller HF. Chloramphenicol, erythromycin, carbomycin and vernamycin protect overlapping sites in the peptidyl transferase region of 23S ribosomal RNA. Biochemie 1987; 69:879–884.

Synthesis and Evaluation of Polyhydro Derivatives of Tylosin

A. Narandja, Ž. Kelnerić, L. Kolačny-Babić,
B. Šušković, and S. Djokić

PLIVA, Pharmaceutical, Chemical, Food and Cosmetic Industry Research Institute
Zagreb, Croatia

INTRODUCTION

To study the structure–activity relation among 16-membered macrolides to prepare an antibiotic with better antimicrobial or pharmacokinetic properties, 10,11,12,13-tetrahydrotylosin (Fig. 1, structure **2**) was selected as a starting compound. Hydrogenation of conjugated diene of related 16-membered macrolides causes no remarkable change in the activity (1,2). Since, for 10,11,12,13-tetrahydro derivatives of tylosin, there were no data available, preliminary antimicrobial screening of **2** encouraged us to continue investigations of the 10,11,12,13-tetrahydro series.

RESULTS

10,11,12,13-Tetrahydrotylosin (**2**) was prepared by catalytic hydrogenation of the conjugated double bond of tylosin (**1**); no change at the keto or the aldehyde group of tetrahydro compound **2** was detected (3). Depending on the reaction conditions, the keto or the aldehyde group of tetrahydro compound **2** was reduced with a metal hydride, yielding two different hexahydro compounds, **5** and **6**, or the octahydro compound **7**. The second area of our interest was the preparation of the 4'-deoxy compound in the 10,11,12,13-tetrahydro series. Deoxygenation at the C-4' position of related 16-membered macrolides has already been accomplished (4–6). We applied a modified process (7) in the synthesis of 4'

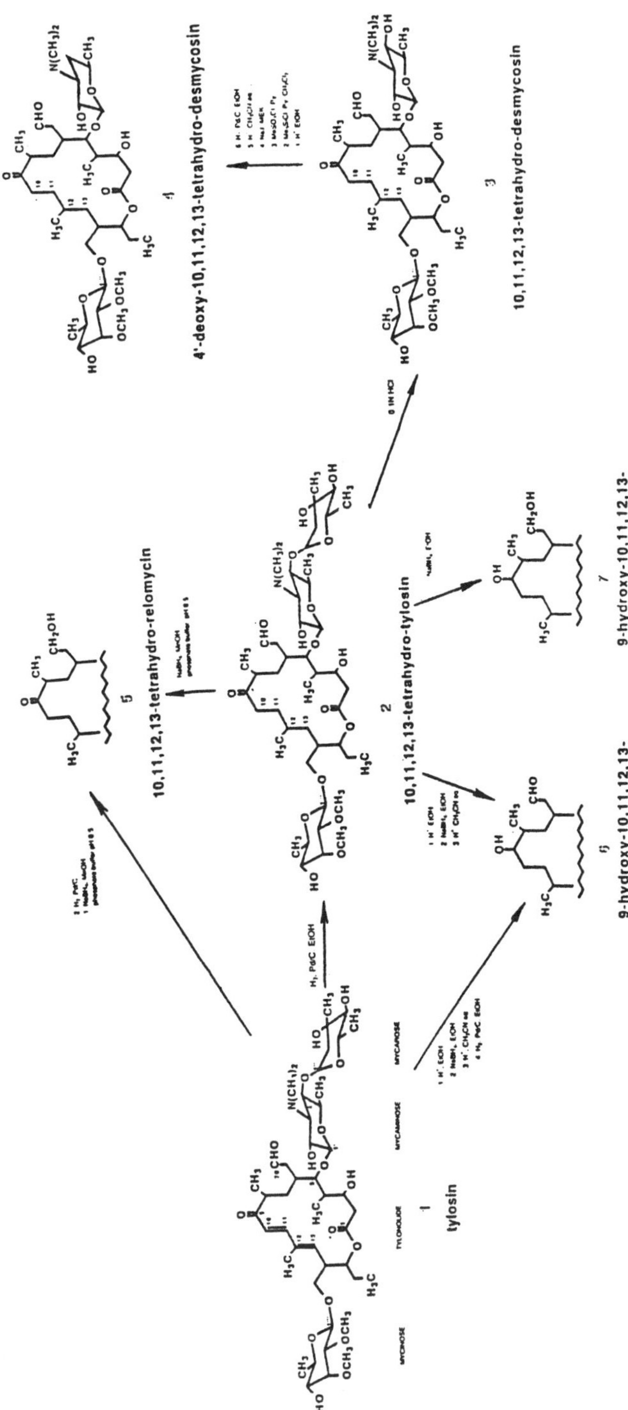

Figure 1 Synthesis scheme of polyhydro derivatives of tylosin.

Table 1 Antimicrobial In Vitro Activity of Polyhydro Derivatives of Tylosin

Organism	MIC(µg/ml)					
	Ty	2	3	4	5	6
Micrococcus luteus ATCC 9341	0.2	0.2	0.39	0.2	25	0.2
M. flavus ATCC 10420	0.78	0.78	0.78	0.78	25	1.56
Staphylococcus aureus ATCC 6538	0.39	0.39	0.78	0.2	12.5	0.78
S. aureus 500 KR[a]	1.56	1.56	3.12		50	3.13
S. epidermidis ATCC 12228	1.56	3.12	6.25	3.12	25	6.25
S. epidermidis 322KR[a]	3.12	3.12	1.56		50	3.12
Bacillus subtilis NCTC 8236	0.78	0.78	1.56	1.56	12.5	1.56
B. cereus ATCC 11778	0.78	1.56	1.56	0.78	6.25	3.12
B. pumilus NCTC 8241	0.78	0.39	0.78		6.25	0.78
Enterococcus faecalis ATCC 8043	1.56	3.12	6.25	6.25	25	6.25
S. pneumoniae (3)[b]	0.39	0.39	0.39	0.39	50	0.39
S. agalactiae (2)[b]	0.39	0.78	1.56		50	1.56
Streptococcus A (2)[b]	0.39	0.39	0.39	0.39	12.5	0.78

Streptococcus B (5)[b]	0.39	0.78	3.12	1.56	25	3.12
Haemophilus influenzae (5)[b]	0.78			0.39		
Corynebacterium pyogenes (1)[b]	1.56			0.39		
Branhamella (Moraxella) catarrhalis (1)[b]	0.2			0.1		
Mycoplasma pneumoniae (1)[b]	0.1	0.5	0.015			
Ureaplasma urealyticum (1)[b]	2	2	0.39			
Pasteurella haemolitica L-314	50	50	25	25	50	50
P. multocida L-315	25	25	12.5	12.5	25	25
Streptococcus suis SS-27[a]	1.56	1.56	6.25		50	3.12
S. suis SS-48[a]	0.78	0.78	3.12		50	1.56
Brucella abortus VB[a]	0.78	50	3.12	1.56		
B. suis-VB[a]	1.56	50	25	12.5		
Klebsiella pneumoniae P[a]	100	100	100	100	100	100
Shigella sonnei 34 Z[a]	100	100	100	100	100	100
Salmonella enteritidis 5 Z[a]	100	100	100	100	100	100
Escherichia coli ATCC 10596	100	100	100	100	100	100

[a]Strains from PLIVA culture collection.
[b]Number of fresh clinical isolates; determined at General Hospital "Sv.DUH," Zagreb.

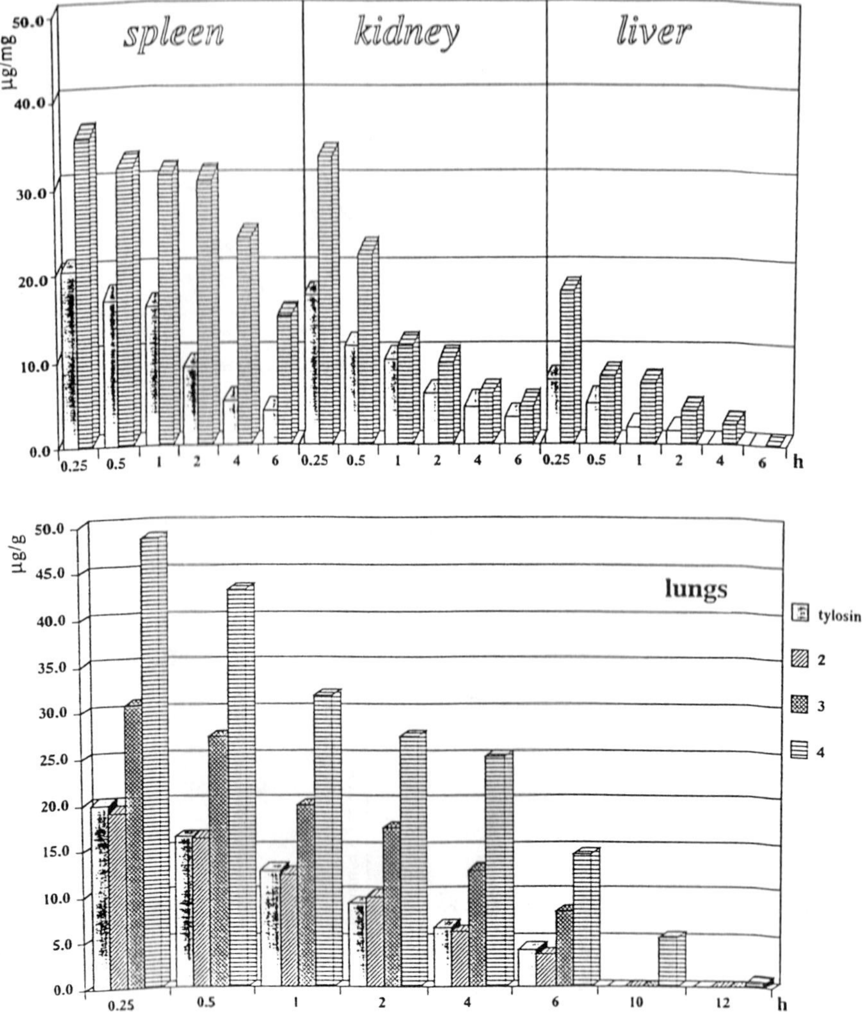

Figure 2   Tissue distribution of compounds **2**, **3**, and **4** in comparison with tylosin (30 mg/kg IV in the rat), by bioassay using *Micrococcus luteus* ATCC 9341.

derivatives, starting from 4′-demycarosyl-10,11,12,13-tetrahydrotylosin (**3**). Protection of concurrent hydroxyl groups was achieved by acetylation and salylation. The C-4′ position was activated by sulfonation and then substituted with iodine. After hydrolysis of the protecting groups, reductive deiodination gave 4′-deoxy-10,11,12,13-tetrahydrodesmycosin (**4**).

Compounds **2–7** were tested against tylosin-sensitive and tylosin-resistant bacteria, including some mycoplasmas, and against veterinary pathogens (Table 1). Compound **7** is inactive, with minimum inhibitory concentration (MIC) values $\geq$ 100 μg/ml.

CONCLUSION

Antimicrobial screening (see Table 1) of new 10,11,12,13-tetrahydro compounds showed that the transformation of the relatively rigid diene structure of the aglycon into a more flexible molecule does not influence the activity. Hydrogenation of the diene does not change in vitro activity, and the tetrahydro compounds **2**, **3**, and **4** retain antimicrobial spectrum of tylosin, with some improvement against mycoplasmas or some clinical isolates, respectively. However, reduction of carbonyls causes small (hexahydro compound **6**) or complete loss of activity (hexahydro compound **5** and octahydro compound **7**).

Pharmacokinetic investigation (30 mg/kg IV rat) of tetrahydro compounds **2**, **3**, and **4** showed very quick distribution from the blood serum into the tissues. The serum concentration of **2**, **3**, and **4** was less than 0.1 μg/ml. The concentration of the tetrahydro compound **2** in the lungs is on the same level as tylosin (Fig. 2), whereas concentrations of demycarosyl-tetrahydro compounds **3** and **4** are about 50–150% greater than those of tylosin. The high concentration of **4** in lung tissue is maintained until the 4th hour, it decreases in the 6th, and is still detectable in the 12th hour. The concentrations of **4** in the kidney and liver are greater than those of tylosin, especially in spleen, where a two- to fourfold increase is maintained for 6 h.

10,11,12,13-Tetrahydrodesmycosin (**3**) and 4′-deoxy-10,11,12,13-tetrahydrodesmycosin (**4**) are promising compounds.

REFERENCES

1. Omura S, Katagiri M, Umezawa I, Komiyama K, Maekawa T, Hata T. Structure–biological activities relationships among leucomycins and their derivatives. J Antibiot 1964; 21:532–538.
2. Maring CJ, Freiberg LA, Grampovnik DJ, Edwards CM, Hardy DJ, Fernandes PB. Synthesis and antimicrobial activities of 9(*S*)-*N*,*N*-dimethylamino-9-deoxo-10,11,12,13-tetrahydroniddamycin. J Antibiot 1991; 44:448–450.
3. Narandja A, Šušković B, Djokićs, Ž. Kelnerić Ž. Structure–activity relationship among polyhydro derivatives of tylosin. J Antibiot (in press).
4. Tanaka A, Watanabe A, Tsuchiya T, Umezawa S. Synthesis of 4′-deoxydemycarosyl tylosin and its analogues. J Antibiot 1981; 34:1381–1383.

5. Sano H, Inou M, Omura S. Chemical modification of spyramycins. J Antibiot 1984; 37:738–749.
6. Fujiwara T, Watanabe H, Kogami Y, Shiritani Y, Sakakibara H. 19-Deformyl-4'-deoxydesmysosin (TMC-016). J Antibiot 42:903–912, 1989
7. Narandja A, Djokic S. EP: 0 490 311 A1

A Comparative NMR and Molecular-Modeling Study Among Some Macrolides and Azalides with Different Antibacterial Properties

Gorjana Lazarevski, Mladen Vinković, Gabrijela Kobrehel, Željko Kelnerić, and Slobodan Dokić

PLIVA, Pharmaceutical, Chemical, Food and Cosmetic Industry, Research Institute
Zagreb, Croatia

Biserka Metelko

Ruder Bosković Institute
Zagreb, Croatia

INTRODUCTION

A Beckmann rearrangement of erythromycin A 9-oxime created a new class of macrolide antibiotics—azalides (1–5). This term has been applied to the group of ring-expanded derivatives of erythromycin A that contain a nitrogen atom embedded within their 15-membered ring system (Fig. 1). Azithromycin (**4**) is a new, and medically the most important member of the azalide-type compounds. Its conformation in solution has been studied by both NMR spectrometry and theoretical calculations (6).

The logical progression of this work was to study the conformational behavior in solution of azalides with different antibacterial activity to determine a possible relation between solution-state conformational preferences of compounds **1–6** and their biological properties. The solution conformations of **1–6** were determined by NMR parameters (^3J analysis, 1D and 2D NOE, T_1 experiments), and molecular mechanics calculations.

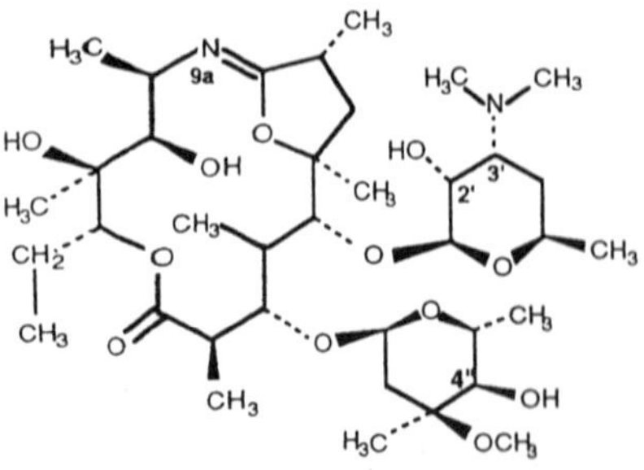

1

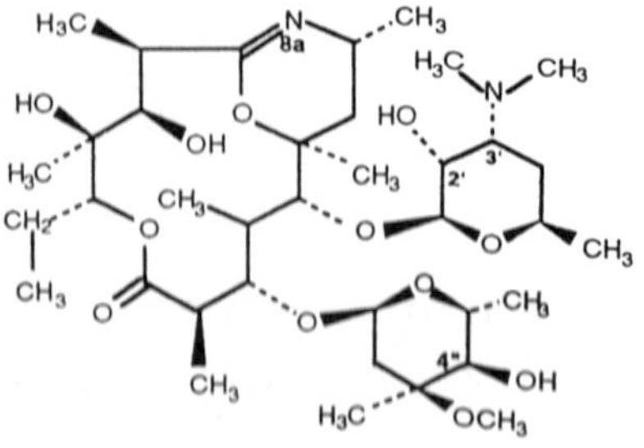

2

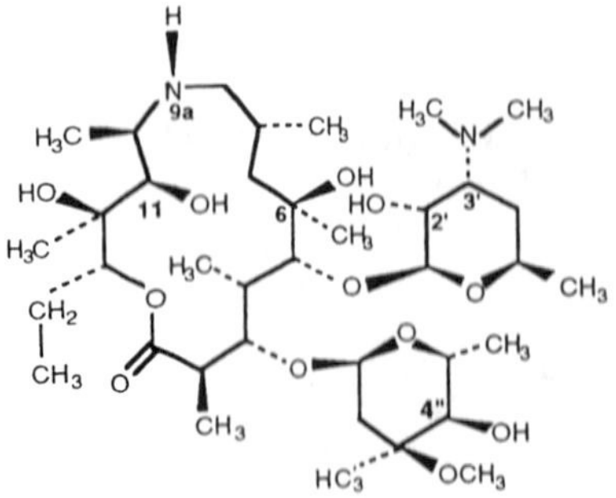

3

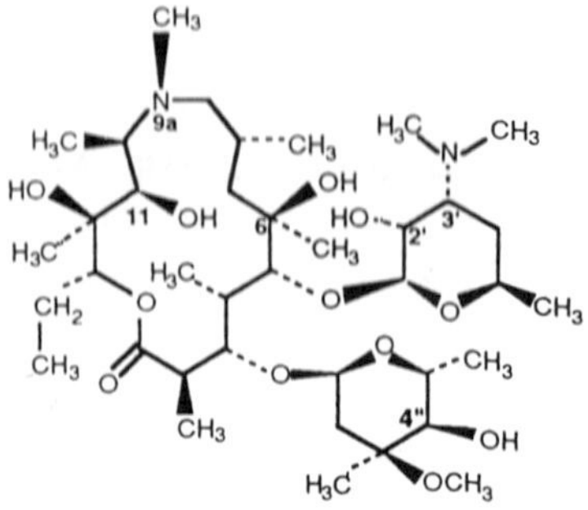

4

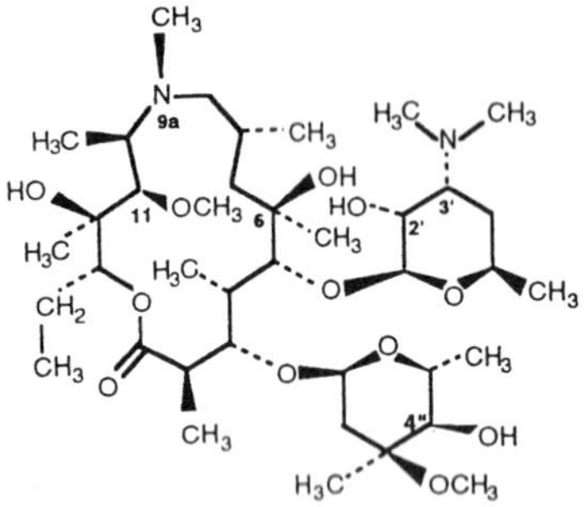

5

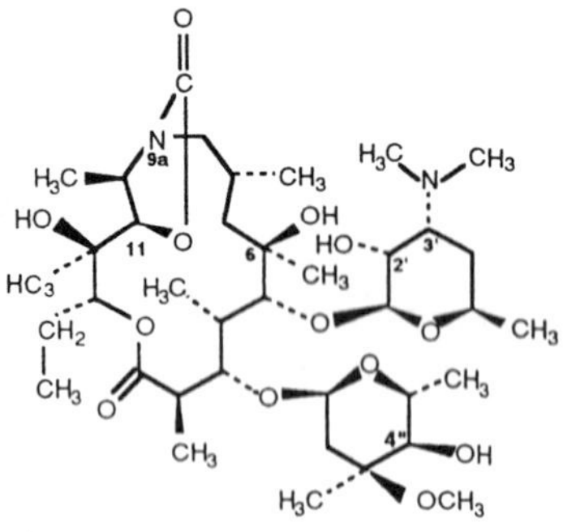

6

Figure 1
(**1**) 9a-Aza-9a-homoerythromycin A 6,9-cyclic iminoether
(**2**) 8a-Aza-8a-homoerythromycin A 6,9-cyclic iminoether
(**3**) 9-Deoxo-9a-aza-9a-homoerythromycin A
(**4**) Azithromycin
(**5**) 11-*O*-Methylazithromycin
(**6**) 9-deoxo-9a-aza-11-deoxy-9a-homoerythromycin A 9a,11-cyclic carbamate

EXPERIMENTAL

The ^{1}H and ^{13}C NMR experiments were performed, as described previously (6), on a Varian Gemini 300 spectrometer, using 5-mm od NMR tubes at ambient temperature and sample concentrations of 30–60 mg cm^{-3}. Molecular mechanics optimization of solution state conformation was performed by using an MMX force field. Calculations of dihedral angles from ^{3}J values were performed using Eq. (1).

$$^3J_{H,H} = P_1 \cos^2\Phi + P_2 \cos\Phi = \Sigma\Delta\chi_i \{P_4 + P_5 \cos^2 (\xi_i\Phi + P_6|\Delta\chi_j|)\} \quad (1)$$

RESULTS AND DISCUSSION

Our study indicated that azalides **1–6** exist preferentially in the conformations shown in Figure 2.

The $^3J_{H,H}$ values of the sugar ring protons, together with intrasugar, intersugar, and sugar-lactone nuclear Overhouser effects (NOEs), indicated that the orientations of the sugar rings relative to one another and relative to the lactone ring were similar for all azalides investigated. For the lactone ring, the main differences were found in C-2/C-5 and C-10/C-11 regions. Table 1 compares ^{1}H-coupling constants found in solutions and corresponding dihedral angles based on experimental and theoretical data. The $^3J_{2,3}$ value suggests that the azalides **1**, **2**, **4**, and **5** are predominantly in a C-3 to C-5 folded-in conformation in which H-3 becomes closer to H-11 (Fig. 3b). Compound **6** in this region has folded-out type of conformation that is characterized by close cross-ring approach of H-4 and H-11 (see Fig. 3a). Compound **3** exists in solution as a mixture of both types of conformations. The NOE experiments confirmed the spatial proximity of H-11 to H-3 for **1**, **2**, **4**, and **5**, and to H-4 for compound **6**, respectively. For compound **3**, NOEs between H-11 and both H-3 and H-4 were found, indicating the presence of both folded-in and folded-out conformations. However, the similarity in $^3J_{3,4}$ and $^3J_{4,5}$ again implies that the orientation of the sugar rings relative to one another is almost the same for **1–6**.

In the region C-10/C-11, azalides **3**, **4**, and **5** have a $^3J_{10,11}$ value similar to that found for most of the erythromycin derivatives. The three bicyclic compounds **1**, **2**, and **6** adopt different conformation in this portion of lactone ring, at least in part, because of the 6,9-oxygen bridge for **1** and **2**, and the 9a,11-cyclic carbamate ring for **6**, respectively, and are similar to that seen in some other bicyclic erythromycin derivatives (7). The NOE 10-Me/6-Me found for compound **2** and MM calculations confirmed this conformation reorganization.

The vicinal proton–proton coupling constants were measured in various solvents to test conformation homogeneity. These values remain invariant relative

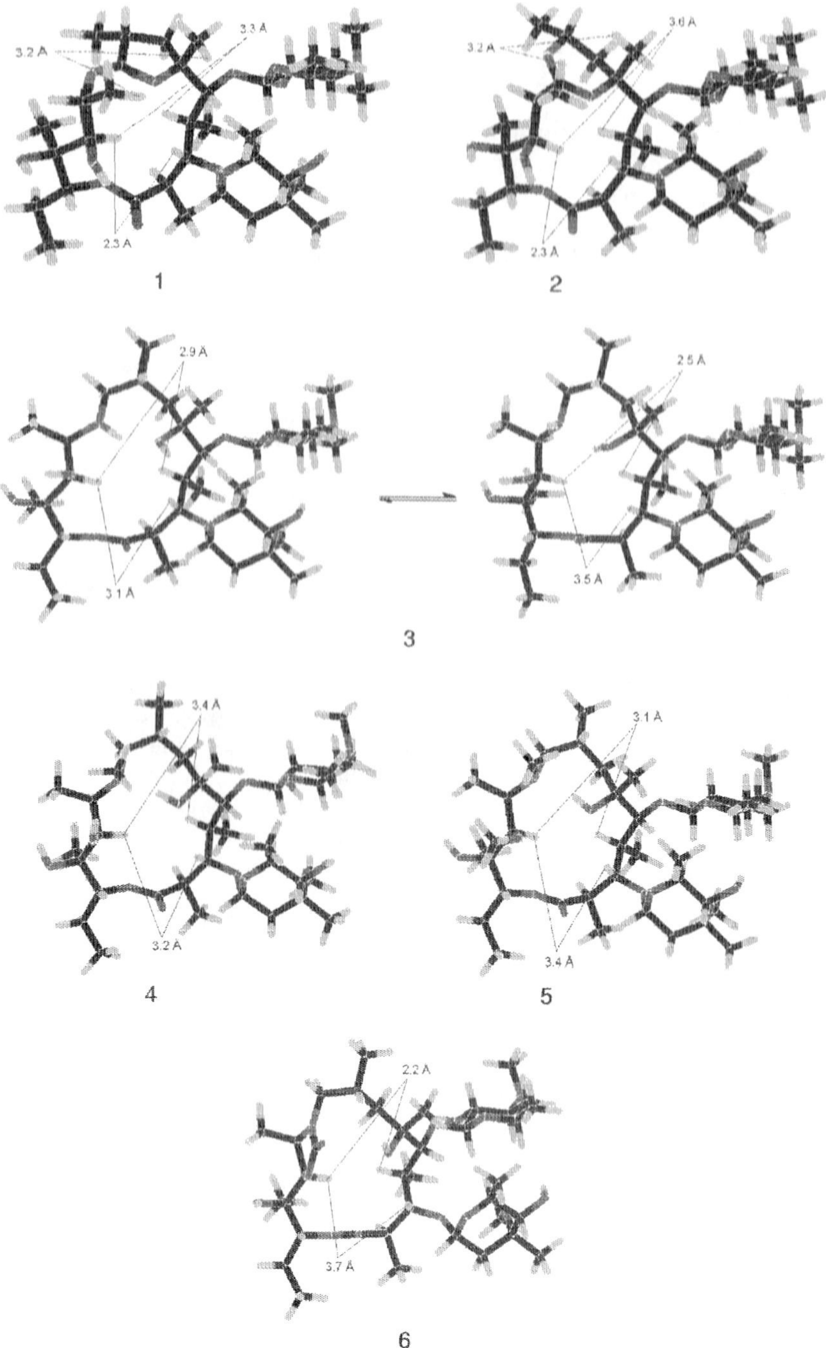

Figure 2 Stick drawing of solution state conformations of azalides **1–6**.

206

Table 1 Diagnostic Coupling Constants for Vicinal Proton Pairs and Corresponding Dihedral Angles for Compounds **1–6**

Vicinal proton pair	1				2				3						4				5				6			
	$^3J^a_{exp}$ (Hz)	ϕ^b_{calc} (°)	ϕ^c MMX (°)	$^3J^d$ MMX (Hz)	$^3J^a_{exp}$ (Hz)	ϕ^b_{calc} (°)	ϕ^c MMX (°)	$^3J^d$ MMX (Hz)	$^3J^a_{exp}$ (Hz)	ϕ^b_{calc} (°)	ϕ^c MMX (°) -in	ϕ^c MMX (°) -out	$^3J^d$ MMX (Hz) -in	$^3J^d$ MMX (Hz) -out	$^3J^a_{exp}$ (Hz)	ϕ^b_{calc} (°)	ϕ^c MMX (°)	$^3J^d$ MMX (Hz)	$^3J^a_{exp}$ (Hz)	ϕ^b_{calc} (°)	ϕ^c MMX (°)	$^{'3}J^d$ MMX (Hz)	$^3J^a_{exp}$ (Hz)	ϕ^b_{calc} (°)	ϕ^c MMX (°)	$^3J^d$ MMX (Hz)
2–3	2.4	107	104	1.9	2.8	111	108	2.4	5.5	126	109	140	2.5	7.9	3.6	116	110	2.7	3.5	115	120	4.3	8.8	146	146	8.9
3–4	2.4	−68	−66	2.6	2.8	−64	−68	2.3	1.8	−57	−69	−67	0.9	1.0	1.7	−60	−74	0.7	2.1	−57	−75	0.6	1.2	−65	−72	0.7
4–5	6.9	134	129	6.0	7.3	136	136	7.3	7.3	136	139	135	7.8	7.0	7.4	137	143	8.5	7.3	136	141	8.2	7.7	138	140	7.9
10–11	9.4	160	169	9.9	10.1	153	168	11.4	1.3	61	66	67	1.5	1.2	1.9	59	75	0.8	1.4	65	62	1.7	6.0	28	29	5.9

[a] Experimental values in $CDCl_3$ at 293 K.
[b] Dihedral angles ϕ_{calc} were calculated from $^3J_{exp}$ using Eq. (1).
[c] Dihedral angles of solute state conformation predicted on base MMX calculation.
[d] Coupling constants calculated for MMX solution state geometry using Eq. (1).

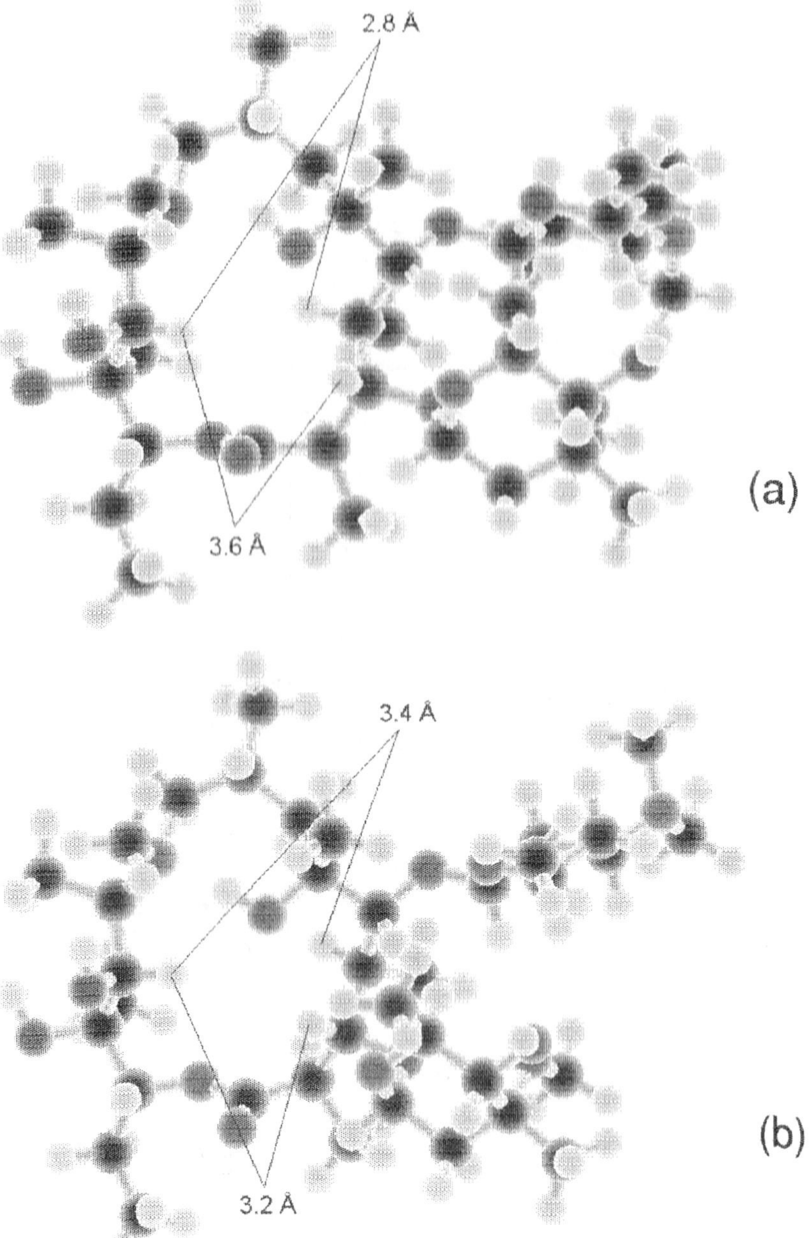

Figure 3 Ball and stick drawing of azithromycin (**4**): (a) C-3/C-5 folded-out (solid state) and (b) C-3/C-5 folded-in (solution state) conformations.

Table 2 Comparative In Vitro Activities of Azalides **1–6** and Erythromycin on Clinical Isolates

Type of C-3/C-5 conformation	Erythromycin folded-out			1 Folded-in			2 Folded-in			3 Mixture of folded- in and out			4 Folded-in			5 Folded-in			6 Folded-out		
Organism (No)	Range	MIC 50%	MIC 90%	Range	MIC 50%	MIC 90%	Range	MIC 50%	MIC 90%	Range	MIC 50%	MIC 90%	Range	MIC 50%	MIC 90%	Range	MIC 50%	MIC 90%	Range	MIC 50%	MIC 90%
Staphylococcus spp. (23)	1–>128	>128	>128	16–>128	>128	>128	16–>128	>128	>128	0.125–>128	64	>128	1–>128	>128	>128	2–>128	>128	>128	8–>128	>128	>128
Enterococcus spp. (14)	0.5–>128	32	>128	16–>128	>128	>128	8–>128	16	>128	1–>128	8	>128	1–>128	64	>128	1–>128	32	>128	2–>128	>128	>1228
Salmonella spp. (8)	16–>128	>128	>128	64–>128	>128	>128	>128	>128	>128	2–16	4	8	1–8	2	2	8–64	16	16	16–>128	64	>128
Acinetobacter spp. (7)	2–16	4	8	32–>128	64	>128	8–>128	64	>128	8–>128	32	>128	16–32	16	32	2–64	16	16	8–64	16	16
Streptococcus pneumoniae spp. (7)	0.06–0.125	0.125	0.125	2–4	4	4	1–4	2	2	0.125–1	0.5	0.5	0.125–0.5	0.25	0.5	0.06–0.25	0.125	0.25	0.25–1	1	1

to solvent changes for the less active compounds **1**, **2**, and **6** (Table 2), indicating that they exist in solution in a single, stable conformation.

The conformational behavior of azithromycin was also compared with other macrolide antibiotics (erythromycin, roxithromycin, clarithromycin, and dirithromycin). Although these antibiotics in solution retain predominately their crystal state conformations, azithromycin in its crystal state exists in a folded-out, and in solution in a folded-in conformation.

CONCLUSION

No simple correlation between solution state, conformational behavior, and antibacterial activity for azalides **1–6** was found. However, the less active compounds **1**, **2**, and **6** exist in solution exclusively in one of the two types of C-3/C-5 conformations. Azalides with a monocyclic aglycone ring were superior to bicyclic ring azalides in activity, which is in agreement with the erythromycin series (8). In contrast with the other macrolide antibiotics, the conformational study has shown that azithromycin in solution does not retain its crystal state conformation.

Each of the newer semisynthetic macrolides, particularly azithromycin, has a characteristic pharmacokinetic profile that differs from the others, rather than in mechanism of action and antimicrobial spectrum. Therefore, other factors (lipid solubility, pH-partition, degradations and transformations, interaction with hepatic enzymes, metabolic pathways, and such) should also be studied to explain some of significant differences in biological properties among them.

REFERENCES

1. Dokić S, Kobrehel G, Lazarevski G, Lopotar N, Tamburašev Z, Kamenar B, Nagl A, Vicković I. J Chem Soc Perkin Trans 1 1986; 1986:1881–1890.
2. Dokić S, Kobrehel G, Lazarevski G. J Antibiot 1967; 40:1006–1015.
3. Dokić S, Kobrehel G, Lopotar N, Kamenar B, Nagl A, Mrvoš D. J Chem Res 1988; (S) 1988:152–153; (M) 1988:1239–1261.
4. Bright GM, Nagel AA, Bordner J, Desai KA, Dibrino JN, Nowakowska J, Vincent L, Watrous RM, Sciavolino FC, English AR, Retsema JA, Anderson MR, Brennan LA, Borovoy RJ, Cimochowski CR, Faiella JA, Girard AE, Girard D, Herbert C, Manousos M, Mason R. J Antibiot 1988; 41:1029–1047.
5. Wilkening RR, Ratcliffe RW, Doss GA, Bartizal KF, Graham AC, Herbert CM. Bioorg Med Chem Lett 1993; 3:1287–1292.
6. Lazarevski G, Vinković M, Kobrehel G, Dokić S, Metelko B, Vikić-Topić D. Tetrahedron 1993; 49:721–730.

7. Everett JR, Hatton JK, Hunt E, Tyler JW. J Chem Soc Trans 2 1989; 1989:1719–1728.
8. Kirst HA. Antibiotics and antiviral compounds. In: Krohn K, Kirst H, Mass H, (eds.) Chemical Synthesis and Modification. Weinheim: VCH, 1993: 143–151.

Antibacterial Activity of Clarithromycin, 14-Hydroxyclarithromycin and Five Other Oral Agents Against Respiratory Pathogens from Outpatients Within the United States

Arthur L. Barry and Trixi Schultheiss

The Clinical Microbiology Institute
Tualatin, Oregon

Orally administered antibacterial agents are particularly useful for chemotherapy on an outpatient basis. When treating respiratory tract infections, bacterial cultures and susceptibility tests are rarely helpful because of difficulties in obtaining adequate cultures and because of the delay before any results are available. Consequently, initial therapy is usually selected empirically, and the choice of drugs is based on the physician's experience in treating other patients with similar diseases. Also, the choice of empiric therapy should be based on in vitro studies documenting the prevalence of bacterial resistance among the more commonly encountered species that are likely to be involved in that patient population (3,5,6,10). Most in vitro surveillance programs study isolates recovered from hospitalized patients, although it is often assumed that resistant strains are less prevalent among noninstitutionalized patients.

This manuscript represents a preliminary report of an ongoing study in which we are evaluating respiratory tract isolates from outpatients attending clinics in 11 different cities spread throughout the continental United States. Each of eleven microbiology laboratories gathered consecutive clinical isolates of *Streptococcus pneumoniae*, *S. pyogenes*, *Moraxella catarrhalis*, and *Haemophilus influenzae*. The respiratory tract isolates were submitted to a central reference laboratory for in vitro susceptibility tests by standardized procedures (9).

Table 1 Description of Outpatient Isolates Evaluated

Medical center city and state	Number of strains contributed					
	H. influenzae β-lactamase		*S. pneumoniae* penicillin		*Streptococcus pyogenes*	*Moraxella catarrhalis*
	Neg.	Pos.	Sensit.	Resist.		
Berkeley, CA	20	7	17	4	30	18
St. Louis, MO	0	0	4	3	28	0
Indianapolis, IN	24	9	20	11	34	6
Galveston, TX	20	9	14	14	28	20
New York, NY	10	7	12	2	28	6
Detroit, MI	25	8	15	6	32	10
Salt Lake City, UT	19	11	16	15	32	17
Renton, WA	16	14	24	4	28	20
Morgantown, WV	16	5	6	2	0	16
Boston, MA	19	9	16	0	35	4
Clearwater, FL	10	1	4	3	0	5
All centers						
Pediatric	52	37(42%)	52	35(40%)	158	63
Adults	127	43(25%)	96	29(23%)	107	59
Total	179	80(31%)	148	64(30%)	265	122

Some characteristics of the 858 isolates that have now been studied are described in Table 1. Approximately half (54%) of the isolates were recovered from adults (12 years or older) and 46% were from pediatric populations (younger than 12 years). Isolates from children contained a larger proportion of penicillin-resistant or relatively resistant *S. pneumoniae* and of ampicillin-resistant *H. influenzae*. Overall, 31% of *H. influenzae* were resistant to ampicillin (42% in the pediatric group). Also 30% of the *S. pneumoniae* strains demonstrated decreased susceptibility to penicillin (40% in the pediatric group). The 212 *S. pneumoniae* isolates included 50 strains with intermediate susceptibility to penicillin (MIC 0.12 –1.0 µg/ml) and 14 strains that were penicillin-resistant (MIC ≥ 2.0 µg/ml). Resistance to two macrolides was evaluated by standardized disk diffusion tests (Table 2). Erythromycin and clarithromycin showed essentially complete cross-resistance. Clarithromycin disk tests showed only minor discrepancies with MIC categories described in Tables 1 and 3. Approximately 1% of *S. pyogenes* isolates displayed macrolide resistance. All 124 *M. catarrhalis* strains were susceptible to both macrolides. Only 2% of the penicillin-susceptible *S. pneumoniae* isolates were resistant to the macrolides. However, 14–15% of the penicillin-intermediate strains and 50% of the penicillin-resistant strains were

Table 2 Prevalence of Macrolide Resistance Among Outpatient Isolates Tested with Standard 15-μg Erythromycin and 15-μg Clarithromycin Disks

Microorganism	% with the following disk test results[a]					
	Susceptible		Intermediate		Resistant	
(no. tested)	Eryth	Clar	Eryth	Clar	Eryth	Clar
S. pyogenes (270)	97.4	98.5	1.5	0.7	1.1	0.7
M. catarrhalis						
β-Lactamase– negative (12)	100	100				
β-Lactamase– positive (112)	100	100				
S. pneumoniae						
Penicillin- susceptible (148)	98.3	98.3	0.7	0.7	1.0	1.0
Penicillin- intermediate (50)	83.7	85.4	2.0	0	14.3	14.6
Penicillin- resistant (14)	50	50	0	0	50	50
H. influenzae[b]						
β-Lactamase– negative (179)		89.5		7.7		2.8
β-Lactamase- positive (80)		88.7		10.0		7.5

[a]Breakpoints for susceptible, intermediate, and resistant categories are as follows:
    Erythromycin ≥23, 14–22, and ≤13 mm, respectively.
    Clarithromycin ≥18, 14–17, and ≤13 mm, respectively or when testing.
    H. influenzae, ≥13, 11–12, and ≤10 mm, respectively.
[b]Erythromycin disk tests of *H. influenzae* could not be interpreted, since there are no interpretive criteria comparable with those used for clarithromycin.

resistant to erythromycin and to clarithromycin. Among *H. influenzae* isolates, clarithromycin resistance was more common among β-lactamase–producing strains.

In vitro studies were performed with broth microdilution methods, using cation-adjusted Mueller–Hinton broth with 2–3% lysed horse blood. The 828 isolates were tested against clarithromycin, the 14-hydroxyclarithromycin metabolite, and a combination of three parts clarithromycin and one part metabolite (expressed as the total amount of drug in the combination). The macrolides were compared with three oral cephalosporins (cefaclor, cefprozil, and cefuroxime axetil) and also against amoxicillin and amoxicillin plus clavulanic acid (2:1 ratio). The results are summarized in Table 3.

Among the *S. pneumoniae* isolates, penicillin-susceptible strains were all susceptible to the β-lactam drugs, and 98% were susceptible to clarithromycin and its metabolite. Against penicillin-resistant or relatively resistant strains, the potencies of the β-lactams were compromised (7,8), whereas 83% of those strains remained susceptible to clarithromycin.

The 79 β-lactamase–producing *H. influenzae* isolates also showed decreased susceptibility to cefaclor and cefprozil, as well as to amoxicillin. One strain was β-lactamase–negative, but ampicillin-resistant, and that strain was relatively resistant to all of the β-lactams that were studied (2). The majority (> 90%) of *H. influenzae* isolates were susceptible to clarithromycin. The 14-hydroxy metabolite was twice as potent as the parent compound. In the blood and tissues of treated patients, both forms of clarithromycin can be found in different ratios. We tested a 3:1 combination and expressed the results as the total amount of drug inhibiting growth, rather than the concentration of clarithromycin in the combination. In that test system, the bioactive metabolite did indeed improve the clarithromycin activity against *H. influenzae* (1). Against other species, the metabolite and its parent compound were essentially identical in the in vitro potency; the metabolite was somewhat less potent than the parent compound against *S. pyogenes* and *S. pneumoniae*, but the 3:1 combination was similar to the parent compound alone.

Among common respiratory tract pathogens that are currently encountered among outpatients in the United States, *S. pneumoniae* strains have developed a relative resistance to penicillin by virtue of altered penicillin-binding sites and thus other β-lactam drugs are also less effective. Whether that relative resistance correlates with a loss of clinical efficacy remains to be seen, but all strains that are not susceptible to penicillin are assumed to be resistant to most other β-lactams. Consequently, non–β-lactam alternative drugs are needed. Clarithromycin and other macrolides are possible options that might be considered (4). Erythromycin-resistant isolates display cross-resistance to clarithromycin and other macrolides. Macrolide resistance is fairly uncommon (1–2%) among *S. pyogenes* and penicillin-susceptible *S. pneumoniae*. Unfortunately, half of the penicillin-resistant pneumococci that are of concern tend to be resistant to the macrolides.

β-Lactamase production and altered penicillin-binding sites among respiratory pathogens are compromising the usefulness of β-lactam drugs for treatment of community-acquired respiratory tract infections, especially in children. In most communities within the United States, penicillin-resistant pneumococci are relatively uncommon. Clarithromycin should be an effective alternative oral agent for treating patients in those communities.

Table 3 Comparative Activity of Antimicrobial Agents Against Respiratory Pathogens from U.S. Outpatients

Microorganism (no. tested)	Antimicrobial agent	MIC (µg/ml)			% susceptible[a]	
		Range	50%	90%		to (µg/ml)
S. pneumoniae penicillin-susceptible (148)	Clarithromycin	≤0.016–4.0	≤0.016	0.03	98	≤2.0
	14-OH clarithro	≤0.016–8.0	0.03	0.06	98	≤2.0
	Clar+14-OH clar[b]	≤0.016–8.0	0.03	0.03	98	≤2.0
	Cefaclor	0.12–2.0	1.0	1.0	100	≤8.0
	Cefprozil	0.06–0.25	0.12	0.25	100	≤8.0
	Cefuroxime axetil	≤0.03–0.25	≤0.03	≤0.03	100	≤4.0
	Amoxicillin	≤0.016–0.06	≤0.016	0.03	100	≤0.12
	Amox+clav acid[c]	≤0.016–0.06	≤0.016	0.03	100	≤8/4
S. pneumoniae penicillin-resistant[d] (64)	Clarithromycin	≤0.016–>32	0.03	>32	83	≤2.0
	14-OH clarithro	≤0.016–>32	0.06	>32	81	≤2.0
	Clar+14-OH Clar[b]	≤0.016–>32	0.03	32	83	≤2.0
	Cefaclor	0.25–>32	2.0	>32	66	≤8.0
	Cefprozil	0.12–32	1.0	16	67	≤8.0
	Cefuroxime axetil	≤0.03–16	0.5	8.0	73	≤4.0
	Amoxicillin	≤0.016–8.0	0.25	2.0	44	≤0.12
	Amox+clav acid[c]	≤0.016–8.0	0.25	2.0	44	≤8/4
H. influenzae β-lactamase-negative (178)	Clarithromycin	0.25–16	8.0	8.0	94	≤8.0
	14-OH clarithro	0.5–16	4.0	8.0	98	≤8.0

	Clar+14-OH clar[b]	0.25–16	8.0	8.0	97	≤8.0
	Cefaclor	1.0–32	4.0	8.0	92	≤8.0
	Cefprozil	0.25->32	4.0	16	88	≤8.0
	Cefuroxime axetil	0.12–8.0	1.0	4.0	96	≤4.0
	Amoxicillin	0.12–2.0	0.5	1.0	99	≤1.0
	Amox+clav acid[c]	0.12–2.0	0.5	1.0	100	≤4/2
H. influenzae β-lactamase-positive (80)	Clarithromycin	2.0->32	8.0	16	90	≤8.0
	14-OH clarithro	2.0->32	4.0	8.0	95	≤8.0
	Clar+14-OH clar[b]	2.0->32	8.0	8.0	91	≤8.0
	Cefaclor	1.0->32	8.0	>32	62	≤8.0
	Cefprozil	1.0->32	8.0	>32	60	≤8.0
	Cefuroxime axetil	0.25–32	1.0	4.0	87	≤4.0
	Amoxicillin	8.0->32	>32	>32	0	≤1.0
	Amox+clav acid[c]	0.5–4.0	1.0	2.0	100	≤4/2
M. catarrhalis β-lactamase-positive (79)	Clarithromycin	≤0.016–0.12	0.06	0.06	100	≤2.0
	14-OH clarithro	≤0.016–0.12	0.06	0.06	100	≤2.0
	Clar+14-OH clar[b]	≤0.016–0.12	0.06	0.12	100	≤2.0
	Cefaclor	1.0–32	4.0	8.0	94	≤8.0
	Cefprozil	2.0->32	4.0	16	85	≤8.0
	Cefuroxime axetil	0.5–4.0	2.0	4.0	100	≤4.0
	Amoxicillin	0.5->32	8.0	32	0	≤0.25
	Amox+clav acid[c]	0.03–0.5	0.25	0.25	100	≤8/4

(continued)

Table 3 (*Continued*)

Microorganism (no. tested)	Antimicrobial agent	MIC (μg/ml)			% susceptible[a] to (μg/ml)	
		Range	50%	90%		
M. catarrhalis β-lactamase-negative (12)	Clarithromycin	≤0.016–0.06	0.03	0.06	100	≤2.0
	14-OH clarithro	≤0.016–0.06	0.03	0.06	100	≤2.0
	Clar+14-OH clar[b]	≤0.016–0.06	0.03	0.06	100	≤2.0
	Cefaclor	0.12–0.5	0.25	0.5	100	≤8.0
	Cefprozil	0.25–0.5	0.5	0.5	100	≤8.0
	Cefuroxime axetil	0.12–1.0	0.25	1.0	100	≤4.0
	Amoxicillin	≤0.016–0.12	≤0.016	0.06	100	≤0.25
	Amox+clav acid[c]	≤0.016–0.12	≤0.016	0.06	100	≤8/4
S. pyogenes (275)	Clarithromycin	≤0.016–>32	0.03	0.03	99	≤2.0
	14-OH clarithro	≤0.016–>32	0.06	0.06	98	≤2.0
	Clar+14-OH clar[b]	≤0.016–>32	0.03	0.06	99	≤2.0
	Cefaclor	0.06–0.25	0.12	0.25	100	≤8.0
	Cefprozil	≤0.03–0.06	≤0.03	≤0.03	100	≤8.0
	Cefuroxime axetil	≤0.03–≤0.03	≤0.03	≤0.03	100	≤4.0
	Amoxicillin	≤0.016–0.03	≤0.016	≤0.016	100	≤0.12
	Amox+clav acid[c]	≤0.016–0.03	≤0.016	≤0.016	100	≤8/4

[a]Percentage of strains inhibited by the designated breakpoint concentrations for susceptible according to the NCCLS. For tests with amoxicillin, ampicillin breakpoints were used.
[b]Three parts clarithromycin plus one part 14-hydroxyclarithromycin, MICs are expressed as the sum of both components.
[c]Two parts amoxicillin plus one part clavulanic acid, MICs are expressed as the concentration of amoxicillin in the 2:1 combination.
[d]Includes 14 penicillin-resistant and 50 relatively resistant strains.
[e]Excludes one (1) ampicillin-resistant, β-lactamase-negative strain.

REFERENCES

1. Barry AL, Fuchs PC, Pfaller MA. Susceptibility of *Haemophilus influenzae* to clarithromycin alone and in combination with its 14-hydroxy metabolite. Eur J Clin Microbiol Infect Dis 1991; 10:1080–1081.

2. Barry AL, Fuchs PC, Pfaller MA. Susceptibility of β-lactamase-producing and -nonproducing ampicillin-resistant strains of *Haemophilus influenzae* to ceftibuten, cefaclor, cefuroxime, cefixime, cefotaxime and amoxicillin–clavulanic acid. Antimicrob Agents Chemother 1993; 37:14–18.

3. Collignon PJ, Bell JM, MacInnes SJ, Gilbert GL, Toohey M, the Australian Group for Antimicrobial Resistance (AGAR). A national collaborative study of resistance to antimicrobial agents in *Haemophilus influenzae* in Australian hospitals. J Antimicrob Chemother 1992; 30:153–163.

4. Hardy DJ, Hensey DM, Beyer JM, Vojtko C, McDonald ET, Fernandes PB. Comparative activity of 14-, 15- and 16-membered macrolides. Antimicrob Agents Chemother 1988; 32:1710–1719.

5. Jorgensen JH, Doern GV, Maher LA, Howell AW, Redding JS. Antimicrobial resistance among respiratory isolates of *Haemophilus influenzae*, *Moraxella catarrhalis* and *Streptococcus pneumoniae* in the United States. Antimicrob Agents Chemother 1990; 34:2075–2080.

6. Kayser FH, Morenzoni G, Santanam P. The second European collaborative study on the frequency of antimicrobial resistance in *Haemophilus influenzae*. Eur J Clin Microbiol Infect Dis 1990; 9:810–817.

7. Linares J, Alonso T, Perez JL, Ayats J, Dominquez MA, Pallares R, Martin R. Decreased susceptibility of penicillin-resistant pneumococci to twenty-four β-lactam antibiotics. J Antimicrob Chemother 1992; 30:279–288.

8. Mason EO, Kaplan SL, Lamberth LB, Tillman J. Increased rate of isolation of penicillin-resistant *Streptococcus pneumoniae* in a children's hospital and in vitro susceptibilities to antibiotics of potential therapeutic use. Antimicrob Agents Chemother 1992; 36:1703–1707.

9. National Committee for Clinical Laboratory Standards. Methods for dilution antimicrobial susceptibility tests for bacteria that grow aerobically. Approved standard M7-A3, NCCLS, Villanova, PA, 1993.

10. Powell M, McVey D, Kassim MH, Chen HY, Williams JO. Antimicrobial susceptibility of *Streptococcus pneumoniae*, *Haemophilus*, and *Moraxella* (*Branhamella*) *catarrhalis*, isolated in the U.K. from sputa. J Antimicrob Chemother 1991; 28:249–259.

The In Vitro Activity of Clarithromycin Alone and in Combination with 14(*R*)-Hydroxy Metabolite Against *Haemophilus influenzae* Isolated in 1993 in New York City

N. X. Chin, P. Della-Latta, S. Whittier, and Harold C. Neu

Columbia University
New York, New York

INTRODUCTION

There is concern about the use of macrolides to treat infections caused by *Haemophilus influenzae*. Clarithromycin, a 6-*O*-methylerythromycin, has shown excellent activity against the common respiratory pathogens. The in vitro activity of clarithromycin against *Streptococcus pyogenes* and *S. pneumoniae* was equal to or twice as active as that of erythromycin, similar to that of ampicillin, and superior to those of cefcalor and doxycycline (1,2). However, clarithromycin is more active than erythromycin against *Haemophilus influenzae* in in vitro and in animal studies when combined with its human metabolite, 14-hydroxyclarithromycin (4). Clarithromycin has a better pharmacokinetic profile than erythromycin, owing to its gastric acid stability and excellent tissue distribution, especially in the lung (3). Several clinical trials have demonstrated that clarithromycin has good clinical efficacy with less frequent dosage compared with erythromycin in treating patients with upper and lower respiratory tract infections. Recent studies have shown that clarithromycin may be a useful drug to treat atypical mycobacterial infections. We determined the in vitro activity of clarithromycin alone and in combination with 14-hydroxyclarithromycin against 115 isolates of *H. influenzae*. The activity of clarithromycin–14-hydroxyclarithromycin was compared with that of erythromycin and ampicillin.

In addition, the effects of the medium on the MICs of antimicrobial agents against *H. influenzae* were also studied.

MATERIALS AND METHODS

Antibiotics

Clarithromycin, 14-hydroxyclarithromycin, and erythromycin were provided by Abbott Laboratories, Chicago, Illinois. Ampicillin was purchased from Sigma Chemical Co.

Bacteria

Clinical isolates were collected between January and November 1993 from patients seen at the Columbia–Presbyterian Medical Center in New York City, a 1500 bed facility hospital. All 115 isolates of *H. influenzae* were cultured from sputum.

Susceptibility Testing

The MICs were determined by the agar dilution method using a 10^4 CFU/ml inoculum, according to M7-A2 NCCLS. The MICs for *H. influenzae* were tested on both haemophilus test medium agar (HTM) and 2% hemoglobin GC chocolate agar (HbC). The combination of clarithromycin and 14-OH-clarithromycin was at a ratio of 3:1, which corresponds to serum concentrations in humans. All plates were incubated in ambient air at 35°C for 20–24 h.

RESULTS AND DISCUSSION

The MICs and cummulative percentage for clarithromycin, 14-OH-clarithromycin alone and in combination compared with other antimicrobial agents against *H. influenzae* are shown in Tables 1 and 2. Clarithromycin alone against *H.*

Table 1 MICs of Clarithromycin–14-Hydroxyclarithromycin (Cl/14OH) for clinical isolates of *H. influenzae* in 1993 Upper New York City

Medium	Cumulative number (%) of isolates at concentration (µg/ml) of						
	0.19/0.06	0.38/0.13	0.75/0.25	1.5/0.5	3/1	6/2	≥12/4
HTM	1 (0.8)	2 (1.7)	6 (5,2)	24 (20.9)	83 (72.2)	111 (96.5)	115 (100)
HbC			3 (2.6)	13 (11.3)	56 (48.7)	101 (87.8)	115 (10)

Table 2 MICs of Clarithromycin (Cl), 14-Hydroxyclarithromycin (14OH), Erythromycin (Ery), and Ampicillin (Amp) Against 115 Isolates of *H. influenzae* in HTM Agar and Hb Chocolate (HbC) Agar

Organism (no. tested)	Medium	Cumulative no. (%) of isolates inhibited at concentration (μg/ml) of								
		0.12	0.25	0.5	1	2	4	8	16	$\geq$32
Cl	HTM					8	33	96	114	115
						(7)	(28.7)	(83.5)	(99.1)	(100)
	HbC					2	23	75	107	115
						(1.5)	(20)	(65.2)	(93)	(100)
14OH	HTM			4	17	74	110	115		
				(3.5)	(14.8)	(64.3)	(95.6)	(100)		
	HbC		1	6	17	70	104	114	115	
			(0.8)	(5.2)	(14.8)	(60.9)	(90.4)	(99.1)	(100)	
Ery	HTM				6	22	78	113	115	
					(5.2)	(19.1)	(67.8)	(98.3)	(100)	
	HbC				2	16	62	99	113	115
					(1.7)	(13.9)	(53.9)	(86.1)	(98.3)	(100)
Amp[a]	HTM	21	73	87	88		93	101	108	115
		(18.3)	(63.5)	(75.6)	(76.5)		(80.9)	(87.8)	(93.9)	(100)
	HbC	1	11	73	84	88		90	94	115
		(0.8)	(9.6)	(63.5)	(73)	(76.5)		(78.2)	(81.7)	(115)

[a]The incidence of ampicillin-resistant isolates of *H. influenzae* (23.5%) was defined as MIC $\geq$2 μg/ml on HTM agar medium. Of 27 Amp-R, β-lac+ strains, 6 were inhibited by $\geq$6:2 μg/ml of Cl/14OH, compared with 26 strains out of 88 (29.5%)Amp-S, β-lac(–) strains ($p > 0.05$).

Table 3 The Effect of HTM and HbC Medium on the MICs of Clarithromycin (Cl), 14-Hydroxyclarithromycin (14OH), Clarithromycin/14-Hydroxyclarithromycin (Cl/14OH), and Erythromycin (Ery) Against *H. influenzae*

		MIC (μg/ml)				
Organism[a]	Medium	Amp	Cl/14OH	Ery	Cl	14OH
H. influenzae						
B-3276	HTM	0.5	3:1	4	4	2
	HbC	2	3:1	4	8	4
B-3280	HTM	0.5	6:2	4	8	2
	HbC	2	3:1	4	4	4
B-3217	HTM	0.5	0.75:0.25	4	8	1
	HbC	2	6:2	4	8	4
B-3218	HTM	0.5	1.5:0.5	2	4	0.5
	HbC	2	1.5:0.5	8	8	2

[a]The MIC of ampicillin and the β-lactamase production were repeated three times. β-Lactamase was absent using nitrocefin.

influenzae was twofold less active than erythromycin. When combined with 14-hydroxyclarithromycin, a significant increase in activity was observed: 72.2% of the *H. influenzae* isolates were inhibited by 3:1 μg/ml of Cl/14OH, compared with 67.8% by 4 μg/ml of erythromycin. Furthermore, the activity of clarithromycin was unaffected by the production of β-lactamase. Of 115 strains tested, 27 (23.5%) were ampicillin-resistant and β-lactamase–positive (25 nontypeable, 1b,1e); 21 (77.8%) of the 27 β-lactamase–positive and 62 (70.1%) of the 88 β-lactamase–negative isolates were inhibited by 3:1 μg/ml of Cl/14OH ($p > 0.05$). In general, the MICs in HTM were two- and fourfold lower than MICs obtained in HbC. As a result, 72.2% strains were inhibited by 3:1 μg/ml of Cl/14OH in HTM, whereas only 48.7% were inhibited in the chocolate medium. In addition, the ampicillin-resistance rate in HTM was 23.5% and was 27% in chocolate agar. This correlates with our previous report (abstract no. 468, 33th ICAAC). Table 3 shows that four β-lactamase–negative strains of *H. influenzae* were resistant to ampicillin on chocolate agar, with MICs of 2 μg/ml, but they were susceptible in HTM with an MIC of 0.5 μg/ml. The same discrepancy was found for other agents. In summary, this study demonstrated the in vitro activity of clarithromycin in the presence of 14-OH-clarithromycin is excellent against *H. influenzae*. Most strains of *H. influenzae* are inhibited by the 3:1 Cl/14OH combination, which is an achievable level in humans (6). In addition, clarithromycin provides a longer postantibiotic effect than erythromycin and favorable pharmacokinetics: that is, acid stability, longer half-life, and high levels in the lung (17.4 + 3.29 μg/ml; 5). Recently, we showed that clarithromycin was as effective as cefixime in the treatment of bronchitis (7). It is clear from this study that clarithromycin is an appropriate agent to treat suggested *H. influenzae* infection of the lung, bronchi, or sinus. Why we consistently have lower MICs in HTM medium is unclear, since only two strains of *H. influenzae* failed to grow in this medium.

REFERENCES

1. Chin NX, Neu NM, Labthavikul P, Saha G, Neu HC. Activity of A-56268 compared with that of erythromycin and other oral agents against aerobic and anaerobic bacteria. Antimicrob Agents Chemother 1987; 31:463–466.
2. Neu HC. The development of macrolides: clarithromycin in perspective. J Antimicrob Chemother 1991; 27(suppl A):1–9.
3. Chu SY, Wilson DS, Guay D, Craft C. Clarithromycin pharmacokinetics in healthy young and elderly volunteers. J Clin Pharmacol 1992; 32:1045–1049.
4. Hardy DJ, Swanson RN, Rode RA, Shipkositx NL, Clement JJ. Enhancement of the in vitro and in vivo activities of clarithromycin against *Haemophilus influenzae* by 14-hydroxy-clarithromycin, its major metabolite in humans. Antimicrob Agents Chemther 1990; 34:1407–1413.
5. Sorgel F, Kinzig M, Naber KG. Physiology disposition of macrolides. In: Bryskier A, Butzler JP, Neu HC, Tulkens PM, eds. Macrolides, Chemistry, Pharmacology and Clinical Uses. Paris: Arnette-Blackwill, 1993:421–435.
6. Gu GW, Scully BE, Neu HC. Bactericidal activity of clarithromycin and its 14-hydroxy metabolite against *Haemophilus influenzae* and streptococcal pathogens. J Clin Pharmacol 1991; 31:1146–1150.
7. Neu HC, Chick TW. Efficacy and safety of clarithromycin compared to cefixime as treatment of outpatient lower respiratory tract infections. Chest 1993; 104:1393–1399.

New and "Unusual" Antimicrobial Properties of Clarithromycin

S. K. Tanaka

Abbott Laboratories
Abbott Park, Illinois

R. N. Jones and P. Lartey

University of Iowa College of Medicine
Iowa City, Iowa

INTRODUCTION

Clinical experience with clarithromycin has clearly established its usefulness in the treatment of respiratory diseases and skin or skin structure diseases caused by the most common organisms, including *Streptococcus pneumoniae*, *S. pyogenes*, *Haemophilus influenzae*, *Moraxella catarrhalis*, *Mycoplasma pneumoniae*, and *Staphylococcus aureus*. The efficacy of clarithromycin in diseases caused by these organisms was predicted by in vitro activity and efficacy in animal models. Although clinical data are lacking or still being investigated for many other pathogens, in vitro and in vivo data reported in the literature suggest that clarithromycin may have utility in infections caused by many other organisms.

The in vivo and clinical activity of clarithromycin may also reflect the activity contribution of the major bioactive metabolite of clarithromycin: 14-OH-clarithromycin. This compound is generated by metabolism of clarithromycin by the liver and is present in humans, but is not generated by many animal species. Although less active in vitro against some gram-positive organisms, 14-OH clarithromycin is substantially active against *H. influenzae* and may contribute to the clinical efficacy of clarithromycin in infections caused by this pathogen.

MATERIALS AND METHODS

A variety of methods have been employed for in vitro and in vivo experiments. Standardization of in vitro susceptibility methods has been only recently established by the National Committee for Clinical Laboratory Standards

(NCCLS) for clarithromycin against the more routine bacterial pathogens. These standards are based on reproducibility of methods, standardization of procedures, and predictability of clinical outcome. Standards for testing of many nonroutine pathogens, particularly those with complex in vitro growth requirements, have not yet been established as predictable indicators of clinical outcome.

The in vitro activity of clarithromycin is affected by testing conditions, particularly the pH of the testing medium. As with all macrolides, this effect is generally not a reflection of chemical structure stability, but rather, the ionization at acidic pH. This ionization apparently reduces the permeability of macrolides through the cytoplasmic membranes of bacteria. This effect is particularly apparent against organisms in which growth (and, therefore, testing) requires increased concentrations of CO_2 in the incubation atmosphere. In many instances this accounts for variations in reported in vitro activity of clarithromycin.

Classic macrolide resistance (MLS) is apparent in some species. This resistance often is overrepresented in test populations resulting in high $MIC_{90}s$. The $MIC_{50}s$ generally indicate the intrinsic susceptibility of the species (Tables 1–8).

Table 1 In Vitro Activity of Clarithromycin Against Gram-Positive Human Pathogens

| | Reported ranges of (μg/ml) | | |
Organism	MIC_{50}	MIC_{90}	Ref.
Staphylococcus aureus (Ery S)	0.1–0.2	0.1–0.5	cgjk
S. aureus (Ery R)	>100	>128	cjk
S. aureus (MRSA)	8.0–>128	>32–>128	defgj
S. epidermidis	0.06–>64	0.2–>128	fg
Streptococcus pyogenes	≤0.06–0.25	≤0.06–2.0	bcefgjk
S. pneumoniae	≤0.06–0.25	≤0.06–>64	cefgjk
S. agalactiae	≤0.06–0.12	≤0.06–0.25	cefgjk
Viridans group streptococci	≤0.06–0.5	≤0.06–>64	efgjk
Group C streptococci	0.05–0.12	0.05–0.25	ah
Group G streptococci	0.12	0.25–4.0	ah
Listeria monocytogenes	0.06–0.25	0.06–2.0	defij
Corynebacterium spp.	0.12–1.0	0.25–32	dfi

[a]Barry AL, et al. Antimicrob Agents Chemother 1987; 31:343–345
[b]Barry AL. Eur J Clin Microbiol Infect Dis 1992; 11:867–869
[c]Benson C. Antimicrob Agents Chemother 1987; 31:328–330
[d]Benson C, et al. Eur J Clin Microbiol 1987; 6:173–178
[e]Chin NX, et al. Antimicrob Agents Chemother 1987; 31:463–466
[f]Eliopoulos GM, et al. J Antimicrob Chemother 1987; 20:671–675
[g]Fass RJ. Antimicrob Agents Chemother 1993; 37:2080–2086
[h]Floyd-Reising, S. et al. Antimicrob Agents Chemother 1987; 31:640–642
[i]Hardy DJ, et al. Antimicrob Agents Chemother 1988; 32:1710–1719
[j]Loza E, et al. Eur J Clin Microbiol Infect Dis 1992; 11:856–866
[k]Sefton AM, et al. Eur J Clin Microbiol Infect Dis 1988; 7:798–802

Table 2 In Vitro Activity of Clarithromycin Against Gram-Negative Human Pathogens

| | Reported ranges of (μg/ml) | | |
Organism	MIC$_{50}$	MIC$_{90}$	Ref.
Haemophilus influenzae	1.0–8.0	2.0–16	acdefghil
Moraxella catarrhalis	≤0.06–0.12	≤0.06–1.0	bcefil
Legionella spp.	≤0.06–0.25	≤0.06–0.5	ghijkl
Neisseria gonorrhoeae	≤0.1–2.0	0.1–2.0	bdehi

[a]Barry AL, et al. Antimicrob Agents Chemother 1988; 32:752–754.
[b]Barry AL, et al. Antimicrob Agents Chemother 1987; 31:343–345.
[c]Barry AL. Eur J Clin Microbiol Infect Dis 1992; 11:867–869.
[d]Benson C, et al. Eur J Clin Microbiol 1987; 6:173–178.
[e]Chin NX, et al. Antimicrob Agents Chemother 1987; 31:463–466.
[f]Fass RJ. Antimicrob Agents Chemother 1993; 37:2080–2086.
[g]Fernandes PB et al. Antimicrob. Agents Chemother 1986; 30:865–873.
[h]Floyd-Reising S, et al. Antimicrob. Agents Chemother 1987; 31:640–642.
[i]Hardy DJ, et al. Antimicrob Agents Chemother 1988; 32:1710–1719.
[j]Johnson DM, et al. Eur J Clin Microbiol Infect Dis 1992; 11:751–754.
[k]Jones RN, Barry AL. J Antimicrob. Chemother 1987; 19:841–842.
[l]Loza E, et al. Eur. J Clin Microbiol Infect Dis 1992; 11:856–866.

Table 3 In Vitro Activity of Clarithromycin Against Atypical Human Pathogens

| | Reported ranges of (μg/ml) | | |
Organism	MIC$_{50}$	MIC$_{90}$	Ref.
Mycoplasma pneumoniae	≤0.004–0.05	0.02–0.05	hj
M. hominis	32–>256	64–>256	hj
Ureaplasma urealyticum	0.05–0.2	0.1–>256	fhj
Chlamydia pneumoniae	—	0.03	cdgi
C. trachomatis	—	0.008–0.12	abe

[a]Benson C, et al. Eur J Clin Microbiol 1987; 6:173–178.
[b]Bowie W, et al. Antimicrob Agents Chemother 1987; 31:470–472.
[c]Fenelon LE, et al. J Antimicrob Chemother 1990; 26:763–767.
[d]Hammerschlag MR, et al. Antimicrob Agents Chemother 1992; 36:1573–1574.
[e]Lefevre JC, et al. Pathol Biol 1993; 41:313–315.
[f]Loza E, et al. Eur J Clin Microbiol Infect Dis 1992; 11:856–866.
[g]Qumei M, et al. 1st Intern Conf Macrolides, Azalides, Streptogramins. 1992: abstr 147.
[h]Renaudin H, Bebear C. Eur J Clin Microbiol Infect Dis 1990; 9:838–841.
[i]Segreti J, et al. 1st Intern Conf Macrolides, Azalides, Streptogramins. 1992: abstr 148.
[j]Waites KB, et al. Antimicrob Agents Chemother 1988; 32:1500–1502.

Table 4 In Vitro Activity of Clarithromycin Against *Mycobacterium* spp.

Organism	Reported ranges of (μg/ml)		
	MIC range	MIC_{90}	Ref.
Mycobacterium tuberculosis	1.3->10	>10	ae
M. *avium-intracellulare*	≤0.1->8.0	≤0.25->8.0	bcdhi
M. *fortuitum*	≤0.06-4.0	0.5-32	bg
M. *chelonae*	≤0.06-1.0	0.12-2.0	bg
M. *kansasii*	—	0.25-1.0	ac
M. *paratuberculosis*	0.25-0.5	—	j
M. *leprae*	12.5-50 mg/kg/d		f

[a]Berlin OGW, et al. Eur J Clin Microbiol 1987; 6:486-487.
[b]Brown B, et al. Antimicrob Agents Chemother 1992; 36:180-184.
[c]Brown B, et al. Antimicrob Agents Chemother 1992; 36:1987-1990.
[d]Fernandes PB, et al. Antimicrob Agents Chemother 1989; 33:1531-1534.
[e]Gorzynski EA, et al. Antimicrob Agents Chemother 1989; 33:591-592.
[f]Ji B, et al. Antimicrob Agents Chemother 1991; 35:579-581.
[g]Loza E, et al. Eur J Clin Microbiol Infect Dis 1992; 11:856-866.
[h]Naik S, Ruck R. Antimicrob Agents Chemother 1989; 33:1614-1616.
[i]Rastogi N, LaBrousse V, Antimicrob Agents Chemother 1991; 35:462-470.
[j]Rastogi N, et al. Antimicrob Agents Chemother 1992; 36:2843-2846.

Table 5 In Vitro Activity of Clarithromycin Against Anaerobic Human Pathogens

Organism	Reported ranges of (μg/ml)		
	MIC_{50}	MIC_{90}	Ref.
Bacteroides fragilis group	1.0-4.0	2.0->64	abcdefg
Fusobacterium spp.	0.12->8.0	2.0->256	bdfg
Prevotella spp.	0.5	4.0	d
Clostridium spp.	0.25-2.0	0.4->256	abdfg
Peptostreptococcus spp.	0.06-2.0	0.25->256	cdf
Proprionibacterium spp.	≤0.06	0.03-0.25	b

[a]Barry AL, et al. Antimicrob Agents Chemother 1987; 31:343-345.
[b]Chin NX, et al. Antimicrob Agents Chemother 1987; 31:463-466.
[c]Eliopoulos GM, et al. J Antimicrob Chemother 1987; 20:671-675.
[d]Fass RJ, Antimicrob Agents Chemother 1993; 37:2080-2086.
[e]Hardy DJ, et al. Antimicrob Agents Chemother 1988; 32:1710-1719.
[f]Hodinka RL, et al. Eur J Clin Microbiol 1987; 6:103-108.
[g]Wexler HM, Finegold S. Eur J Clin Microbiol 1987; 6:492-494.

Table 6 In Vitro Activity of Clarithromycin Against Newly Recognized Pathogens

| Organism | Reported ranges of (μg/ml) | | Ref. |
	MIC$_{50}$	MIC$_{90}$	
Helicobacter pylori	0.015–0.03	0.015–0.03	bd
Borrelia burgdorferi	0.007–≤0.03	0.015–≤0.03	ac

[a]Dever LL, et al. Antimicrob Agents Chemother 1993; 37:1704–1706.
[b]Hardy DJ, et al. J Antimicrob Chemother 1988; 22:631–636.
[c]Levin JM, et al. Antimicrob Agents Chemother 1993; 37:1444–1446.
[d]Malanoski GJ, et al. Eur J Microbiol Infect Dis 1993; 12:131–133.

Table 7 In Vitro/In Vivo Activity of Clarithromycin Against Eukaryotic Pathogens

Organism	Effective dose	Ref.
Toxoplasma gondii	300 mg/kg/d	bc
Plasmodium falciparum	60–100 μg/ml in vitro	
	75 mg/kg/d (*P. berghi*)	f
Pneumocystis carinii	50 mg/kg/d+sulfamethoxazole	ad
Giardia lamblia	0.5–100 μg/ml in vitro	e

[a]Alder J, et al. 1st Intern. Conf. Macrolides, Azalides, Streptogramins. 1992: abstr 179.
[b]Araujo FG, et al. Antimicrob Agents Chemother 1992; 36:2454–2457.
[c]Chang HR, et al. J. Antimicrob Chemother 1988; 22:359–361.
[d]Hughes WT, Kilmer JT. 1st Intern. Conf. Macrolides, Azalides, Streptogramins. 1992: abstr 179, 180.
[e]Ikerd TR, Koletar SL. J. Antimicrob Chemother 1993; 31:615–617.
[f]Torres J, et al. 33rd Intersci Confer Antimicrob Agents Chemother 1993: abstr 754.

Table 8 In Vitro Activity of 14-OH-Clarithromycin Against Various Organisms

Organism	Reported ranges of (μg/ml)		
	MIC_{50} 14-OH	MIC_{50} Clari	Ref.
Staphylococcus aureus (MSSA)	0.12	0.06–0.12	ad
S. aureus (MRSA)	>128	>128	a
Steptococcus pneumoniae	≤0.015–0.12	≤0.015–0.12	acd
S. pyogenes	0.012–0.03	≤0.015–0.06	acd
S. agalactiae	0.06	0.06–0.12	ad
Haemophilus influenzae	1.0–2.0	1.0–4.0	ac
Legionella spp.	0.25	0.12	a
Moraxella catarrhalis	0.03–0.06	0.03–0.06	ac
Helicobacter pylori	0.06	0.03	b

[a]Hardy DJ, et al. Antimicrob Agents Chemother 1988; 32:1710–1719.
[b]Hardy DJ, et al. J Antimicrob Chemother 1988; 22:631–636.
[c]Hoover WW, et al. Diag Microbiol Infect Dis 1992; 15:259–266.
[d]Logan MN, et al. J Antimicrob Chemother 1991; 27:161–170.

CONCLUSIONS

1. Clarithromycin is highly active in vitro against a wide variety of gram-positive bacteria, including *S. aureus* (excluding MRSA), and the *Streptococcus* spp. (see Table 1). Macrolide resistance is apparent in some organism collections and tends to mask the intrinsic susceptibility of these species (MIC_{50} vs. MIC_{90}).

2. Clarithromycin is active in vitro against several common gram-negative pathogens (typical and atypical) including *H. influenzae*, *M. catarrhalis*, *Legionella* spp., and *Chlamydia* spp. (see Tables 2 and 3). In addition, clarithromycin is active against *M. pneumoniae* and *N. gonorrhoeae*.

3. Clarithromycin is active in vitro against gram-negative and gram-positive anaerobes, although not uniformly for the population. Many *B. fragilis* group and the gram-positive anaerobes appear sensitive (see Table 5).

4. Clarithromycin is active in vitro against the nontuberculosis *Mycobacterium* spp. (see Table 4). In vitro and in vivo efficacy has been demonstrated for *M. avium–intracellulare*, *M. leprae*, and other *Mycobacterium* spp.

5. Clarithromycin has exhibited in vitro activity against *H. pylori* and *B. burgdorferi* (see Table 6).

6. The 14-OH metabolite of clarithromycin is slightly more active than clarithromycin against *H. influenzae* and slightly less active against other bacterial pathogens (see Table 8).

7. Clarithromycin exhibits activity against the eukaryotic parasites, *T. gondii*, *P. carinii*, *P. falciparum*, and *G. lamblia* (see Table 7). The basis for this activity is as yet unknown.

Bacteriostatic and Bactericidal Activity of Roxithromycin Against *Haemophilus influenzae* Isolated from Infants and Adults with Respiratory Tract Infections

G. Tome, M. Goldberg, M. Jugo, E. M. D'Andrea, Y. Farinati, and J. M. Casellas

Universidad Catolica Argentina
Buenos Aires, Argentina

INTRODUCTION

Roxithromycin is one of a new generation of orally active macrolides, with improved pharmacokinetic characteristics and excellent bioavailability. Activity of roxithromycin against *Streptococcus pneumoniae* and *Branhamella catarrhalis* has been demonstrated (1). However, its activity against *Haemophilus influenzae* strains is controversial, raising questions about the usefulness of this compound for the empirical treatment of acute sinusitis and exacerbations of chronic bronchitis. A study was initiated to determine the bacteriostatic and bactericidal activity of roxithromycin against *H. influenzae* isolated from outpatients or inpatients at the Sanatorio San Lucas, in Argentina, who had respiratory tract or otorhinolaryngeal infections.

PATIENTS AND METHODS

Patients aged 2 months to 66 years were admitted to the study. Fifty consecutive *H. influenzae* strains were isolated from patients with otitis media (14), acute sinusitis (3), acute exacerbations of chronic bronchitis (24), and community-acquired pneumonia (9). The strains were identified according to Killian (2) and serotyped when possible with Difco antisera.

Minimum inhibitory concentrations were determined by broth macrodilution tests performed in HTM broth. A final inoculum of 5×10^5 cfu/ml was used. The range of antibiotic dilutions was 0.015–64 μg/ml. Tubes were incubated for 20–24 h at 35°C. *Staphylococcus aureus* ATCC 29213 and *H. influenzae* ATCC 49247 were used as controls for MIC, and *H. influenzae* ATCC 10211 as a quality control test strain of HTM medium.

Determination of MBCs on 15 strains was performed on aliquots of 0.01 ml from clear tubes, subcultured into chocolate agar plates supplemented with Polyvitex, incubated in 5% CO_2 atmosphere for 20–24 h. The MBC on 15 strains was defined as a 99.9% reduction in colony-forming units (CFU) compared with the original culture.

Five strains were selected for estimation of time-kill curves with roxithromycin. Concentrations of roxithromycin equivalent to the MIC and to twice the MIC were tested in 20-ml volumes of HTM broth using an inoculum of 5×10^5 to 2×10^{16} CFU/ml. Aliquots of the antibiotic-containing and antibiotic-free control broths were removed initially and after 4, 8, and 24 h of incubation at 35°C, and quantitative plate counts were made in supplemented chocolate agar incubated in 5% CO_2. The lack of a significant antibiotic carryover effect was demonstrated by comparing plate counts of the strains at inocula of approximately 10^2 to 10^3 CFU/ml in antibiotic-free broth and in broth containing the antibiotic concentrations used for the kinetic time-kill studies (4).

All strains were tested for β-lactamase production by the nitrocefinase method.

RESULTS

The distribution of MICs and MBCs for the 50 strains included in the study is shown in Table 1. The range of MICs was $\leq$0.016–16 μg/ml and of MBCs 0.06–64 μg/ml, an MBC/MIC ratio of 1:4. The MBC/MIC relation for 90% of the strains is 2 (MBC_{90}:16/MIC_{90}:8), which is characteristic of bactericidal activity.

Table 1 Distribution of MICs and MBCs for the 50 Strains Tested

	Concentration of roxithromycin (μg/ml)												
	<0.015	0.03	0.06	0.12	0.25	0.5	1	2	4	8	16	32	64
MIC	2	2	3	3	3	2	6	8	15	4	2	0	0
MBC	0	0	2	1	5	3	3	3	9	10	10	3	1

The percent of strains susceptible to roxithromycin at concentrations of 4 μg/ml was 88% and at 8 μg/ml it was 96%.

Against the 12 β-lactamase-producing strains, roxithromycin MICs of $\leq$0.015–2 μg/ml were demonstrated against seven strains and MICs of 4–64 μg/ml were demonstrated against five strains.

Results of the time-killing curve studies with roxithromycin against five strains are shown in Table 2. At 2 × MIC, at 8 h, there was a reduction of the inoculum of 3 log^{10} for four strains and of 2 log^{10} for one strain.

CONCLUSIONS

In adults after a single oral dose of 150 mg roxithromycin, serum levels are 6.6 μg/ml at 1.5 h and average 4 μg/ml at 7 h. Levels in bronchial secretions are 6.2 μg/ml at 4 h after dosing, and in maxillary sinus secretions levels of 4.1 μg/ml are achieved at 4 h (5). Consequently this dosage is probably useful for the treatment of *H. influenzae* infections.

In adults, roxithromycin peak serum levels after a single oral dose of 300 mg have been shown to range from 9.1 to 10.8 μg/ml (6,7). Values are sustained over 4 μg/ml until 14 h after administration of the drug. Bronchial secretion and maxillary sinus secretion levels represent 96% and 60% of the serum level, respectively.

Those data suggest that at an MIC of 4 μg/ml roxithromycin should eradicate strains of *H. influenzae* in cases of acute sinusitis and exacerbations of chronic bronchitis.

Erwin and Jones (8) recently suggested that the roxithromycin MIC breakpoint against *H. influenzae* should be changed to $\geq$16 μg/ml to ensure reproducibility with in vivo results. With this breakpoint, 100% of our strains would show susceptibility to roxithromycin in terms of MICs.

MBCs were not substantially different from MICs in the strains tested. This bactericidal capacity is confirmed by the time-killing curves. Therefore, we can conclude that roxithromycin has bactericidal activity for most of the *H. influenzae* strains included in our study. Similar studies measuring MBC, serum bactericidal titers, and time-killing curves should be conducted to confirm these results.

In view of MIC, MBC, and time-killing curve data, roxithromycin could be recommended in acute sinusitis, exacerbations of chronic bronchitis, and mild respiratory infections due to *H. influenzae* in normoimmune, nonsevere patients.

Our results are in agreement with previous reports of 80% clinical cure rates in the treatment of acute sinusitis and mild respiratory tract infections due to *H. influenzae* in normoimmune outpatients (9,10).

A caution should, however, be noted: In hospitalized, severely ill, or neutropenic patients, knowledge of susceptibility data for *H. influenzae* is

Table 2 Results of Time-Killing Curve Studies with Roxithromycin Against Five Strains of *H. influenzae*

Antibiotic concentration	Range of CFU/ml determined at			
	0 h	4 h	8 h	24 h
Control	$1.4 \times 10^5 - 1.7 \times 10^6$	$7 \times 10^5 - 2.2 \times 10^6$	$1.1 \times 10^6 - 2 \times 10^7$	$1.1 \times 10^7 - 5 \times 10^8$
$1 \times$ MIC		$3 \times 10^4 - 7 \times 10^5$	$8 \times 10^3 - 5 \times 10^5$	$4 \times 10^3 - 2 \times 10^5$
$2 \times$ MIC		$7 \times 10^3 - 4 \times 10^5$	$7 \times 10^2 - 6 \times 10^3$	$<3 \times 10^2 - 3 \times 10^3$

advisable whenever possible and is necessary in any case if the treatment is not followed by rapid improvement.

REFERENCES

1. Casellas JM, Goldberg H, Arduino S, Farinati I, Iribarren MA. Comparative MIC and MBC of roxithromycin, A56286 and erythromycin against 600 clinical isolates. 15th International Congress of Chemotherapy, Istanbul, July 19–24, 1987.

2. Killian M. *Haemophilus*. In: Lennette et al, eds. Manual of Clinical Microbiology. Washington: American Society for Microbiology, 1985.

3. Jorgensen JH, Rodding JS, Mahor HA, Howell AW. Improved medium for antimicrobial susceptibility testing of *H. influenzae*. J Clin Microbiol 1987; 25:2105.

4. Jorgensen JH, Maher MA, Howell AW. Activity of clarithromycin and its principal human metabolite against *H. influenzae*. Antimicrob Agents Chemother 1991; 35:1524.

5. Wilsen OG, Zahlsen K, Svarva P. Macrolide pharmacokinetic and dose scheduling of roxithromycin. Diag Microbiol Infect Dis 1992; 15:715.

6. Boeckh M, Lode H, Hoffken G, Daeschlein S, Koeppe P. Pharmacokinetics of roxithromycin and influence of H_2-blockers and antacids in gastrointestinal absorption. Eur J Clin Microbiol Infect Dis 1992; 11:465.

7. Nilsen OG. Roxithromycin, a new molecule, a new pharmacokinetic profile. Drug Invest 1991; 3(Suppl 3):28–32, 190.

8. Erwin ME, Jones RN. Roxithromycin in vitro testing of *H. influenzae* by NCCLS method. J Antimicrob Chemother 1993; 32:652–654.

9. Stamboulian D, MacLoughlin FGJ, Lancel JL, Sarachian B. Clinical evaluation of roxithromycin in 101 children. Br J Clin Pract 1988; 42:115.

10. Grassi BR, de Rose V, Manara G, Mangiarotti P. Roxithromycin (RU28965) in the treatment of respiratory tract infections. Chemioterapia 1987;6:41.

11. Rimoldi, Mangiarotti P, de Rose V, Nonis A, Bertoletti R. Penetration of roxithromycin into bronchial secretions. Br J Clin Pract 1988; 42:74.

Comparative Antipneumococcal Activity of Penicillin G, RP 59500, Erythromycin, Sparfloxacin, Ciprofloxacin, and Vancomycin by Time–Kill Methodology

G. A. Pankuch and P. C. Appelbaum

Hershey Medical Center
Hershey, Pennsylvania

M. R. Jacobs

Case Western Reserve University
Cleveland, Ohio

INTRODUCTION

The past two decades, and in particular the last few years, have witnessed an alarming increase in *Streptococcus pneumoniae* strains resistant to penicillin, as well as other antimicrobials, all over the world (1,5,7). Pneumococcal suscep-tibility to all classes of macrolides and azalides is similar: a strain resistant to erythromycin will also be resistant to azithromycin, clarithromycin, roxithromycin, and other members of this group; the reverse also obtains (4,9). RP 59500, a new streptogramin (2,4,8,9), is the only member of the macrolide–lincosamide–streptogramin group that is active against both erythromycin-sus-ceptible and erythromycin-resistant strains (irrespective of their penicillin sus-ceptibility status), with MIC$_{90}$ of 1.0 μg/ml and 1.0–2.0 μg/ml, respectively (4,9). Available quinolones, such as ciprofloxacin and ofloxacin, are marginally active against pneumococci (MIC$_{90}$, 2.0–4.0 μg/ml; 3,9). Sparfloxacin is a new fluoroquinolone (3,9) with increased activity against these strains, irrespective of their penicillin susceptibility status (9).

In the current study, we have employed time–kill methodology to examine the susceptibility of eight pneumococcal strains (three penicillin-susceptible, two penicillin–intermediate-resistant, three penicillin-resistant) to penicillin G, RP 59500, erythromycin, ciprofloxacin, sparfloxacin, and vancomycin.

MATERIALS AND METHODS

Eight clinical isolates of *S. pneumoniae* obtained from blood, cerebrospinal fluid, nasopharynx, or sputum were tested. These comprised three penicillin-susceptible (MIC <0.1 μg/ml), two penicillin–intermediate-resistant (MIC 0.1–1.0 μg/ml), and three penicillin-resistant (MIC $\geq$ 2.0 μg/ml) organisms. Antimicrobial agents were obtained from their respective manufacturers. The MICs were determined by the agar dilution method recommended by the National Committee on Clinical Laboratory Standards using Mueller–Hinton agar (BBL Microbiology Systems, Cockeysville, MD), supplemented with 5% sheep blood. For time–kill experiments, glass tubes containing 5 ml cation-adjusted Mueller–Hinton broth (Difco Laboratories, Detroit, MI) plus 5% lysed horse blood (cleared of debris by prior sedimentation at 12,000 g for 20 min), and doubling antibiotic concentrations were inoculated with approximately 5×10^5 CFU/ml (range 1×10^5–1×10^6 CFU/ml) of organisms, and incubated at 35°C in a shaking water bath. Antibiotic concentrations were chosen to comprise three dilutions above and four dilutions below the agar dilution MIC. Bacterial inoculum concentration was calibrated by performing viability counts on broth suspensions (medium as in foregoing) of organisms incubated for 16 h at 35°C in ambient air. Viability counts of antibiotic-containing suspensions were performed at 0, 6, 12, and 24 h, respectively, by plating tenfold dilutions of 0.1-ml aliquots from each tube in Mueller–Hinton broth onto trypticase soy 5% sheep blood agar plates (BBL). Plates were incubated for up to 48 h, and colony counts performed on plates yielding 30–300 colonies. In addition, one penicillin-resistant strain was tested for viable bacteria after 0, 1, 2, and 3 h, respectively. Growth controls, containing organisms but no antibiotic, were included in each run. Antibiotics were considered to be bactericidal if the original inoculum was reduced by $\geq$2 $\log_{10}$ CFU/ml after $\geq$6 h, and bacteriostatic if the original inoculum was reduced by <2 $\log_{10}$ CFU/ml or growth increased by $\leq$1 $\log_{10}$ CFU/ml. Regrowth was defined as an increase $\geq$2 $\log_{10}$ CFU/ml after $\geq$6 h.

RESULTS

Agar dilution MICs of penicillin-susceptible strains were 0.015 μg/ml, those of penicillin–intermediate-resistant strains 0.125–0.25 μg/ml, and those of penicillin-resistant strains 2.0–4.0 μg/ml. All strains were susceptible to RP 59500 (preliminary breakpoint 4.0 μg/ml), with MICs of 0.5–1.0 μg/ml. Erythromycin MICs for penicillin-susceptible, intermediate-resistant and resistant strains were 0.06, 0.06–32, and 8.0–32.0 μg/ml, respectively. Ciprofloxacin MICs ranged between 0.5 and 4.0 μg/ml, and sparfloxacin MICs between 0.125 and 0.25 μg/ml. All strains were susceptible to vancomycin, with MICs $\leq$0.5 μg/ml.

Results of time–kill experiments for one representative penicillin-resistant strain are depicted graphically in Figure 1. Antibiotic concentrations higher than the MIC were bactericidal for each strain, with the exception of erythromycin, which was bactericidal for two resistant strains after 6 and 12 h, respectively, with regrowth after 24 h. One penicillin-susceptible strain was bacteriostatically inhibited by erythromycin at concentrations at or higher than the MIC by 6 h. Erythromycin was bactericidal at concentrations one to threefold less than the MIC for two of three susceptible strains only. Ten minutes after inoculation, a 1–3 $\log_{10}$ reduction (90–99.9%) of the original inoculum was seen with RP 59500 for six of eight strains. This rapid bactericidal effect was seen with RP 59500 concentrations at or greater than the MIC (Table 1). This effect was not found with any of the other compounds tested. A bactericidal effect was found with RP 59500 at 6 and 12 h at concentrations that were 1–2 twofold doubling dilutions below the MIC, with regrowth at 24 h. Regrowth of strains at ciprofloxacin concentrations equal to or one to two dilutions lower than the MIC was found. For sparfloxacin, regrowth, with colony counts equal to 0 h, occurred at the MIC after 24 h with one susceptible and one resistant strain. One susceptible and one resistant strain were bacteriostatically inhibited by this compound. Vancomycin was bactericidal at concentrations higher than the MIC, with regrowth at lower concentrations.

Results of time–kills at 0, 1, 2, and 3 h for one penicillin-resistant strain are depicted graphically in Figure 2. As can be seen, RP 59500, at concentrations one to twofold dilutions lower than the MIC, was bactericidal within 1 h. This phenomenon was not seen with the other antimicrobials tested.

DISCUSSION

Although many reports on the in vitro susceptibility of pneumococci to various agents using MIC techniques have been published, few have studied this problem by time–kill methods. Yourassowsky and co-workers (10) have reported high kill rates for cefdinir and cefaclor against penicillin-susceptible pneumococci. Jacobs et al. (6) have reported a paradoxical increase in viability count compared with the drug-free control for four of the eight strains tested, and of temafloxacin for two of the eight strains. This phenomenon was not observed in our study. Fremaux et al. (4) have reported a 4–5 $\log_{10}$ decrease in colony counts of pneumococci with RP 59500 for erythromycin-susceptible and -resistant strains, at MICs 0.5 to 4.0-fold the MIC. Similarly, we have found excellent bactericidal activity of RP 59500 against all eight strains, irrespective of their erythromycin susceptibility status. An additional feature of the killing effect of RP 59500, was

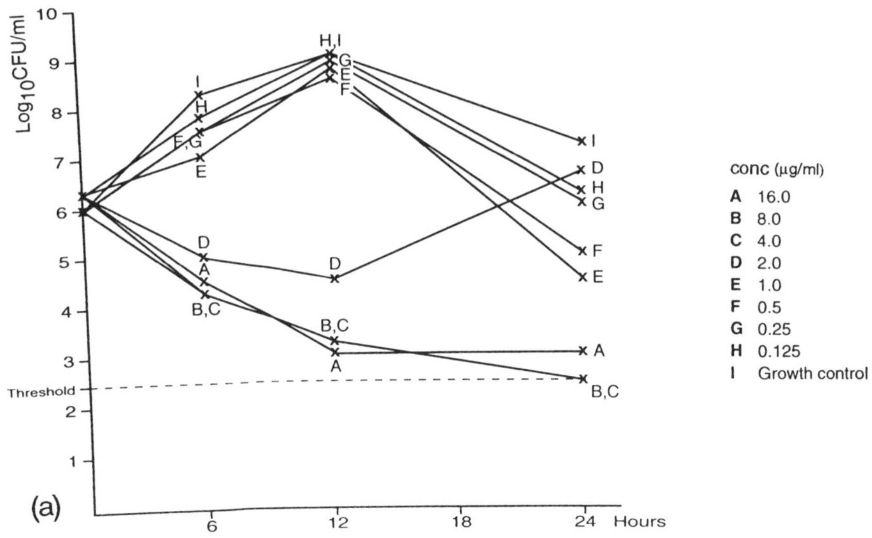

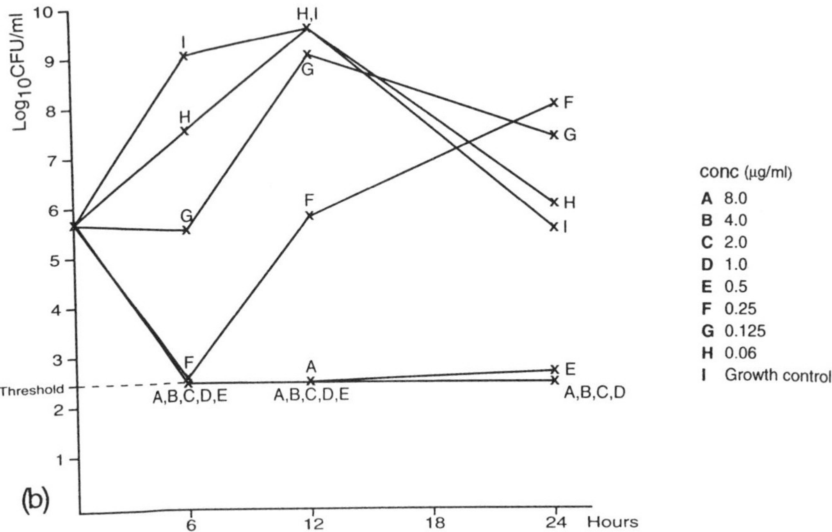

Figure 1 Time–kill experiments at 0, 6, 12, and 24 h for one penicillin-resistant strain: (a) penicillin G pneumo #228(R); (b) RP 59500 pneumo #228(R); (c) erythromycin pneumo #228(R); (d) ciprofloxacin pneumo #228(R); (e) sparfloxacin pneumo #228(R); (f) vancomycin pneumo #228(R).

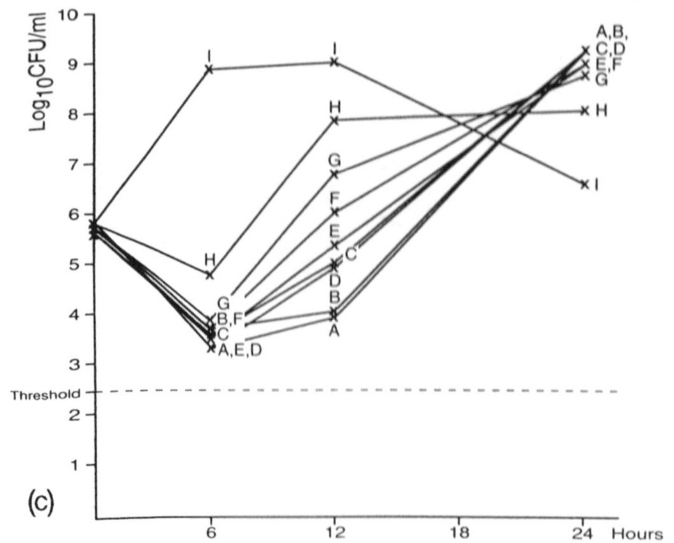
10
9
8
7
6
5
4
3
2
1
Log10CFU/ml
I
I
H
H
G
F
E
C
G
B,F
C
A,E,D
D
B
A
A,B,
C,D
E,F
G
H
I
Threshold
(c)
6
12
18
24
Hours
conc (µg/ml)
A 64.0
B 32.0
C 16.0
D 8.0
E 4.0
F 2.0
G 1.0
H 0.5
I Growth control

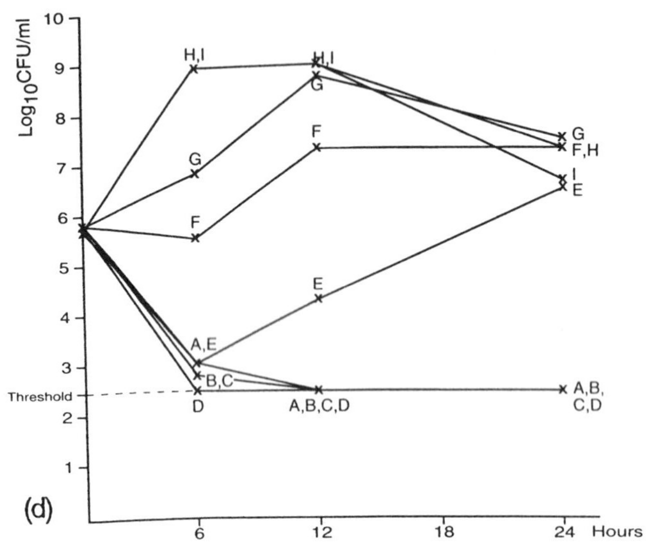
10
9
8
7
6
5
4
3
2
1
Log10CFU/ml
H,I
H,I
G
G
F
F
F
E
E
A,E
B,C
D
A,B,C,D
G
F,H
I
E
A,B,
C,D
Threshold
(d)
6
12
18
24
Hours
conc (µg/ml)
A 4.0
B 32.0
C 16.0
D 8.0
E 2.0
F 1.0
G 0.5
H 0.25
I Growth control

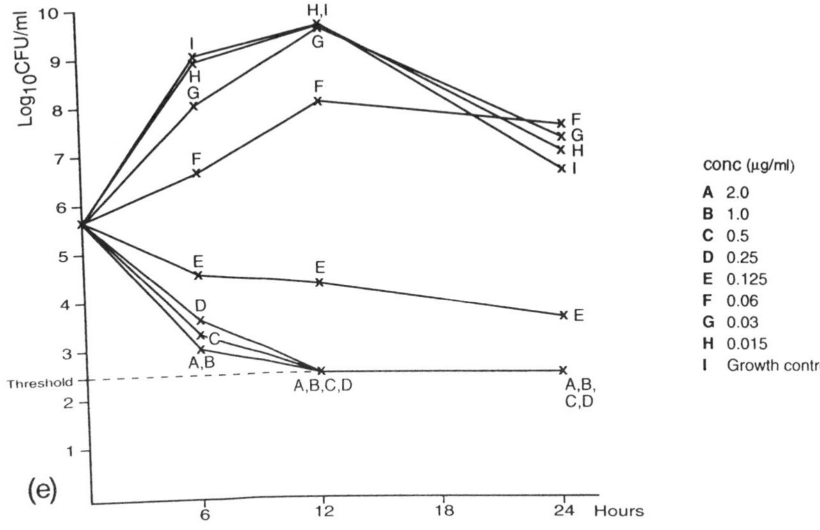
Log10CFU/ml
10
9
8
7
6
5
4
3
2
1
H,I
I
H
G
F
G
F
F
G
H
I
E
E
E
D
C
A,B
A,B,C,D
A,B,
C,D
Threshold
6
12
18
24
Hours
(e)
conc (µg/ml)
A 2.0
B 1.0
C 0.5
D 0.25
E 0.125
F 0.06
G 0.03
H 0.015
I Growth control

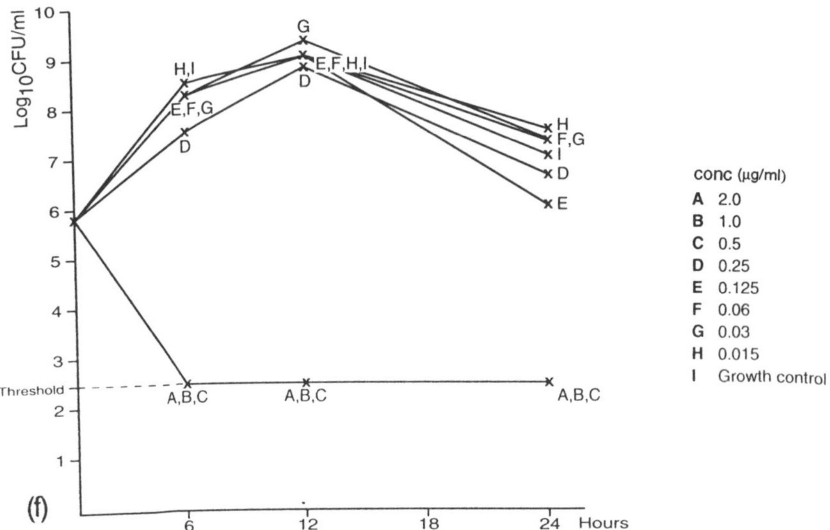
Log10CFU/ml
10
9
8
7
6
5
4
3
2
1
G
E,F,H,I
H,I
D
E,F,G
D
H
F,G
I
D
E
A,B,C
A,B,C
A,B,C
Threshold
6
12
18
24
Hours
(f)
conc (µg/ml)
A 2.0
B 1.0
C 0.5
D 0.25
E 0.125
F 0.06
G 0.03
H 0.015
I Growth control

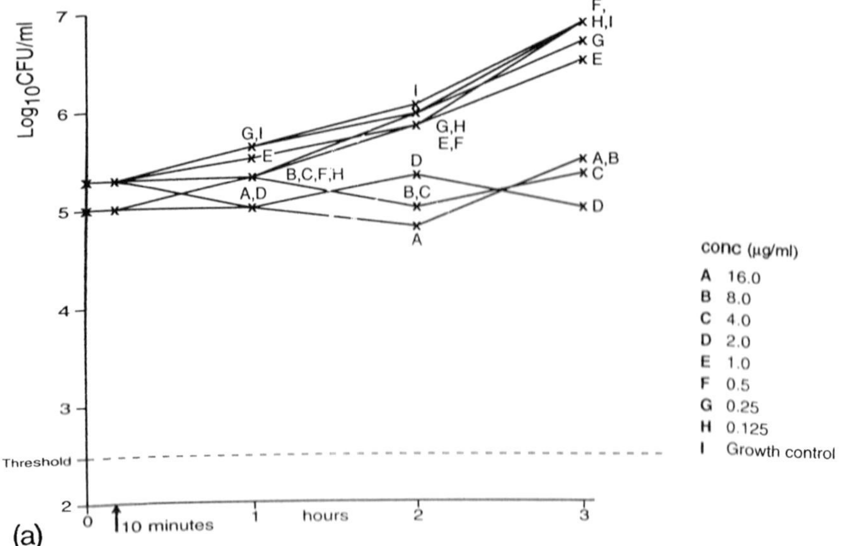

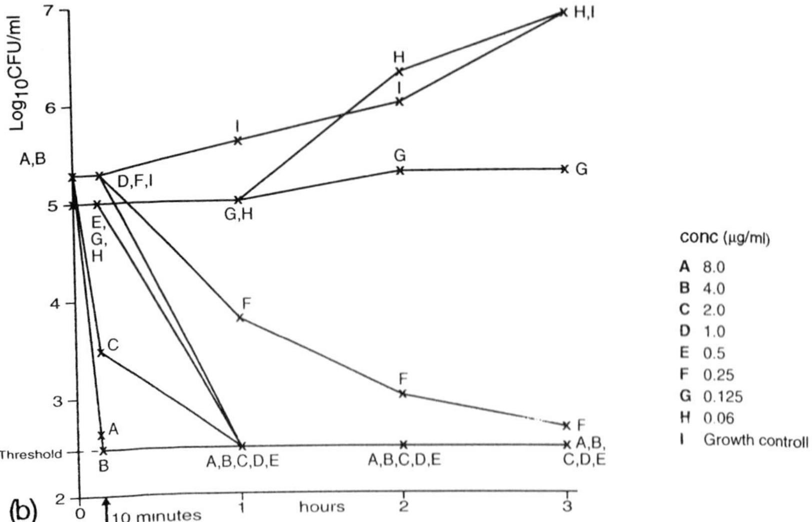

Figure 2 Time–kill experiments at 0, 1, 2, and 3 h for one penicillin-resistant strain: (a) penicillin G pneumo #228(R); (b) RP 59500 pneumo #228(R); (c) erythromycin pneumo #228(R); (d) ciprofloxacin pneumo #228(R); (e) sparfloxacin pneumo #228 (R); (f) vancomycin pneumo #228(R).

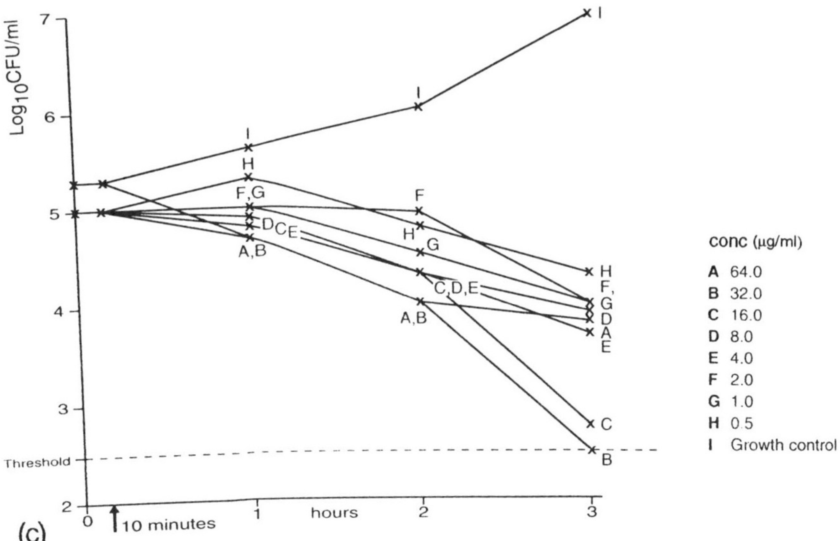
Log10CFU/ml
7
6
5
4
3
2
I
H
F,G
D C E
A,B
F
H
G
C,D,E
A,B
H
F,
G
D
A
E
C
B
Threshold
0 10 minutes 1 hours 2 3
(c)
conc (µg/ml)
A 64.0
B 32.0
C 16.0
D 8.0
E 4.0
F 2.0
G 1.0
H 0.5
I Growth control

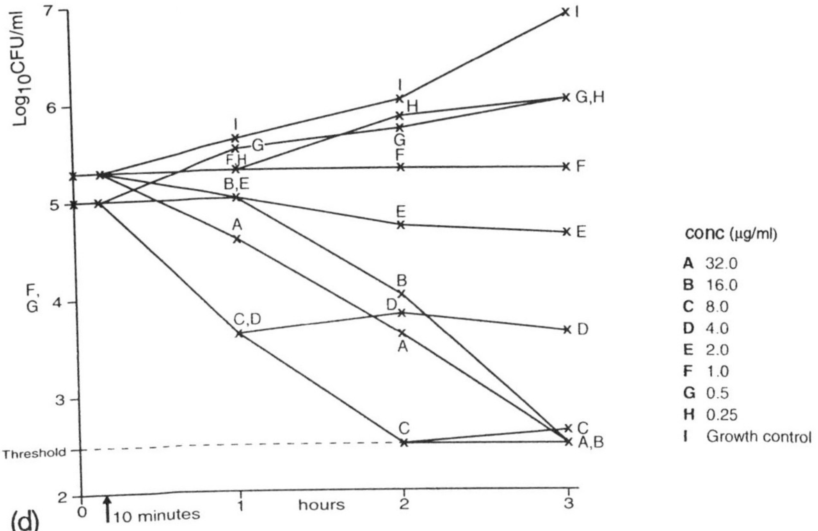
Log10CFU/ml
7
6
5
4
3
2
I
I
G
F H
B,E
A
F,
G
C,D
I
H
G
F
E
B
D
A
C
G,H
F
E
D
C
A,B
Threshold
0 10 minutes 1 hours 2 3
(d)
conc (µg/ml)
A 32.0
B 16.0
C 8.0
D 4.0
E 2.0
F 1.0
G 0.5
H 0.25
I Growth control

Log₁₀CFU/ml
H
G,
I
G,I
H
I
G
F
F
H
E
C,E,F
E
B
A,D
A,D
C
B,
C,
D
A
Threshold
10 minutes
hours
conc (µg/ml)
A   2.0
B   1.0
C   0.5
D   0.25
E   0.125
F   0.06
G   0.03
H   0.015
I   Growth control

(e)

Log₁₀CFU/ml
I
F,H
D,G
I
G,H
E
F
E
G,H
A,D,E,F
D
A,C
B,C
B
B
A,C
Threshold
10 minutes
hours
conc (µg/ml)
A   2.0
B   1.0
C   0.5
D   0.25
E   0.125
F   0.06
G   0.03
H   0.015
I   Growth control

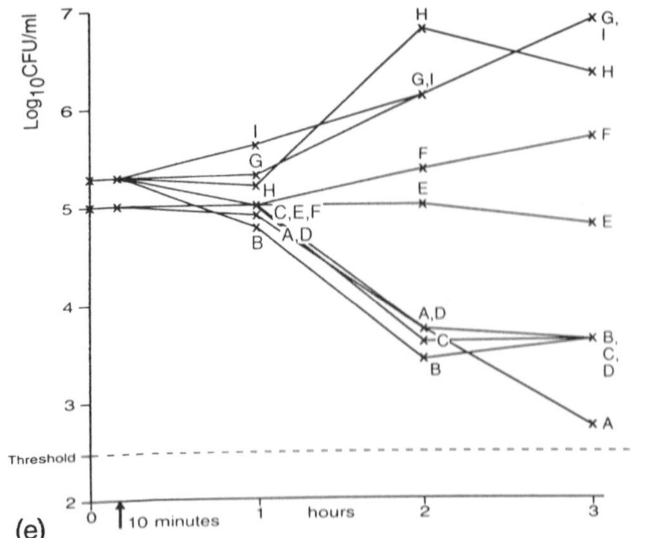

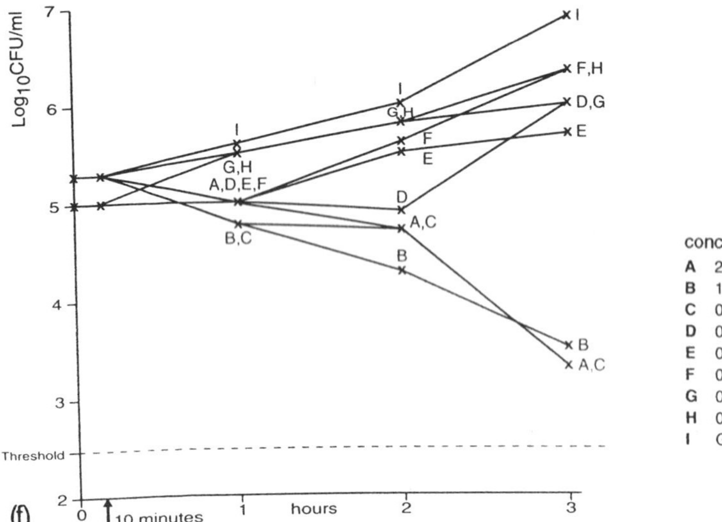

(f)

Table 1 Effect of RP 59500 on Eight Pneumococci Within 10 min of Addition of Antimicrobial to Organisms

Drug concentration	Penicillin-susceptible			Penicillin-intermediate		Penicillin-resistant		
	WRU 294[a]	64	60	114B	5	114	227	228
8 × MIC	−3[b]	−2	−2	−1	−3	0	0	−2
4 × MIC	−3	−2	−2	0	−3	0	0	−2
2 × MIC	0	−2	−2	0	−2	0	0	−1
MIC	0	0	0	0	−2	0	0	0
0.5 × MIC	0	0	0	0	0	0	0	0

[a]Strain number.
[b]Log_{10} colony count lower than time zero without antimicrobial.
  $-1 = \Delta\text{log}_{10}$ CFU/ml = 90% killing
  $-2 = \Delta\text{log}_{10}$ CFU/ml = 99% killing
  $-3 = \Delta\text{log}_{10}$ CFU/ml = 99.9% killing

the very rapid bactericidal activity, which began within 10 min in six of eight of strains. This was not found with any other compound tested. Berthaud and colleagues (2), using an in vitro pharmacokinetic model, have reported a similar rapid decrease of 3.9–4.3 Δlog_{10} CFU/ml within 2 h for three pneumococcal strains. This very rapid killing by RP 59500 may have therapeutic implications and requires clinical trials to validate this in vitro finding. Activity of RP 59500 against erythromycin-susceptible and -resistant pneumococci has been described before (4,9).

Sparfloxacin was very active against all strains. However, regrowth occurred at the MIC after 24 h with two strains; additionally, two strains were bacteriostatically inhibited by this compound. Anti-pneumococcal activity of sparfloxacin in our study was superior to that of ciprofloxacin by both MIC and time–kill methodology. Clinical studies are required to delineate the in vivo significance (if any) of the regrowth/bacteriostatic phenomena in the foregoing four strains.

The bacteriostatic activity of erythromycin was mirrored in results of time–kill experiments, in which regrowth occurred after 24 h in two strains, and one strain was bacteriostatically inhibited after 6–24 h. Vancomycin was very active against all strains by both MIC and time–kill methods.

CONCLUSIONS

Results of this study indicate that, of the new compounds tested, both RP 59500 and sparfloxacin show promise in therapy of nonmeningitic infections caused by penicillin-susceptible and -resistant pneumococci. The significance of the very rapid bactericidal activity of RP 59500 deserves further study, and must be tested in clinical studies.

REFERENCES

1. Appelbaum PC. Antimicrobial resistance in *Streptococcus pneumoniae*: an overview. Clin Infect Dis 1992; 15:77–83.
2. Berthaud N, Gouin AM, Rousseau J, Desnottes JF. 33rd Interscience Conference on Antimicrobial Agents and Chemotherapy. 1993:abstr 1048.
3. Chin N-X, Gu J-W, Yu K-W, Zhang Y-X, Neu HC. In vitro activity of sparfloxacin. Antimicrob Agents Chemother 1991; 35:567–571.
4. Fremaux A, Sissia G, Cohen R, Geslin P. In-vitro antibacterial activity of RP 59500, a semisynthetic streptogramin, against *Streptococcus pneumoniae*. J Antimicrob Chemother 1992; 30(suppl A):19–23.
5. Jacobs MR. Treatment and diagnosis of infections caused by drug-resistant *Streptococcus pneumoniae*. Clin Infect Dis 1992; 15:119–127.
6. Jacobs MR, Bajaksouzian S, Appelbaum PC. 31st Interscience Conference on Antimicrobial Agents Chemotherapy. 1991:abstr 193.
7. Liñares J, Pallares R, Alonso T, Perez JL, Ayats J, Gudiol F, Viladrich PF, Martin R. Trends in antimicrobial resistance of clinical isolates of *Streptococcus pneumoniae* in Bellvitge hospital, Barcelona, Spain (1979–1990). Clin Infect Dis 1992; 15:99–105.
8. Soussy CJ, Acar JF, Cluzel R, Courvalin P, Duval J, Fleurette J, Megraud F, Meyran M, Thabaut A. A collaborative study of the in-vitro sensitivity to RP 59500 of bacteria isolated in seven hospitals in France. J Antimicrob Chemother 1992; 30(suppl A):53–58.
9. Spangler SK, Jacobs MR, Appelbaum PC. Susceptibilities of penicillin-susceptible and -resistant strains of *Streptococcus pneumoniae* to RP 59500, vancomycin, erythromycin, PD 131628, sparfloxacin, temafloxacin, Win 57273, ofloxacin, and ciprofloxacin. Antimicrob Agents Chemother 1992; 36:856–859.
10. Yourassowsky E, van der Linden MP, Crokaert F. Comparative kill and growth rates determined with cefdinir and cefaclor and with *Streptococcus pneumoniae* and β-lactamase–producing *Haemophilus influenzae*. Antimicrob Agents Chemother 1992; 36:46–49.

Serum Bactericidal Activity of RP 57669/54476: RP 59500 Against *Streptococcus pneumoniae*

B. Pangon, P. Bray, B. Couzon, P. Allouch, and J. C. Ghnassia

C. H. de Versailles
Le Chesnay, France

R. Panis-Rouzier

C. H. de Nîmes
Nîmes, France

S. Etienne

Rhône-Poulenc Rorer
Antony, France

INTRODUCTION

RP 59500, a semisynthetic injectable streptogramin, consists of two components: RP 57669 (quinupristine) and RP 54476 (dalfopristin) in a 30:70% weight ratio. These two compounds have a synergistic activity against gram-positive bacteria:staphylococci, streptococci, enterococci, and pneumococci (1).

The emergence of penicillin-resistant strains of *Streptococcus pneumoniae* is becoming a therapeutic problem. In vitro studies and animal models demonstrated antipneumococcal activity of this drug (2,3).

The aim of our study was to evaluate the serum bactericidal activity of RP 59500 against *S. pneumoniae*, using serum samples taken from healthy volunteers who received a single IV dose of RP 59500.

MATERIALS AND METHODS

Subjects

Twelve healthy volunteers were included in this study.

Serum Samples

At the end of a 1-h infusion of 15 mg/kg RP 59500, the time of expected peak serum concentration, blood samples were collected into a citrate tube. After centrifugation, the upper phase was stored at $-70°C$ before the serum bactericidal assay.

Strains

Two strains of *S. pneumoniae* isolated from blood cultures were tested. One strain was erythromycin-susceptible (Er S) and the other strain was erythromycin-resistant (Er R). Susceptibility of RP 59500 and erythromycin was determined using a broth macrodilution method (inoculum size: 10^6 CFU/ml).

Serum Bactericidal Assay

Serum bactericidal activity of each sample was evaluated, as previously described (4). Serum was serially diluted twofold from 1:4 to 1:512, in Mueller–Hinton broth (Sanofi-Diagnostics Pasteur), in glassware tubes with an inoculum size of 10^6 CFU/ml of a log phase culture of *S. pneumoniae*. Cultures were incubated at 37°C in 5% CO_2 atmosphere. A sample of each serum dilution and control (Mueller–Hinton broth) was removed after 1, 3, and 5 h incubation and plated onto Mueller–Hinton agar supplemented with 5% horse blood. Surviving bacteria were counted using a spiral system (Interscience; lower limit of detection: 10^2 CFU/ml).

RESULTS

The minimum inhibitory concentration (MIC) of erythromycin was 0.125 mg/L and >16 mg/L, respectively, for the susceptible and resistant strains. The MIC and minimum bactericidal concentration (MBC) of RP 59500 of each strain was 1 mg/L; this agrees with the results previously reported in other studies (1).

Table 1 Bactericidal Activity of Serum after 5 h Incubation (mean $\log_{10}$ CFU/ml $\pm$ SD)

Serum dilution	ER S strain	ER R strain
1:4	≤ 2	1.97 ± 0.16
1:8	1.99 ± 0.03	2.06 ± 0.33
1:16	1.99 ± 0.06	2.05 ± 0.26
1:32	1.97 ± 0.11	2.22 ± 0.33
1:64	1.99 ± 0.17	2.82 ± 0.68
1:128	3.44 ± 0.88	4.28 ± 0.78
1:256	5.42 ± 0.66	5.70 ± 0.37
1:512	>6	>6

The mean bactericidal activity of serum for the 12 subjects after 5 h incubation is reported in Table 1.

Kinetics of serum bactericidal activity is shown in Figure 1, for dilutions 1:4 and 1:32.

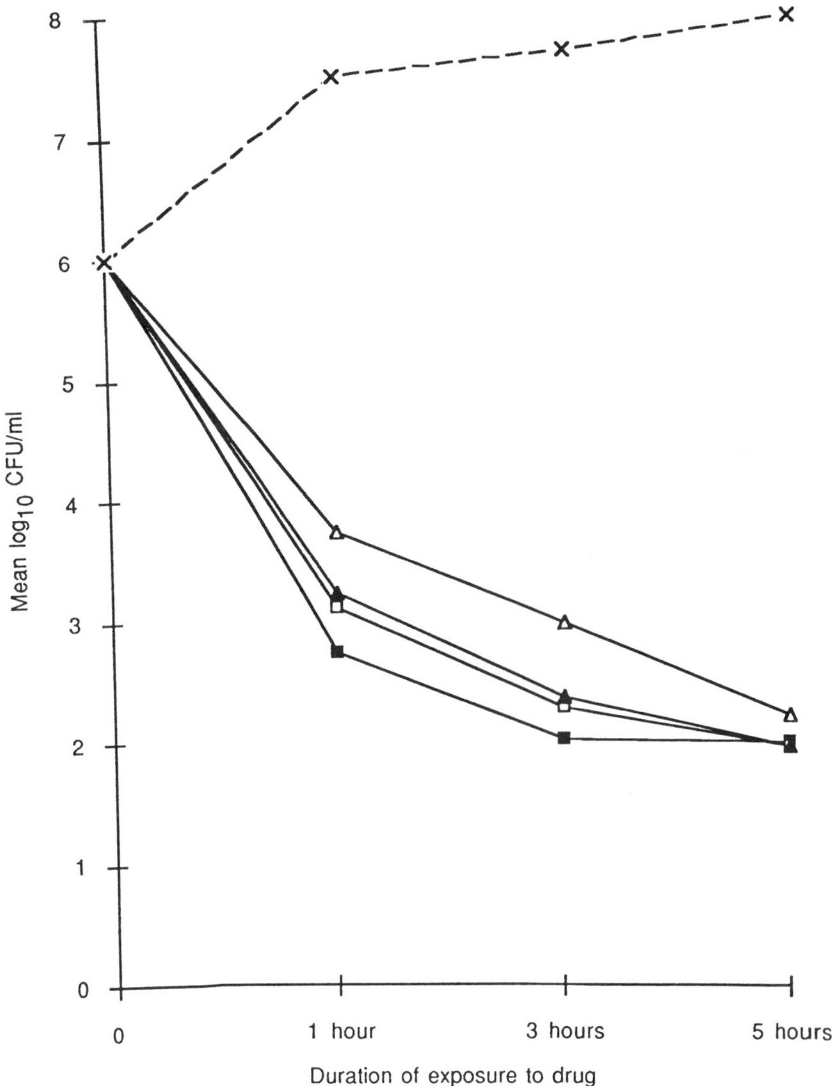

Figure 1 Kinetics of serum bactericidal activity against erythromycin-resistant and susceptible strains of *S. pneumoniae* (control: x; erythromycin-susceptible strain dilution 1:4 ■, dilution 1:32 □; erythromycin-resistant strain dilution 1:4 ▲, dilution 1:32 △)

DISCUSSION

The in vitro activity of RP 59500 against *S. pneumoniae* was reported by Fremaux to have an MIC_{90} of 1 mg/L, whatever the erythromycin susceptibility (2). In an experimental model of pneumonia, this efficacy was confirmed against an erythromycin-resistant strain (MIC = 32 mg/L), with 100% of animals surviving after six IV injections (3). An in vitro model mimicking human pharmacokinetics after a 7-mg/kg IV injection demonstrated the rapid bactericidal activity of RP 59500 against an erythromycin-resistant strain of *S. pneumoniae* (5).

In our study, samples were taken at the end of a 15-mg/kg infusion at the time of expected peak concentration. The serum concentration was 3.4 and 9.5 mg/L respectively, for RP 57669 and RP 54476 (HPLC method; unpublished data). Serum bactericidal titer (3 $\log_{10}$ decrease) was 1:64 after 5 h incubation, for the two strains. A bactericidal activity was observed for the erythromycin-susceptible strain after 1-h incubation, at the 1:16 dilution and after 3-h incubation, at the 1:64 dilution. For the erythromycin-resistant strain, there was no bactericidal activity at 1:4 serum dilution after 1 h, but a bactericidal activity was observed after 3-h incubation, at the 1:32 dilution.

CONCLUSION

These results demonstrate the synergistic activity of the two compounds and confirm the strong activity of RP 59500 against *S. pneumoniae*.

REFERENCES

1. Pechère JC. In vitro activity of RP 59500, a semisynthetic streptogramin, against staphylococci and streptococci. J Antimicrob Chemother 1992; 30(suppl A):15–18.
2. Fremaux A, Sissia G, Cohen R, Geslin P. In vitro antibacterial activity of RP 59500, a semisynthetic streptogramin, against *S. pneumoniae*. J Antimicrob Chemother 1992; 30(suppl A):19–23.
3. Azoulay-Dupuis E, Vallée E, Veber B, Pocidalo JJ. Efficacy of RP 59500, a new semisynthetic streptogramin, against penicillin-resistant and multi-resistant strains of *Streptococcus pneumoniae*. 32th Interscience Conference on Antimicrobial Agents Chemotherapy, 1992: abstr 1311.
4. Pangon B, Bray P, Etienne S, Bougon N, Manfredi R, and Garaud JJ. Striving for a standardized serum bactericidal activity assay for RP 59500:testing different diluents and materials. 32th Interscience Conference Antimicrobial Agents Chemotherapy, 1992: abstr 1313.
5. Berthault N, Desnottes JF. RP 59500: in vitro and in vivo killing kinetics against *Streptococcus pneumoniae*. 13th Interdisciplinary Meeting on Anti-infectious Chemotherapy, 1993: abstr 149.

The Activity of Streptogramin RP 59500 Against Methicillin-Sensitive and -Resistant Staphylococci

I. Raad, M. Sacilowski, R. Hachem and G. P. Bodey

University of Texas M. D. Anderson Cancer Center
Houston, Texas

INTRODUCTION

Staphylococci are the most common cause of nosocomial primary bacteremia (1–5). They are also being encountered with increasing frequency in cancer patients. Because methicillin resistance is high among *S. epidermidis* and is increasing in frequency among *S. aureus*, vancomycin remains the frontline intravenous antibiotic used in the treatment of catheter-related bacteremia. The catheter-related staphylococcal organisms (especially *S. epidermidis*) tend to be slime producing.

Several recent studies have shown that *S. epidermidis* extracted slime inhibits the antimicrobial action of vancomycin and teicoplanin (glycopeptide antibiotics). Farber et al. (6) showed that this phenomenon is not observed for rifampin, cephalosporins, and daptomycin. In this study, the in vitro activity of several nonglycopeptide antibiotics (streptogramin, minocycline, and rifampin) against staphylococci causing nosocomial infections was determined. In addition, the emergence and susceptibility profiles of quinolone-resistant staphylococci were determined at our center.

METHODS

Between January 1983 and January 1989, 97 staphylococcal bloodstream isolates from febrile cancer patients with nosocomial bacteremia were obtained. Each isolate belonged to one patient. The susceptibility profiles of these isolates were compared with those of another 100 staphylococcal bacteremic isolates obtained from another 100 patients during a period of heavy quinolone use (January 1990 to January 1992).

Staphylococcus aureus and *S. epidermidis* were identified by standard microbiological methods (Gram stain, colony morphology, coagulase production, hemolysis, novobiocin resistance) and were speciated using the API Staph-Ident system.

Standard antibiotic powders for laboratory use were obtained for the following antibiotics: minocycline, novobiocin, teicoplanin, streptogramin RP 59500 (RP), rifampin, oxacillin, penicillin, vancomycin, temafloxacin, ciprofloxacin, and clindamycin.

Susceptibility testing was performed using a microtiter broth dilution method. Cation (Ca^{2+}, Mg^{2+})-supplemented Mueller–Hinton broth, containing 2% NaCl was used as the test medium. Antibiotic solutions were dispensed and serially diluted in a 96-well microtiter plate. Appropriate dilutions were made so that final inoculum was 10^5 CFU/ml. The MIC's were read as the lowest concentration without visible growth after 24 h of incubation at 37°C.

The MBCs were performed by subculturing 0.1 ml of material from the MIC plate wells on sheep agar plates and incubating for 24 and 48 h. The MBC was read as the lowest concentration of antibiotic preventing bacterial growth (99.9% kill).

RESULTS

The 97 staphylococcal bloodstream isolates from 1983–1989 consisted of 47 methicillin-sensitive *S. aureus* (MSSA), 20 methicillin-resistant *S. aureus* (MRSA), and 30 methicillin-resistant *S. epidermidis* (MRSE). The 100 staphylococcal bloodstream isolates from the 1990–1992 period consisted of 48 MSSA, 22 MRSA, and 30 MRSE. At least 90% of all *S. aureus* and *S. epidermidis* isolates from the 1980s (including the methicillin-resistant) isolates were inhibited by streptogramin RP 59500 (RP), minocycline (MIN), teicoplanin (TEI), rifampin (RIF), vancomycin (VA), ciprofloxacin, and novobiocin (Table 1).

Similarly, 90% of MSSA, MRSA, and MRSE isolates from the 1990s were inhibited by RP 59500, MIN, RIF, VA, and NOV (Table 2). However, resistance to ciprofloxacin emerged because of excessive use of this drug at M. D. Anderson between 1988 and 1990. Table 2 shows the emergence of quinolone resistance in the early 1990s among methicillin-resistant staphylococci. This occurred after heavy use of ciprofloxacin in the prophylaxis of neutropenic cancer patients. However, quinolone- and methicillin-resistant isolates remained susceptible to RP 59500, novobiocin, minocycline, rifampin, and vancomycin.

Table 1 In Vitro Susceptibility of Staphylococcal Isolates Between 1983 and 1989 (97 Isolates)

Antibiotic	Susceptibility level (μg/ml)	MIC$_{90}$/MBC$_{90}$ (μg/ml) MRSE $n = 30$	MRSA $n = 20$	MSSA $n = 47$
RP 59500	≤2	0.25/0.5	1.0/2.0	0.5/1.0
Cefamandole	≤8	2/8	3/32	1/8
Ciprofloxacin	≤1	2/2	0.25/0.25	0.25/0.25
Minocycline	≤4	2/64	1/32	0.5/64
Novobiocin	≤4	0.12/1	0.25/0.5	0.12/2.0
Oxacillin	≤2	>64/>64	>64/>64	0.5/1
Rifampin	≤2	0.06/2	2/2	0.06/2
Teicoplanin	≤8	4/8	0.5/2	1/16
Vancomycin	≤4	2/4	1/1	1/4

DISCUSSION

Streptogramin RP 59500, minocycline, novobiocin, and rifampin showed equivalent bacteriostatic activity to glycopeptide antibiotics (vancomycin and teicoplanin) against oxacillin-sensitive and -resistant staphylococci causing nosocomial bacteremia.

Streptogramin RP 59500, novobiocin, and rifampin had bactericidal activity similar to vancomycin. RP 59500 bactericidal activity was superior to that of teicoplanin.

Table 2 In Vitro Susceptibility of Staphylococcal Isolates Between 1990 and 1992 (100 Isolates)

Antibiotic	Susceptibility level (μg/ml)	MIC$_{90}$/MBC$_{90}$ (μg/ml) MRSE $n = 30$	MRSA $n = 22$	MSSA $n = 48$
RP 59500	≤2	0.25/0.5	0.15/0.5	0.5/1.0
Cefamandole	≤8	32/32	16/64	1/1
Clindamycin	≤0.5	>64/>64	>64/>64	0.06/0.125
Ciprofloxacin	≤1	32/>64	16/32	0.25/0.25
Minocycline	≤4	0.25/2	1/2	0.25/1
Novobiocin	≤4	0.125/0.5	0.02/0.25	0.06/0.25
Rifampin	≤2	0.03/0.25	0.5/0.5	0.03/0.06
Vancomycin	≤4	1/2	1/1	0.5/1

With recent data showing that the *S. epidermidis* slime extract inhibits the antimicrobial action of glycopeptide antibiotics streptogramin RP 59500 should be further investigated in the therapy of resistant staphylococcal catheter-related infections.

Quinolone resistance emerged among methicillin-resistant staphylococci after excessive use of ciprofloxacin. Quinolone- and methicillin-resistant staphylococci remained susceptible to streptogramin RP 59500, novobiocin, vancomycin, rifampin, and minocycline. Streptogramin (RP 59500) should be considered as an alternative antibiotic in the treatment of resistant staphylococci.

REFERENCES

1. Maki DG, Weise CE, Sarafin HW. A semiquantitative culture method for identifying intravenous catheter-related infection. N Engl J Med 1977; 296:1305–1309.
2. Sherertz RJ, Raad II, Balani A, et al. Three year experience with sonicated vascular catheter cultures in a clinical microbiology laboratory. J Clin Microbiol 1990; 28:76–82.
3. Cleri DJ, Corrado ML, Seligman SJ. Quantitative culture of intravenous catheters and other intravascular inserts. J Infect Dis 1980; 141:781–786.
4. Moyer MA, Edwards LD, Farley L. Comparative culture methods on 101 intravenous catheters. Arch Intern Med 1983; 143:66–69.
5. Linares J, Sitges-Serra A, Garau J, Perez JL, Martin R. Pathogenesis of catheter sepsis: a prospective study with quantitative and semiquantitative cultures of catheter hub and segments. J Clin Microbiol 1985; 21:357–360.
6. Farber BF, Kaplan MH, Clogston AG. *Staphylococcus epidermidis* extracted slime inhibits the antimicrobial action of glycopeptide antibiotics. J Infect Dis 1990; 161:37–40.

Comparative Activity of RP 59500, Ciprofloxacin, and Erythromycin on *Staphylococcus epidermidis* in Biofilm

J. M. T. Hamilton-Miller and W. Brumfitt

Royal Free Hospital and School of Medicine
London, England

INTRODUCTION

Several medically important bacteria, notably coagulase-negative staphylococci, form biofilm in vivo (1). This complicates the therapy of infections of indwelling devices (2). The matrix of biofilm prevents antibiotic access to the infecting bacteria, and sessile organisms within the biofilm are often much less sensitive to antibiotics than planktonic organisms. These factors may explain the disappointing cure rates obtained in patients with infected indwelling lines when treated with antibiotics to which the infecting strains are apparently fully sensitive.

Here we investigate the activity of antibiotics on sessile bacteria growing in biofilm on Silastic catheter material. This model may provide a better predictor of antibiotic success or failure than conventional testing.

METHODS AND MATERIALS

Bacterial Strains

Staphylococcus epidermidis, with different genotypes of susceptibility to erythromycin (sensitive, inducibly resistant, and constitutively resistant), that tested either positive or negative for slime and adhesion were chosen (Table 1). The latter properties were tested for by culturing overnight in tryptone soya broth

Table 1   Properties of *Staphylococcus epidermidis* Strains

Strain no.	Slime and adherence	MIC (mg/L)		
		Ciprofloxacin	RP 59500	Erythromycin
53	−	0.5	0.25	0.5
1966	−	0.25	0.13	>128 (inducible)
6967	−	0.25	0.25	>128 (constitutive)
N15	+	0.5	0.13	1
N10	+	0.25	0.25	>128 (inducible)
0303	+	4	0.13	>128 (constitutive)

(TSB, Oxoid) in two glass tubes. The broth was discarded, and one tube stained with safranin for adhering bacteria and the other with alcian blue for slime.

Formation of Biofilm

The model was based on that described by Prosser et al. (3): 8-mm disks, cut from Silastic sheeting (Dow Corning), sterilized by autoclaving in water, were layered with 10^7 colony-forming units (CFU) of *S. epidermidis* in 0.1 ml phosphate-buffered saline (PBS). After incubation at 37°C for 4 h, disks were rinsed twice with PBS to remove nonadhering (planktonic) bacteria, covered with TSB, and incubated for 48 h at 37°C.

Killing of Bacteria in Biofilm

"Two-day" biofilms made, as outlined in the foregoing, were washed in PBS, and one was placed in each well of a 25-compartment polystyrene dish, 2 ml of TSB plus antibiotic added, and the plates incubated at 37°C. At times 0, 24, and 48 h, four disks were removed, washed twice in PBS, then sequentially sonicated and vortexed in 5 ml TSB plus 0.3% Tween 80; viable counts were made from the resulting suspensions.

Times for 99.9% kill (3 log reduction in viable counts) were determined by interpolation or extrapolation from time–kill plots.

Killing of Planktonic Bacteria

One hundred milliliters of TSB in a 500-ml conical flask was inoculated with 10^7 CFU from an overnight broth culture, and antibiotic was added. Flasks were shaken at 100 rpm at 37°C, and viable counts made at intervals up to 24 h. Times for 99.9% kill were determined as before.

Antibiotics

The compounds tested were [concentration of active material in micrograms per milliliter (μg/ml) in parentheses]: RP 59500 (30), ciprofloxacin (10), and erythromycin (75).

RESULTS

Growth of Sessile Organisms

Two-day biofilms of slime-producing strains of *S. epidermidis* yielded between 1×10^7 and 3×10^7 CFU per disk, whereas strains that did not make slime produced only about 0.01 of these numbers per disk. Yields per disk were quite consistent, with a variance of about 25%.

Killing of Sessile Organisms

The activities of the three antibiotics against *S. epidermidis* in biofilm are summarized in Table 2, in which the times (in hours) required to bring about 99.9% kill for the six strains are shown. There was considerable variation between the strains, but statistical analysis of the individual data showed that killing of slime-negative strains was no more rapid than that of slime-positive strains ($0.5 > p < 0.4$), and that ciprofloxacin and RP 59500 were not significantly different in their speed of killing ($0.3 > p < 0.2$). Both ciprofloxacin and RP 59500 seemed to kill more quickly than erythromycin; the latter antibiotic, not surprisingly, did not kill any of the four strains that were resistant to it. There was no correlation between erythromycin sensitivity status and rate of killing by RP 59500.

Killing of Planktonic Organisms

Results from time–kill plots against planktonic *S. epidermidis* are summarized in Table 2, in which the times (in hours) required to bring about 99.9% kill for the six strains are shown. For ciprofloxacin and RP 59500, rates of kill were rather similar for both sessile and planktonic bacteria. Erythromycin, again, had a bactericidal effect only on the two sensitive strains (N15 and N53), and this was slower than the observed killing rates of RP 59500 and ciprofloxacin.

DISCUSSION

The strains tested in these experiments came from our collection of coagulase-negative staphylococci isolated from significant infections. Many such strains (especially *S. haemolyticus*) are multiresistant, and selecting an appropriate

Table 2 Killing Activities of Ciprofloxacin and RP 59500 Against *S. epidermidis* in Planktonic and Sessile Modes

Strain no. (slime production)	Erythromycin susceptibility status	Growth modality	Time (h) for 99.9% kill	
			Ciprofloxacin	RP 59500
53 (−)	Sensitive	Planktonic	17	18
		Sessile	21	17
1966 (−)	Inducible resistance	Planktonic	27	>48
		Sessile	11	25
6967 (−)	Constitutive resistance	Planktonic	15	19
		Sessile	19	17
N15 (+)	Sensitive	Planktonic	18	38
		Sessile	21	23
N10 (+)	Inducible resistance	Plankonic	15	19
		Sessile	21	37
0303 (+)	Constitutive resistance	Planktonic	19	13
		Sessile	17	15

antibiotic can present problems. Therefore, the development of a novel, active agent, such as RP 59500 is welcome.

We have shown that clinical isolates of *S. epidermidis*, growing in the form of biofilm on the surface of a polymer (Silastic), identical with that used in Tenckhoff catheters, are killed by RP 59500 at rates similar to those found with ciprofloxacin. It is encouraging that biofilms from strains of differing genotypes in terms of antibiotic resistance and slime or adhesion production were equally susceptible.

The concentrations of antibiotics we used were based on the following: for ciprofloxacin, on that used successfully (4) to treat peritonitis in continuous ambulatory peritoneal dialysis; for erythromycin, on the recommendations of a U.S. Peritonitis Management Advisory Committee (5); and for RP 59500, for which no clinical data are yet available, on a reasonable achievable concentration in dialysis fluid.

We consider that our results justify the use of RP 59500 for the treatment of infections of indwelling lines.

ACKNOWLEDGMENT

We are grateful to Rhone-Poulenc Rorer for financial support.

REFERENCES

1. Denyer SP, Gorman SP, Sussman M, eds. Microbial Biofilms: Formation and Control. Oxford: Blackwell, 1993.
2. Raad II, Bodey GP. Infectious complications of indwelling vascular catheters. Clin Infect Dis 1992; 15:197–210.
3. Prosser BLT, Taylor D, Dix BA, Cleeland R. Method of evaluating effects of antibiotics on bacterial biofilm. Antimicrob Agents Chemother 1987; 31:1502–1506.
4. Ludlam HA, Barton I, White L, McMullin C, King A, Phillips I. Intraperitoneal ciprofloxacin for the treatment of peritonitis in patients receiving continuous ambulatory peritoneal dialysis (CAPD). J Antimicrob Chemother 1990; 25:843–851.
5. Keane WF, Everett ED, Fine RN, Golper TA, Vas SI, Peterson PK. CAPD related peritonitis management and antibiotic therapy recommendations. Peritoneal Dial Bull 1987; 7:56–62.

Suppression of the *Pseudomonas aeruginosa*-Induced Biofilm Formation on Epithelial Cells by Roxithromycin

Eiji Kita, Masayoshi Sawaki, Keiichi Mikasa, and Nobuhiro Narita

Nara Medical University

Nara, Japan

INTRODUCTION

Once established on the mucus lining of the airways, pathogenic bacteria can form microcolonies. Development of a glycocalyx-enclosed microcolony leads to a confluent autochthonous bacterial biofilm (1). Bacteria within the biofilms can persist and grow, eventually resulting in masses resembling those seen in the lung in cystic fibrosis (2). Erythromycin inhibits production of a mucin-like glycoprotein by human epithelial cells (3) and of exoenzymes by *Pseudomonas aeruginosa* (4). Roxithromycin inhibits only glycoprotein production by host cells. The present study compared the effect on biofilm formation of roxithromycin and erythromycin.

MATERIALS AND METHODS

Microorganisms

A temperature-sensitive mutant (Ts25) of *P. aeruginosa* N-42, which can grow at 25°C, but not at 37°C, was used. This mutant produces pyocyanin, elastase, exoenzyme A, leukocidin, and protease at 37°C, without multiplication.

260

Cell Culture

Ishikawa cells (human endometrial adenocarcinoma cell line) (5) produce a mucin-like glycoprotein that is physicochemically similar to mucoproteins produced in the human airway. Cells were plated in 24-well, flat-bottomed plates at a density of 10^4/ml in 1 ml of minimal essential medium (MEM), containing 5% fetal bovine serum, at 37°C in 5% CO_2, until confluent monolayers were formed. Then, the monolayers were treated with mitomycin (50 μg/ml) at 37°C for 30 min, washed, and then, incubated in the same medium for 24 h.

Biofilm Formation

Mitomycin-treated Ishikawa cells were cultured in MEM containing 10% human plasma and 10^7 colony-forming units (CFU) of strain Ts25, at 37°C for 24 h, in 5% CO_2. After washing with Hanks' balanced salt solution, the cells were cultured in MEM, containing 10% human plasma, at 37°C for 14 days, in the presence or absence of the antibiotics tested. The number of biofilms was measured under an Olympus inverted microscope. Usually, 38–45 microcolonies or biofilms per well were formed after 14 days of incubation without antibiotics (Fig. 1).
F1

Measurement of Glycoproteins and Bacterial Enzymes

Glycoproteins produced by Ishikawa cells and bacterial exoenzyme A were measured by rocket immunoelectrophoresis (IEF), using rabbit polyclonal antibodies to these antigens. Glycoprotein contents of the purified Ishikawa's glycoprotein were expressed as the content of hexose, whereas exoenzyme A was determined by the Authrone reaction. Purified exoenzyme A was purchased from Biological Laboratories, Inc. (Campbell, CA). These were used to construct standard curves in the assay of rocket IEF.

Enumeration of Viable Bacterial Counts

Each monolayer was treated with 0.1% Triton X and sonicated at the end of culture. Several dilutions were plated on tryptic soy agar, and the number of CFU was determined 48 h after incubation at 25°C.

RESULTS

Table 1 shows the effect of different concentrations of the two antibiotics on formation of biofilms. Roxithromycin suppressed biofilm formation at concentrations both lower and higher than erythromycin. Roxithromycin inhibited the adhesion to Ishikawa cells of *P. aeruginosa* and its subsequent colonization of

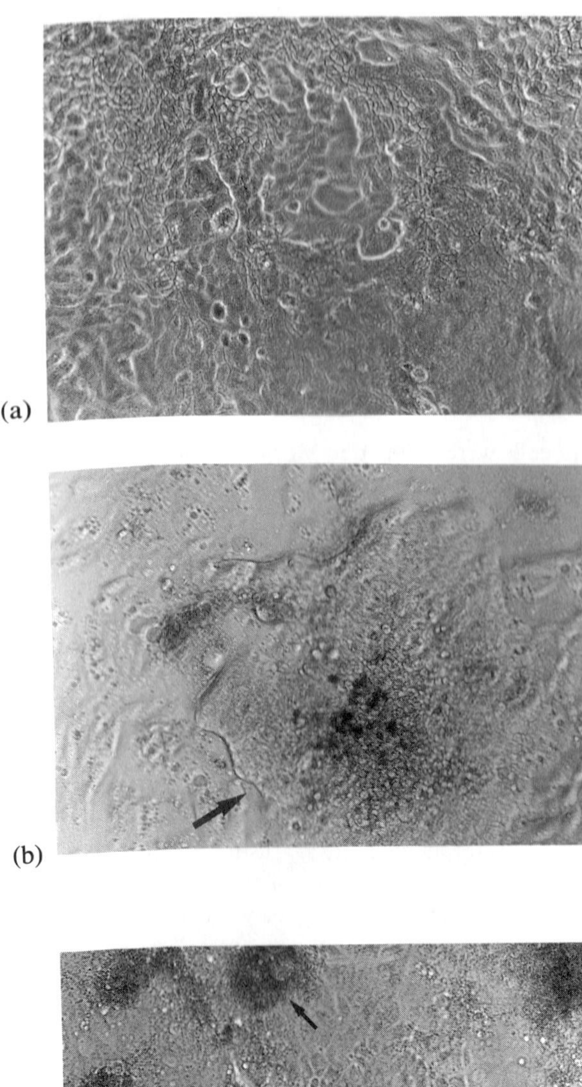

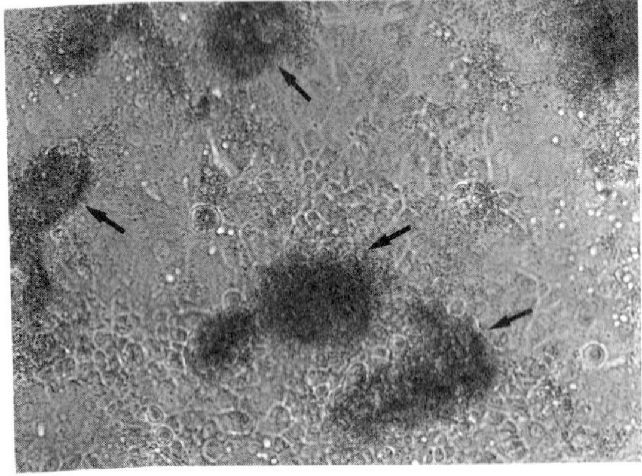

Figure 1 (a) Normal appearance of Ishikawa cells; (b) initial formation of biofilms consisting of mucin and bacteria; (c) multiple biofilm colonies.

Table 1 Effects of Roxithromycin and Erythromycin on Biofilm Formation in Culture of Ishikawa Cells

Concentratio ns (µg/ml)	No. of biofilms per well	
	Roxithromycin	Erythromycin
0	43 ± 15	
0.05	21 ± 6	Not tested
0.2	6 ± 3	18 ± 6
0.5	<2	12 ± 4
1	0	3 ± 2
2	0	<2
5	0	0
10	0	5 ± 2

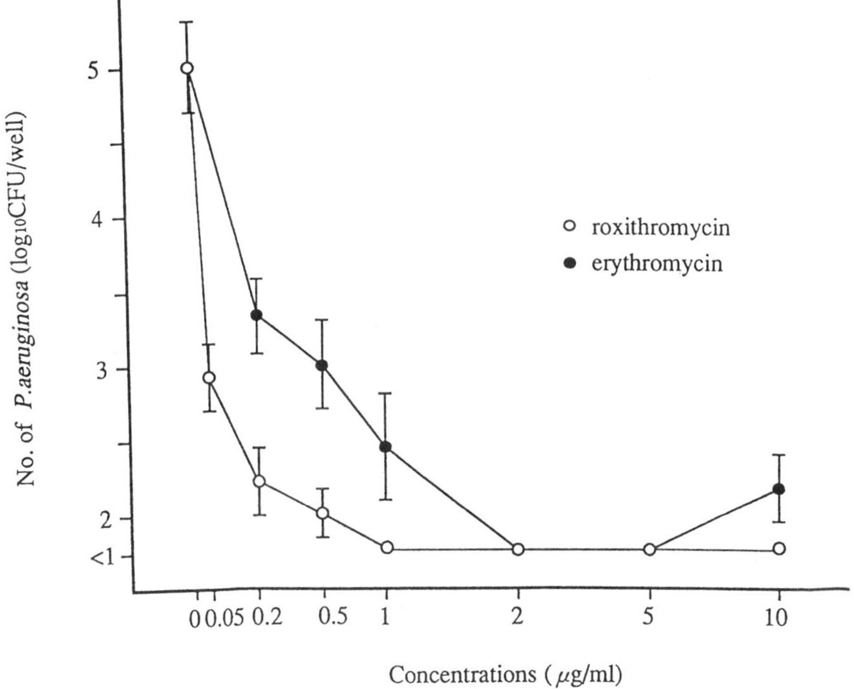

Figure 2 The number of *P. aeruginosa* Ts colonizing the monolayers of Ishikawa cells in the presence of roxithromycin or erythromycin.

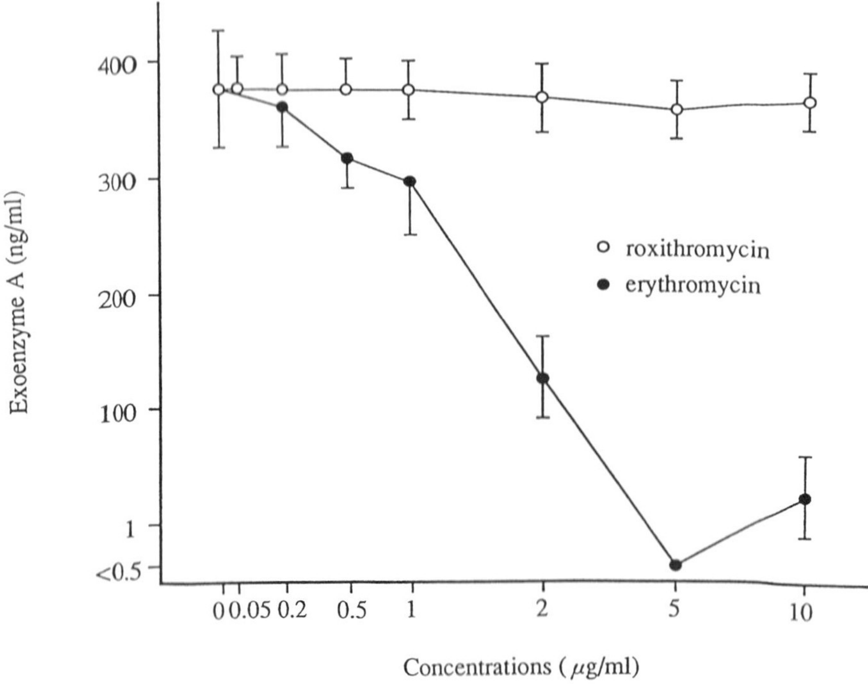

Figure 3   Effects of roxithromycin and erythromycin on exoenzyme A production by *P. aeruginosa* Ts in culture with Ishikawa cells.

the cells at concentrations lower than those of erythromycin that are required for the same level of suppression (Fig. 2). Erythromycin suppressed exoenzyme A production by *P. aeruginosa* in the dose range of 2–5 µg/ml, whereas roxithromycin did not affect the production (Fig. 3).

Both antibiotics exhibited a suppressive effect on the production of glycoproteins by Ishikawa cells. However, roxithromycin exerted its suppressive effect at lower doses than did erythromycin; even at 0.2 µg/ml, roxithromycin inhibited glycoprotein production almost completely (Fig. 4). In contrast, maximal suppression by erythromycin was achieved at 5 µg/ml.

DISCUSSION

Roxithromycin did not affect the enzyme production by *P. aeruginosa*. However, inhibition of the biofilm formation by roxithromycin became stronger as suppression of the glycoprotein production increased, whereas higher doses of erythromycin were required to inhibit biofilm formation, despite the suppressive

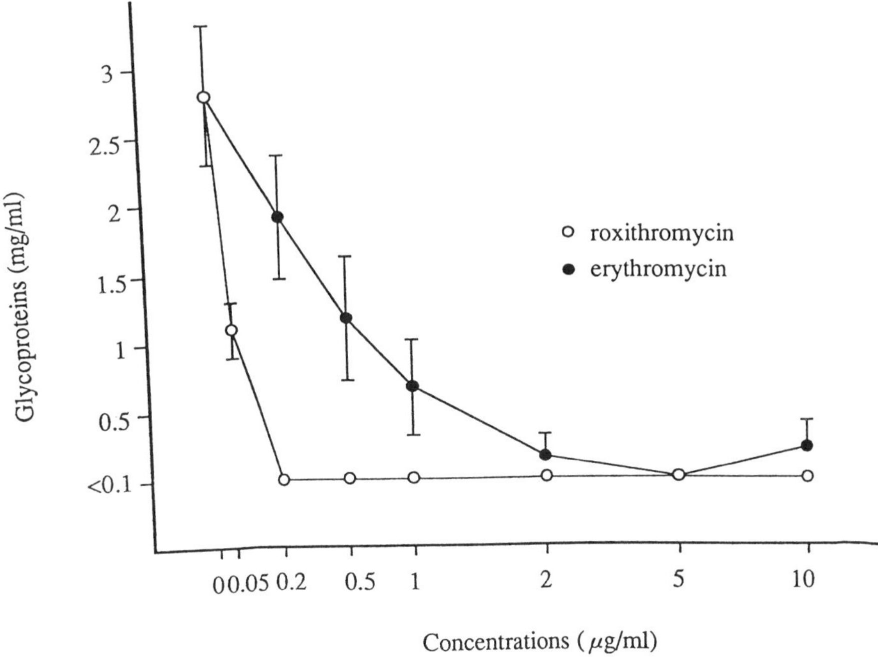

Figure 4   Effects of roxithromycin and erythromycin on glycoprotein production by Ishikawa cells cultured with *P. aeruginosa* Ts.

effect on production of bacterial enzymes. Therefore, biofilm formation in cultures of human epithelial cells and *P. aeruginosa* may be attributed to host cell-derived factors, rather than bacterial products.

The present data strongly suggest that inhibition of glycoprotein production by human epithelial cells is more effective for prevention of biofilm formation by macrolide antibiotics than their suppressive effects on bacterial enzyme production. Moreover, roxithromycin exhibits such an effect at a lower dose than erythromycin.

REFERENCES

1. Costerton JW, Cheng K-J, Geesey GG, Ladd TI, Nickel JC, Dasgupta M, Marrie TJ. Bacterial biofilms in nature and disease. Annu Rev Microbiol 1987; 41:435–464.

2. Lam JS, Chan R, Lam K, Costerton JW. The production of mucoid microcolonies by *Pseudomonas aeruginosa* within infected lungs in cystic fibrosis. Infect Immun 1980; 28:546–556.

3. Amin DN, Goswami S, Klein T, Maayani S, Marom Z. Functional antagonism between hormone receptor systems: modulation of glycoprotein secretion in secretory epithelial cells. Am J Respir Cell Mol Biol 1991; 4:135–139.
4. Kita E, Sawaki M, Oku D, Hamuro A, Mikasa K, Konishi M, Emoto M, Takeuchi S, Narita N, Kashiba S. Suppression of virulence factors of *Pseudomonas aeruginosa* by erythromycin. J Antimicrob Chemother 1991; 27:273–284.
5. Nishida M, Kasahara K, Kaneko M, Iwasaki H. Establishment of a new human endometrial adenocarcinoma cell line, Ishikawa cells, containing estrogen and progesterone receptors. Acta Obstet Gynecol Jpn 1985; 37:1103–1111.

Review of the Antilegionella Activity of Roxithromycin and the Use of the E Test to Determine Potency

R. N. Jones and M. E. Erwin

University of Iowa College of Medicine
Iowa City, Iowa

INTRODUCTION

Roxithromycin is an acid-stable oxime-esterified macrolide possessing significant activity against *Legionella spp.*, which remain one of the most important lower respiratory tract pathogens, presenting both as community-acquired and as nosocomial infection. Erythromycin and rifampin, which have good penetration into phagocytic cells, are also effective against legionella (1), but sometimes lack clinical efficacy (2,3). Macrolides, with or without concomitant rifampin, are the drugs most frequently used, but other compounds with documented clinical efficacy are the fluoroquinolones, some carbapenems, tetracycline, and some β-lactamase inhibitor combinations. Macrolides vary in their antilegionella potency and their ability to concentrate in pulmonary macrophages and lung cells. This presentation reviews the comparative features of roxithromycin tested against *Legionella* spp. strains and infections (4–10).

MATERIALS AND METHODS

Details of the tests used to establish medium drug-binding characteristics and antimicrobial activity of the various agents are given in the papers listed in the references.

RESULTS

The studies demonstrate a mean roxithromycin 50% minimum inhibitory concentration (MIC$_{50}$) value of 0.12 µg/ml with an MIC$_{90}$ of 0.25 µg/ml against *L. pneumophila*. Potency was generally twofold greater than erythromycin in direct comparisons, but 10- to 100-fold less than rifampin. Comparison of the in vitro activity of 13 antimicrobial agents against 103 strains of *L. pneumophila* is shown in Table 1.

Various media were used in the different studies, and the highest roxithromycin MICs have been reported on charcoal-containing agar (BCYE). On BSYE or in broth formulations (RPMI, BSYE, ACES-yeast extract), the MICs were two- to fourfold lower. Roxithromycin legionellacidal concentrations were usually at or within fourfold of the measured MIC. The E test MICs correlated well with reference agar results and were simple to perform, even on charcoal-containing media (data not shown).

Legionella spp. clinical isolates can be tested in vitro simply and accurately by the E test method, producing results equal to reference agar dilution methods within 48–72 h of initial culture.

Table 1 In Vitro Activity of 13 Antimicrobial Agents Tested on Agar (No Charcoal) Against 103 Strains of *Legionella pneumophila*

	MIC (µg/ml)		
Antimicrobial agents by group	50%	90%	Range
Macrolide–lincosamine–streptogramins			
Roxithromycin	0.12	0.25	0.03–0.5
Azithromycin	0.5	1	0.03–4
Dirithromycin	1	4	0.25–4
Erythromycin	0.25	0.5	≤0.015–1
Clindamycin	4	8	2–>8
RP 59500	0.5	1	0.06–2
Fluoroquinolones			
Ciprofloxacin	0.03	0.06	0.015–0.06
Fleroxacin	0.06	0.06	0.015–0.06
Lomefloxacin	0.06	0.12	0.03–0.12
Ofloxacin	0.06	0.06	0.03–0.12
Other Compounds			
Doxycycline	1	2	0.12–2
TMP/SMX[a]	0.5	0.5	≤0.03–1
Rifampin	0.004	0.008	≤0.002–0.03

[a]Includes the trimethoprim–sulfamethoxazole combination at a 1:19 ratio. Only the trimethoprim concentration of that ratio is listed.

Source: From Ref. 7.

Table 2 Minimum Extracellular Concentration (MIEC) Inhibiting Intracellular Multiplication of *Legionella pneumophila* in Peritoneal Macrophages

Antimicrobial	MIEC (μg/ml)
Roxithromycin	0.01
Erythromycin	0.5
Ofloxacin	0.03
Rifampin	0.001

Maximal intracellular concentrations are exhibited by roxithromycin compared with other macrolides, and in vivo animal models demonstrate excellent eradication of *Legionella* organisms at doses below that used for erythromycin. *Legionella pneumophila* and several other species are equally susceptible to roxithromycin.

The relation between the MIEC and the MIC of 13 antibiotics against *L. pneumophila* was calculated (10). Lower ratios are indicative of a high rate of drug penetration into the macrophages (Table 2). On this basis, the greatest penetration rates were obtained with roxithromycin (0.16), rifampin (1), ofloxacin (1.9), AT-4140 (2.5), and ciprofloxacin (3.8).

In vivo animal model results demonstrate comparable protective effects for

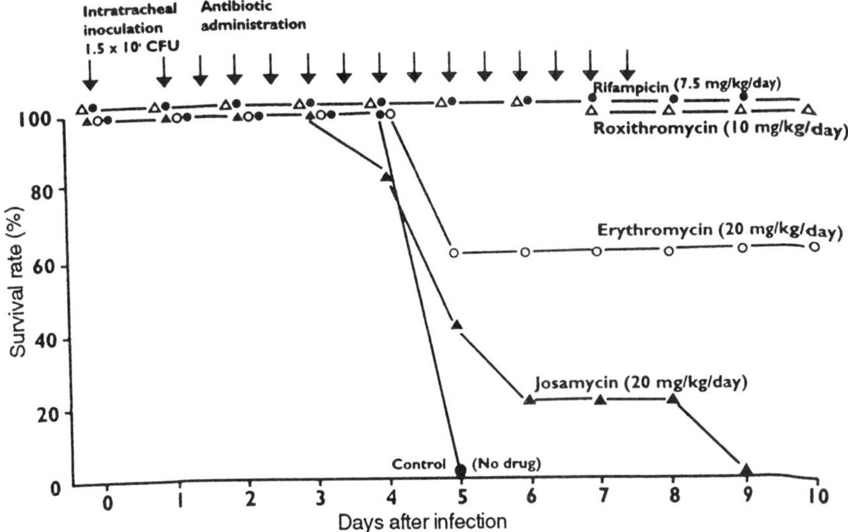

Figure 1 The effect of three macrolides and rifampin regimens in experimental guinea pigs infected with *L. pneumophila*. (From Ref. 11.)

rifampin and roxithromycin. These rates were superior to erythromycin and josamycin (Fig. 1).

In conclusion, roxithromycin is generally more potent against *Legionella* spp. than erythromycin, azithromycin, dirithromycin, clindamycin, or RP 59500. Roxithromycin MICs for *Legionella* spp. are modified (increased two- to fourfold) by the medium charcoal content, but the E test MICs may be influenced to a lesser extent. Roxithromycin MBCs versus *Legionella* spp. are similar to MICs. Roxithromycin MICs, favorable bioavailability, and intracellular concentrations produce the lowest MIEC among tested macrolides and fluoroquinolones.

REFERENCES

1. Greenwood D, Laverick A. Activities of newer quinolones against *Legionella* group organisms. Lancet 1983; 2:279–280.
2. Kurz RW, Graninger W, Egger TP, Pichler H, Tragl KH. Failure of treatment of legionella pneumonia with ciprofloxacin. J Antimicrob Chemother 1988; 22:389–391.
3. Miller AC. Erythromycin in legionnaires' disease: a reappraisal. J Antimicrob Chemother 1981; 7:217–222.
4. Fleurette J, Bornstein N. Susceptibility of *Legionella* spp. to roxithromycin. 15th International Congress of Chemotherapy, Istanbul, July 19–24, 1987.
5. Fournet M-P, Xini R, Deforges L, Duval J, Tillement J-P. Determination of binding parameters of macrolides, lincosamides, and streptogramins to *Legionella pneumophila*. J Pharmaceut Sci 1987; 76:153–156.
6. Hara J, et al. Activity of macrolides against organisms responsible for respiratory infections with emphasis on *Mycoplasma* and *Legionella*. J Antimicrob Chemother 1987; 20(suppl B):75–80.
7. Johnson et al. Antimicrobial activity of ten macrolide, lincosamine and streptogramin drugs tested against *Legionella* spp. Eur J Clin Microbiol Infect Dis 1992; 11:751–755.
8. Jones RN, Barry AL, Fuchs PC, Thornsberry C. Disk diffusion susceptibility testing of two macrolide antimicrobial agents: revised interpretive criteria for erythromycin and preliminary guidelines for roxithromycin (RU965). J Clin Microbiol 1986; 24:233–9.
9. Jones RN, et al. The antimicrobial activity of A-56268 (TE-301) and roxithromycin (RU965) against legionella using broth microdilution method. J Antimicrob Chemother 1987; 19:841–842.
10. Kitsukawa K, Hara J, Saito A. Inhibition of *Legionella pneumophila* in guinea pig peritoneal macrophages by new quinolone, macrolide and other antimicrobial agents. *J Antimicrob Chemother* 1991; 27:343–353.
11. Saito A. Treatment of severe respiratory infection, *Legionella* pneumonia. Nippon Kyobu Shikkan Gakkai Zasshi 1989; 27:281–285.

Antimicrobial Susceptibility of *Haemophilus ducreyi* in Rwanda

Eddy Van Dyck

Institute of Tropical Medicine
Antwerp, Belgium

Jos Bogaerts

Centre Hospitalier de Kigali and Belgo-Rwandan Medical Cooperation
Kigali, Rwanda

Chancroid, caused by *Haemophilus ducreyi*, is a common cause of genital ulcer disease (GUD) in many developing countries. The current primary treatment regimen recommended by the World Health Organization (WHO) is erythromycin, with ceftriaxone, ciprofloxacin, spectinomycin, and trimethoprim–sulfamethoxazole (TMP–SMZ) as alternative recommended regimens (10). Single-dose azithromycin therapy appears another promising alternative. Treatment with TMP–SMZ has long been poorly effective in Asia and, more recently, has also become less effective in East Africa (6,9).

Current methods of GUD diagnosis, including the isolation of *H. ducreyi*, are beyond the capacity of most settings in developing countries. Generally, cases of *H. ducreyi* infection are treated empirically as part of syndromic GUD case management. However, the therapeutic efficacy of recommended treatment regimens for GUD may change over time, as a consequence of an increase in antimicrobial resistance of local *H. ducreyi* strains. Therefore, periodic surveillance of the clinical efficacy of treatment, of the etiology of GUD, and of in vitro antimicrobial susceptibility of local *H. ducreyi* isolates is recommended.

TMP–SMZ has been the treatment of choice for chancroid in Rwanda for a long time, but treatment failure has recently been increasingly reported in the country. The present study was undertaken to determine the in vitro susceptibility to recommended drugs of clinical isolates of *H. ducreyi* obtained between 1986 and 1991 in Kigali, capital of Rwanda.

Between 1986 and 1992, 112 clinical isolates of *H. ducreyi* were collected. They were obtained during three GUD studies performed in 1986 (18 isolates), 1988 (23 isolates), and 1991 (71 isolates). An agar dilution technique was used to determine minimal inhibitory concentrations (MICs) for azithromycin, ceftriaxone, ciprofloxacin, erythromycin, TMP, and TMP–SMZ. Antimicrobial agents were obtained as standard powders from different pharmaceutical companies. Serial twofold dilutions of the antimicrobials were added to the test medium consisting of GC agar (Difco Laboratories, Detroit, MI), 1% hemoglobin (Becton Dickinson, Cockeysville, MD), 5% fetal bovine serum, 0.1% glucose, 0.01% L-glutamine, and 0.025% L-cysteine hydrochloride. The growth from 48-h *H. ducreyi* cultures on GC agar (Difco), enriched with 1% hemoglobin (Becton Dickinson), 1% IsoVitaleX (Becton Dickinson), and 5% fetal bovine serum, was suspended in Mueller–Hinton broth (Difco), vortexed, and allowed to sediment for 20 min. The supernatant was transferred to another tube and adjusted to a bacterial concentration of 10^8/ml by comparison with the 0.5 McFarland standard. With a multipoint replicator, inocula of 10^5 colony forming units (CFU) were spotted on the test media. The MIC results were read after a 48-h incubation of the test plates at 35°C in 5% CO_2 atmosphere.

The MIC ranges, MIC_{50}, and MIC_{90} results are shown in Table 1. All *H. ducreyi* isolates were susceptible to azithromycin, ceftriaxone, ciprofloxacin, and erythromycin. Overall, 51 (46%) isolates were resistant to TMP (MIC $\geq$ 4.0 mg/L), and 36 (32%) were resistant to TMP–SMZ (MIC $\geq$ 4.0/76 mg/L). Between the groups of *H. ducreyi* isolates of the three periods, no differences in susceptibilities to azithromycin, ceftriaxone, ciprofloxacin, and erythromycin were observed. However, for TMP and for TMP–SMZ a significant increase of MICs occurred over time. All 18 isolates of 1986 were susceptible to both antimicrobials; among the isolates of 1988 39% (9/23) and 9% (2/23) were resistant to TMP (MIC $\geq$ 4.0 mg/L) and to TMP–SMZ (MIC $\geq$ 4.0/76 mg/L), respectively; this resistance rate further increased to 59% (42/71) for TMP and to 48% (34/71) for TMP–SMZ among the isolates of 1991 (χ^2 for trend: $p <$ 0.0001 for both antimicrobials).

The activities observed for azithromycin, ceftriaxone, ciprofloxacin, and erythromycin for *H. ducreyi* isolates in the present study are very similar to those reported elsewhere (1,2,4,5). The changing susceptibility patterns for TMP and TMP–SMZ observed between 1986 and 1991 suggest that this type of resistance has occurred recently. Most *H. ducreyi* isolates in Africa and Asia are resistant to SMZ, although many SMZ-resistant strains have remained susceptible to the combination TMP–SMZ (7,8). Resistance to TMP–SMZ develops more slowly in vitro than to either component alone, and TMP–SMZ-resistant organisms are generally resistant to both components of the mixture. In this study, all 36

Table 1 Antimicrobial Susceptibility of 112 *Haemophilus ducreyi* Isolates, Obtained in Rwanda Between 1986 and 1991

	MIC (mg/L)		
Antimicrobial	MIC range	MIC_{50}	MIC_{90}
Azithromycin	0.002–0.125	0.004	0.008
Ceftriaxone	0.001–0.06	0.001	0.002
Ciprofloxacin	0.002–0.06	0.015	0.015
Erythromycin	0.004–0.25	0.015	0.03
Trimethoprim	0.06–32	2.0	32
Trimethoprim–sulfamethoxazole (1:19)	0.6–320	20	320

TMP–SMZ-resistant isolates were resistant to TMP (MIC $\geq$ 4.0 mg/L), and 15 of the 51 TMP-resistant isolates (29%) were still susceptible to the combination TMP–SMZ (MIC $\leq$ 2.0/38 mg/L). The modes of action of TMP and SMZ are complementary, affecting different stages in folate metabolism, a potent synergistic effect exists between both antimicrobials, and this may result in an increase of up to about tenfold in antibacterial activity and to a frequently bactericidal action of the combination, whereas the components individually are generally bacteriostatic.

The data in the present study strongly suggest that the appearance of TMP–SMZ-resistant *H. ducreyi* isolates in Rwanda is a consequence of a recent emergence of TMP resistance. Resistance to TMP may be due to several mechanisms. It is often due to plasmid-mediated dihydrofolate reductases that may become incorporated into the chromosome by transposons. It may also be due to overproduction of dihydrofolate reductase, changes in cell permeability, or bacterial mutants that are intrinsically resistant to TMP because they depend on exogenous thymine and thymidine for growth (3).

Our in vitro antimicrobial susceptibility study suggest that TMP–SMZ should no longer be recommended for treatment of chancroid in Rwanda, and possibly elsewhere in Central Africa. Erythromycin is now recommended as the primary treatment regimen, although single-dose treatment with ceftriaxone, ciprofloxacin, and potentially azithromycin, may offer attractive alternatives.

REFERENCES

1. Aldridge KE, Commarata C, Martin DH. Comparison of the in vitro activities of various parenteral and oral antimicrobial agents against endemic *Haemophilus ducreyi*. Antimicrob Agents Chemother 1993; 37:1986–1988.
2. Dangor Y, Ballard RC, Miller SD, Koornhof HJ. Antimicrobial suscepti-

bility of *Haemophilus ducreyi*. Antimicrob Agents Chemother 1990; 34:1303–1307.

3. Foster TJ. Plasmid-determined resistance to antimicrobial drugs and toxic metal ions in bacteria. Microbiol Rev 1983; 47:361–409.

4. Knapp JS, Back AF, Babst AF, Taylor D, Rice RJ. In vitro susceptibility of isolates of *Haemophilus ducreyi* from Thailand and the United States to currently recommended and newer agents for treatment of chancroid. Antimicrob Agents Chemother 1993; 37:1552–1555.

5. Motley M, Sarafian SK, Knapp JS, Zaidi AA, Schmid G. Correlation between in vitro antimicrobial susceptibilities and β-lactamase plasmid contents of isolates of *Haemophilus ducreyi* from the United States. Antimicrob Agents Chemother 1992; 36:1639–1643.

6. Plourde JP, D'Costa LJ, Agoki E, Ombette J, Ndinya-Achola JO, Slaney LA, Ronald AR, Plummer FA. A randomized, double blind study of the efficacy of fleroxacin versus trimethoprim–sulfamethoxazole in men with culture-proven chancroid. J Infect Dis 1992; 165:949–952.

7. Plummer FA, Nsanze H, D'Costa LJ, Karasira P, MacLean IW, Ellison RH, Ronald AR. Single-dose therapy of chancroid with trimethoprim–sulfametrole. N Engl J Med 1983; 309:67–70.

8. Schmid GP. Treatment of chancroid. Rev Infect Dis 1989; 12(suppl 6):S580–589.

9. Taylor DN, Pitarangi C, Echeverria P, Panikabutra K, Suvongse C. Comparative study of ceftriaxone and trimethoprim–sulfamethoxazole for the treatment of chancroid in Thailand. J Infect Dis 1985; 152:1002–1006.

10. World Health Organization. Recommendations for the management of sexually transmitted diseases. WHO/GPA/STD/93.1, 1993.

Antibiotic Susceptibility of *Ureaplasma urealyticum*

Z. Samra, S. Rosenberg, and L. Kaufman

Beilinson Medical Center
Petah Tiqva, Israel
Tel Aviv University
Tel Aviv, Israel

INTRODUCTION

Ureaplasma urealyticum is considered a sexually transmitted pathogen responsible for some pathological conditions of the urogenital tract in males and females (1), as well as other infections, particularly in immunosuppressed patients (2) and newborn infants (3). Cassel et al. (4) and Israeli et al. (5) have recently shown that *U. urealyticum* is the most common organism isolated from the lower airways of premature infants. Its presence has been associated with a higher incidence of chronic lung disease and increased mortality in extremely low birth weight infants. Infection with *U. urealyticum* is often treated with tetracycline and erythromycin (6). Resistance and side effects to these antibiotics indicate that alternative active chemotherapeutic agents are important (7). The aim of the present study was to compare the activity of roxithromycin, a new macrolide, with that of tetracycline, doxycycline, and erythromycin against clinical isolates of *U. urealyticum*.

MATERIALS AND METHODS

The antibiotic susceptibility of 143 *U. urealyticum* clinical isolates from genital and respiratory specimens was tested by the agar dilution method (8). The minimal inhibitory concentration (MIC) of roxithromycin (Rulid, Roussel, France), tetracycline, doxycycline, and erythromycin was determined. A7 agar plates were prepared with antibiotic dilutions as a twofold series, ranging from 0.125–128 μg/ml. The inoculum was prepared by inoculating A7 broth medium with tenfold dilutions of the organism. The dilution that just showed a color change after an 18-h incubation was used as the inoculum. This culture was diluted 1:100 and 1:1000 in A7 broth, and 20 μl of the two dilutions were spotted onto duplicate A7 agar plates with antibiotics. Control plates without antibiotics were included. In addition, to ensure the reproducibility of the results, some isolates were tested on different days. Plates were incubated at 37°C and examined microscopically after 3 and 4 days. The MIC was defined as the lowest antibiotic concentration that completely inhibited visible microscopic growth.

RESULTS

The MICs of the four antibiotics for the 143 *U. urealyticum* clinical isolates are given in Table 1 and Figure 1. Growth of 97.9% of the isolates was inhibited by ≤4 μg/ml roxithromycin (ROX); in 60.8% of these isolates, the MIC values was ≤2 μg/ml. Doxycycline (DOX), tetracycline (TC), and erythromycin (ERY), in concentrations of ≤4 μg/ml, inhibited 90.9, 69.9, and 27.3% of the isolates, respectively. The highest MIC observed for ROX was 8 μg/ml, for only three isolates (2.1%). One of them was very resistant to the other three antibiotics and was inhibited by 32 μg/ml ERY, 64 μg/ml DOX, and 128 μg/ml TC. The other two isolates were inhibited by 16 μg/ml ERY, 8 μg/ml DOX, and 16 μg/ml TC. The highest MIC observed for DOX was 64 μg/ml (five isolates), and for TC, 128 μg/ml (six isolates). No difference was observed between the incubation periods or the two inoculum dilutions. The test method

Table 1 Minimal Inhibitory Concentration (MIC) of Four Antibiotics for 143 *Ureaplasma urealyticum* Isolates

	MIC/(μg/ml)	No. isolates (%)	
Roxithromycin	1–4	140	(97.9)
	8	3	(2.1)
Erythromycin	4	39	(27.3)
	8	76	(53.1)
	16–32	28	(19.6)
Doxycycline	0.5–4	130	(90.9)
	8	5	(3.5)
	16–64	8	(5.6)
Tetracycline	1–4	100	(69.9)
	8	24	(16.8)
	16–128	19	(13.3)

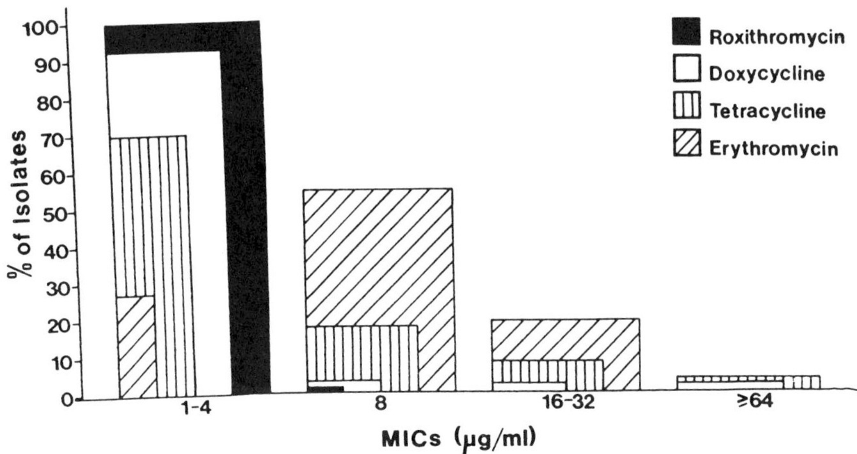

Figure 1 Activity (MIC) of four antibiotics against 143 *Ureaplasma urealyticum* clinical isolates.

showed excellent reproducibility between the duplicates tested on the same day and between assays done on different days.

DISCUSSION

Tetracycline and erythromycin are the drugs of choice in the treatment of *U. urealyticum* infections (6). However, side effects and resistance to these antibiotics indicate the need for an alternative chemotherapeutic agent (7). In this study, the in vitro activity of ROX, a new macrolide, was compared with that of ERY, DOX, and TC. The results indicate that ROX shows the best activity. Of the isolates, 97.9% were inhibited by ≤4 µg/ml ROX, and 60.8% of them by ≤2 µg/ml. The remaining 2.1% were inhibited by 8 µg/ml. A high resistance was observed for TC and DOX in 4.2 and 3.5% of the isolates, respectively, with MIC ≥64 µg/ml. The testing method showed excellent reproducibility between the duplicates tested on the same day and between assays done on different days. The recommended adult oral dosage of ROX is 150 mg twice daily. After a single dose of 150 mg, the mean plasma concentration is approximately 7 µg/ml after 2 h. This compares with a maximum of 1.8 µg/ml following administration of a single dose of 500 mg ERY.

Roxithromycin is well tolerated and is extensively distributed throughout tissue and body fluids, with a corresponding plasma concentration that is higher and greater than the MIC for susceptible bacteria (9). The percentage of the drug recovered was 12% in urine and 88% in feces. The excellent penetration of ROX into the respiratory and genital tissues (10) indicates that this drug may prove useful in the treatment of respiratory and genitourinary tract infections.

REFERENCES

1. Samra Z, Borin M, Bukowsky Y, Lifshitz Y, Sompolinsky D. Nonoccurrence of *Mycoplasma genitalium* in clinical specimens. Eur J Clin Microbiol Infect Dis 1988; 7:49–51.

2. Haller M, Forst H, Ruckdeshel G, Denecke H, Peter K. Peritonitis due to *Mycoplasma hominis* and *Ureaplasma urealyticum* in a liver transplant recipient. Eur J Clin Microbiol Infect Dis 1991; 10:172.

3. Waites KB, Rudd PT, Crouse DT. Chronic *Ureaplasma urealyticum* and *Mycoplasma hominis* infections of the central nervous system in preterm infants. Lancet 1988; 1:17–21.

4. Cassel GH, Waites KB, Crouse DT. Association of *Ureaplasma urealyticum* infection of the lower respiratory tract with chronic lung disease and death in very low birthweight infants. Lancet 1988; 2:240–245.

5. Izraeli S, Samra Z, Sirota L, Merlob P, Davidson S. Genital mycoplasmas in preterm infants: prevalence and clinical significance. Eur J Pediatr 1991; 150:804–807.

6. Rylander M, Hallander HO. In vitro comparison of the activity of doxycycline, tetracycline, erythromycin and a new macrolide CP-62993, against *Mycoplasma pneumoniae*, *Mycoplasma hominis* and *Ureaplasma urealyticum*. Scand J Infect Dis [Suppl] 1988; 3:12–17.

7. Taylor-Rubinson D, Furr PM. Clinical antibiotic resistance of *Ureaplasma urealyticum*. Pediatr Infect Dis 1986; 5:S335–337.

8. Kenney GE, Cartwright FD, Roberts MC. Agar dilution method for determination of antibiotic susceptibility of *Ureaplasma urealyticum*. Pediatr Infect Dis 1986; 5:S332–334.

9. Young RA, Gonzalez JP, Sorkin EM. Roxithromycin. A review of its antibacterial activity, pharmacokinetic properties and clinical efficacy. Drugs 1989; 37:8–41.

10. de Grandi P, Conte R, von Moss G, Grutter F, Pechere JC. Concentration of roxithromycin in plasma and gynaecological tissues following repeated oral administration. Br J Clin Pract 1988; 42; 55(suppl):84–85.

In Vitro Susceptibility of *Mycoplasma hominis* and *Ureaplasma urealyticum* to Virginiamycin

P. Sednaoui and S. Kowalski-Foray

Institut Alfred Fournier
Paris, France

INTRODUCTION

Mycoplasmas are small prokaryotes, classified as mollicutes among the bacteria, characterized by the absence of a cell wall. Their particular structure influences their cultural properties as well as their resistance to some antibiotics. Five species can be found as normal components of the genital flora in about 20–50% of healthy carriers: *Ureaplasma urealyticum, Mycoplasma hominis, M. genitalium, M. fermentans, M. penetrans.*

Only *U. urealyticum, M. hominis,* and *M. genitalium* are associated with infectious disorders, including urethritis, epididymitis, vaginosis, endometritis, salpingitis, infertility, postpartum sepsis, and neonatal infections. Their role as pathogens is considered when bacterial counts are $\geq 10^4$ unit color change organisms per milliliter (UCC/ml).

Since mycoplasmas are devoid of a bacterial wall, they are naturally resistant to β-lactams, rifamycin, polymyxin, and glycopeptides. Some species are naturally resistant to macrolides and lincosamides. For instance, *M. hominis* and *M. fermentans* are always resistant to 14-carbon macrolides (e.g., erythromycin), but generally susceptible to 16-carbon macrolides (e.g., josamycin) as well as to lincosamides; *U. urealyticum* is always resistant to lincosamides. In vitro mycoplasmas are mostly susceptible to tetracyclines, macrolides, synergistines, fluoroquinolones, and fusidic acid. Obviously, acquired plasmid-mediated resistance may occur, such as resistance to tetracycline in 5% of *U. urealyticum* and *M. hominis* (*tetM* transposable element). Resistance to erythromycin or fluoroquinolones may also occur. Thus, pathogenic mycoplasmas must be systematically checked for susceptibility to these antibiotics.

PURPOSE OF THE STUDY

The purpose of our study was to compare the in vitro activities of eight antimicrobial agents—erythromycin (Abbott), josamycin (Roger Bellon), lincomycin (Upjohn), pristinamycin (Rhone-Poulenc), virginiamycin (Smith Kline Beecham), doxycycline (Pfizer), minocycline (Lederle), and ofloxacin (Roussel Uclaf)—against 37 *U. urealyticum* and 15 *M. hominis* clinical isolates from 42 women attending the sexually transmitted disease clinic at the Institut Alfred Fournier in Paris.

PATIENTS AND METHODS

The 42 patients had urethral and cervical samples investigated routinely for the presence of known and potential pathogens (*Neisseria gonorrhoeae*, *Chlamydia trachomatis*, *Trichomonas vaginalis*, *Candida albicans*, *U. urealyticum*, *M. hominis*) and had vaginal samples collected for semiquantitative analysis of the aerobic and anaerobic bacterial flora. Most of the strains were isolated from the exoendocervical junction and, less frequently, from the urethra, as shown in Table 1. Only titers values of 10^4 UCC/ml or higher were retained in the study, as shown in Table 2.

Table 1 Sources of the Mycoplasma Isolates

Site	*U. urealyticum*	*M. hominis*	*U. urealyticum* + *M. hominis*
Cervix	28	9	4
Urethra	4	1	1

Table 2 Bacterial Counts of *U. urealyticum* and *M. hominis* Clinical Isolates

Titer (UCC/ml)	*U. urealyticum* (no. strains)	*M. hominis* (no. strains)
10^4	18	6
10^5	11	3
10^6	6	4
10^7	1	0
10^8	1	2

Table 3 Organisms Associated with Mycoplasma Isolates

Organism	No. cases (%)
Anaerobes including	22 (42.3)
Prevotella bivia	7
Mobiluncus spp.	3
Gardnerella vaginalis	4
Trichomonas vaginalis	3 (5.8)
Candida albicans	2 (3.8)
Chlamydia trachomatis	1 (1.9)

Positive mycoplasma isolation was often associated with other organisms, mostly *T. vaginalis* and anaerobic bacteria commonly found in vaginosis (Table 3). Although genital samples were systematically checked for the presence of *N. gonorrhoeae*, no positive detection was obtained.

Antibiotic susceptibility testing was performed by the broth dilution technique in microtiter plates, using M42 broth (supplemented with 10 mM arginine) for *M. hominis* and U9 broth (supplemented 10 mM urea, 20% horse serum, and 10% fresh yeast extract) for *U. urealyticum*. Bacterial inoculum ranged from 10^3 to 10^4 UCC/ml, according to the recommendation of the Antibiogram French Committee. Results were scored after a 24- 48-h incubation at 37°C in a microaerophilic atmosphere.

RESULTS

Table 4 shows that 76% *U. urealyticum* strains were resistant or intermediate to erythromycin, 35% intermediate to ofloxacin, and 8% resistant or intermediate

Table 4 Antibiogram of *U. urealyticum* Isolates

Antibiotics	Critical concentrations (mg/L)		Susceptible No. strains (%)		Intermediate No. strains (%)		Resistant No. strains (%)	
Erythromycin	1	>8	9	(24)	27	(73)	1	(2.7)
Josamycin	1	>8	37	(100)	0	(0)	0	(0)
Lincomycin	2	>8	0	(0)	0	(0)	37	(100)
Pristinamycin	2	>2	37	(100)	0	(0)	0	(0)
Virginiamycin	2	>2	37	(100)	0	(0)	0	(0)
Doxycycline	4	>8	33	(89.2)	1	(2.7)	2	(5.4)
Minocycline	4	>8	33	(89.2)	1	(2.7)	2	(5.4)
Ofloxacin	1	>4	24	(64.9)	13	(35.1)	0	(0)

Table 5 Antibiogram of *M. hominis* Isolates

Antibiotics	Critical concentrations (mg/L)		Susceptible No. strains (%)		Intermediate No. strains (%)		Resistant No. strains (%)	
Erythromycin	1	>8	0	(0)	0	(0)	15	(100)
Josamycin	1	>8	15	(100)	0	(0)	0	(0)
Lincomycin	2	>8	15	(100)	0	(0)	0	(0)
Pristinamycin	2	>2	15	(100)	0	(0)	0	(0)
Virginiamycin	2	>2	15	(100)	0	(0)	0	(0)
Doxycycline	4	>8	15	(100)	0	(0)	0	(0)
Minocycline	4	>8	15	(100)	0	(0)	0	(0)
Ofloxacin	1	>4	15	(100)	0	(0)	0	(0)

to doxycycline and minocycline. All *U. urealyticum* isolates were susceptible to josamycin, pristinamycin, and virginiamycin. The 15 *M. hominis* isolates that expressed natural resistance to erythromycin, were susceptible to josamycin, lincomycin, pristinamycin, virginiamycin, doxycycline, minocycline, and ofloxacin as shown in Table 5. The MIC_{50} and MIC_{90} to virginiamycin of *U. urealyticum* and *M. hominis* were determined from the data shown in the Table 6. The MIC_{50} and MIC_{90} of virginiamycin to *M. hominis* strains were 0.25 and 0.39 mg/L, respectively; MIC_{50} and MIC_{90} of virginiamycin to *U. urealyticum* strains were 0.6 and 1.1 mg/L, respectively.

CONCLUSION

Genital mycoplasmas (37 *U. urealyticum* and 15 *M. hominis*) in our study were all associated with pathogenic conditions, as assessed by the bacterial burden in the various samples and frequent association with agents of vaginosis. Only *U. urealyticum* isolates were resistant to erythromycin, doxycycline, minocycline, and fluoroquinolone. But all *U. urealyticum* and *M. hominis* isolates were susceptible to virginiamycin. Thus, the use of synergistins in the treatment of genital infections caused by mycoplasma must be considered highly efficient.

Table 6 In Vitro Susceptibility of *U. urealyticum* and *M. hominis* to Virginiamycin

Antibiotic concentration (mg/L)		0.1	0.2	0.4	0.8	1.56	3.12	6.25
U. urealyticum	No. strains	0	1	1	26	9	0	0
	% cumulated	0	2.7	5.4	75.7	100	100	100
M. hominis	No. strains	0	4	10	1	0	0	0
	% cumulated	0	26.7	93.3	100	0	0	0

ACKNOWLEDGMENTS

We thank M. C. Wallez for technical assistance and J. M. Alonso for critical review of the manuscript.

REFERENCES

1. Shepard MC. Culture medium for mycoplasma. In: Tully JG, Razin S, eds. Methods in Mycoplasmology. 1983; 1:37–46.
2. Senterfit LB. Antibiotic sensitivity testing mycoplasmas. In: Tully JG, Razin S, eds. Methods in Mycoplasmology 1983; 2:397–401.
3. Bebear C. Les infections à mycoplasmes génitaux. Rev Eur Dermatol MST 1991; 3:307–314.
4. Bebear C, de Barbeyrac B, Dewilde A, Edert D, Janvresse C, Layani MP, Le Faou A, Lefevre JC, Mendel I, Renaudin H, Sanson Le Pors, MJ, Thouvenot D, and the Groupe MST. Étude multicentrique de la sensibilité in vitro des mycoplasmes génitaux aux antibiotiques. Pathol Biol 1993; 41:289–293.
5. Bebear C, Renaudin H, Maugein J, De Barbeyrac B, Clerc MT. Pristinamycin and human mycoplasmas: in vitro activity compared with macrolides and lincosamides, in vivo efficacy in *Mycoplasma pneumoniae* experimental infection. Zentralbl Bacteriol, 1990, 20(suppl):77–82.
6. Cassell GH, Cole BC. Mycoplasmas as agents of human diseases. N Engl J Med 1981; 304:80–89.
7. Kenny GE, Cartwright FD. Susceptibilities of *Mycoplasma hominis* and *Ureaplasma urealyticum* to two new quinolones, sparfloxacin and Win 57273. Antimicrob Agents Chemother 1991; 35:1515–1516.
8. Palu G, Valisena S, Barile MF, Meloni GA. Mechanism of macrolide resistance in *Ureaplasma urealyticum*: a study on collection and clinical strains. Eur J Epidemiol 1989; 5:146–153.
9. Renaudin H, Bebear C, Robertson JA. In vitro susceptibility of tetracycline-resistant strains of *Ureaplasma urealyticum* to newer macrolides and quinolones and a streptogramin. Eur J Clin Microbiol Infect Dis 1991; 10:984–986.

Rate of Intracellular Killing of Chlamydiae by Clarithromycin and Erythromycin

J. Segreti and K. Kapell

Rush Medical College
Chicago, Illinois

INTRODUCTION

Chlamydiae are strict intracellular bacteria that are important causes of respiratory and genital tract infections. Effective therapy is possible only with agents that achieve adequate intracellular concentrations. Although clarithromycin and erythromycin achieve high intracellular concentrations, there is no information on how rapidly these drugs kill chlamydiae. We performed time–kill studies to determine the rate of killing of one strain each of *Chlamydia pneumoniae* and *Chlamydia trachomatis* with erythromycin and clarithromycin.

MATERIALS AND METHODS

Chlamydia trachomatis serovar D (ATCC VR-885) and *C. pneumoniae* AR-388 were used in the study. *Chlamydia trachomatis* was cultivated in McCoy cell monolayers and *C. pneumoniae* was cultivated in HL cells. The antibiotics tested included erythromycin and clarithromycin obtained from Abbott Laboratories, North Chicago, Illinois. We used 96-well microtiter plates as previously described (Segreti et al. *Antimicrobial Agents and Chemotherapy*, 31:100). Briefly, 24-h-old McCoy cell monolayers and HL cell monolayers grown in antibiotic-free medium were inoculated with a dilution of either *C. trachomatis* or *C. pneumoniae* known to yield 100–1000 inclusions per well. These were centrifuged at 1000 $\times$ *g* at 25°C for 60 min and then overlaid with 0.1 ml of each drug to yield appropriate twofold dilutions. Cultures were then incubated

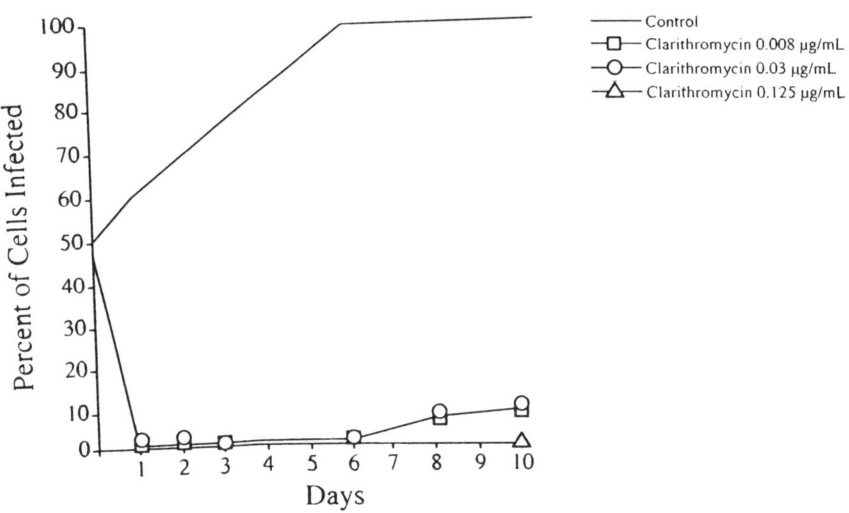

Figure 1 Time–Kill curves of clarithromycin against *C. trachomatis* ATCC VR-885.

at 37°C in 5% CO_2. Cells were fixed with absolute ethanol and stained with fluorescein-conjugated mouse monoclonal antibody to *C. trachomatis* and *C. pneumoniae* (Kallestad, Chaska, MN) at 24, 48, and 72 hr. At 72 hr after addition of antibiotics, the medium was removed and infected cells were washed three times, then refed with fresh antibiotic-free medium. The percentage of infected cells after removal of antibiotics was evaluated on day 3 after antibiotic removal and then also on days 5 and 7 after antibiotic removal. The MIC was defined as the lowest concentration capable of preventing the growth of chlamydiae, as reflected by the portion of infected cells at 72 h posttreatment. The MBC was defined as the lowest concentration capable of reducing the number of chlamydiae present in the cells by day 3 after removal of antibiotics. Bactericidal effect of the antibiotic was confirmed by the lack of regrowth of chlamydiae by day 6 postantibiotic removal.

Under these conditions, *C. trachomatis* was highly susceptible to clarithromycin and less susceptible to erythromycin. In clarithromycin-treated cells, the proportion of infected cells decreased from 50 to 5% during the first 24 h of treatment (Fig. 1). The MIC and MBC were < 0.08 µg/ml. Between days 3 and 5 after antibiotic removal, there was a slight increase in the number of infected cells. There was slight regrowth of *C. trachomatis* at lower concentrations; however, at 0.125 µg/ml, there was no regrowth of *C. trachomatis*.

Erythromycin was significantly less effective against *C. trachomatis* with

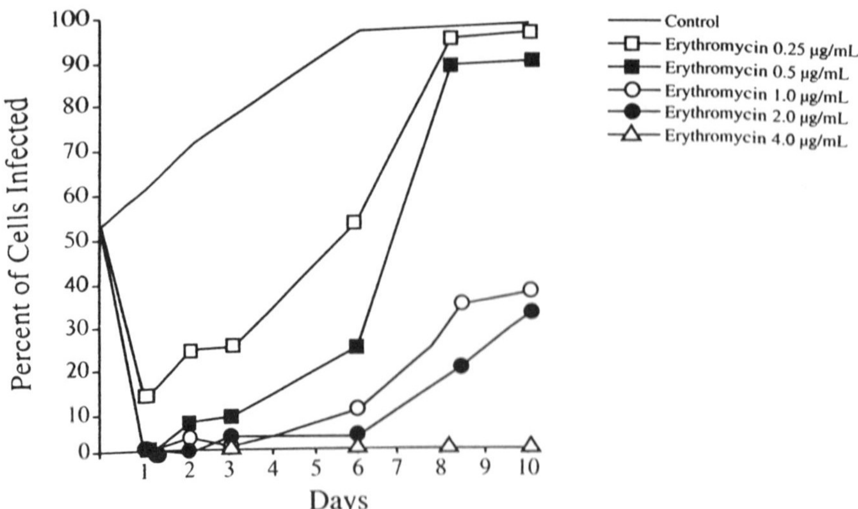

Figure 2   Time–kill curves of erythromycin against *C. trachomatis* VR-885.

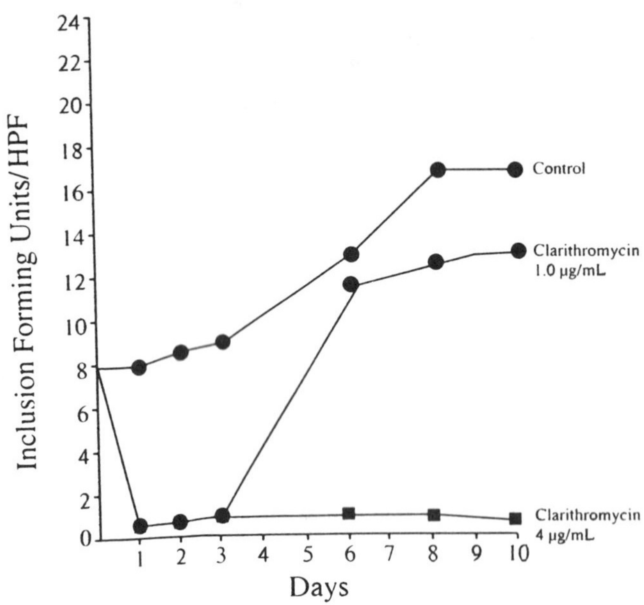

Figure 3   Time–kill curves of clarithromycin against *C. pneumoniae* AR-388.

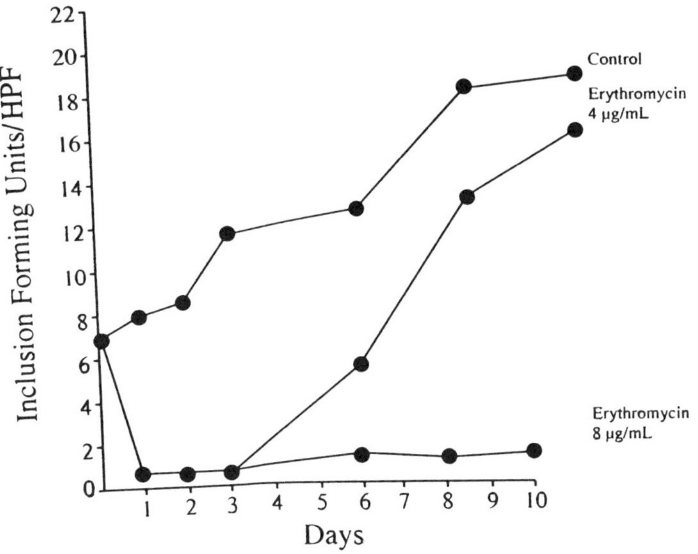

Figure 4   Time–kill curves of erythromycin against *C. pneumoniae* AR-388.

an MBC of 1 µg/ml (Fig. 2). After removal of erythromycin, there was regrowth of *C. trachomatis* at all concentrations < 4 µg/ml.

The results with *C. pneumoniae* were somewhat different (Figs. 3 and 4). Although there was a decline in number of inclusion-forming units by 3 days of exposure to antibiotic with both clarithromycin and erythromycin, there was regrowth of *C. pneumoniae* at postantibiotic removal days 3, 5, and 7 for clarithromycin at 1 µg/ml and for erythromycin at 4 µg/ml. There was no regrowth in cells treated with clarithromycin, 4 µg/ml, and erythromycin, 8 µg/ml.

CONCLUSIONS

Clarithromycin was significantly more effective than erythromycin in killing *C. trachomatis* and in inhibiting its regrowth after removal of antibiotic. Both erythromycin and clarithromycin were bacteriostatic at lower concentrations against *C. pneumoniae*. Clarithromycin was bactericidal at 4 µg/ml, and erythromycin was bactericidal at 8 µg/ml.

Given these results, clarithromycin would be expected to be significantly better than erythromycin in the treatment of *C. trachomatis* infections, and as good as, or possibly slightly better than, erythromycin in the treatment of *C. pneumoniae* infections.

In Vitro Activity of Ten Antibiotic Agents Against *Chlamydia psittaci*

J. Orfila, F. Haider, and A. Bryskier

Centre Hospitalier Regional d'Amiens
Amiens, France

INTRODUCTION

Chlamydia psittaci appears to be involved in about 5% of cases of primary pneumonia requiring hospitalization in the United Kingdom (1) and in 2.3% of cases in Sweden (2). However, these data were derived from complement fixation testing and a serological survey carried out in 1982 in northern France, using a microimmunofluorescence test that gave a prevalence rate of 25% for *C. psittaci* in a population sample of 433 subjects, 38.8% in the subgroup of bird breeders, and 40% in the subgroup of coal miners. The specific antibody titer, ranged from 10 to 128^3. These results were obtained before the introduction of serological testing for *C. psittaci*.

The usual symptoms of infection are pulmonary manifestations, ranging from a "flu-like" syndrome, to potentially fatal hypoxemic pneumonia. The diversity of clinical signs, the possibly life-threatening nature of the infection, and the difficulty of obtaining a rapid etiological diagnosis means that empiric therapy is usually warranted. The aim of our study was to assess the antibacterial activity of ten antibiotics against *C. psittaci*.

MATERIALS AND METHODS

Bacterial Strains

Chlamydia psittaci Loth was isolated from a sick pigeon. McCoy cells were cultured in Eagle's medium, containing fetal calf serum, in 24-well plates. The suspension of *C. psittaci* Loth, titrated at 120×10^6 IFU/ml, was added; the plates were centrifuged for 1 h at 3000 rpm. Antibiotics were added 6 h after inoculation.

Four dilutions of each antibiotic were studied: 0.05, 0.5, 5, and 50 mg/L, with three wells per dilution. The first plate was read after 24 h of contact with the antibiotics, and the second after 48 h. The plates were read by indirect immunofluorescence, with a monoclonal antibody specific for the genus *Chlamydia*. The inclusions were counted in each well by fluorescence microscopy, and the results were calculated as mean for the three wells (as the percentage of infected cells) relative to antibiotic-free control culture.

Fifty-four hours after infection, all the control cells were infected by the second cycle of chlamydia multiplication, and the inclusions were too numerous to count; by convention, the percentage of inclusions in control culture is taken as 100%, corresponding to 200 cells coating the bottom of each well.

Antibiotics

The following antibiotics were tested: roxithromycin, erythromycin, josamycin, spiramycin, minocycline, doxycycline, tetracycline, pristinamycin, pefloxacin, and ofloxacin.

RESULTS

The results are summarized in Table 1.

DISCUSSION

Doxycycline is the most active compound against *C. psittaci* Loth, followed by minocycline (MIC, 0.05 mg/L), roxithromycin (MIC, 0.025 mg/L), and eryth-

Table 1 Percentages of Residual Inclusions Relative to Control (100%)

Antibiotic	0.05 mg/L		0.5 mg/L		5 mg/L		50 mg/L	
Erythromycin	70	8.3	0	0	0	0	0	0
Josamycin	69	8.5	7.1	0.6	5.4	1.2	3.8	0.2
Spiramycin			7.4	2.5	7.4	6.5	8.6	7
Roxithromycin	76.2	0.26	0.	0	0	0	0	0
Tetracycline	72	60	52.28	9.76	47.7	9.1	42.85	5.19
Minocycline	65.3	7.9	0	0.9	0	0	0	0
Doxycycline	10.4	12.5	0	0	0	0	0	0
Ofloxacin	40.3	100	13.8	9.9	0	0.6	0	0.5
Pefloxacin	75.7	100	78.9	100	7.4	3.3	87.3	1.2
Pristinamycin			52.7	8.5	6.9	0.2		

romycin (MIC, 0.1 mg/L). Among the macrolides, spiramycin (MIC, 5 mg/L) and josamycin (MIC, 10 mg/L) are the less active molecules. Ofloxacin (MIC, 0.5 mg/L) shows a better activity than pefloxacin (MIC > 10 mg/L). The MIC value of pristinamycin is 5 mg/L.

Previously published data show good activity for azithromycin (MIC, 0.025 mg/L) and clarithromycin (MIC, 0.05 mg/L), but not for miokamycin (MIC, 2 mg/L), spiramycin (MIC, 5 mg/L), dirithromycin (MIC, 2.5 mg/L), or josamycin (MIC, 10 mg/L), (4).

CONCLUSION

Roxithromycin and azithromycin have similar in vitro activities. Clarithromycin and erythromycin also display good activity. Sixteen-membered ring macrolides exhibit poor activity, and 14-membered ring macrolides are more active than standard fluoroquinolones.

These macrolides offer an alternative therapy to tetracyclines in the treatment of respiratory tract infections caused by *C. psittaci*.

REFERENCES

1. McFarlane JT, Ward MJ, Finch RG, Macrae AD. Hospital study of adult community acquired pneumonia. Lancet 1982; 2:225–228.
2. Berntsson E, Blomberg J, Lagergard T, Trollfors B. Etiology of community-acquired pneumonia in patients requiring hospitalization. Eur J Clin Microbiol 1985; 4:268–272.
3. Orfila J, Pinault J-F, Loisier E, Thomas D. Etude epidemiologique de l'infection a *Chlamydia psittaci* en milieu minier du nord de la France. Rev Roum Med Vir 1982; 33:23–33.
4. Orfila J. Chlamydial infections. In: Bryskier A, Butzler J-P, Neu HC, Tulkens PM, eds. Macrolides, Chemistry, Pharmacology and Clinical Uses. Paris: Arnette Blackwell, 1993:241–252.

Evaluation of Antirickettsial Activity
of Azithromycin and Clarithromycin
in In Vitro Systems

Gershon Keren and Ethan Rubinstein

Sheba Medical Center, Tel-Hashomer Hospital
Tel Aviv, Israel

Avi Keysary, Avi Itzhaki, and Chaya Oron

Israel Institute for Biological Research
Ness-Ziona, Israel

Tel-Aviv University
Tel-Aviv, Israel

INTRODUCTION

Rickettsia conorii, *R. typhi*, and *Coxiella burnetii* are intracellular organisms that cause Mediterranean spotted fever, endemic typhus, and Q-fever, respectively.

Presently, tetracyclines and chloramphenicol serve as the antibiotics of choice for the treatment of these infections (1). However, since tetracyclines are deposited in calcifying tissues, such as teeth and bones, they should not be administered to pregnant or nursing women, or to children younger than 8 years of age. Chloramphenicol use is restricted owing to its most devastating side effect—aplastic anemia. Since macrolides reach effective concentrations in many tissues and penetrate into cells (2–4), their activity against pathogens, such as mycobacteria, chlamydia, and legionella is of great interest (3–5).

The demonstration of antirickettsial activity of macrolides may lead to their use in treating human rickettsioses in patients in whom tetracycline or chloramphenicol cannot be used.

MATERIALS AND METHODS

Antibiotics

1. Azithromycin (AZ, Pfizer Laboratories, USA).
2. Clarithromycin (CL, Abbott Laboratories, USA)
3. Tetracycline: minocycline hydrochloride (Minocin; Lederle, USA).

Rickettsiae

Rickettsia conorii (Moroccan strain), *R. typhi* (Wilmington strain), and *C. burnetii* (phase I, Ohio 314 strain) were used. Rickettsiae were propagated in embryonated yolk sacs. The infected yolk sacs were triturated by Ultra-Thorax, and rickettsiae were partially purified by three differential centrifugation cycles. In each cycle the cell debris pellet was removed by centrifugation at $210 \times g$ for 10 min, and the rickettsiae were sedimented at $17,300 \times g$ for 1 h. The partially purified rickettsiae were suspended in SPG (218 mM sucrose, 37.6 mM KH_2PO_4, 7.1 mM K_2HPO_4, 4.9 mM potassium glutamate; pH 7.0), kept at $-70°C$ and were used to infect the tissue culture cells.

Tissue Cultures

A Vero cell line was used. Cells were grown in Dulbecco's modified minimal essential medium supplemented with 10% fetal calf serum. Cells were grown at 34°C in a CO_2 humidified incubator.

Determination of Antirickettsial Activity of Antibiotics

Vero cells were seeded in 96-well plates, 5×10^4 cells per well in 0.1 ml medium, 1 day before infection. On the day of infection, cells were washed once with Hanks' balanced salt solution plus glucose (HBSSGG) solution and then inoculated with a rickettsial suspension that yielded 0.5–1.5 rickettsiae per cell at zero time, counted microscopically. For *R. conorii* and *R. typhi*, plates were centrifuged at $600 \times g$ for 15 min at room temperature and then incubated for an additional 45 min at 34°C in a humidified CO_2 incubator. *Coxiella burnetii*-inoculated plates were centrifuged for 60 min without further incubation. Then, plates were washed three times with growth-medium containing 1 μg/ml cycloheximide. The *R. conorii*- and *R. typhi*-inoculated cells were incubated at 34°C in a humidified CO_2 incubator for 3 days; *C. burnetii*-inoculated cells were incubated at 37°C in a humidified CO_2 incubator for 6 days.

Rickettsial Growth Determinations

Rickettsial growth determinations were performed by two methods, rickettsial counts and enzyme-linked immunosorbent assay (ELISA). Rickettsial counts were performed as described previously (6). The number of rickettsiae in the infected cells was determined using a modification of the Gimenez stain, as described by Wisseman et al. (7). The medium was aspirated and cells were harvested by addition of 0.1% trypsin solution, and suspended in 15–20 μl phosphate-buffered saline (PBS). A drop of cell suspension was applied onto a slide and dried at room temperature, and slides were kept desiccated until staining. The number of intracellular rickettsiae at each treatment were counted in duplicate. Fifty cells were counted from each well. When there were more than 30 rickettsiae per cell, a value of 30 rickettsiae per cell was assigned.

The ELISA procedure used was a modification of existing methods in which various rickettsial antigens sensitize the solid phase (8,9). This assay was performed in four wells from each treatment. Following aspiration of the medium, cells were fixed with 0.1 ml 80% acetone for 15 min at room temperature, the fixative was aspirated, and the dried plates were kept at 4°C until assayed. Wells were washed once with TST (0.05 M tris pH 7.6; 0.85% NaCl; 0.05% Tween 20), then 0.1 ml of antirickettsial-specific guinea pig serum (1:3000 titer in immunofluorescence assay) at a dilution of 1:100 was applied into each well. Following a 1-h incubation at 37°C, a 1:400 dilution of anti-guinea–IgG:peroxidase conjugate, 0.05 ml/well was added. After similar incubation, ABTS (Sigma) reagent was added for 20 min at room temperature, and the plates were read at 405 nm. Wells containing sham-infected cells served as blank controls.

Evaluation of Antibiotic Activity

Inhibition of rickettsial growth was studied in four to five concentrations of each antibiotic. Since all wells contained the same number of cells, rickettsial growth was derived from the average number of rickettsiae per cell, as determined from rickettsial counts and from the average ELISA value per well.

Rickettsial counts and ELISA determination from control wells (no antibiotics) were considered as 0% inhibition. Values from wells in which 10 μg/ml minocycline, a known inhibitor of rickettsial growth, was present were considered as 100% inhibition. Inhibition rates for each concentration were determined in duplicate.

RESULTS

On inoculation, the number of *R. conorii* per cell was 1.5 ± 0.3 increasing to 27.3 ± 3.0 over a 3-day period. *Rickettsia typhi* multiplied from 1.5 ± 0.6 to 26.6 ± 3.2 organisms per cell over the same period; *C. burnetii* multiplied 27-fold from 0.5 ± 0.2 to 13.7 ± 2.3 over a 6-day period.

The ELISA results were in accordance with rickettsial counts and are presented in Tables 1–3. The ranges of antibiotic concentrations that caused a 50% growth-inhibition (growth IC$_{50}$) for the three rickettsial species are shown

Table 1 Inhibition of *R. conorii* Growth in Vero Cells by Antibiotics

Method	Antibiotic concentration (μg/ml)	% inhibition[d]	
		Azithromycin	Clarithromycin
Count[a,b]	0.001	3 ± 4	
	0.01	7 ± 9	0 ± 0
	0.1	22 ± 9	23 ± 32
	1.0	100 ± 0	89 ± 14
	10.0		100 ± 0
ELISA[c]	0.001	1 ± 1	
	0.01	3 ± 4	0 ± 0
	0.1	45 ± 2	14 ± 9
	1.0	92 ± 11	76 ± 32
	10.0		86 ± 10

[a]Number of rickettsiae per cell was 1.5 ± 0.03 at infection.
[b]Numbers of rickettsiae per cell on day 3 in control and in minocycline-treated cells were 27.3 ± 3.0 and 0.3 ±0.3, respectively.
[c]ELISA values on day 3 in control and minocycline-treated cells were 0.249 ± 0.07 and 0.008 ± 0.008, respectively.
[d]Values are expressed as means ± standard deviation.

Table 2 Inhibition of *R. typhi* in Vero Cells by Antibiotics

Method	Antibiotic concentration (μg/ml)	% inhibition[d]	
		Azithromycin	Clarithromycin
Count[a,b]	0.03	0 ± 4	
	0.01	32 ± 34	15 ± 1
	0.05	100 ± 0	
	0.1		96 ±6
	1.0		100 ±0
ELISA[c]	0.03	11 ± 7	
	0.01	57 ± 20	2 ± 2
	0.05	100 ± 0	
	0.1		84 ± 4
	1.0		90 ±7

[a]Number of rickettsiae per cell was 1.5 ± 0.6 at infection.
[b]Numbers of rickettsiae per cell on day 3 in control and in minocycline-treated cells were 26.6 ± 3.2 and 0.3 ± 0.1, respectively.
[c]ELISA values on day 3 in control and minocycline-treated cells were 0.330 ± 0.09 and 0.069 ± 0.033, respectively.
[d]Values are expressed as means ± standard deviation.

Table 3 Inhibition of *C. burnetii* Growth in Vero Cells by Antibiotics[a,b]

Antibiotic concentration (μg/ml)	% inhibition[c]	
	Azithromycin	Clarithromycin
0.001	24 ± 34	0 ± 0
0.01	56 ± 11	0 ± 0
0.1	58 ± 21	23 ± 32
1.0	63 ± 18	76 ± 4
10.0	81 ± 2	100 ± 3

[a]Number of rickettsiae per cell was 0.5 ± 0.2 upon infection.
[b]Numbers of rickettsiae per cell on day 6 in control and in minocycline-treated cells were 13.7 ± 2.3 and 0.2 ± 0.1, respectively.
[c]Values are expressed as means ± standard deviation.

in Table 4. Growth IC_{50} of all antibiotics were less than 1.0 μg/ml, but azithromycin and clarithromycin had growth IC_{50}s of less than 0.1 μg/ml against *R. typhi*. The growth IC_{50} range for clarithromycin against *C. burnetii* was 0.1–1.0 μg/ml. Azithromycin showed moderate activity over the range of 0.01–1.0 μg/ml.

DISCUSSION

The antirickettsial activity of two novel antibiotics, belonging to the macrolide family, on the growth of *R. conorii*, *R. typhi*, and *C. burnetii* was studied in Vero cells. Azithromycin and clarithromycin largely inhibited the growth of the three studied rickettsial species at a concentration of less than 1.0 μg/ml. This concentration is commonly achieved in humans after conventional dosages and is known to be therapeutic for other infections. An ELISA had not been developed for *C. burnetii* growth determination at the time of the study.

The demonstration of the antirickettsial activity of these new antibiotics encourages their clinical evaluation.

Table 4 Range of Antibiotic Concentration Inhibiting 50% of Rickettsial Growth (Growth IC_{50}) in Vero Cells

Rickettsia	Azithromycin	Clarithromycin (μg/ml)
R. conorii	0.1–1.0	0.1–1.0
R. typhi	0.01–0.05	0.01–0.1
C. burnetii	0.01–0.1	0.1–1.0

REFERENCES

1. Conte JE Jr, Barriere SL. Tetracycline. In: Conte JE Jr, Barriere SL, eds. Manual of Antibiotics and Infectious Diseases. Philadelphia: Lea & Febiger, 1992:60–61.

2. Hand WL, King-Thompeson NL. Uptake of antibiotics by human polymorphonuclear leukocyte cytoplasts. Antimicrob Agents Chemother 1990; 34:1189–1193.

3. Lambert HP, O'Grady FW. Macrolides. In: Lambert HP, O'Grady FW, eds. Antibiotics and Chemotherapy. Edinburgh: Churchill Livingstone, 1992: 168–179.

4. Tulkens PM. Intracellular pharmacokinetics and localization of antibiotics as predictors of their efficacy against intraphagocytic infections. Scand J Infect Dis [Suppl] 1991; 74:209–217.

5. de Lalla FR, Maserati R, Scaprellini P, Marone P, Nicolin R, Caccamo F, Rigoli R. Clarithromycin–ciprofloxacin–amikacin for therapy of *Mycobacterium avium–Mycobacterium intracellulare* bacteremia in patients in AIDS. Antimicrob Agents Chemother 1992; 36:1567–1569.

6. Turco J, Winkler HH. Differentiation between virulent and avirulent strains of *Rickettsia prowazekii* by macrophage-like cell lines. Infect Immun 1982; 35:783–791.

7. Wisseman CL Jr, Waddel AD, Walsh WT. In-vitro studies of the action of antibiotics on *Rickettsia prowazekii* by two basic methods of cell culture. J Infect Dis 1974; 130:564–574.

8. Halle S, Dasch GA, Weiss E. Sensitive enzyme-linked immunosorbent assay for detection of antibodies against typhus rickettsiae *Rickettsia prowazekii* and *Rickettsia typhi*. J Clin Microbiol 1979; 6:101–110.

9. Yamamoto S, Minamishima Y. Serodiagnosis of tsutsugamushi (scrub-typhus) disease by the indirect immunoperoxidase technique. J Clin Microbiol 1982; 15:1128–1132.

Potential Role of Roxithromycin Against the *Mycobacterium avium* Complex

C. B. Inderlied

Children's Hospital of Los Angeles and USC School of Medicine
Los Angeles, California

Lowell S. Young, L. E. Bermudez, and M. Wu

Kuzell Institute for Arthritis and Infectious Diseases
California Pacific Medical Center
San Francisco, California

INTRODUCTION

Infections caused by atypical mycobacteria, such as organisms of the *Mycobacterium avium* complex (MAC) and *M. kansasii*, are common in patients with acquired immunodeficiency syndrome (AIDS; 1–3). In the past, macrolides have not been considered valuable antimycobacterial agents. However, studies of some of the newer compounds have revealed that both azithromycin and clarithromycin are therapeutically active against MAC infections in both animals and humans (4–6). Since roxithromycin shares similar properties with azithromycin and clarithromycin several studies have been undertaken to determine the potential usefulness of this compound for similar indications.

An earlier study reported that roxithromycin, combined with tumor necrosis factor alpha (TNF-α) in a test system, exerted a bactericidal effect against MAC (7). The combination of TNF and an antibiotic in the in vitro test system may, in fact, parallel the situation in vivo. The preliminary evidence of roxithromycin activity against MAC and its activity in the test system with TNF have led to the present series of experiments in which the activity of roxithromycin was reexamined at different pHs against isolates from AIDS patients.

MATERIALS AND METHODS

The activity of roxithromycin was compared with that of azithromycin, flurithromycin, and clarithromycin at concentrations varying from 0.5 to 128 μg/ml against MAC strains. All MAC strains were isolated from patients with AIDS and disseminated MAC disease. A broth radiometric macrodilution method was used to measure the in vitro activity of the antimicrobial agents (8). Roxithromycin activity was measured over 7 days and compared with four controls: no drug, inoculum heat-killed before testing, inoculum diluted 1:100, and inoculum diluted 1:1000. The MIC was determined by generating a dose–response curve of drug concentration versus growth inhibition. The MIC was defined as the lowest concentration of drug that would suppress the cumulative growth index to below 100, compared with the 1:100 or 1:1000 control.

A modified checkerboard assay was used to measure the activity of combinations of drugs, based on the radiometric broth macrodilution assay.

Monolayers containing approximately 10^5 cells were used in the assays. Monolayers infected with MAC were treated with antibiotics for 4 days and then lysed. The lysate was plated onto agar plates and the number of viable intracellular bacteria determined by quantitative plate counts.

RESULTS

Roxithromycin was tested against 24 strains of MAC. In a broth dilution system, with a pH of approximately 6.8, the range of activity was <2–32 μg/ml.

The comparison of roxithromycin activity with that of azithromycin, clarithromycin, and flurithromycin against 15 isolates of MAC is shown in Figure 1. Strains of *M. avium* were less well inhibited by azithromycin and flurithromycin than by clarithromycin and roxithromycin.

Since macrolide activity is known to be influenced by pH, the effect of pH on roxithromycin activity against MAC was tested. Activity was measured at pH 6.9 and 7.4 against all 24 strains. There was a significant shift in the MICs (lower) from pH 6.9 to 7.4 for most strains. This observation agrees with that of Rastogi (9). However, we also observed that at pH 7.4, some MAC strains grew more slowly than at pH 6.9.

Ethambutol is known to potentiate the activity of many antimycobacterial agents (10); therefore, roxithromycin was tested at a low (0.015–0.25 μg/ml) and a high (2–32 μg/ml) concentration range against two MAC strains. In each instance the fractional inhibitory concentrations were 0.56 and 0.38, suggesting that the drugs are additive or synergistic.

Results in the macrophage test system showed roxithromycin activity to be strain-dependent. Against MAC 100 roxithromycin was bactericidal at

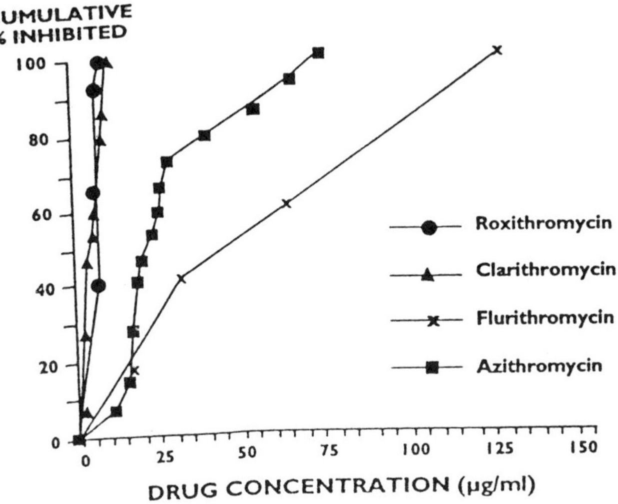

Figure 1   The percentage of MAC strains inhibited at various concentrations of four macrolides: roxithromycin, clarithromycin, flurithromycin, and azithromycin over a range of 0.5–128 µg/ml.

concentrations of 1–64 µg/ml ($p < 0.05$, compared with control). Against MAC 101 and MAC 109, roxithromycin was bacteriostatic at concentrations equal to or greater than 8 µg/ml (MAC 101) and 32 µg/ml (MAC 109).

CONCLUSIONS

On a weight basis alone, the in vitro activity of roxithromycin is most comparable with clarithromycin and significantly more active than either azithromycin or flurithromycin.

The activity of macrolides, including roxithromycin, is strongly influenced by pH, macrolides being more active at a slightly alkaline pH. However, the in vitro growth of MAC is also influenced by pH, many strains growing more slowly at a slightly alkaline pH.

Ethambutol in combination with roxithromycin is additive or synergistic and offers potential for increasing the potency of roxithromycin, since the mechanism of action most likely involves the effect of ethambutol on the mycobacterial cell wall and an increased penetration of roxithromycin to the target site of the drug. However, further studies, including in vivo studies, are necessary to confirm these observations.

In a human macrophage assay, roxithromycin demonstrated modest bactericidal activity at only the highest concentrations (i.e., $\geq$ 16 µg/ml). However,

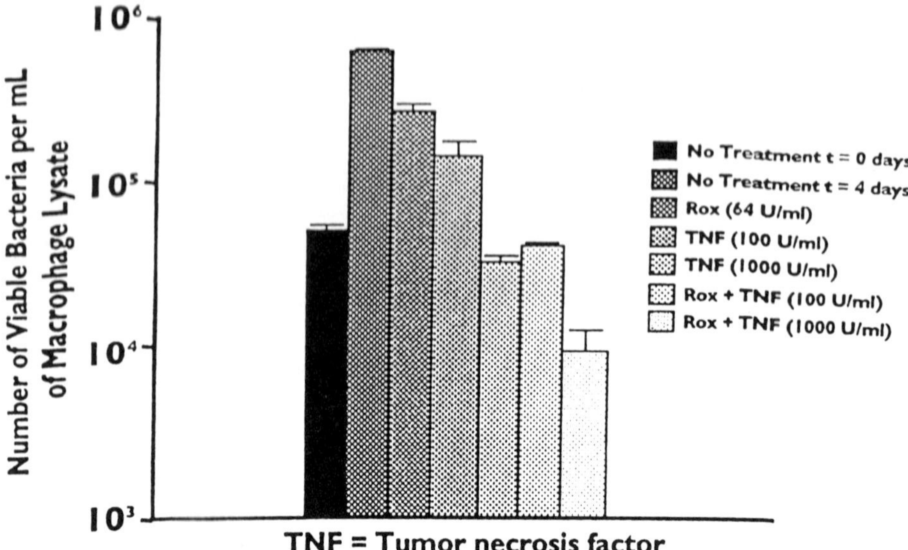

Figure 2   Activity of roxithromycin in combination with TNF against MAC 101 in a human macrophage assay.

the intracellular concentration of roxithromycin was not measured, and the assay was performed using only two MAC strains.

In previous studies with other macrolides, a synergistic interaction between the macrolide and TNF had been observed. Tumor necrosis factor stimulates macrophage mycobactericidal mechanisms. In a test of a single, virulent strain of MAC (101), increased killing of MAC bacilli was seen when roxithromycin, at 64 μg/ml, was added to macrophages stimulated with 100 or 1000 μg/ml TNF (Fig. 2).

The role of macrolides in the treatment of MAC disease is not entirely clear, although in many patients with disseminated MAC disease, treatment with macrolides has been associated with a clinical and microbiological response. The nature of the disease and the pharmacokinetic features of the macrolides certainly suggest that the efficacy of macrolide therapy relates to the pathophysiology of the disease and the ability of these drugs to concentrate in tissues without toxicity.

The correlation of traditional studies of in vitro activity is complicated by factors such as the influence of pH on both the macrolide and the bacterium. Also, although it is known that mycobacteria are capable of inhibiting phagolysosome fusion, thereby possibly promoting the in vivo activity of macrolides, this has never been directly demonstrated.

With an increased understanding of the action of macrolides in the treatment of MAC disease, especially at the mechanistic level, the role of roxithromycin will become clearer, and it is likely that strategies will emerge that will improve the clinical use of this agent. The animal studies of roxithromycin should focus on both assessing its clinical use alone and in combination with other agents, and also on a better understanding of how roxithromycin exerts an antimicrobial effect and how this effect relates to the host–parasite response.

REFERENCES

1. Young LS. *Mycobacterium avium* complex infection. J Infect Dis 1988; 5:863–867.
2. Horsburgh CR Jr. *Mycobacterium avium* complex in the acquired immunodeficiency syndrome (AIDS). N Engl J Med 1991; 324:1332–1338.
3. Levine B, Chaisson RE. *Mycobacterium kansasii*: a cause of untreatable pulmonary disease associated with advanced human immunodeficiency virus infection. Ann Intern Med 1991; 114:861–868.
4. Naik S, Ruck R. In vitro activities of several new macrolide antibiotics against *Mycobacterium avium* complex. Antimicrob Agents Chemother 1989; 33:1616.
5. Young LS, Wiviott L, Wu M, Kolonski PT, Bolan R, Inderlied CB. Azithromycin for treatment of *Mycobacterium avium intracellulare* complex infection in patients with AIDS. Lancet 1991; 338:1107–1109.
6. Dautzenberg B, Truffot C, Legris S, et al. Activity of clarithromycin against *Mycobacterium avium* in patients with the acquired immune deficiency syndrome. Am Rev Respir Dis 1991; 144:564–569.
7. Bermudez LE, Young LS. Activities of amikacin, roxithromycin and azithromycin alone or in combination with tumor necrosis factor against *Mycobacterium avium* complex. Antimicrob Agents Chemother 1988; 32:1149–1553.
8. Inderlied CB. Antimycobacterial agents in vitro susceptibility testing, spectrums of activity, mechanisms of action and resistance, and assays for activity in biological fluids. In: Lorian V, ed. Antibiotics in Laboratory Medicine. Baltimore: Williams & Wilkins, 1991:134–197.
9. Rastogi N, Goh KS, Bryskier A. In vitro activity of roxithromycin against 16 species of atypical mycobacteria and effect of pH on its radiometric MICs. Antimicrob Agents Chemother 1993; 37:1560–1562.
10. Hoffner SE, Kratz M, Olsson-Liljequist B, Svenson SB, Kallenius G. In vitro synergistic activity between ethambutol and fluorinated quinolones against *Mycobacterium avium* complex. J Antimicrob Chemother 1989; 24:317–324.

Activity of Clarithromycin Against *Mycobacterium avium* Complex Determined in Bactec Broth: Effect of pH

D. Moinard, P. Bemer-Melchior, and F. Raffi

G. & R. Laënnec University Hospital
Nantes, France

INTRODUCTION

Mycobacterium avium complex (MAC) is responsible for frequent and severe infections in acquired immunodeficiency syndrome (AIDS) patients. Resistant to many antibiotics and disseminated throughout the body, MAC are very difficult to eradicate. However, there is increasing evidence that treatment of MAC does prolong life and improves the survival quality (4). Currently, clarithromycin (CLA) appears to be one of the most active antibiotics against these bacteria (2,7); its in vitro activity must be evaluated under the best conditions. Macrolides are more active at a basic pH, but commercially available media for mycobacterial cultures have a pH of 6.6–6.7. In this study, the in vitro activity was investigated in Bactec broth at different pHs.

MATERIALS AND METHODS

Strains

The 24 MAC strains used were isolated from the blood of AIDS patients.

Drugs

Clarithromycin (Abbott Laboratories) was dissolved in methanol and further diluted in sterile distilled water to reach a range of final concentrations from 0.125 to 16 mg/L.

Media

Bactec broth (Becton Dickinson) was used at a standard pH of 6.7 and at the physiological pH of 7.4 prevailing in plasma. The broth pH was adjusted to 7.4 by the addition of 120 μl of Na_2HPO_4 solution to the Bactec vials; Na_2HPO_4 was chosen because of its role in the buffered system of the Bactec broth.

Middlebrook agar was supplemented with 10% Middlebrook OADC enrichment and was used at a standard pH of 6.7.

Determination of MICs According to the Bactec Radiometric Procedure (3)

Cultures with a recent growth index (GI) of 999, containing 10^7 CFU/ml, were diluted as follows: 10^{-4} to seed drug-free control vials and 10^{-2} to seed drug-containing vials. The vials were incubated at 37°C and the GIs were recorded daily. In each instance, the values were compared with those of the control vial containing the 1:100 diluted inoculum. The radiometric MIC was the lowest drug concentration that produced a daily GI increase lower than that in the 1% control. This drug concentration was considered to have inhibited more than 99% of the bacterial population. The MICs were determined after comparing the growth of the MAC strains at the two pH values.

Determination of MBCs

The MBCs were determined by subculturing on Middlebrook 7H11 agar. At time zero, the drug-free Bactec vials were plated onto 7H11 Middlebrook agar. After MIC determinations, the vials containing the drug at concentrations $\geq$ MICs were plated onto 7H11 agar. All the plates were incubated at 37°C for 7 days, and the bacterial colonies were counted. The MBC was defined as the minimal concentration of drug that reduced the bacterial count compared with that of drug-free control at time zero.

RESULTS

The MICs determined in Bactec broth at pH 6.7 ranged from 1 to 8 mg/L; 87.5% of the strains were inhibited by 4 mg/L of CLA, and one strain was inhibited by 1 mg/L of CLA (Table 1). In Bactec broth at a pH adjusted to 7.4, MICs ranged from 0.25 to 2 mg/L; 79% of the strains studied were inhibited by 0.5 mg/L of CLA and 95.8% by 1 mg/L. The MBCs were close to MICs (Table 2). The MBC/MIC ratio was similar whether plating cultures onto agar from broth at pH 6.7 or from broth at pH 7.4. The ratio was 1 or 2 against 87.5% of the strains.

Table 1 MICs of Clarithromycin Determined in Bactec Broth Against 24 *Mycobacterium avium* Complex Strains: pH Effect

Bactec broth pH	Clarithromycin (mg/L)						
	0.12	0.25	0.5	1	2	4	8
6.7				1	5	15	3
7.4	1	6	12	4	1		

DISCUSSION AND CONCLUSION

The MICs of CLA against MAC strains varied significantly according to the pH of the medium. The MICs obtained at pH 7.4 were four- to eightfold lower than those measured at pH 6.7. Truffot et al. (5), using two agar media at a standard pH, reported that MICs of CLA obtained on OADC-enriched Mueller–Hinton at pH 7.3 were two dilutions lower than those obtained in the 7H11 agar medium at pH 6.6. At a physiological pH, MICs of CLA against the 24 strains studied were below the C_{max} of the drug in human serum. Clarithromycin is concentrated in cells; but, as with all macrolides, it is less potent at an acidic pH, which was thought to be present within macrophages. However, recently, Crowle et al. (1) demonstrated that the environment of live *M. tuberculosis* and *M. avium* in macrophagic vesicles was not acidic. If that is true, the efficacy of macrolides against MAC should be reassessed.

This in vitro study does not allow the determination of the true activity of a cell-concentrated drug against intracellular bacteria. However, the in vitro tests can suggest great sensitivity of the bacteria or resistance surpassing any cell concentration of a drug. Currently, the Bactec radiometric method appears to be an adequate, easy, and rapid way to determine the in vitro activity of drugs against mycobacteria, but the pH of commercially available Bactec broth appears unsuitable for testing macrolides.

Table 2 MBCs of Clarithromycin Determined from Bactec Broth at pH 6.7 and at pH 7.4 Against 24 *Mycobacterium avium* Complex Strains

Bactec broth pH	Clarithromycin (mg/L)						
	0.25	0.5	1	2	4	8	16
6.7				1	6	15	2
7.4	1	7	8	8			

SUMMARY

By using Bactec broth at pH 6.7 and 7.4, the MICs of clarithromycin against ten *M. avium* complex strains ranged from 1 to 8 mg/L and from 0.25 to 2 mg/L respectively, the MICs obtained at pH 6.7 were four- to eightfold higher than those obtained at pH 7.4. At a physiological pH, MICs were significantly below the C_{max} levels of clarithromycin in human serum. The pH of commercially available Bactec broth appears unsuitable for testing macrolides.

REFERENCES

1. Crowle AJ, Ross R, May MH. Evidence that vesicles containing living, virulent *Mycobacterium tuberculosis* or *Mycobacterium avium* in cultured human macrophages are not acidic. Infect immun 1991; 59:1823–1831.
2. Dautzenberg BS, Legris S, Truffot C, Grosset J, for the Clarithromycin Trial Group. Double blind study of the efficacy of clarithromycin versus placebo in *Mycobacterium avium–intracellulare* infection in AIDS patients [abstract]. World Conference on Lung Health Supplement, Am Rev Respir Dis 1990: 141:A615.
3. Heifets L. MIC as a quantitative measurement of the susceptibility of *Mycobacterium avium* strains to seven antituberculosis drugs. Antimicrob Agents Chemother 1988; 32:1131–1136.
4. Horsburgh CR Jr. *Mycobacterium avium* complex infection in the acquired immunodeficiency syndrome. N Engl J Med 1991; 324:1332–1338.
5. Truffot-Pernot C, Ji B, Grosset J. Effect of pH on the in vitro potency of clarithromycin against *Mycobacterium avium* complex. Antimicrob Agents Chemother 1991; 35:1677–1678.
6. Yajko DM. In vitro activity of antimicrobial agents against the *Mycobacterium avium* complex inside macrophages from HIV-infected individuals: the link to clinical response to treatment? Res Microbiol 1992; 143:411–419.
7. Young LS, Bermudez LE, Inderlied CB. Mycobacteria and AIDS: treatment, prevention and future prospects. Res Microbiol 1992; 143:420–422.

Interaction of Macrolides with Human Neutrophils in Vitro

Marie Thérèse Labro, Houria Abdelghaffar, and El Mostafa Mtairag

INSERM U294
Paris, France

INTRODUCTION

In the past 20 years, the panorama of infectious diseases has been greatly modified by the emergence of new pathogens, the increased resistance of microorganisms to anti-infective drugs, and the growing number of patients with congenital or acquired immune deficiencies. All these aspects should intensify in the near future and result in increased therapeutic problems. Also, the understanding of the host defense system as an ambivalent weapon in infectious diseases, with both beneficial (pathogen destruction) and deleterious (host tissue destruction) responses, has suggested that anti-infectious therapy should involve host response "modulators." Parallel to the combination of antibacterial agents, substances recognized as pure "immunodulators" (e.g., G-, GM-CSFs, cytokines, and others), the possibility that some antimicrobial drugs also interfere with the host defense responses is raising new hopes for the therapeutic armamentarium of the future (1).

Among the many drugs that have been studied extensively in vitro, ex vivo, and to a lesser extent, in vivo, macrolide antibiotics appear to be good candidates in this area of research. Interest in this class of drugs stems mainly from their outstanding ability to concentrate within host cells, particularly phagocytes (2), a property that may partly explain their activity against intracellular pathogens. However, such intracellular accumulation may not be neutral to cell function. Indeed, a large body of evidence demonstrates that macrolides interfere with phagocyte functions (reviewed in 3). Since these cells are crucial effectors in the anti-infectious responses, both at the level of microbial killing and tissue damage, the understanding of mechanism(s) governing the macrolide-induced modification of phagocyte function is an area of active investigation.

Here, we summarize some of our recent data comparing the effects of three 14-membered ring macrolides (roxithromycin, dirithromycin, and its hydrolysis product, erythromycylamine) which are all semisynthetic derivatives of erythromycin as a result of modification at the C-9 position of the lactone ring.

First, we studied the uptake of dirithromycin and erythromycylamine by human neutrophils and then analyzed the consequences of this cellular accumulation on two important neutrophil functions: degranulation and oxidant production.

DIRITHROMYCIN AND ERYTHROMYCYLAMINE UPTAKE BY HUMAN NEUTROPHILS IN VITRO

These data have been recently published (4). Radiolabeled drugs ([^{3}H]dirithromycin, 20 mCi/mg, solution 0.05 mg/ml in ethanol/water, 7:3; and [^{14}C]erythromycylamine, 4.8 μCi/mg) were provided by Eli Lilly Research Laboratories (Indianapolis, IN). Drug uptake was measured by a classic velocity gradient centrifugation method through a water-impermeable silicone–paraffin oil barrier. Cell-associated drugs were first expressed as nanograms per 2.5 $\times$ 10^6 neutrophils. After measurement of the intracellular water space (0.6 $\pm$ 0.06 μl/2.5 $\times$ 10^6 cells: ten experiments) and assessment of the greater than 90% intracellular location of the drugs (fractionation of macrolide-loaded cells), we also determined the cellular/extracellular concentration ratio (C/E).

The degree of drug association with neutrophils was linearly related to extracellular drug concentration, without saturation over the concentration range 0.25–500 mg/L (Fig. 1). Accordingly, the C/E values were constant whatever the extracellular concentration. Uptake was rapid and increased with time, with no saturation up to 180 min (Fig. 2), and erythromycylamine uptake was always significantly lower than that of its parent compound. A point of interest was the extreme interindividual variability observed for the uptake kinetics (Fig. 3), a phenomenon already reported with azithromycin (5), but not with other macrolides.

Drug uptake was not influenced by any metabolic inhibitors assessed (NaN$_3$, 2,4-dinitrophenol, sodium cyanide—after buffering the solution to pH 7.4—, or sodium fluoride) and possible competitive inhibitors of known active transport systems (D-glucose, nucleosides, or amino acids). Only ouabain (an inhibitor of Na$^+$, K$^+$-ATPase) impaired drug uptake by about 30%. Lastly, as observed with other macrolides, extracellular acidic pH decreased and basic pH (up to 9) increased the uptake of both drugs. Activation energy was greater than

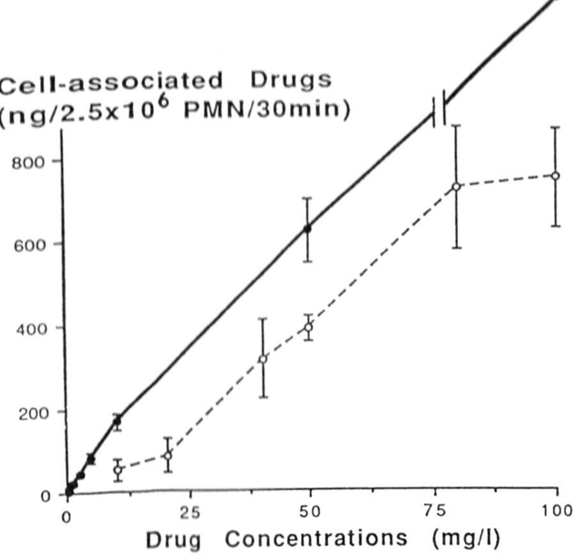

Figure 1 Comparison of dirithromycin (solid circles) and erythromycylamine (open circles) uptake by neutrophils; at an extracellular concentration of 500 mg/ml, cell-associated dirithromycin was 5400 ± 606.1 ng/2.5×10^6 cells per 30 min.

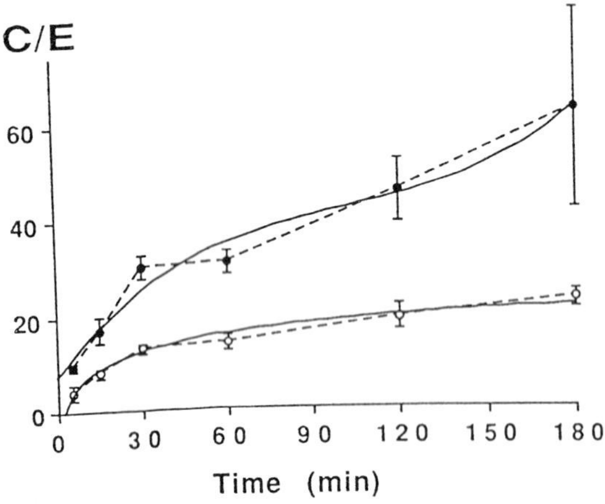

Figure 2 Time-dependent accumulation of dirithromycin (solid circles) and erythromycylamine (open circles). Experimental curves (dotted lines); theoretical curves (solid lines).

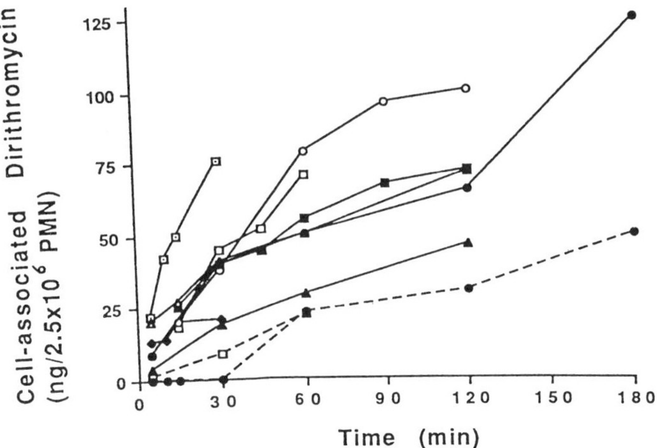

Figure 3 Interindividual variability for kinetics of uptake (dirithromycin: neutrophils from ten different volunteers).

100 kj/mol for both drugs, and as proposed for azithromycin (5), this could be related to the preferential (intragranular) location of these drugs that requires the crossing of two (cytoplasmic and granular) membranes. Accordingly, chloroquine, a lysosomotropic weak base, which alkalinizes intragranular compartments, impaired drug uptake.

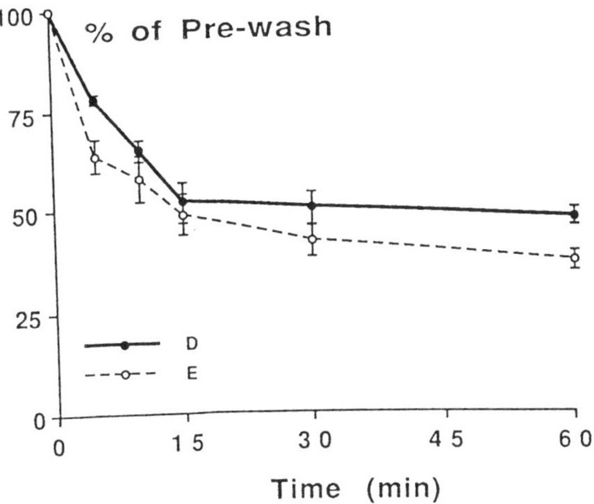

Figure 4 Efflux of dirithromycin (solid circles) and erythromycylamine (open circles) from drug-loaded cells placed in drug-free medium.

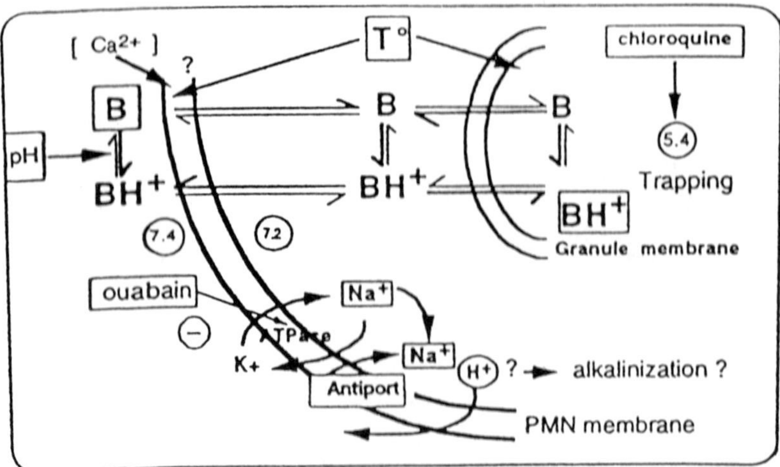

Figure 5   Summary of factors affecting macrolide uptake.

Furthermore, preliminary experiments in our laboratory suggest that about 60–70% of the drugs are located within neutrophil granules, a value largely greater than that reported with roxithromycin and erythromycin (6). In addition, consistent with the hypothesis of ion trapping inside the acidic granules, was that both drugs, at a variance from classic macrolides (6), were released slowly from loaded cells placed into drug-free medium (Fig. 4). This phenomenon further reinforces the similarity of dirithromycin and erythromycylamine with azithromycin, which also egresses slowly from loaded cells (7). Unlike other macrolides, these three molecules possess two basic amine groups, which may favor greater ionization and, consequently, trapping within neutrophil granules.

Figure 5 summarizes the essential mechanism for the intracellular accumulation (granular trapping) of dirithromycin and erythromycylamine (represented as B, for base). The first step, intracellular penetration of the unprotonated (B) form through the cytoplasmic membrane, is far less understood. Although the lipophilicity of the molecules certainly plays a nonnegligible role, other factors seem to be involved. In particular, we recently demonstrated in intact cells and cytoplasts (enucleated granule-poor neutrophils) that extracellular calcium is required for optimal uptake of dirithromycin, erythromycin, and roxithromycin (8). We are currently investigating the link between this cation and macrolide uptake.

EFFECT OF DIRITHROMYCIN, ERYTHROMYCIN, ERYTHROMYCYLAMINE, AND ROXITHROMYCIN ON NEUTROPHIL FUNCTIONS

Degranulation

That macrolides concentrate within neutrophil granules and possibly alkalinize this acidic compartment, prompted us to analyze the consequences of this trapping on neutrophil exocytosis. Dirithromycin and, to a lesser extent, erythromycylamine and erythromycin, directly induced the release of three intragranular enzymes: β-glucuronidase, a marker of azurophilic granules; lactoferrin, a marker of specific granules; and lysozyme, contained in both subsets (9). The macrolide-induced release was dependent on the incubation time (30–180 min; Fig. 6) and drug concentration. The lowest macrolide concentrations that induced significant enzyme release were 10, 100, and 25 mg/L, respectively, for dirithromycin, erythromycylamine, and erythromycin. Interestingly, although roxithromycin and clarithromycin displayed similar "prodegranulating" effects, this was not true for various 16-membered ring macrolides (josamycin, spiramycin, rokitamycin; 10; manuscript in preparation). The biochemical mechanism underlying this effect is under investigation.

Our data raise interesting hypotheses on the intracellular bioactivity of macrolides (mainly located within cell granules), particularly relative to pathogens that inhibit phagolysosomal fusion, such as chlamydiae, *Mycobacterium avium*, *Legionella* spp., and others).

The possibility that the prodegranulating activity of some macrolides counteracts the inhibitory effect of some pathogens on the process of phagolysosomal fusion and, thereby, permits the access both of the antibiotic and the bactericidal granular components to the pathogen-containing endosome, should be further investigated. Such a hypothesis is reinforced by the observation that chloroquine (which also possesses prodegranulating activity) reverses the inhibition of phagolysosomal fusion by some pathogens.

Oxidant Production

Another facet of the functional activity of phagocytes, particularly the neutrophils, is the generation of reactive oxygen species that contribute to both pathogen and host tissue destruction. We and others have previously reported that roxithromycin impairs the human neutrophil oxidative burst (11,12). Preliminary data from our laboratory have shown that dirithromycin, roxithromycin, and erythromycylamine exerted a similar inhibitory effect on the production of oxidant by PMA- and opsonized zymosan-stimulated neutrophils (13). This

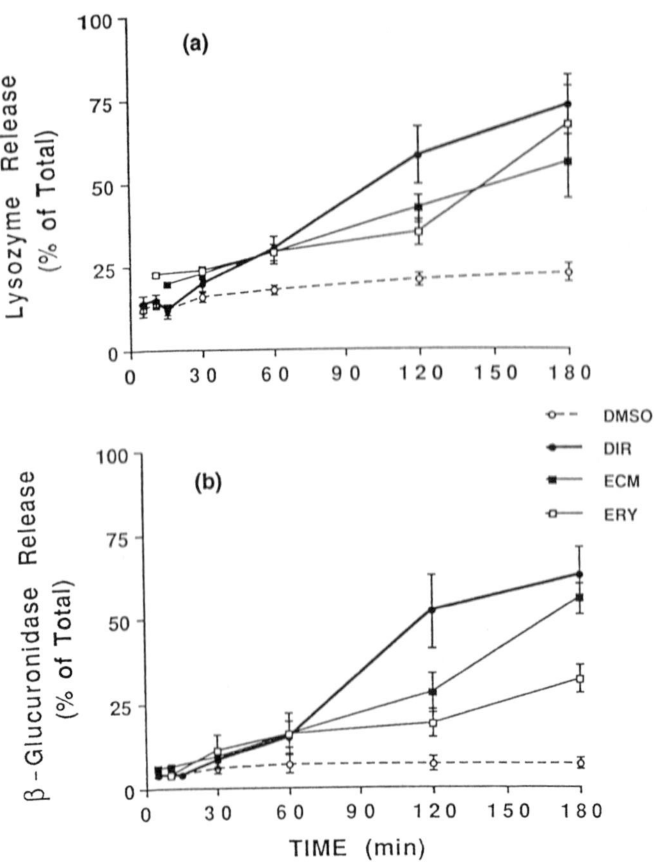

Figure 6 Macrolide-induced neutrophil exocytosis. (From Ref. 9.)

inhibition is time- and concentration-dependent and, as already observed for drug uptake, there is clear interindividual variability in sensitivity to drug-induced effects. In further experiments and in agreement with the literature (14), we demonstrated that macrolide-induced inhibition is not stimulus-specific.

Furthermore, although the underlying mechanism is not completely clear, macrolide-induced inhibition seems to be related to alteration of the reconstitution (not the activity) of an active NADPH oxidase system (manuscript in preparation).

The in vivo relevance of these data remains to be demonstrated. However, our data and those of Jooné et al. (14) show that the antioxidant effect of the macrolides is obtained in vitro at concentrations therapeutically achievable in the serum or tissues (2.5–10 mg/L). That this property sustains the anti-inflammatory activity of macrolides reported in vivo in some experimental models (15,16) requires further investigation.

CONCLUSION

Although macrolides have been used for more than 40 years, only recently has this old class of antibiotics revealed new and stimulating features. Their property of accumulating within host cells, particularly the mobile phagocytes, has been proposed to sustain the modern pharmacokinetic concept of infected tissue-targeted transport and delivery, accounting for the characteristic pharmacokinetic profile of these drugs.

On the other hand, it is quite clear that the C/E parameter does not completely explain the intravascular bioactivity of macrolides, and some of our data may raise interesting prospects for deepening our understanding of macrolide antimicrobial effects.

Lastly, the possibility of using some of the side effects of these molecules to modulate the host inflammatory response is one of the most attractive hypotheses concerning this class of molecules.

It is likely that, in the forthcoming century, this class will continue to expand and that the optimization of the properties mentioned earlier will permit new clinical indications (17).

REFERENCES

1. Labro MT. Immunomodulation by antibacterial agents. Is it clinically relevant? Drugs 1993; 45:319–328.
2. Labro MT. Intraphagocytic penetration of macrolide antibiotics. In: Bryskier AJ, Butzler JP, Neu HC, Tulkens PM, eds. Macrolides: Chemistry, Pharmacology and Clinical Use. Paris: Arnette-Blackwell, 1993: 379–388.
3. Labro MT. Effects of macrolides on host natural defences. In: Bryskier AJ, Butzler JP, Neu HC, Tulkens PM, eds. Macrolides: Chemistry, Pharmacology and Clinical Use. Paris: Arnette-Blackwell, 1993:389–408.
4. Mtairag EM, Abdelghaffar H, Labro MT. Investigation of dirithromycin and erythromycylamine uptake by human neutrophils in vitro. J Antimicrob Chemother 1994; 33:523–536.
5. Laufen H, Wildfeuer A, Lack P. Mechanism of azithromycin uptake in human polymorphonuclear leucocytes. Arzneimittelforschung 1990; 40:686–689.
6. Carlier MB, Zenebergh A, Tulkens PM. Cellular uptake and subcellular distribution of roxithromycin and erythromycin in phagocytic cells. J Antimicrob Chemother 1987; 20(suppl B):47–56.

7. Gladue RP, Bright GM, Isaacson RE, Newborg MF. In vitro and in vivo uptake of azithromycin (CP-62,993) by phagocytic cells: possible mechanism of delivery and release at sites of infection. Antimicrob Agents Chemother 1989; 33:277–282.

8. Labro MT, Abdelghaffar H, Mtairag EM. Extracellular Ca^{2+} is required for macrolide uptake by human neutrophil (PMN) and subsequent PMN exocytosis. Programme and Abstracts of the 93rd General Meeting of the American Society for Microbiology, Las Vegas, 1994: abstr E110.

9. Abdelghaffar H, Mtairag EM, Labro MT. Effect of dirithromycin and erythromycylamine on human neutrophil degranulation. Antimicrob Agents Chemother 1994; 39:1548–1554.

10. Labro MT, Abdelghaffar H, Bryskier A. Effect of macrolides on human neutrophil degranulation. 33rd Interscience Conference on Antimicrobial Agents Chemotherapy, New Orleans, 1993: abstr 309.

11. Labro MT, El Benna J, Babin-Chevaye C. Comparison of the in-vitro effect of several macrolides on the oxidative burst of human neutrophils. J Antimicrob Chemother 1989; 24:561–572.

12. Anderson R. Erythromycin and roxithromycin potentiate human neutrophil locomotion in vitro by inhibition of leukoattractant-activated superoxide generation and autooxidation. J Infect Dis 1989; 159:966–973.

13. Labro MT, El Benna J, Abdelghaffar H. Modulation of human polymorphonuclear neutrophil function by macrolides: preliminary data concerning dirithromycin. J Antimicrob Chemother 1993; 31(suppl C):51–64.

14. Jooné GK, Van Rensburg CEJ, Anderson R. Investigation of the in-vitro uptake, intra-phagocytic biological activity and effects on neutrophil superoxide generation of dirithromycin compared with erythromycin. J Antimicrob Chemother 1992; 30:509–523.

15. Mikasa K, Kita E, Sawaki M, et al. The antiinflammatory activity of erythromycin in zymosan-induced peritonitis of mice. J Antimicrob Chemother 1992; 30:339–348.

16. Agen C, Danesi R, Costa M, Stacchini P, Favini P, Del Tacca M. Macrolide antibiotics as antiinflammatory agents: roxithromycin in an unexpected role. Agents Action 1993; 38:85–90.

17. Bryskier A, Agouridas C, Chantot JF. New medical targets for macrolides. Exp Opinion Invest Drugs 1994; 3:405–410.

Prevalence of Streptogramin Resistance by Acetylation Among Streptogramin-Resistant Staphylococcal Clinical Isolates in France

Roland Bismuth

Centre Hospitalier et Universitaire Pitié-Salpêtrière
Paris, France

François Jehl, Laurence Linger, Christophe Kœchlin, and Henri Monteil

Centre Hospitalier et Universitaire
Strasbourg, France

INTRODUCTION

Pristinamycin (PR) and virginiamycin are antibacterial agents belonging to the streptogramin family, which have been used in Europe as oral and topical agents. They are a mixture of two chemically unrelated molecules (streptogramin A, compound SgA; and streptogramin B, compound SgB) that act synergistically in vivo and in vitro (5). SgA and SgB are present in a respective ratio of 65:25. SgA (or PIIA) is a polyunsaturated cyclic peptolide and SgB (or PIB) a cyclic hexadesipeptide. A novel semisynthetic injectable streptogramin (RP 59500) made of a mixture of SgA and SgB compounds is presently being studied. The resistance of staphylococci to macrolides (M), lincosamides (L), and to SgB compound (S_B) (MLS_B pattern) by target modification has emerged since the introduction of erythromycin use. Expression of MLS_B resistance, encoded by the *erm* gene (6) is constitutive (cons) or inducible (ind) by subinhibitory concentration of drug. In contrast, staphylococci remained susceptible to SgA and to PR, the synergy between SgA and SgB being maintained (4). In France, resistance to PR was first encountered among staphylococci in 1975 (7,8). The prevalence of PR resistance still remains low ($\leq 3\%$) and is detected essentially among methicillin-resistant strains (8).

Resistance to streptogramins owing to modification of both factors, was first described in 1975 in *Staphylococcus aureus* (7). The resistant strains harbored a large plasmid containing genes encoding streptogramin A acetyl transferase (SgA-AC) and streptogramin B hydrolase (SgB-H) (10). This resistant pattern was easily detected by disk diffusion (4,10). The genes *vat* (3) and *vgb* (2) encoding SgA-AC and SgB-H, respectively, were recently isolated and sequenced. Resistance to SgA and to L has been described (8; LS_A pattern). Some strains inactivated SgA (8). These enzymatic resistances were, or were not, associated with MLS_B resistance (4–10).

The aim of this study was to analyze the prevalence of enzymatic inactivation of SgA and SgB among PR-resistant staphylococci collected in different French hospitals. We used high-performance liquid chromatography (HPLC) procedures (9) that allowed the detection of inactivation of SgA and SgB and the appearance of transformation products SgA-AC.

MATERIAL AND METHODS

Bacterial Strains

Eighty-nine MLS-resistant clinical isolates of staphylococci (50 *S. aureus* and 39 coagulase-negative staphylococci, CNS) were selected in 25 French university hospitals during 1992 and 1993. The distribution of the strains among the different resistance patterns is summarized in Table 1.

Methods

The susceptibility to MLS was tested by the diffusion method, using disks of erythromycin (Em), spiramycin, lincomycin, pristinamycin (PR) SgA (20 μg), and SgB (40 μg). The enzymatic inactivation of SgA and SgB was detected by Gots test. The MICs of Em, PR, SgA, and SgB were determined by the agar dilution method. The inactivation of SgA and SgB and the appearance of SgA-AC were measured by SgA- and SgB-selective HPLC assay procedures as described previously (9).

Two reference strains were tested: RN 450-susceptible *S. aureus* and STE *S. aureus*, which harbored a plasmid encoding *vga*, *vgb*, and *vat* genes (1–3). Ten susceptible and ten MLS_B staphylococci were also tested.

Table 1 Main Patterns of Resistance of Staphylococci to MLS

| | | MLS_B | | | | | MLS_B-ind | MLS_B-cons | |
	Susceptible	ind[a]	cons	LS_A	LS_A–S_B	L[b]	+ LS_A	+LS_A	+ LS_A – S_B
Erythromycin	S[c]	R	R	S	S	S	R	R	R
Spiramycin	S	S	R	S	S	S	S	R	R
Lincomycin	S	S	R	I/R	I/R	I/R	I/R	R	R
Streptogramin A	S	S	S	R	R	S	R	R	R
Streptogramin B	S	S	R	S	R	S	S	R	R
Pristinamycin	S	S	S	I/S	I/R	S	I/S	I/R	I/R
65% SgA + 25% SgB)									
Genes	–	*ermA/ermC*		*vat/vga*	*vat/vga* +*vgb*	*linA*		+ *vat/vga*	*ermA/ermC* + *vat/vga* +*vgb*
No. strains	10	10		23	4	None tested	10	48	4

[a]ind, inducible; cons, constitutive.
[b]Not tested in this study.
[c]S, susceptible; 1, intermediate; R, resistant.

RESULTS

The inactivation of SgA and the appearance of acetyl SgA were detected in 36 strains (26 *S. aureus* and 10 CNS; Tables 2 and 3).

Four LS_A–S_B *S. aureus*
Four MLS_B plus LS_A–S_B strains: three *S. aureus* and one *S. epidermidis*
Five LS_A strains: four *S. aureus* and one *S. epidermidis*
Twenty-three MLS_B plus LS_A strains: 15 *S. aureus*, 8 CNS

All the eight LS_A–S_B ($\pm$ MLS_B) strains hydrolyzed SgB and the Gots test was positive for SgA and SgB. Among LS_A strains ($\pm$ MLS_B; 19 *S. aureus*, 9 CNS), the Gots test for SgA was positive for only 16 strains.

The MIC values for PR varied according to the pattern of the strains the MICs of PR ranged from 0.25 mg/L among susceptible strains, to 0.75 mg/L when one compound of PR was modified (MLS_B-cons, LS_A, MLS_B-ind + LS_A). The MIC was 10 mg/L when two compounds were modified (LS_A–S_B and MLS_B + LS_A) and increased to 32 mg/L in strains harboring the composite pattern MLS_B + LS_A–S_B. The genes contributed qualitatively and quantitatively to the PR resistance level of the host.

No activation of SgA was detected in 53 strains (24 *S. aureus* and 29 CNS; see Tables 2 and 3).

18 LS_A strains (13 *S. aureus* and 5 CNS)
8 MLS_B-ind + LS_A strains (6 *S. aureus* and 2 CNS)
27 MLS_B-cons + LS_A strains (5 *S. aureus* and 22 CNS)

The Gots test for SgA was negative. The MIC values of PR varied, as previously according to the pattern of the strains: the MICs of PR passed from 0.7 mg/L among LS_A or MLS_B-ind + LS_A strains to 4 mg/L among MLS_B-cons + LS_A strains. The other(s) mechanism(s) involved in SgA-resistant strains as active efflux (*vga* gene) did not modify the PR-resistance level.

DISCUSSION AND CONCLUSION

1. The acetylation of SgA demonstrated by Dublanchet et al. (7) was probably the main mechanism imparting resistance to SgA and PR in clinical isolates of staphylococci. This mechanism was detected in 40% of the strains tested.
2. This mechanism was detected among *S. aureus* and CNS strains and was combined with SgB hydrolase, as described in STE strains (17), or alone, as described recently (8). Contrary to SgA, SgB was never detected alone. This phenomenon produced a different segregation of the two genes from the same original plasmid.

Table 2 Activity of Streptogramins, Percentage of Inactivation of Streptogramin A and Appearance of Acetyl Streptogramin A Among MLS$_B$ + LS$_A$ or LS$_A$–S$_B$ Staphylococcal Strains

Resistance patterns	No. strains	Em[a]	PR	SgA	SgB	SgA (SgB) inactivation (%)	SgA–Ac[b] appearance (%)	Gots test SgA	Gots test SgB
SgA–Ac-positive strains									
MLS$_B$-cons+LS$_A$–S$_B$ *S. aureus*	3	>128	32	128	>128	−38(−63)	+62	+	+
MLS$_B$-cons+LS$_A$–S$_B$ CNS[c]	1	>128	32	64	>128	−90(−55)	+47	+	+
MLS$_B$-ind[d]+LS$_A$ *S. aureus*	2	>128	0.5	48	8	−20	+4.3	−	−
MLS$_B$-cons+LS$_A$ *S. aureus*	13	>128	14.8	128	>128	−77	+17.4	+	−
MLS$_B$-cons+LS$_A$ CNS	8	>128	6	89	>128	−35.6	+23.8	+ (3/8)	−
Sg A–Ac-negative strains									
MLS$_B$-ind[d]+LS$_A$ *S. aureus*	6	>128	0.7	48	14.6	−1.7	+1.3	−	−
MLS$_B$-ind+LS$_A$ CNS	2	32	0.5	32	12	−	+1.3	−	−
MLS$_B$-cons+LS$_A$ *S. aureus*	5	>128	4	51	>128	−2.8	+1.7	−	−
MLS$_B$-cons+LS$_A$ CNS	22	>128	4	56	>128	−1.5	+1	−	−

[a]Em, erythromycin; PR, pristinamycin; SgA, streptogramin A; SgB, streptogramin B.
[b]SgA-Ac, acetyl streptogramin A.
[c]CNS, coagulase-negative staphylococci.
[d]MLS$_B$-ind, MLS$_B$ inducible; MLS$_B$-cons; MLS$_B$-constitutive.

Table 3 Activity of Streptogramins, Percentage of Inactivation of Streptogramin A and Appearance of Acetyl Streptogramin A Among LS_A and LS_A–S_B Staphylococcal Strains

Resistance patterns	No. strains	Geometric MICs (mg/L)				SgA (SgB) inactivation (%)	SgA–Ac[b] appearance (%)	Gots test	
		Em^a	PR	SgA	SgB			SgA	SgB
SgA–Ac-positive strains									
LS_A–S_B *S. aureus*	4	0.75	10	48	32	−36 (−70)	+23.6	+	+
LS_A *S. aureus*	4	1	0.75	56	7	−20	+6	−	−
LS_A *S. epidermidis*	1	0.25	0.5	32	8	−29	+6	−	−
SgA–Ac-negative strains									
LS_A *S. aureus*	13	0.85	0.55	44	9.2	−0.2	+2.6	−	−
LS_A CNS[c]	5	0.8	0.7	57	7.2	−6.6	+1.1	−	−
Reference strains									
RN 450	1	0.5	0.25	2	8	−	−	−	−
Susceptible strains	10	0.37	0.21	2.2	8.7	−	−	−	−
MLS_B-cons[d] strains	10	>128	0.7	2	>128	−	−	−	−
STE strain (LS_A + S_B)	1	0.25	4	128	32	−73 (−72)	+17	+ +	+ +

[a]Em, erythromycin; PR, pristinamycin; SgA, streptogramin A; SgB, streptogramin B.
[b]SgA–Ac, acetyl streptogramin A.
[c]CNS, coagulase-negative staphylococci.
[d]MLS_B-cons, MLS_B-constitutive.

3. These enzymatic resistance mechanisms were, or were not, associated with MLS$_B$ resistance.
4. The Gots test was positive for SgB for all the strains hydrolyzing the SgB compound. To the contrary, this test was not reliable for the detection of acetylation of the SgA compound (7).
5. Other mechanisms were implicated among SgA resistant strains. Probably, active efflux by the ATP-binding protein encoded by the *vga* gene was involved. DNA–DNA hybridization with the intragenic probes described previously (1,3) would allow the determination of other mechanisms if present in the expression of SgA resistance.
6. The presence of SgA-resistance determinants conferred a low level resistance to PR, not easily detected by the diffusion method or MIC determination. The association with SgB-resistance determinants (*erm* or *vgb* genes) conferred high level resistance to PR.

REFERENCES

1. Allignet J, Loncle V, El Solh N. Sequence of a staphylococcal plasmid gene *vga* encoding a putative ATP-binding protein involved in resistance to virginiamycin A-like antibiotics. Gene 1992; 117:45–51.
2. Allignet J, Loncle V, Mazodier P, El Solh N. Nucleotide sequence of staphylococcal plasmid gene *vgb* encoding a hydrolase inactivating the B components of virginiamycin-like antibiotics. Plasmid 1988; 20:271–275.
3. Allignet J, Loncle V, Simenel C, Dellepierre M, El Solh N. Sequence of a staphylococcal gene, *vat*, encoding an acetyltransferase inactivating the A-type compounds of virginiamycin-like antibiotics. Gene 1993; 130:91–98.
4. Bismuth R, Vermee F, Grosset J. Activité bactériostatique et bactéricide des streptogramines sur *S. aureus* en fonction des phénotypes de résistance aux macrolides, lincosamides et streptogramins (MLS). In: Pocidalo JJ, Vachon F, Coulaud JP, Vilde JL, eds. Macrolides et Synergistines. Paris: Arnette, 1988:187–193.
5. Coccito C. Antibiotics of the virginiamycin family, inhibitors which contains synergistic components. Microbiol Rev 1979; 43:145–198.
6. Courvalin P, Ounissi H, Arthur M. Multiplicity of macrolide–lincosamide–streptogramin antibiotic resistance determinants. J Antimicrob Chemother 1985; 16(suppl A):91–100.
7. Dublanchet A, Soussy CJ, Squinazi F, Duval J. Résistance de *Staphylococcus aureus* aux streptogramines. Ann Microbiol (Inst Pasteur) 1977; 128A:277–287.
8. El Solh N, Bismuth R, Allignet J, Fouace JM. Resistance à la pristinamycine (ou virginiamycine) des souches de *Staphylococcus aureus*. Pathol Biol 1984; 32:362–368.
9. Koechlin C, Jehl F, Monteil H. Determination of PIA and PIIA, the two

main components of pristinamycin, by high performance liquid chromatography in plasma. J Chromatogr 1988; 425:197–202.

10. Leclercq R, Courvalin P. Intrinsic and unusual, resistance to macrolide, lincosamide and streptogramin antibiotics in bacteria. Antimicrob Agents Chemother 1991; 35:1273–1276.

Multiple Dose Pharmacokinetics and Pharmacodynamics of RP 57669–RP 54476 in Preinfected Fibrin Clots

M. G. Bergeron, André Turcotte, and N. J. Morin

Centre Hospitalier de l'Université Laval and Université Laval
Laval, Quebec, Canada

INTRODUCTION

RP 59500 (RP) belongs to a group of families called MLS (i.e., macrolides–lincosamides–streptogramins). RP 59500 is derived from a combination of two soluble semisynthetic derivatives of the purified natural pristinamycin produced by fermentation of *Streptomyces pristinaespinalis* compound PI (quinupristin, RP 57669) and compound PII (dalfopristin, RP 54476) that are present in a proportion of 30:70% (w:w), respectively. The antibiotics of the streptogramin family are inhibitors of protein biosynthesis through their irreversible blocking action on the ribosome. RP 59500 is active against a range of gram-positive pathogenic bacteria. Included in this group are methicillin-susceptible and methicillin-resistant *Staphylococcus aureus* and *S. epidermidis*, erythromycin-resistant *Streptococcus pneumoniae*, other streptococci, and clostridia (1). It also has activity against *Neisseria* spp., *Moraxella catarrhalis*, *Haemophilus influenzae*, *Legionella* spp., *Mycoplasma* spp., and *chlamydia* spp. As it is the first formulation of an injectable streptogramin, it may, if proved effective, have great clinical importance for the treatment of gram-positive infections.

The present investigation was undertaken to study the efficacy and penetration of RP 59500, given at 50 mg/kg tid q8h, in preinfected fibrin clots. Fibrin is one of the main constituents of the inflammatory process, and bacteria located within the core of fibrin clots are protected from host defenses and the action of the antibiotics, as they often interact with and adhere to major constituents of clots. Moreover, penetration of antimicrobials within the clots is quite variable. New antibiotics that can penetrate fibrin and control gram-positive infections are needed. The experimental model of the preinflamed, preinfected, implanted fibrin clots in subcutaneous (s.c.) pockets in rabbits was used to evaluate the pharmacodynamic interaction between RP 59500 and gram-positive bacteria infecting these clots.

MATERIAL AND METHODS

Bacterial Strains

Four strains were used: methicillin-resistant *Staphylococcus epidermidis* (SE 1130; MRSE) and *S. aureus* (ATCC 43350; MRSA), methicillin-susceptible *S. aureus* (STA 560; MSSA), and *S. epidermidis* (SE 438; MSSE). Noninfected and infected fibrin clots were prepared as follows: a sterile solution of 3% bovine fibrinogen (Sigma Chemical Co., St. Louis MO) was supplemented with 5% Mueller–Hinton broth [sterile or infected with an inoculum of 10^2–10^{-3} colony forming units (CFU) of the appropriate strain per milliliter] and distributed in a 2-ml volume into siliconized test tubes. Thrombin was added, and following a 1-h incubation at 37°C, the clots were removed, washed in sterile water, and inserted s.c. in rabbits.

Rabbit Model

As described previously (2), New Zealand white female rabbits (weight 1.8–2.2 kg) were given an intramuscular injection of 20 mg/kg of chlorpromazine. Both flanks were shaved and swabbed with povidone–iodine. The skin was anesthetized with 2% lidocaine, and a 4-cm incision was made on each side. After blunt dissection of the skin, four to six infected or noninfected clots were placed in each s.c. pocket to limit clumping. Autoclips (18 mm) were applied to close the incision. After monitoring the well-being of the rabbits for 1–2 h, they were returned to their cage for 24 h. This allowed sufficient time to induce the preinfection and preinflammatory state. Water and feedings were given ad libitum. The next morning, after IM injection of ketamine-xylazine, a scalp-vein needle (23 gauge) was inserted in the central vein of the left ear for infusion of the antibiotic. A Harvard infusion pump was used to ensure a steady flow rate. Another scalp vein needle (25 gauge) inserted in the central vein of the right ear was used to collect blood samples.

Antibiotic Regimen

Three doses of 50 mg/kg of RP were infused over 30 min in each rabbit at 8-h intervals. Four rabbits were used for each bacterial strain studied and for the experiments in which sterile clots were inserted. Blood and fibrin clots were removed aseptically before the administration of antibiotic and for blood at 0.08, 0.25, 0.5, 1, 2, 4, 6 h after the last bolus, and for the clot at 0, 0.5, 1, 8, 8.5, 9, 16, 16.5, 17, 18, 20, 22, 24, and 40 h after the beginning of the first infusion.

RP 59500 Assay

Clots were weighed and homogenized in a 1% solution of trypsin (Difco) in a volume equal to the weight of the clot. Trypsin had no effect on antibiotic activity and did not influence the bacterial count. Dissolved clots and serum samples were assayed by seeded antibiotic medium no. 1 using *Micrococcus luteus* (*Sarcina lutea*) ATCC 9341 as the assay organism. Standard solution of RP were diluted in rabbit serum for serum assay and in dissolved clot for clot assay. The regression parameters were always between $r = 0.994$ and 0.999, with limit of sensibility at 0.4 μg/ml both for serum and clot.

The degree of protein binding of RP 59500 to rabbit serum was determined for different concentrations. Protein binding was determined by ultrafiltration using Centrifree Micropartition System (Amicon Canada, Mississauga, Ont).

In Vivo Efficacy

The efficacy of the regimen was evaluated by analysis of the bacterial content of infected clots at each timed interval. Appropriate dilutions of trypsinized clots were inoculated on blood agar, followed by incubation at 37°C for 24 h.

RESULTS AND DISCUSSION

The MICs of RP against the four gram-positive pathogens was ≤ 1 μg/ml. Although the inoculum did not modify the minimum inhibitory concentration (MIC), the minimum bactericidal concentration (MBC) was greatly affected by the high inoculum (Table 1).

The third 50-mg/kg dose of RP yielded serum levels higher than those observed in humans (3; Fig. 1). The elimination half-life of RP in serum, at the third infusion, was shorter than that observed in humans (Table 2), and at 6 h the mean serum levels were below the MIC of the staphylococcal strains tested (two *S. aureus* and two *S. epidermidis*; see Table 1). As we have observed previously, the half-life of RP in fibrin clots was much longer than that observed in serum (see Table 2).

Although fibrin is hard to penetrate, the concentration and area under the concentration–time curve (AUC) of RP increased considerably between the final and third doses. Interestingly, protein binding was saturable, and at a concentration of 250 μg/ml, the percentage binding was at least 20% less than at a

Table 1 MICs and MBCs of RP 59500 with Inoculum Effect

Strains	Inoculum (CFU/ml)	MIC (μg/ml)	MBC (μg/ml)
Methicillin–susceptible *S. aureus*	10^3	0.5	0.5
	10^5	0.5	1.0
	10^7	1.0	2.0
Methicillin-resistant *S. aureus*	10^3	0.5	0.5
	10^5	1.0	1.0
	10^7	1.0	>16
Methicillin-susceptible *S. epidermidis*	10^3	0.25	0.5
	10^5	0.25	1.0
	10^7	0.5	>16
Methicillin-resistant *S. epidermidis*	10^3	0.25	0.5
	10^5	0.5	1.0
	10^7	0.5	>16

concentration of 25 μg/ml (91.2%). The RP levels were not influenced by the presence of the pathogens, and concentrations in the infected versus the control (not infected) clots were identical. The inoculum of all pathogens detected at initiation of therapy was more than 10^8 CFU/g of fibrin clots. Even in the presence of such high inoculum, RP was able to reduce the number of CFU in fibrin clots of the staphylococci studied (Fig. 2). At such high inoculum for MSSA, MRSA, and MRSE it took three injections to observe reduction in colony counts (Figs. 3–5). Regrowth of the pathogens was observed between 4 and 6 h after cessation of therapy, at which time levels of the drug in the fibrin were equal or less than the MIC. The MSSE behaved differently, and the pharmacodynamic activity of RP was maintained for more than 24 h after cessation of therapy (Fig. 6). Morever, in contrast with the other pathogens, it responded rapidly to the first dose of the antibiotic. This was followed by a rapid regrowth between the second and third dose, whereas the colony counts were markedly reduced following the third dose.

The overall in vivo antibacterial activity of RP was important, with reduction in colony counts varying between 10^6 and 10^9 CFU/g for MSSA, MSSE, and MRSE. As for the MRSA the reduction observed was $10^{1.5}$ CFU/g. The MBC of RP against this strain was >16 μg/ml. We are now evaluating the in vivo response to RP of other MRSA infecting fibrin clots.

In contrast to our previous observations in noninflamed fibrin clots, for which the in vivo response of RP, in general, was more rapid, the presence of a very high inoculum in inflamed clots was probably partly responsible for the

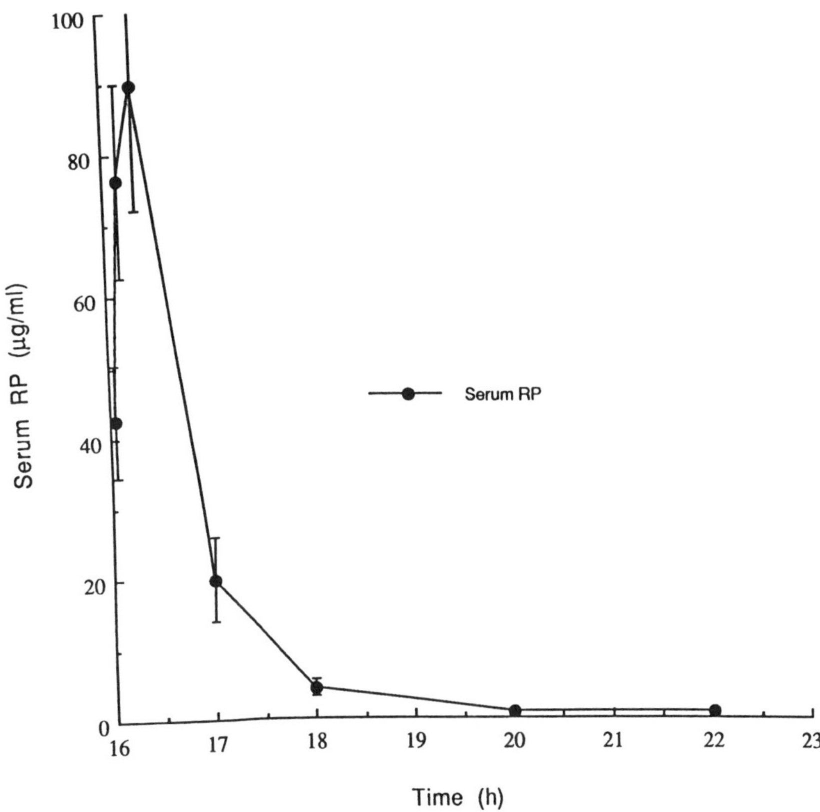

Figure 1 Serum RP concentration vs. time after the third injection.

Table 2 RP Pharmacokinetic Parameters

Parameter[a]	Serum (3rd bolus)	Clot (3rd bolus)
$AUC_{0\rightarrow t}(\mu g/ml\cdot h^{-1})$	76.8	8.8
$AUC_{0\rightarrow\infty}(\mu g/ml\cdot h^{-1})$	77.5	13.9
$\beta 1/2$ life (h)	0.8	6.9
AUC_c/AUC_s	0.18	

[a]AUC, area under the concentration versus time curve.

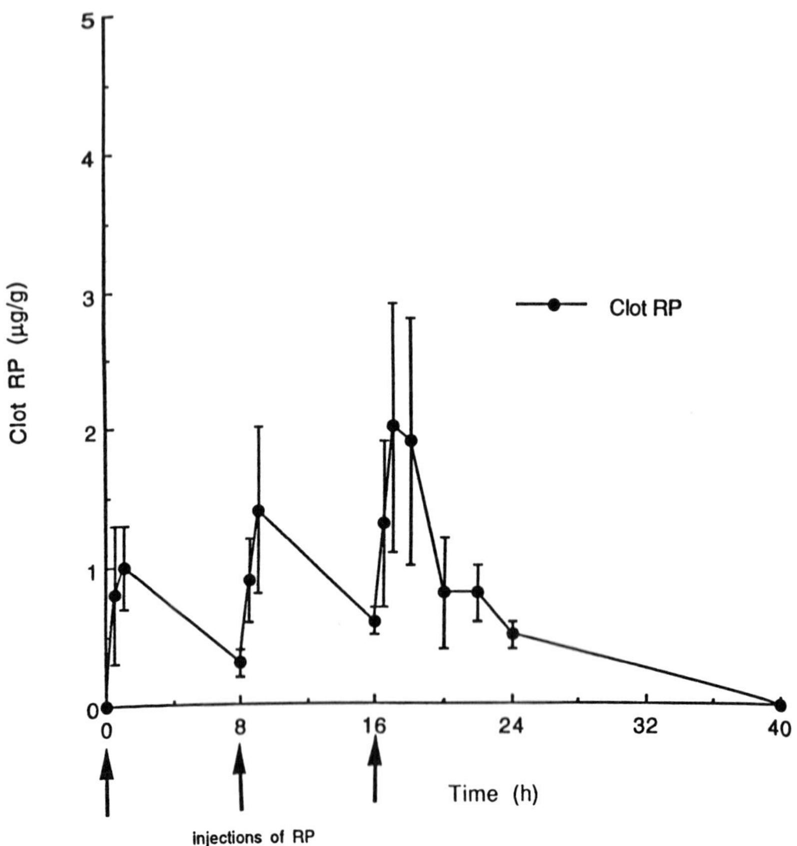

Figure 2   Clot RP concentration vs. time.

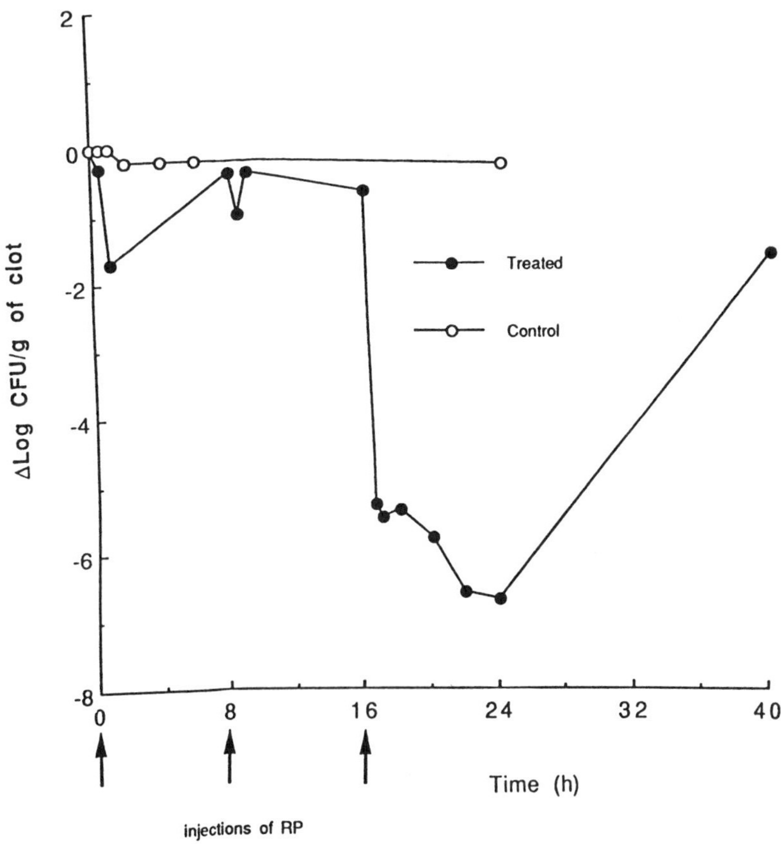

Figure 3 Viability of methicillin-sensitive *S. aureus* embedded in fibrin clot.

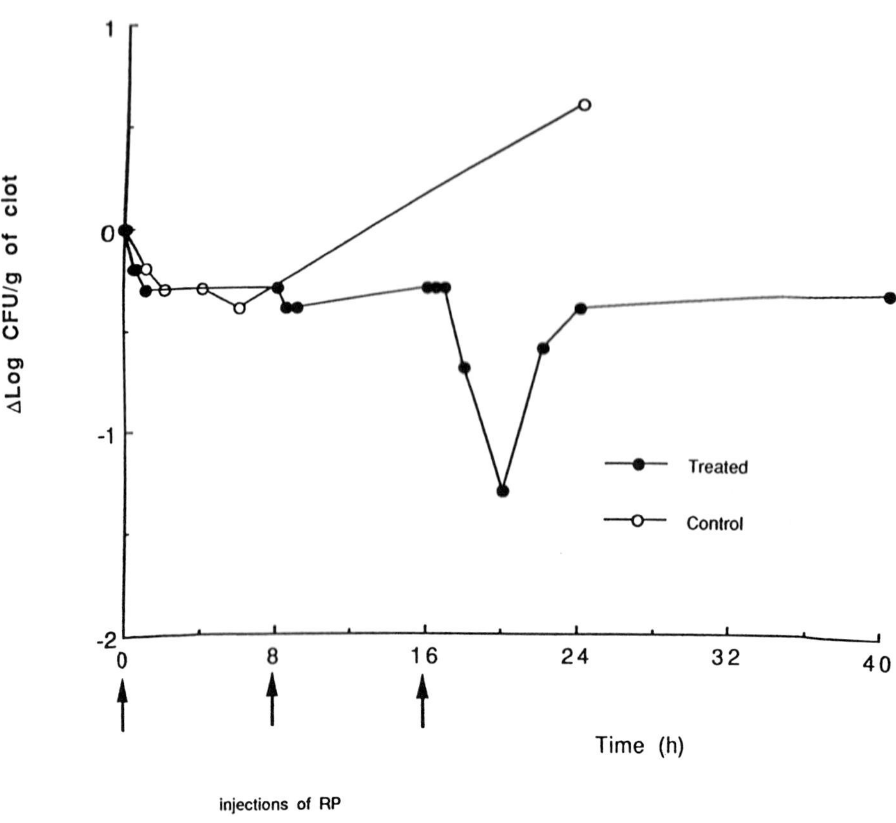

Figure 4 Viability of methicillin-resistant *S. aureus* embedded in fibrin clot.

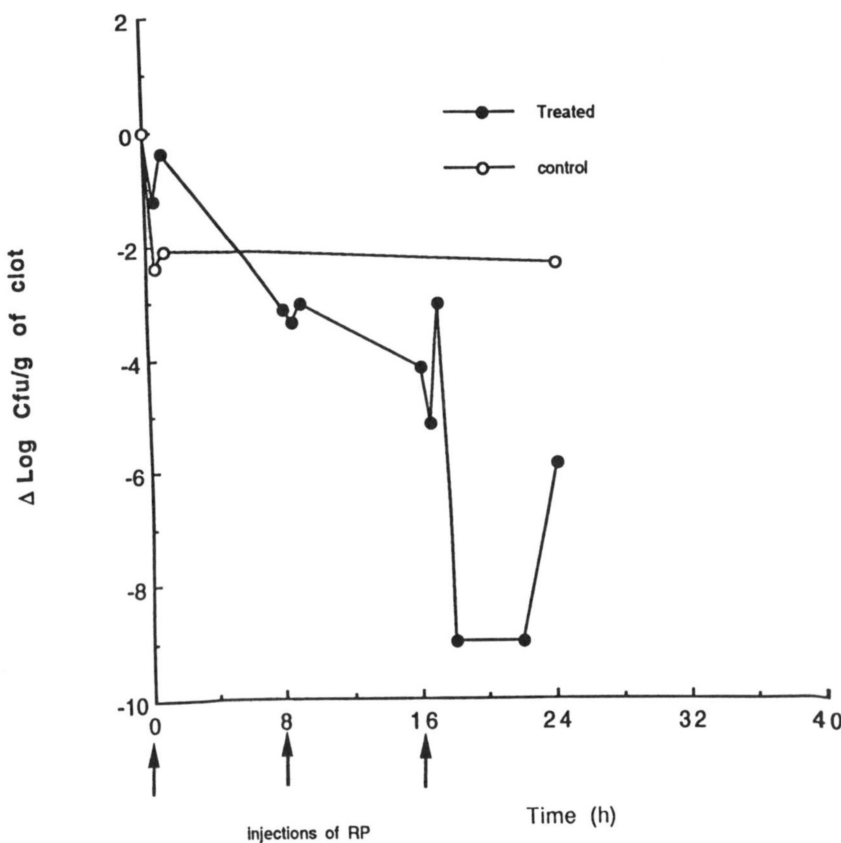

Figure 5 Viability of methicillin-resistant *S. epidermidis* embedded in fibrin clot.

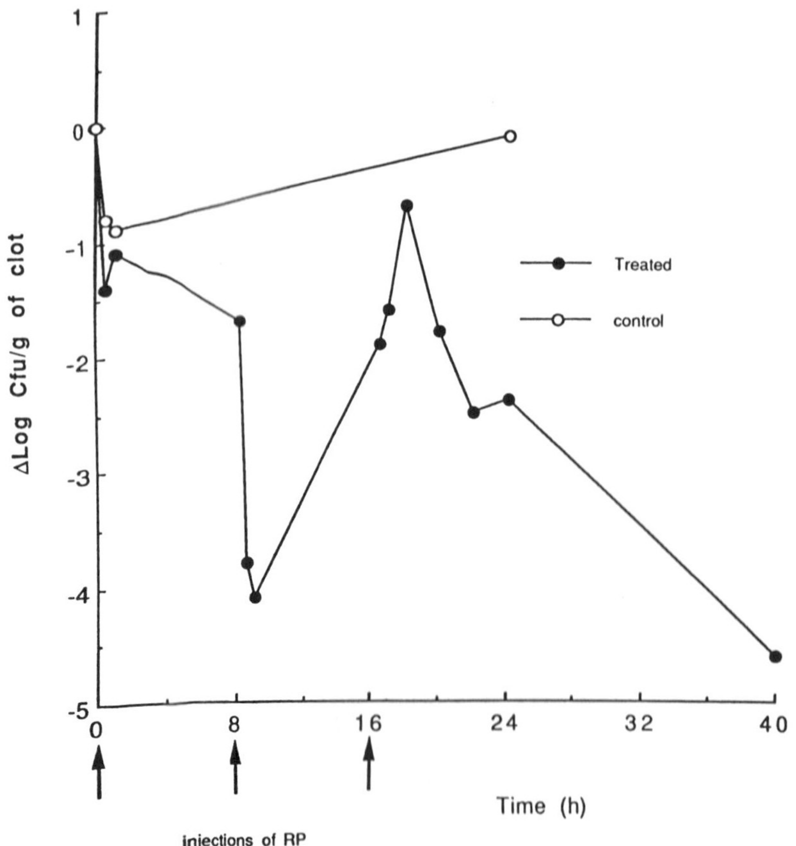

Figure 6   Viability of methicillin-susceptible *S. epidermidis* embedded in fibrin clot.

slower, but good, response. Diffusion of antibiotics within these inflamed clots was also lower than that observed in acute experiments. Whether this decrease penetration was due to tissue repair, which might interfere with diffusion of antibiotics, or to physicochemical interaction between the drug and the inflamed fibrin clots needs to be further explored.

REFERENCES

1. Fass RJ. In vitro activity of RP 59500, a semi-synthetic injectable pristinamycin, against staphylococci, streptococci, and enterococci. Antimicrob Agents Chemother 1991; 35:553–559.

2. Lavole GY, Bergeron MG. Influence of four modes of administration or penetration of aztreonam, cefuroxime, and ampicillin into interstitial fluid and fibrin clots, and an in vivo efficacy against *Haemophilus influenzae*. Antimicrob Agents Chemother 1985; 28:404–412.

3. Turcotte A, Bergeron MG. Pharmacodynamic interaction between RP 59500 and gram positive bacteria infecting fibrin clots. Antimicrob Agents Chemother 1992; 36:2211–2215.

Synergism of Roxithromycin and Pyrimethamine or Sulfadiazine Against *Toxoplasma gondii*

S. Romand and F. Derouin

Hôpital Saint-Louis
Paris, France

INTRODUCTION

Since the treatment of disseminated toxoplasmosis with the standard regimen of pyrimethamine–sulfonamides has been associated with a high incidence of intolerance, there is now an urgent need to evaluate new alternative therapies for this major opportunistic infection (3). Several studies have shown that among new macrolides, roxithromycin alone has limited efficacy in treatment of acute toxoplasmosis in humans and animals (1,2). However, its excellent diffusion and concentration in tissues, as well as its good tolerance are in favor of its use in combined therapies with other antitoxoplasma drugs, which could possibly result in a significant increase in activity (7). In this study, we examined the activity of roxithromycin (ROX) alone and in combination with pyrimethamine (PYR) and sulfadiazine (SDZ) against *Toxoplasma gondii*, both in vitro and in an experimental model of acute murine toxoplasmosis, enabling the sequential determination of parasitic burdens in tissues.

MATERIAL AND METHODS

In vitro experiments were carried out using MRC5 fibroblast tissue cultures as previously described (4). Briefly, confluent monolayers, prepared in 96-well tissue culture plates, were inoculated with 1500 tachyzoites of the RH strain.

After 4 h, antimicrobial agents at various concentrations were added into the medium and the cultures were incubated for an additional 72 h. Toxoplasmal growth was assessed by an enzyme-linked immunoassay performed directly on the fixed cultures. Roxithromycin alone was studied at eight different concentrations, and each concentration was studied in eight replicate wells in two different culture plates. Combinations of three concentrations of ROX and four concentrations of PYR or SDZ were also tested in a two-way design. Each experiment comprised five replicate plates in which each drug or drug combination was tested in four replicate wells.

In vivo experiments were performed in Swiss albino mice infected intraperitoneally with 10^4 tachyzoites of the RH strain. Parasitic burdens in blood, brain, and lungs were determined by subcultures, as previously described (8). Briefly, from each blood and organ suspension, serial fourfold dilutions were prepared in the culture medium, and then inoculated into duplicate wells of tissue culture plates. After 72 h of incubation at 37°C, cultures were fixed and examined for *Toxoplasma* organisms by using an indirect immunofluorescence assay. The number of parasites per gram or per milliliter (parasitic burden) was calculated as the reciprocal titer in tissue culture–volume (μl) or weight (mg) $\times$ 1000. Studies were performed with ROX administered at 50 and 200 mg/kg per day in combination with PYR at 12.5 mg/kg per day or SDZ at 100 mg/kg per day. Twenty mice were not treated (controls) and 40 were used for each drug regimen. Treatments were administered individually by tube feeding for 10 days from day 1 after infection. Mice were studied for 30 days after infection and parasitic burdens were determined in five mice of each group at days 4, 7, 10, 14, 21, and 30 after infection.

RESULTS

In vitro, ROX exhibited a significant inhibitory effect on the RH strain at concentrations higher than 0.02 mg/L, and the dose–response relation yielded a progressive increase in inhibition of *T. gondii*. The IC_{50} was estimated at 1.34 mg/L (range, 1.30–1.38 mg/L). When combined with PYR or SDZ at different concentrations, no significant interacting effect could be demonstrated between ROX and PYR or SDZ for all ratios of drug concentrations.

The results of in vivo experiments are summarized in Table 1 and Figures 1 and 2.

All control mice died within 7 days, showing a predominant parasitic involvement of lungs and brain. With ROX at 50 mg/kg per day, survival was not significantly prolonged compared with controls, and no effect of treatment was observed on blood and tissue burdens. With ROX at 200 mg/kg per day, survival was slightly prolonged, but parasitemia and tissue infection remained at a high level. A marked improvement of survival was obtained with both doses

Table 1 Survival of Mice Treated with ROX Alone or in Combination with PYR or SDZ

Treatment (mg/kg/day)	% Survival[a] on following day after infection						Mean survival (days)
	4	7	10	14	21	30	
Control[b]	100	0	0	0	0	0	5.8
Roxithromycin (50)[b]	100	10	0	0	0	0	6.3
Roxithromycin (200)[b]	100	45	0	0	0	0	7.3
Pyrimethamine (12.5)	100	76	31	31	0	0	8.5
Sulfadiazine (100)	100	100	100	100	20	0	19.3
Roxithromycin (50) + Pyrimethamine (12.5)	100	88	68	64	49	49	20
Roxithromycin (200) + Pyrimethamine (12.5)	100	92	63	63	45	45	20
Roxithromycin (50) + Sulfadiazine (100)	100	100	100	100	33	33	19.8
Roxithromycin (200) + Sulfadiazine (100)	100	100	100	100	87	87	>30

[a]Survival was estimated at the date of examination of parasitic burden in blood and tissues.
[b]Mean of two experiments.

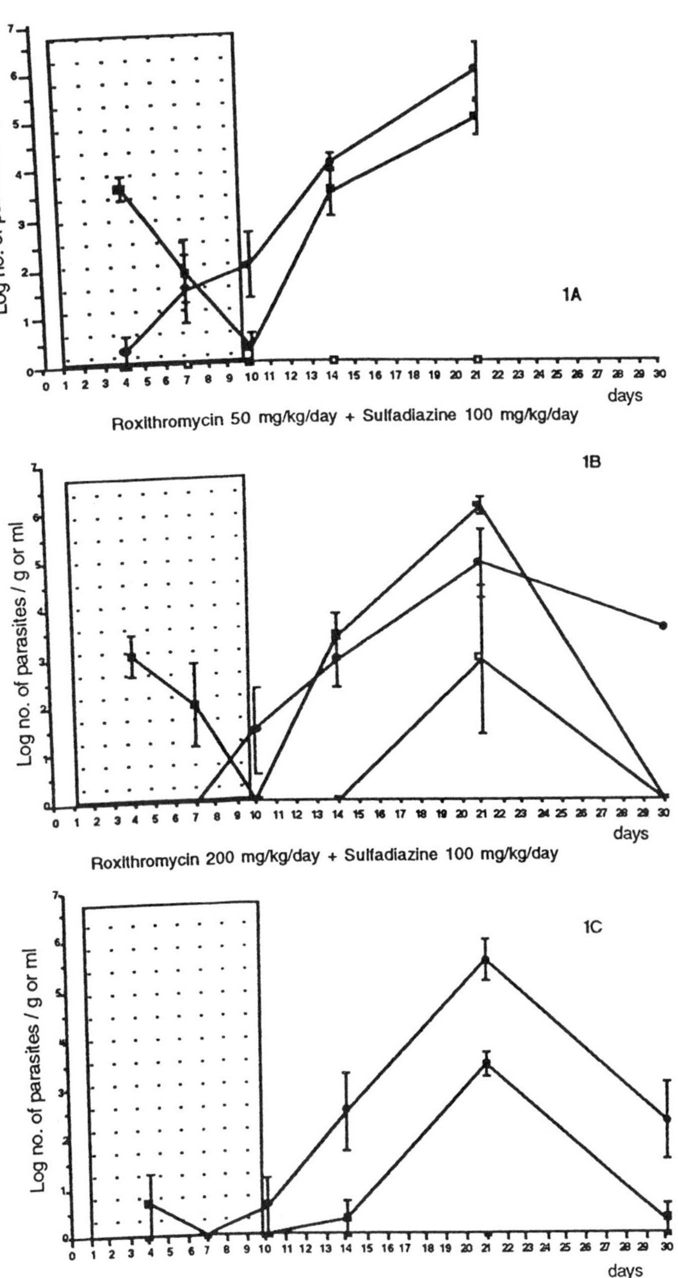

Figure 1 Kinetics of infection in blood, lungs, and brain of control and treated mice. SDZ alone (A) + ROX (B and C). Shaded areas represent period of drug administration. Each point represents the mean (±S.E.M.) of parasitic burdens in five mice in blood (□), lungs (■), and brain (●).

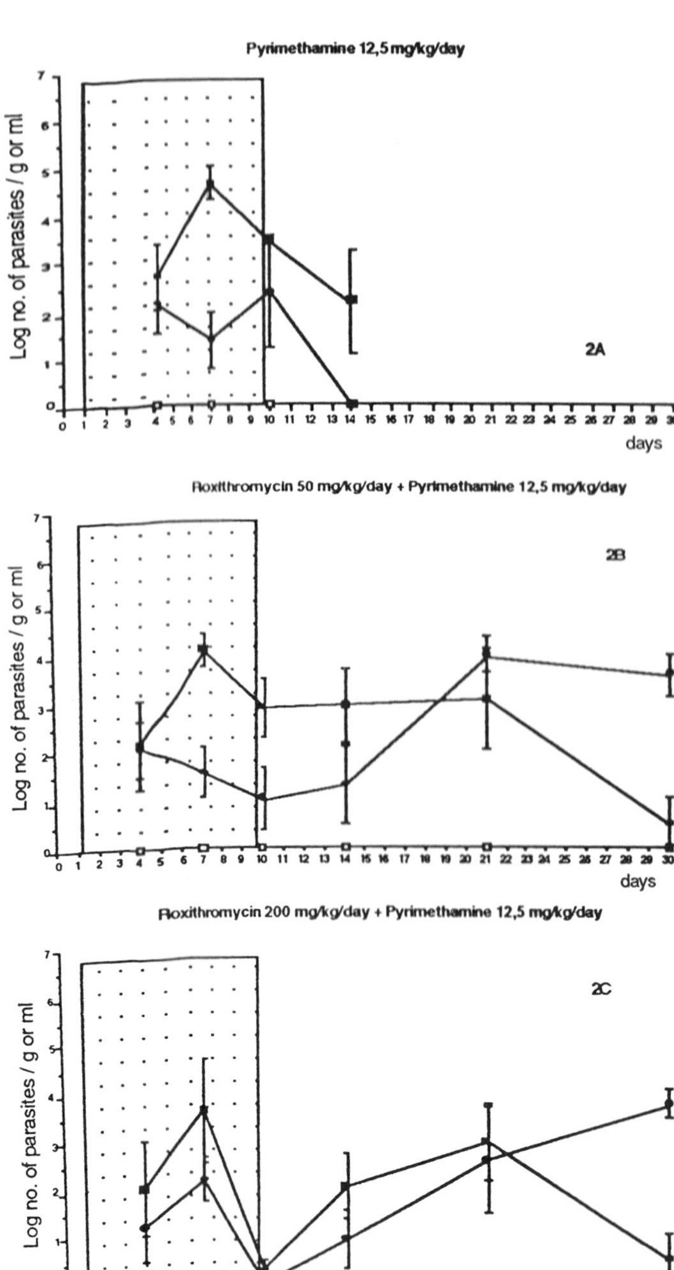

Figure 2 Kinetics of infection in blood, lungs, and brain of control and treated mice. PYR alone (A) + ROX (B and C). Shaded areas represent period of drug administration. Each point represents the mean (±S.E.M.) of parasitic burdens in five mice in blood (□), lungs (■), and brain (●).

of ROX combined with PYR. Comparable kinetics and levels of brain and lung infection were observed with the combined regimens, but relapses followed soon after cessation of therapy. Compared with ROX or SDZ administered alone, a synergistic effect was observed on survival rates in mice treated with ROX at 200 mg/kg per day combined with SDZ. Relapse of parasitemia occurred at day 21 in only two mice treated with ROX 50 mg/kg plus SDZ. While mice were under therapy, brain burdens were negative with both combined therapies and compared with other mice; lung infection was much lower in mice treated with ROX 200 mg/kg plus SDZ.

DISCUSSION

In vitro, our results confirm the significant in vitro activity of ROX against *T. gondii*. The dose–response relation shows, as with other macrolides, a progressive and linear dose-dependant inhibitory activity of ROX on *T. gondii*, with final inhibition being achieved only at high concentrations. These data suggest a parasitostatic effect of ROX on *T. gondii*. The minimum inhibitory concentration (0.02 mg/L) and the IC_{50} (1.34 mg/L) were in the range of values observed in previous experiments (6). The total inhibition of *T. gondii* is obtained at concentrations greater than 100 mg/L, much higher than the usual peak serum levels in humans. However, unlike other macrolides, ROX achieves high and continued serum concentrations that largely exceed the IC_{50} value (7). In addition, the excellent tissue and intracellular penetration of ROX should also be considered for its activity against *T. gondii* (9). A mild additive effect was demonstrated when ROX was combined with either pyrimethamine or SDZ. These results are consistent with other experiments that also failed to demonstrate a synergistic effect between azithromycin or clarithromycin and PYR (5).

In vivo, ROX administered alone was of limited efficacy, since survival rates and kinetics of parasitic infection did not show marked differences with untreated mice, even with a high dose of drug. However, since almost all mice survived when treated with ROX at 200 mg/kg per day and SDZ at a noncurative dose, a strong synergistic activity could be demonstrated between these drugs. In the same way, a milder, but real, synergistic activity was also observed between ROX and PYR, in terms of survival. This synergistic activity was partially confirmed by analyses of the kinetics of infection in blood and organs. With the combination of ROX and SDZ, parasitic burdens were markedly reduced during treatment, compared with that observed in mice treated by one agent alone. After treatment, parasites were still detectable and maintained at a nonlethal level in organs. Of note, at day 30, parasite burdens in brain and lungs of mice treated with ROX at 200 mg/kg per day plus SDZ were reduced to a low level. With the combination of ROX and PYR, we observed a moderate effect during treatment, compared with that observed with PYR or ROX alone, but after treatment, parasitic burdens were controlled at a moderate level and parasitemia was not detectable.

CONCLUSIONS

Although parasites were not eradicated from tissues during and after treatment, synergistic activities between ROX and PYR or SDZ were clearly evidenced by the prolonged survival of mice that received combined therapies. Hence, ROX in combination with PYR or SDZ may represent a new advance in the search for alternative therapies for toxoplasmic encephalitis in patients intolerant to one of the compounds of the standard regimen of PYR–SDZ.

REFERENCES

1. Araujo FG, Shepard RM, Remington JS. In vivo activity of the macrolide antibiotics azithromycin, ROX and spiramycin against *Toxoplasma gondii*. Eur J Clin Microbiol Infect Dis 1991; 10:519–524.
2. Chang HR, Pechère JC. Effect of ROX on acute toxoplasmosis in mice, Antimicrob Agents Chemother 1987; 31:1147–1149.
3. Dannemann B, McCutchan JA, Israelski D, et al. Treatment of toxoplasmic encephalitis in patients with AIDS. Ann Intern Med 1992; 116:33–43.
4. Derouin F, Chastang C. Enzyme immunoassay to assess effect of antimicrobial agents on *Toxoplasma gondii* in tissue culture. Antimicrob Agents Chemother 1988; 32:303–307.
5. Derouin F, Chastang C. Activity in vitro against *Toxoplasma gondii* of azithromycin and clarithromycin alone and with PYR. J Antimicrob Chemother 1990; 25:708–711.
6. Derouin F, Nalpas J, Chastang C. Mesure in vitro de l'effet inhibiteur de macrolides, lincosamides et synergestines sur la croissance de *Toxoplasma gondii*. Pathol Biol 1988; 36:1204–1210.
7. Lassman HB, Puri SK, Ho I, Sabo R, Mezzino MJ. Pharmacokinetics of ROX (RU 965). J Clin Pharmacol 1988; 28:141–152.
8. Piketty C, Derouin F, Rouveix B, Pocidalo JJ. In vivo assessment of antimicrobial agents against *Toxoplasma gondii* by quantification of parasites in the blood, lungs, and brain of infected mice. Antimicrob Agents Chemother 1990; 34:1467–1472.
9. Williams JD, Sefton AM. Comparison of macrolide antibiotics. J Antimicrob Chemother 1993; 31(suppl C):11–26.

Influence of Azithromycin, an Azalide Antibiotic, on Intestinal Bacterial Flora in Gnotobiotic Mice Infected by Four Bacterial Strains

S. Iwata

Kasumigaura National Hospital
Ibaraki, Japan

H. Akita

Yamato City Hospital
Kanagawa, Japan

Y. Sato

Ota General Hospital
Gunma, Japan

K. Sunakawa

The Second Tokyo National Hospital
Tokyo, Japan

I. Kobayashi

Mitsubishi-Yuka Bio Clinical Lab
Tokyo, Japan

INTRODUCTION

The influence of an azalide antibiotic azithromycin (AZM) on intestinal bacterial flora of gnotobiotic mice infected by four bacterial strains, was the objective of this study.

MATERIAL AND METHODS

Four- to six-week-old ICR germ-free male mice, orally inoculated with four organisms, *Escherichia coli*, *Enterococcus faecalis*, *Bacteroides fragilis*, and *Bifidobacterium breve*, in the GI tract were prepared. The mice then received a 10 mg/kg or 20 mg/kg dose of AZM once daily for 3 consecutive days, or 10 mg/kg of clarithromycin (CAM) once daily for 7 consecutive days as a comparative control agent. Cell counts of viable bacteria in feces were done daily. On the seventh day of drug administration, viable bacteria in internal contents of the stomach; upper, middle, and lower parts of the small intestine; and the large intestine of the mice were counted. In addition, AZM and CAM levels in the feces and internal contents were measured, and minimum inhibitory concentration (MIC) determinations were performed for the bacterial strains before, during, and after the administration period. Drug level determinations were conducted by a bioassay method, and the MIC determinations were performed in accordance with the Japan Chemotherapy Society standard procedure.

RESULTS

The study showed a marked decrease in *B. breve* counts and a transient, mild decrease in *B. fragilis* in the feces and internal contents, whereas no significant change occurred in the counts of either *E. coli* or *E. faecalis* (Fig. 1). Those alterations were similarly observed in mice receiving either AZM or CAM. The AZM levels found in feces collected from the second day of administration to the second day after drug withdrawal ranged from 0.09 to 1.30 μg/g in the mice receiving the 10-mg/kg dose of AZM, except in one sample, and from 0.09 to 5.90 μg/g in the 20-mg/kg group (Fig. 2).

On the other hand, CAM detected in feces was lower than the detection limit, except in three samples at 0.25–19.1 μg/g level (see the third and sixth days in Fig. 2). CAM was detected in internal GI contents on the seventh day of drug administration, with levels in the large intestine ranging from 7.66 to 23.2 μg/g.

The MIC of AZM before drug administration was 6.25–12.5 μg/ml in *E. coli*, 6.25–12.5 μg/ml in *E. faecalis*, 1.56–3.13 μg/ml in *B. fragilis*, and 0.10 μg/ml in *B. breve*. The MIC in *E. faecalis* and *B. fragilis* after AZM administration showed that few strains developed resistance. The MIC for CAM before the drug administration was 12.5–25 μg/ml in *E. coli*, 1.56 μg/ml in *E. faecalis*, 0.39–0.78 μg/ml in *B. fragilis*, and less than 0.025 μg/ml in *B. breve*, the drug administration induced resistance in the strains of *B. fragilis*. In the other species the difference of MIC was not significant (Fig. 3).

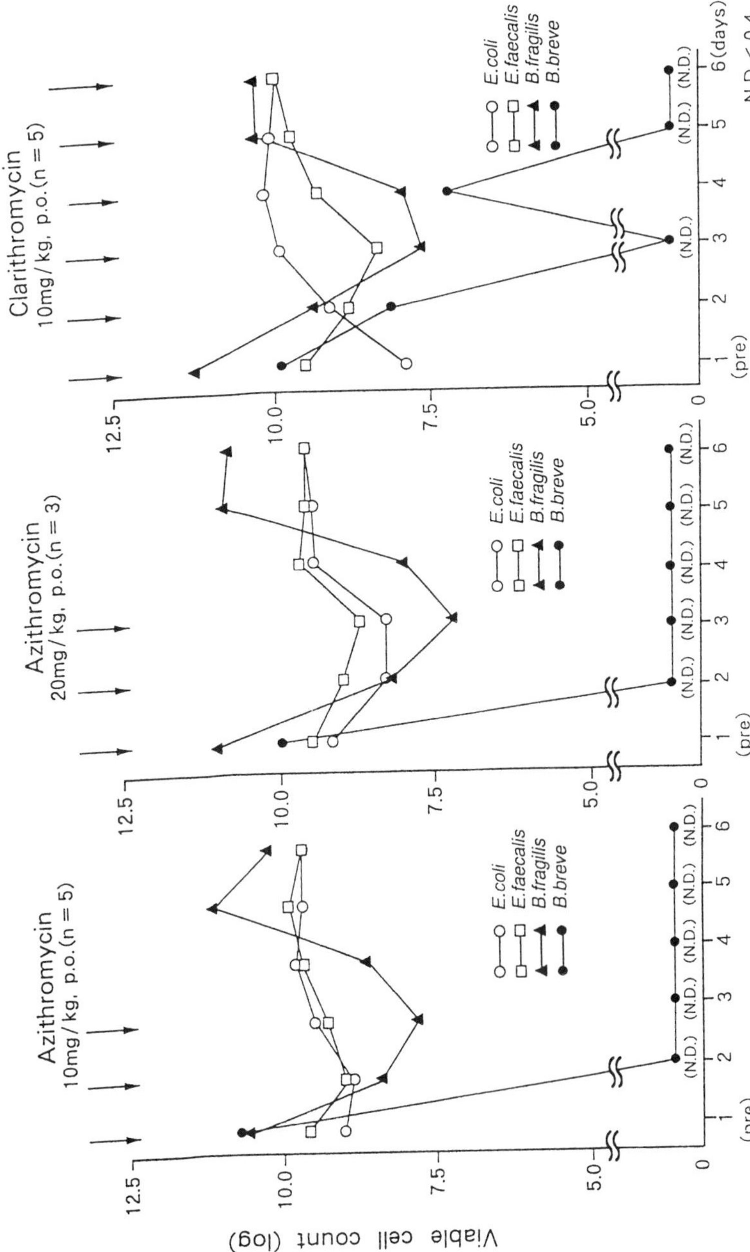

Figure 1 Changes of viable cells in feces following administration of azithromycin and clarithromycin to the tetracontaminated mice. N.D., nondetectable.

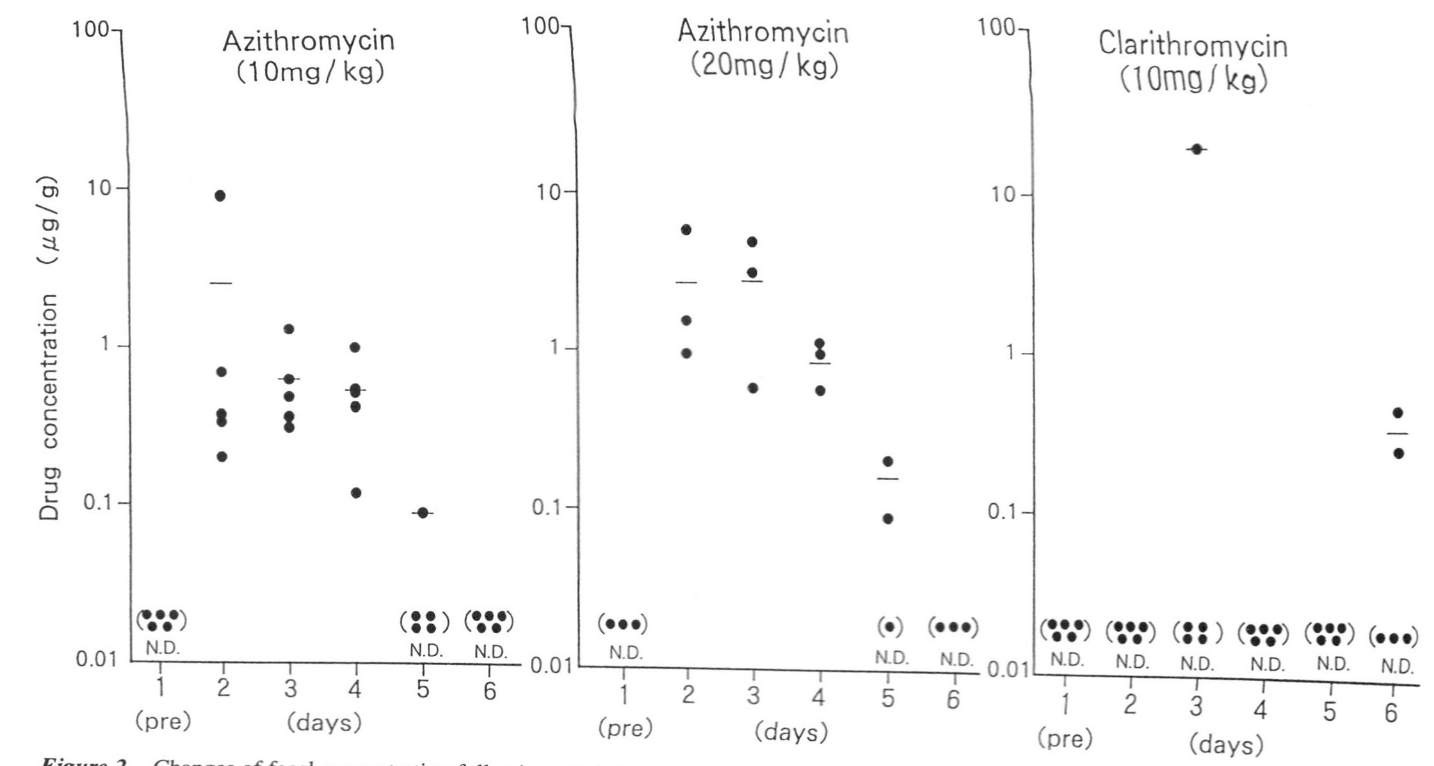

Figure 2   Changes of fecal concentration following administration of azithromycin and clarithromycin to the tetracontaminated mice.

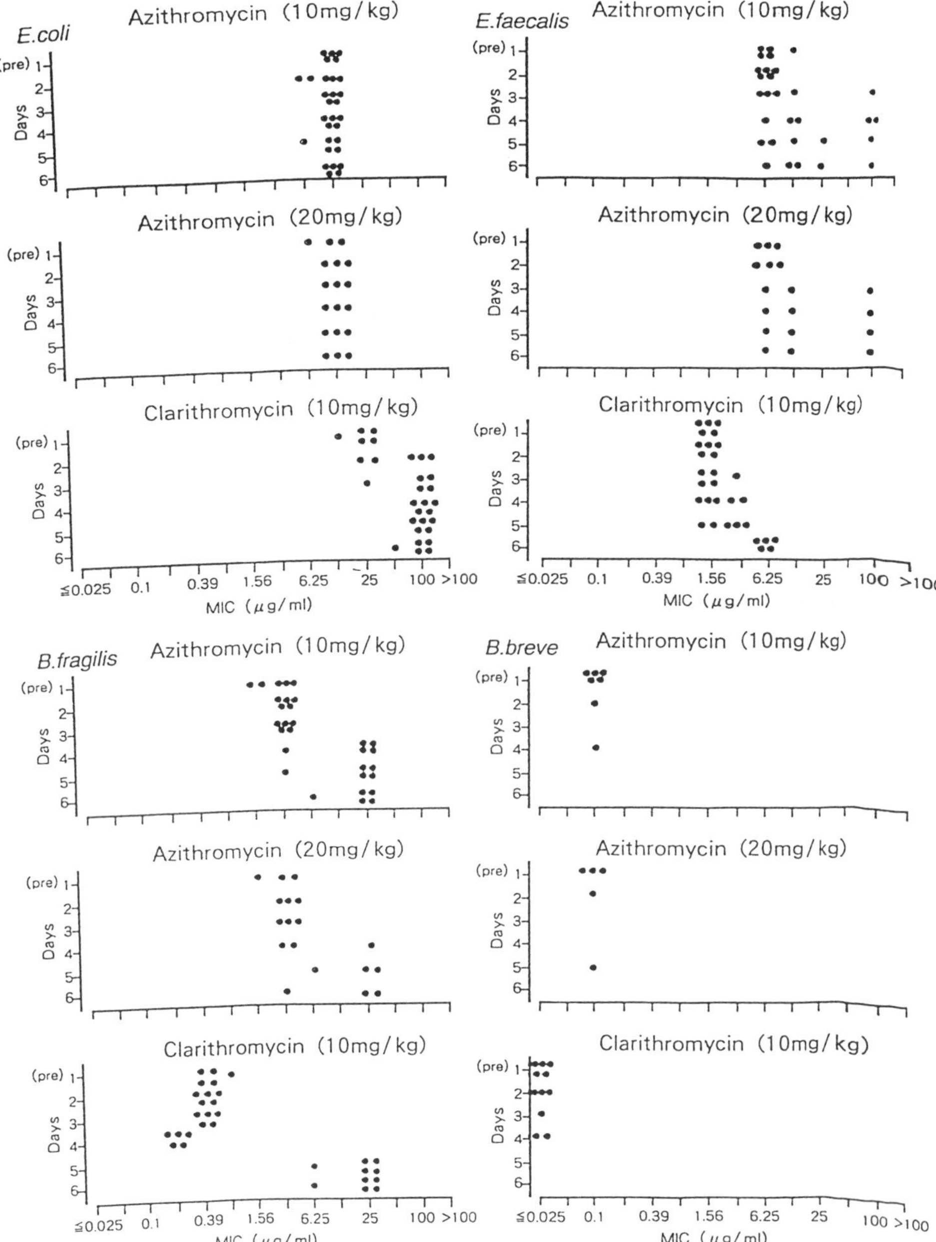

Figure 3 The MIC of azithromycin and clarithromycin against isolated bacteria in feces following their administration to the tetracontaminated mice.

DISCUSSION

Azithromycin has an antibiotic spectrum very similar to other macrolide antibiotics. It has an excellent drug penetration profile in organs and phagocytes, in addition to a very long pharmacological drug half-life: approximately 60–70 h in the human body, approximately 21 h in dogs, and approximately 6 to 7 h in mice. Thus, AZM is expected to show its clinical efficacy at a dose level lower and with a shorter duration of administration than conventional macrolide antibiotic agents. In this study in which gnotobiotic mice were orally inoculated with four bacterial strains, the influence of AZM on the intestinal bacterial flora was examined. AZM was found in a low concentration in feces obtained during the drug administration and for 1–2 days after the withdrawal of the drug. In the same experiment, a significant decrease in the *B. breve* counts and a temporarily decline in those of *B. fragilis* were noted. This finding showed an outcome similar to that of another experiment with CAM in which the same material and conditions had been used and of the study of erythromycin in gnotobiotic mice. Moreover, this AZM study indicated the possibility that the time for AZM detection in feces might be shortened as the duration of AZM administration becomes shorter. Furthermore, the tendency to develop resistance in *E. faecalis* and *B. fragilis* from feces and GI contents had not been noted in the previous studies of various antibiotics. In our study, the resistance to CAM developed in *B. fragilis* must be noted. The mechanism of resistance of bacterial strains will be examined in future studies.

Protective Effect of Roxithromycin on Endotoxin-Mediated Microvascular Leakage and Leukocyte Recruitment in the Airways

Jun Tamaoki, Noritaka Sakai, Etsuko Tagaya, and Kimio Konno

Tokyo Women's Medical College
Tokyo, Japan

INTRODUCTION

Gram-negative bacteria and their cell envelope lipopolysaccharide (LPS) are present in a wide variety of occupational and general environments and have the capacity to interact with the cellular mediator systems of the host, including inflammatory cells and endothelial cells. Through these interactions with the respiratory system, LPS has been shown to contribute to the pathophysiology of pulmonary edema and lung injury (1).

The macrolide antibiotics are widely used as an alternative to β-lactams for the treatment and prevention of airway bacterial infections. There is an increasing evidence that these drugs also modulate the actions of several inflammatory cells, such as polymorphonuclear leukocytes, lymphocytes, and macrophages (2), and directly affect airway secretory cell (3) and epithelial cell functions (4). Thus, these nonantimicrobial effects are proposed to reflect the efficacy of macrolides in the treatment of chronic bronchitis and asthma. In the present experiments, to determine the effects of newly developed macrolide roxithromycin (RXM) on the LPS-induced airway inflammatory reactions, we studied vascular permeability and neutrophil influx in the rat airway mucosa.

METHODS

Pathogen-free male Sprague-Dawley rats, weighing 210–280 g, were divided into four treatment groups, and given placebo or RXM (Roussel Uclaf, Paris,

France) orally at a daily dose of 1, 5, or 10 mg/kg for 1 week. The rats were then anesthetized with urethane and α-chloralose, and injected with Monastral blue pigment (MB; 30 mg/kg, IV) as a tracer to identify the abnormally permeable blood vessels (5). The LPS (*Escherichia coli* 026:B6, 1 mg/kg, Sigma Chemicals, St. Louis, MO) was subsequently administered intravenously, to produce airway inflammation and its associated increase in vascular permeability and neutrophil adherence; control rats were given only the vehicle of LPS (diluted dimethyl sulfoxide). At selected intervals, ranging from 5 min to 12 h after LPS infection, the rats were perfused through the heart with 1% paraformaldehyde, and the trachea and main bronchi were removed.

To quantitate neutrophils and abnormally permeable blood vessels, tissues were stained with a histochemical reaction for myeloperoxidase and prepared as flat transparent whole mounts (6). Neutrophils, identified by the golden brown color, were counted at a magnification of $\times 400$ in 20 square regions of the mucosa located between cartilaginous rings in each section. These values were expressed per square millimeter of the mucosal surface area. The areal density of MB-labeled blood vessels was determined by stereological point counting of 20 intercartilaginous regions and expressed as a percentage of the mucosal surface area.

All values were expressed as means $\pm$ SE. Statistical analysis was performed by ANOVA or Newman-Keuls multiple comparison test, and $p < 0.05$ was considered significant.

RESULTS

As demonstrated in Figure 1, intravenous LPS increased both vascular permeability and neutrophil influx in the airway mucosa of pathogen-free rats, whereas the vehicle alone had no effect. The LPS caused a rapid increase in the number of neutrophils, which were migrating through MB-labeled venules or were located in the perivascular connective tissues. This increase was significant after 5 min of LPS injection (46 ± 6 vs. 12 ± 4 cells/mm^2; $p < 0.01$) and reached a maximum response within 30 min (323 ± 59 cells/mm^2; $p < 0.001$). The increase in the areal density of MB-labeled blood vessels was observed at 60 min after LPS administration (2.7 ± 0.8 vs. $0.5 \pm 0.3\%$; $p < 0.05$) and reached a plateau at 180 min ($7.4 \pm 1.6\%$; $p < 0.01$).

The effect of RXM on airway inflammation was assessed at 180 min after LPS injection. The LPS-induced increase in MB-labeled blood vessels was less in the RXM (10 mg/kg)-treated rats than in those receiving the placebo (6.7 ± 1.5 vs. $0.4 \pm 0.3\%$; $p < 0.01$). Likewise, treatment with RXM (5 and 10 mg/kg) reduced the number of neutrophils present in the airway mucosa in response to LPS (341 ± 48 cells/mm^2 decreasing to 80 ± 17 and 12 ± 3 cells/mm^2; $p < 0.01$ and $p < 0.001$, respectively; Fig. 2).

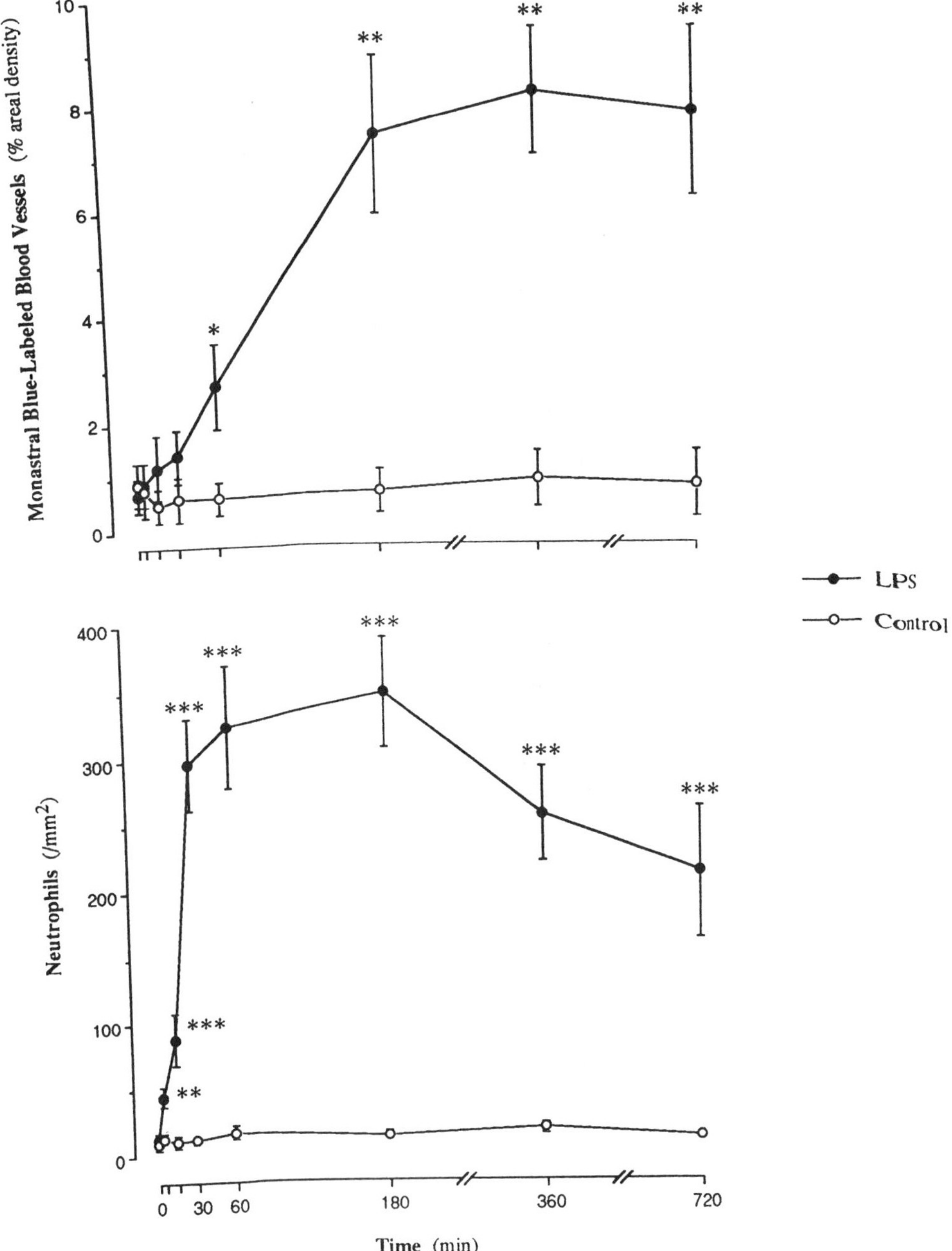

Figure 1 Time course of the effects of LPS (1 mg/kg, IV) on vascular permeability and neutrophil recruitment in the rat tracheal mucosa. The magnitude of vascular permeability was expressed as a percentage of the area occupied by Monastral blue-labeled blood vessels. Data are means $\pm$ SE; $n = 6$ for each point. *$p < 0.05$; **$p < 0.01$; ***$p < 0.001$, significantly different from corresponding control values.

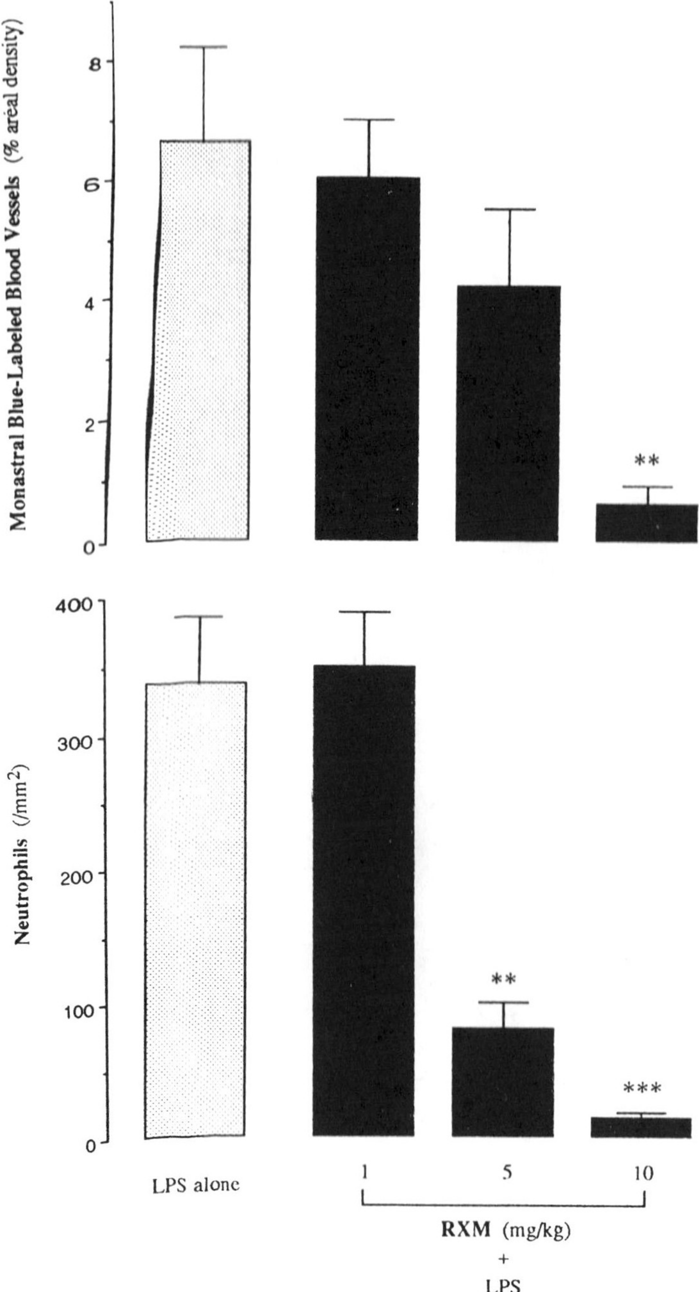

Figure 2 Dose-dependent effect of roxithromycin (RXM) on the LPS-induced increase in vascular permeability and neutrophil recruitment in the rat tracheal mucosa. Vascular permeability and neutrophil recruitment were assessed at 3 h after LPS injection. Values are means ± SE; $n = 6$ for each column. $**p < 0.01$; $***p < 0.001$, significantly different from the response to LPS alone.

DISCUSSION

These studies demonstrate that LPS from *E. coli* increases the number of neutrophils that adhered to the vascular walls and migrated to the mucosal surface, which was followed by a corresponding increase in the area occupied by MB-labeled postcapillary venules and, thereby, increased vascular permeability in the airway mucosa. It has been known that LPS from gram-negative bacteria causes lung injury through endothelial dysfunction in the pulmonary microcirculation (1). Our present findings suggest that LPS may also play a role in the pathogenesis of inflammation in the central airways.

We also found that oral administration of the macrolide RXM for 1 week greatly attenuated each the LPS-induced increase in vascular permeability and neutrophil recruitment, suggesting that this drug might be of value in preventing the development of neutrophil-associated inflammation in the respiratory tract. Macrolide antibiotics possess several biological actions, such as immunomodulation of inflammatory cells (2) and inhibition of airway secretions (3). Although the mechanism of action of RXM in our experimental system is uncertain, it is possible that antioxidant property of RXM could contribute to the protection against the LPS-induced microvascular leakage. This hypothesis is based on the previous studies that LPS is capable of recruiting neutrophils and concomitantly stimulates these cells to release several mediators, including oxygen radicals, thereby causing a dysfunction of endothelial gap and the increased vascular permeability (7), and that macrolide antibiotics can inhibit the release of oxygen radicals from neutrophils (8). Other possibilities would be that RXM could have exerted its action by elevating intracellular contents of cyclic AMP (4), which protects against endothelial dysfunction. As to the effect of macrolide antibiotics on neutrophil migration, there are some conflicting reports. Enhancing effects (9) have been described, whereas others have shown either no effects or inhibition (10). The reason for this disagreement is unknown, but the inhibition of LPS-induced recruitment of neutrophils observed in the present study might be due to the direct inhibitory action of RXM against neutrophil migration, in agreement with the findings by Nelson and colleagues (10). In addition, it has been known that LPS stimulates the expression of adhesion molecules for neutrophils and the generation of inflammatory cytokines, some of which possess neutrophil chemotactic activity. Therefore, the inhibitory action of RXM on these processes could also be involved in the macrolide-induced protection against neutrophil recruitment in the airway.

In conclusion, LPS not only causes lung injury and pulmonary edema, but also increases neutrophil accumulation and microvascular leakage in the central airways. The macrolide RXM can inhibit both of the airway inflammatory reactions, suggesting that this drug may have therapeutic implications for airway inflammation produced by gram-negative bacterial infection.

REFERENCES

1. Brigham KL, Bowers RE, Haynes J. Increased sheep lung vascular permeability caused by *Escherichia coli* endotoxin. Circ Res 1979; 45:292–297.

2. Roche Y, Gougerot-Pocidalo MA, Fay M, Forest N, Pocidalo JJ. Macrolides and immunity: effects of erythromycin and spiramycin on human mononuclear cells proliferation. J Antimicrob Chemother 1986; 17:195–203.

3. Goswami SK, Kivity S, Marom Z. Erythromycin inhibits respiratory glycoconjugate secretion from human airways in vitro. Am Rev Respir Dis 1990; 141:72–78.

4. Takeyama K, Tamaoki J, Chiyotani A, Tagaya E, Konno K. Effect of macrolide antibiotics on ciliary motility in rabbit airway epithelium. J Pharm Pharmacol 1993; 45:756–758.

5. Joris I, DeGirolami U, Worthman K, Majno G. Vascular labeling with Monastral blue B. Stain Technol 1982; 57:177–183.

6. McDonald DM. Neurogenic inflammation in the rat trachea. I. Changes in venules, leucocytes, and epithelial cells. J Neurocytol 1988; 17:583–603.

7. Johanson KJ, Fantone JC, Kaplan J, Ward PA. In vivo damage of rat lungs by oxygen metabolites. J Clin Invest 1981; 67:983–993.

8. Anderson R. Erythromycin and roxithromycin potentiate human neutrophil locomotion in vitro by inhibition of leukoattractant-activated superoxide generation and autooxidation. J Infect Dis 1989; 159:966–973.

9. Dalziel K, Dykes PJ, Marks R. The effect of tetracycline and erythromycin in a model of acute-type inflammation. Br J Exp Pathol 1987; 68:67–70.

10. Nelson S, Summer WR, Terry PB, Warr GA, Jakab GJ. Erythromycin-induced suppression of pulmonary antibacterial defenses: a potential mechanism of superinfection in the lung. Am Rev Respir Dis 1987; 136:1207–1212.

Pharmacokinetics of Macrolides with Reference to Total and Free Concentrations

O. G. Nilsen

University of Trondheim
Trondheim, Norway

INTRODUCTION

Because of a higher stability in acidic environments and prolonged elimination half-lives, the new macrolides azithromycin (1), clarithromycin (2), and roxithromycin (3), all show pharmacokinetic characteristics superior to those of erythromycin (3). Accordingly, more favorable dosage regimens can be applied (4,5). However, among the new macrolides, great differences exist in plasma concentration–time profiles, plasma protein binding, and plasma elimination half-lives. Although the plasma protein-binding characteristics of azithromycin, clarithromycin, and roxithromycin have been established, no direct comparison has been made. This is of interest, as the free concentration in plasma equals the free concentration in tissue at an achieved distribution equilibrium. Thus, the free concentration in plasma would, supplementary to the total plasma concentration, be a good indicator of tissue availability, especially for interstitial fluid. In this study, a single-dose pharmacokinetic comparison is made between the new macrolides relative to total and free plasma concentrations.

MATERIALS AND METHODS

Azithromycin, clarithromycin, and roxithromycin single-dose pharmacokinetics were determined in the same population of 12 healthy subjects, aged from 22 to 37 years (mean, 31.2 ± 4.7 years). The participants were randomly divided into groups of equal size and received the drugs in a Latin square fashion with a

1-week washout period between treatments. Azithromycin (500 mg), clarithromycin (500 mg), and roxithromycin (300 mg) were given orally after fasting overnight. Heparinized plasma was obtained by centrifugation at 1100 × g. Extraction, separation, and detection of azithromycin (6), clarithromycin (5), and roxithromycin (5) were performed as described elsewhere. The quantification limits were 0.01, 0.05, and 0.02 mg/L, respectively.

Azithromycin capsules, 250 mg × 2 (lot 16401 C), were supplied by Norsk Medisinaldepot, Oslo, Norway; clarithromycin tablets, 250 mg × 2 (lot 33065 TF), were supplied by Abbott AB, Stockholm, Sweden; and roxithromycin tablets, 300 mg (lot CR 22731-145), were supplied by Roussel Uclaf, Romainville, France.

RESULTS AND DISCUSSION

The binding of azithromycin (7), clarithromycin (8), and roxithromycin (9) to human plasma proteins has been published by others. All binding experiments have been performed in vitro by equilibrium dialysis and are illustrated graphically in Figure 1.

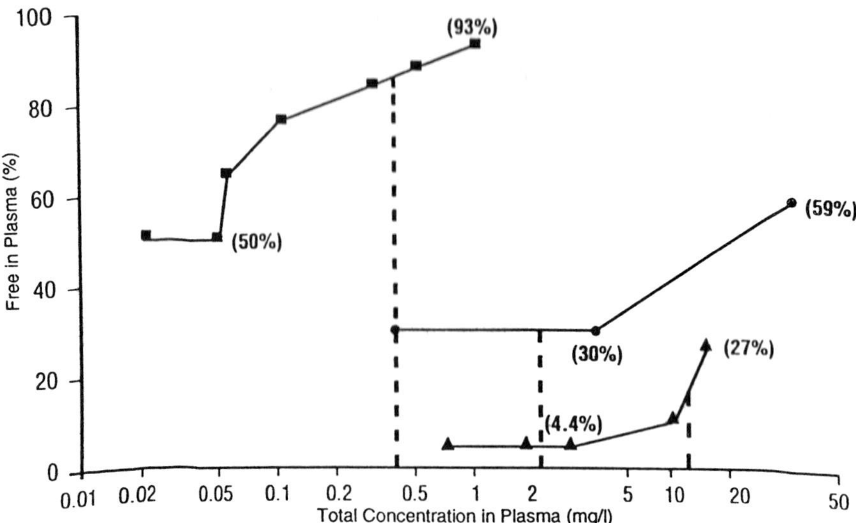

Figure 1 Protein binding of (■) azithromycin, (●) clarithromycin, and (▲) roxithromycin in human plasma expressed as the percentage of free, unbound drug in plasma as a function of the total plasma concentration. The dotted lines indicate the percentage of free, unbound drug in plasma at the maximum total plasma concentrations achieved after a single-dose administration of azithromycin and clarithromycin, 500 mg, and roxithromycin, 300 mg.

Figure 1 shows a decrease in binding (i.e., a relative increase in the free unbound fraction) of all macrolides in plasma when their total concentration in plasma exceeds a certain level. However, this specific level is different for the different macrolides. This saturation phenomenon in binding occurs for azithromycin and roxithromycin within the therapeutic range, whereas the binding of clarithromycin probably is constant over the whole therapeutic range, with about 30% of the total concentration in plasma in the free unbound form. For azithromycin, a decrease in total plasma concentration from 0.4 to 0.05 mg/L will decrease the fraction of free drug from about 85 to 50%. For roxithromycin, a decrease in total plasma concentration from 11 to 3 mg/L will decrease the fraction of free drug from about 20 to 4.4%. Substantial differences thus exist in the binding of the three macrolides, indicating different binding characteristics (association constant and number of binding sites) for the macrolides.

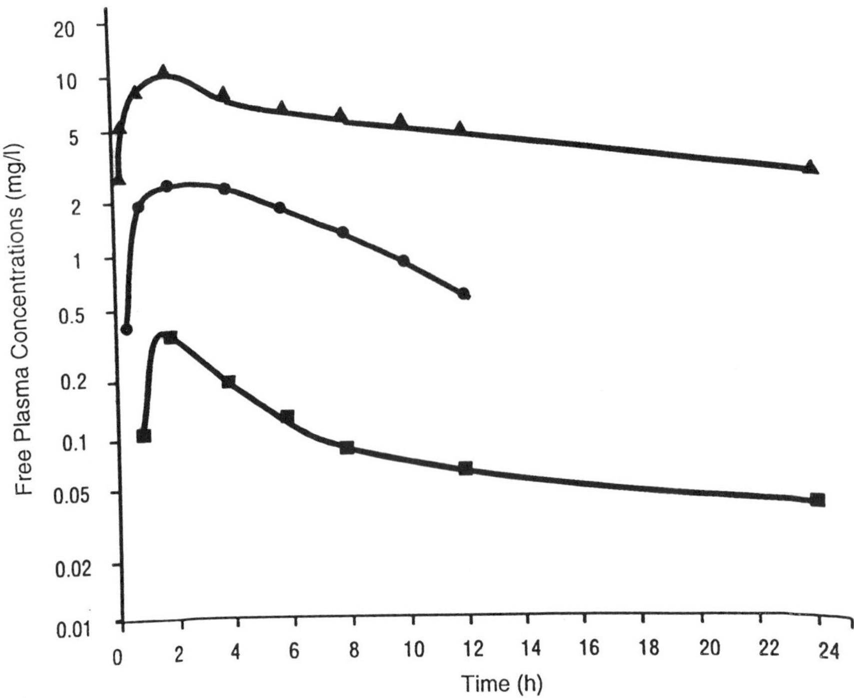

Figure 2 Single-dose plasma pharmacokinetic profiles of total (▲) roxithromycin, 300 mg; (●) clarithromycin, 500 mg; and (■) azithromycin 500 mg, in healthy adult subjects. Each macrolide profile is shown over a time span identical with the dosing frequency recommended for common infections.

The single-dose plasma concentration–time profiles of total concentrations of roxithromycin (300 mg), clarithromycin (500 mg), and azithromycin (500 mg) are presented in Figure 2. The time intervals correspond to the standard therapeutic-dosing frequency used for the three macrolides during repeated dosing. The maximum plasma concentration for the macrolides, in the same order as above, are 11, 2.3, and 0.4 mg/L, respectively, with minimum plasma concentrations of 2.8, 0.5, and 0.04 mg/L. Thus, the percentage decrease in the actual total plasma concentration of the macrolides from maximum to a trough level is highest for azithromycin, followed by roxithromycin, then clarithromycin.

Single-dose plasma concentration–time profiles of free macrolide concentrations, corresponding to the total concentrations presented in Figure 2, are shown in Figure 3. The free concentrations shown are estimated from the measured total plasma concentrations and the total-to-free relations for the macrolides given in Figure 1. Figure 1 is based on earlier published data from

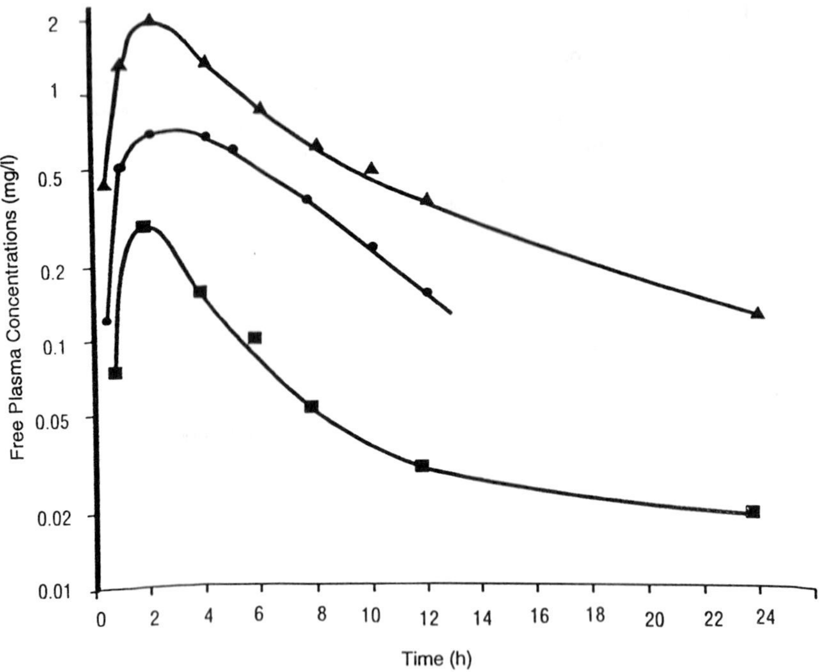

Figure 3 Single-dose plasma pharmacokinetic profiles of free, unbound (▲) roxithromycin, (●) clarithromycin, and (■) azithromycin corresponding to the total plasma concentrations shown in Figure 2.

other laboratories (7–9). Two main characteristics can be observed for the free concentration profiles. (1) The decrease over time in free plasma concentration for roxithromycin and azithromycin is more rapid than that of the corresponding total plasma concentration. (2) Despite possessing the highest degree of plasma protein binding, roxithromycin shows the highest free plasma concentration, followed by clarithromycin and then by azithromycin. The maximum plasma concentrations of free drug are 2.0, 0.7, and 0.35 mg/L, respectively.

The faster initial decline with time of the free concentrations of roxithromycin and azithromycin, as compared with total concentrations, is due to the saturable binding of both compounds within the therapeutic range. A decrease is found in the free fraction of the two drugs from 20 and 85%, respectively, at maximum plasma concentrations to 4.4 and 50%, respectively, at troughs.

No systematic measurements have been performed on the free concentrations of macrolides in tissues, and no conclusive statements can be made relative to differences between the macrolides here. However, by accepted pharmacological principles, the free concentration of drug should be equal in tissues and plasma when equilibrium has been achieved. This may also indicate differences between the macrolides in their free tissue concentrations, with relative levels substantially different from the total tissue concentrations published previously.

REFERENCES

1. Wildfeuer A, Laufen H, Leitold M, Zimmermann T. Comparison of the pharmacokinetics of three-day and five-day regimens of azithromycin in plasma and urine. J Antimicrob Chemother 1993; 31(suppl E):51–56.
2. Hardy DJ, Guay DRP, Jones RN. Clarithromycin, a unique macrolide. A pharmacokinetic, microbiological, and clinical overview. Diagn Microbiol Infect Dis 1992; 15:39–53.
3. Nilsen OG. Roxithromycin. A new molecule, a new pharmacokinetic profile. Drug Invest 1991; 3(suppl 3):28–32.
4. Foulds G, Johnson RB. Selection of dose regimens of azithromycin. J Antimicrob Chemother 1993; 31(suppl E):39–50.
5. Nilsen OG, Aamo T, Zahlsen K, Svarva P. Macrolide pharmacokinetics and dose scheduling of roxithromycin. Diagn Microbiol Infect Dis 1992; 15:71–76.
6. Shepard R, Duthu GS, Ferraina RA, Mullins MA. High performance liquid chromatographic assay with electrochemical detection for azithromycin in serum and tissues. J Chromatogr 1991; 565:321–337.
7. Foulds G, Shepard RM, Johnson RB. The pharmacokinetics of azithromycin in human serum and tissues. J Antimicrob Chemother 1990; 25(suppl A):73–82.

8. Davey PG. The pharmacokinetics of clarithromycin and its 14-OH metabolite. J Hosp Infect 1991; 19(suppl A):29–37.
9. Zini R, Fournet MP, Barre F, Tremblay D, Tillement JP. In vitro study of roxithromycin binding to serum proteins and erythrocytes in humans. Br J Clin Pract 1988; 42(suppl 55):54–55.

The Role of Clarithromycin in Patients with Legionella Pneumonia

J. C. Craft and D. Stamler

Abbott Laboratories
Abbott Park, Illinois

BACKGROUND

Although the first documented epidemic of legionella infection occurred in 1957 at a Minnesota meat-packing plant, it was not until 1976, with an epidemic of pneumonia among American Legion members who were attending a convention in Philadelphia, that legionnaires' disease gained worldwide recognition. Although the infecting organism was initially elusive, the culprit was finally identified and subsequently named *Legionella pneumophila* in honor of those who had the disease as well as the organ infected. Although multiple species and serotypes have been recognized, *L. pneumophila* serogroup 1 remains the most common (approximately 90% of cases). The habitat for legionella is natural and treated waters, and legionnaires' disease is acquired by the inhalation of aerosolized water containing *Legionella* organisms. Even though the spectrum of clinical presentation is wide, the typical presentation involves malaise, low-grade fever, and anorexia. Gastrointestinal complaints, then systemic febrile illness and pneumonia, with few respiratory tract symptoms follow. Estimates suggest 1–5% of all pneumonias in adults are due to *L. pneumophila*. However, average prevalence rates for community-acquired legionnaires' disease range from 10 to 20% in some geographic regions. When the bacterium causes endemic or epidemic nosocomial infections, as many as 20% of hospitalized patients with pneumonia have this infection.

Since neither the clinical presentation nor the radiologic findings of the infection are specific, the diagnosis can be established by laboratory tests: culture or DFA stain of *L. pneumophila* from respiratory secretions and serological detection. Currently available laboratory tests are not completely accurate for the diagnosis of legionnaires' disease; therefore, empirical therapy must often be initiated in the clinical setting. Clarithromycin, an advanced-generation macrolide, is more active ($MIC_{90} = 0.25$ µg/ml) against *L. pneumophila* in vitro and in vivo than erythromycin ($MIC_{90} = 2$ µg/ml), which has been considered the drug of choice for respiratory infections caused by this microorganism.

STUDY OBJECTIVE

The objective of these studies was to evaluate the efficacy and safety of oral clarithromycin in the treatment of outpatients or hospitalized patients with community-acquired legionella pneumonia.

PATIENTS AND METHODS

Study Type

The study was designed as a multicenter, comparative, two double-blind and two open clinical trials.

Inclusions

Patients were at least 12 ($n = 3$ studies) or 18 ($n = 1$ study) years old or more.

Clinical signs and symptoms were consistent with community-acquired pneumonia.

Documentation of pneumonia was by abnormal chest x-ray films

Diagnosis of legionella pneumonia was by serology or bacterial culture or DFA of bronchopulmonary secretions.

Patient had given written informed consent.

Exclusions

($n = 3$ studies) Patients with a history of hypersensitivity to macrolide antibiotics or with significant renal or hepatic impairment were excluded.

Patients treated with a systemic antibiotic within 3–7 days or with a long-acting injectable antibiotic within 6 weeks of study drug administration were also excluded.

Drug Administration

Patients received clarithromycin 250–500 mg bid for 14–36 days.

Evaluations

	Pretreatment	During treatment	Posttreatment	4–6 weeks posttreatment[a]
Medical history	X			
Physical exam	X			
Chest x-ray	X	X	X	
Signs and symptoms	X	X	X	X[a]
LRT culture	X[b]	X[b]	X[b]	X[a]
Legionella titer				X[a]
Clinical response				X[a]

[a]Not all protocols.
[b]If culture material available.

RESULTS

The results are summarized in Table 1 and Figure 1.

Adverse Events

Thirteen of the fifty evaluable patients reported an adverse event. Seven patients (14%) had an adverse event involving the gastrointestinal tract: abdominal pain, diarrhea, nausea, mild dyspepsia, or gastroenteritis. The next most frequently reported adverse event was taste perversion.

Table 1 Summary of Patient Enrollment and Demographic Data

Number of patients enrolled	429
Number of patients with Legionella pneumonia	50
Age (years)	
Mean	47
Range	12–74
Gender	
Female	19
Male	31
History of pulmonary disease	
Yes	30
No	20
Diagnosis of Legionella infection by	
Serology	45
Direct antigen fluorescence of bronchopulmonary secretions	37
Bacterial culture of bronchopulmonary secretions	12

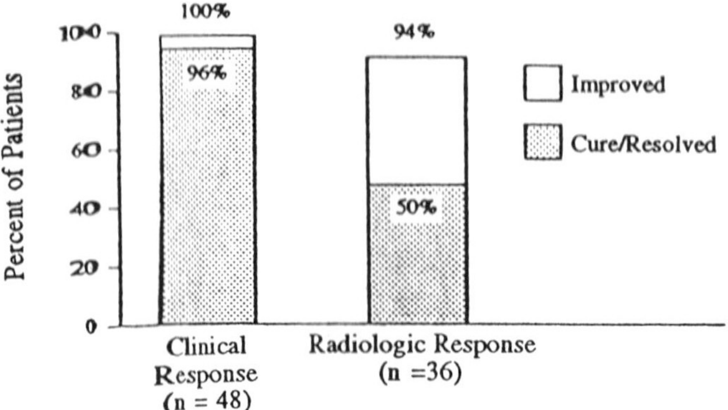

Figure 1   Last evaluable clinical and radiologic response for evaluable patients with legionella pneumonia who received clarithromycin.

CONCLUSION

Given its potent in vitro activity against *L. pneumophila*, its high lung and intracellular concentrations, and its excellent clinical and radiologic response rates among infected patients, clarithromycin is an ideal choice for the empirical treatment of community-acquired legionella pneumonia.

The most appropriate dosage of clarithromycin for treating legionellosis based on present data is 500 mg bid for 14 days. Doses from 250 mg bid to 1000 mg bid have been used with success but over 90% of all successfully treated patients have been given the 500 mg bid dosage of clarithromycin.

Pharmacokinetics of Azithromycin in Patients with Renal Failure

K. Shiba, N. Shindo, and O. Sakai

The Jikei University School of Medicine
Tokyo, Japan

INTRODUCTION

Azithromycin is the prototype of a new subclass of macrolide, the azalides, produced by the insertion of a methyl-substituted nitrogen into the lactone ring of the erythromycin molecule. It is potent against gram-positive, gram-negative, and anaerobic bacteria as well as specific pathogens, such as *Mycoplasma pneumoniae*, *Chlamydia trachomatis*, and *Legionella pneumophila*.

This agent has a remarkable pharmacokinetic profile, characterized by blood levels, very high tissue levels, and slow clearance from the body. The present study made a comparison between pharmacokinetic parameters of renally impaired patients and those with normal renal function, the dosage of AZM was once-daily, 500-mg, single administration. Its concentration was measured by high-performance liquid chromatography (HPLC) and bioassay.

RESULTS

The results are outlined in Figure 1 and Tables 1 and 2.

The patients were classified into the following three groups.

Groups (degree of impairment)	Creatinine clearance	No. of patients
Normal volunteers		6
Mild	$30 < \sim \leq 50\,\mathrm{ml/min}$	1
High	$\leq 30\,\mathrm{ml/min}$	3

CONCLUSION

No appreciable difference was found between healthy and renally impaired patients in C_{max}, AUC, and $T_{1/2}$. Therefore, it is suggested that AZM dosing regimen may not have to be modified in renally impaired patients.

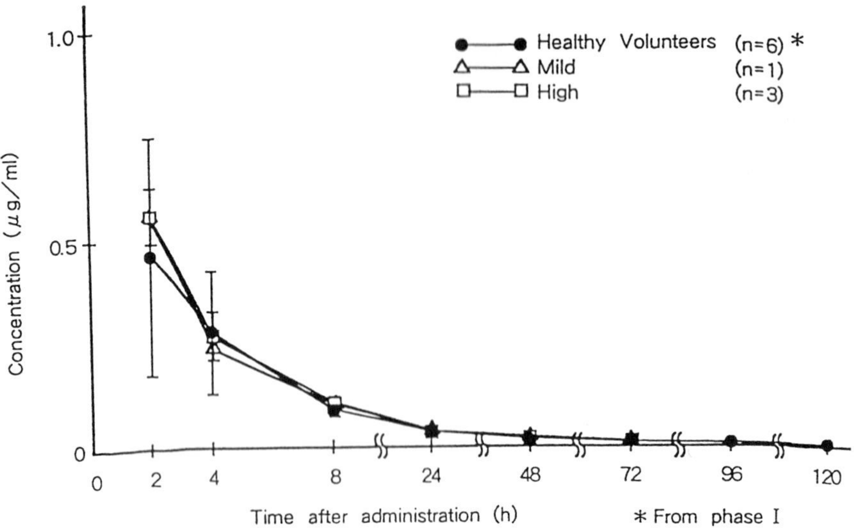

Figure 1   Serum concentration of AZM after oral administration.

Table 1 Serum Concentration and Cumulative Urinary Recovery Rate of Azithromycin After Oral Administration

		Time after administration													
		Serum concentration[a]									Cumulative urinary recovery rate				
		Before	2	4	8	24	48	72	96	120	0~24	~48	~72	~96	~120
Mean serum concentration (μg/ml)	Low ($n=0$)														
	Mild ($n=1$)	N.D.	0.560	0.240	0.104	0.039	0.021	0.014	N.D.	N.D.	3.39	4.32	4.78	5.05	5.35
	High ($n=3$)	N.D.	0.560	0.267	0.108	0.039	0.019	0.013	N.D.	N.D.	1.30	1.19	1.37	1.47	1.54
			±0.069	±0.057	±0.011	±0.008	±0.006	±0.002			±0.90	±0.38	±0.41	±0.46	±0.49
Mean ($n=4$)		N.D.	0.560	0.260	0.107	0.039	0.020	0.013	N.D.	N.D.	1.82	2.23	2.51	2.67	2.81
			±0.056	±0.048	±0.009	±0.006	±0.005	±0.002			±1.27	±1.83	±1.99	2.09	±2.23
					9hr										
Healthy volunteers ($n=6$)[b]			0.464	0.279	0.093	0.038	0.018	0.012	0.009	0.007	5.53	6.86	7.57	8.05	8.42
			±0.284	±0.146	±0.013	±0.006	±0.003	±0.001	±0.002	±0.001	±0.61	±0.83	±0.99	±1.06	±1.19

[a]N.D., <0.01 μg/ml.
[b]From Phase I; ±SD.

Table 2 Pharmacokinetic Parameters of AZM

Group	C_{max} (μg/ml)	$T_{1/2}$ (min)	AUC$_{0\sim72}$ (μg·h/ml)	AUC$_{0\sim\infty}$ (μg·h/ml)	Cumulative urinary recovery rate (%)
Low ($n=0$)					
Mild ($n=1$)	0.56	31.7	4.31	4.92	5.35
High ($n=3$)	0.56 ± 0.07	30.2 ± 1.95	4.40 ± 0.72	4.97 ± 0.80	1.54 ± 0.49
Mean ($n=4$)	0.56 ± 0.06	30.6 ± 1.76	4.38 ± 0.59	4.96 ± 0.65	2.81 ± 2.23
Healthy volunteers ($n=6$)[a]	0.58 ± 0.11	30.5 ± 4.3	3.69 ± 0.47	4.23 ± 0.41	8.42 ± 1.19

[a]From Phase I; ±SD.

Azithromycin Concentrations in Gallbladder, Hepatic Tissue, and Bile Following a 5-Day Regimen in Humans

G. Foulds, R. A. Ferraina, H. G. Fouda, R. B. Johnson, A. M. Kamel, and R. M. Shepard

Pfizer Inc.
Groton, Connecticut

R. Falcone

Grant Medical Center
Columbus, Ohio

C. Hanna

Spartanburg Medical Center
Spartanburg, South Carolina

BACKGROUND

Azithromycin is an azalide antibiotic with pharmacokinetics characterized by modest serum concentrations, but high tissue concentrations (1). These high tissue concentrations appear to be correlated with efficacy in animal models of human infections (2). Following parenteral administration of radiolabeled azithromycin to dogs and rats, approximately two-thirds of the drug-related material recovered in excreta was recovered in feces and about one-third was recovered in urine (3). Following IV administration of azithromycin to a dog with a bile duct cannula, the recovery was 12% azithromycin plus 5% major metabolites in bile and 18% azithromycin plus 2% major metabolites in urine in 19 days (4). However, the excretion of azithromycin and metabolites in human bile has not been reported. During a study to examine the excretion of azithromycin in human bile, we were also able to obtain samples of liver and gallbladder for assay. Although prior studies have examined the pharmacokinetics of azithromycin in tissues following single doses (5–7), tissue concentrations have not been examined following multiple doses, with the exception of leukocytes (8). This paper reports azithromycin concentrations in gallbladder and hepatic tissue from patients undergoing cholecystectomy and examines concentrations of azithromycin and three major metabolites in human bile.

METHODS

Data were obtained from patients receiving azithromycin at three study sites: New London, Connecticut (1 patient), Columbus, Ohio (21 patients), and Spartanburg, South Carolina (14 patients). Samples were also received from 11 placebo-treated subjects. The protocol was approved by ethical review committees before initiation of the study. Informed consent was obtained as part of enrollment into the study. The dose regimen was the standard oral dose regimen used for treatment of respiratory tract and soft-tissue infections in the United States (i.e., 500 mg azithromycin on the first day, followed by 250 mg/day for 4 days). All doses were administered in capsules with water at least 2 h following a meal, or 1 h before a meal. Between 24 and 264 h after the final dose, surgery was performed and samples of serum, gallbladder, liver, and bile from the gallbladder were obtained.

All of the foregoing samples were assayed for azithromycin by high-performance liquid chromatography (HPLC) with electrochemical detection (9). Sample preparation for tissues began with homogenization of 0.1- to 0.5-g samples with acetonitrile and internal standard (9a-*N*-desmethyl,9a-*N*-propargylazithromycin.) Following centrifugation, separation of the layers, and evaporation of the acetonitrile layer to dryness, the residue was extracted with methyl-*t*-butyl ether at alkaline pH. Recovery of azithromycin during the tissue assay was estimated to be 85%. Recovery of the internal standard was 89%. Recoveries of azithromycin and internal standard were 86 and 89%, respectively, during the serum assay. The dynamic range of the assays for azithromycin was 0.1 or 0.2–1000 μg/g in tissues, 0.010–2.0 μg/ml in serum, and 0.05–300 μg/ml in bile. However, standard curves did not usually cover the entire dynamic range. Additionally, 25 bile samples were assayed for the major metabolites of azithromycin, CP-66,458 (descladinose-azithromycin), CP-64,434 (3'-*N*-desmethylazithromycin), and CP-60,273 (9a-*N*-desmethylazithromycin). The LLOQ for each metabolite in bile was 0.05 μg/ml. Additionally, extracts of 20 serum samples from patients receiving azithromycin were analyzed for the three major metabolites by HPLC with selected ion monitoring with a Sciex API III triple quadrapole mass spectrometer (10). The LLOQ for each metabolite in the HPLC/MS/MS assay was about 5 ng/ml.

Depletion rates of azithromycin from tissues were calculated by least-squares regression of log concentration against time. Half-life = 0.6931/slope of the regression.

RESULTS

The concentrations of azithromycin in gallbladder, hepatic tissue, and serum are summarized in Table 1. Concentrations in liver from patients receiving azithromycin were usually two- to threefold those in gallbladder, and concentrations in both tissues were 20-fold, or more, greater than those in serum. The concentrations in tissues were highly variable for each time interval. Concentrations in liver and gallbladder tissue declined slowly following the end of the dose regimen, with estimated depletion half-lives of 2.9 and 2.3 days, respectively.

Table 1 Summary of Concentrations of Azithromycin in Tissues Obtained from Surgical Patients Following a 5-Day Treatment Regimen Consisting of 500 mg on Day 1, Followed by 250 mg Daily on Days 2–5

	Time (h;day) after dose	No. of samples	Tissue conc. (μg/g) Gallbladder	Liver	No. of samples	Serum Conc. (μg/ml)
Mean	26.0	6	27.6	38.1	4	0.05
SEM range			6.9	8.5		0.01
Lower	24		4.0	5.3		0.03
Upper	33		51.8	64.8		0.06
Mean	51.2	5	11.2	22.9	5	0.04
SEM range			2.9	6.1		0.01
Lower	48		5.7	9.4		0.01
Upper	53		21.9	46.0		0.06
Mean	73.8	5	5.68	16.3	4	0.03
SEM range			1.50	4.3		0.01
Lower	72		2.7	8.6		0.01
Upper	76		11.1	28.6		0.04
Mean	99.2	4	3.63	10.6	4	0.06
SEM range			0.96	2.7		0.05
Lower	96		1.7	5.5		0.20
Upper	102		6.0	18.0		0.00
Mean	120.8; day 5	6	3.42	6.83	6	0.02
SEM range			0.71	1.45		0.004
Lower	120		1.1	4.7		0.01
Upper	125		6.2	13.9		0.04
Mean	145.8; day 6	7	2.74	8.90[a]	5	0.02
SEM range			0.63	4.23		0.01
Lower	144		0.9	2.0		0.00
Upper	151		5.9	25.5		0.04
	192; day 8	1	2.8	9.6	1	0.01
	264; day 11	1	2.9	4.5	0	

[a]Five samples.

Table 2 Concentration of Azithromycin and Metabolites in Human Bile from Patients Following Administration of a Dose Regimen of 500 mg on Day 1 and 250 mg Daily on Days 2–5

	Time (h; day) after dose	Conc. (µg/ml) Azith	% of drug-related material analyzed[a]			
			Azith	CP66458	CP64434	CP60273
Mean	27	95.1	65.4	11.9	14.8	8.0
SEM		35.1	12.8	5.1	4.8	3.2
N		4	4	4	4	4
Range						
Lower	24	47.0	27.8	4.1	7.1	3.0
Upper	33	200.0	83.8	26.9	28.2	17.2
Mean	51	115.6	69.0	5.8	17.0	8.2
SEM		43.2	5.9	1.9	4.7	2.7
N		4	3[b]	3	3	3
Range						
Lower	48	34.9	57.2	3.0	10.6	5.0
Upper	53	237	75.1	9.4	26.2	13.5
Mean	74	31.6	61.0	22.3	13.1	3.7
SEM		15.4	7.8	5.4	2.1	1.9
N		5	3[c]	3	3	3
Range						
Lower	72	3.0	46.5	12.0	9.8	0.0
Upper	76	87.0	73.4	30.0	17.1	6.4
Mean	99	35.6	60.1	24.3	10.4	5.2
SEM		17.4	11.4	12.9	1.1	2.8
N		3	3	3	3	3
Range						
Lower	96	2.9	37.5	10.7	9.0	0.0
Upper	102	62.0	73.8	50.0	12.5	9.8
Mean	121; 5 days	19.4	53.8	33.3	8.4	4.7
SEM		4.9	3.5	6.0	2.3	1.2
N		6	6	6	6	6
Range						
Lower	120	2.0	38.2	11.5	0.0	0.0
Upper	125	35.8	63.8	51.2	16.6	8.1
Mean	147	27.2	56.0	16.3	10.0	20.0
SEM		12.4	12.7	2.8	1.8	14.0
N		5	4[a]	4	4	4
Range						
Lower	144; 6 days	5.2	18.8	9.2	5.1	5.4
Upper	151	73.9	75.7	21.6	13.1	61.8
Mean	192; 8 days	7.2	43.3	36.3	13.4	7.0
N		1	1	1	1	1

Table 2 Continued

	Time (h; day) after dose	Conc. (μg/ml) Azith	% of drug-related material analyzed[a]			
			Azith	CP66458	CP64434	CP60273
Mean	264; 11 days	13.6	47.8	26.5	15.7	10.1
N		1	1	1	1	1
SEM			58.8	21.3	12.0	8.3
Range						
Upper			83.8	51.2	28.2	61.8
Lower			18.8	3.0	0.0	0.0

[a]Corrected for molecular weight.
[b]One sample was assayed for only azithromycin
[c]Two samples were assayed for only azithromycin.

Concentrations of azithromycin in bile (Table 2) were usually ≥ 100-fold those in serum and were greater than those in hepatic tissue. Azithromycin itself was the dominant drug-related material (mean 59%; range 19–84%) of the assayed material in bile. Azithromycin represented approximately 65, 69, 61, 60, 54, and 56% of analyzed materials in bile collected approximately 27, 51, 74, 99, 121, and 147 h after the last dose, respectively. Azithromycin constituted less than 40% of the drug-related material in only four samples, one of which contained relatively low concentrations of azithromycin (2.9 μg/ml) or metabolites. Azithromycin was the preponderant drug-related material found in serum. Low concentrations (7–49 ng/ml) of the descladinose metabolite were found in 3 of 20 serum samples; N-desmethyl metabolites were not found (< 5 ng/ml) in serum.

CONCLUSIONS

Following administration of the standard 5-day regimen, azithromycin was the preponderant drug-related material in human serum and bile. The concentrations of azithromycin in bile were much greater than those in serum, suggesting active biliary secretion of drug. The proportion of drug-related material assayed as azithromycin did not change with time following the dose regimen.

Azithromycin concentrations in hepatic tissue and gallbladder tissue were much greater than those in serum. Azithromycin concentrations in liver and gallbladder declined slowly over the 1- to 6-day period following completion of the dose regimen. The estimates of apparent depletion half-lives of 2.3 and 2.9 days are similar to the depletion half-lives of 2.5 to 3.2 days in tonsillar, prostatic, and uterine tissues following single doses (5–7). The standard 5-day regimen of azithromycin produced significant tissue concentrations for at least 6 days following the end of the regimen and at least 10 days from the beginning of the dose regimen.

REFERENCES

1. Foulds G, Shepard RM, Johnson RB. The pharmacokinetics of azithromycin in human serum and tissues. J Antimicrob Chemother 1990; 25(suppl A):73–82.

2. Retsema JA, Girard AE, Girard D, Milisen WB. Relationship of high tissue concentrations of azithromycin to bactericidal activity and efficacy in vivo. J Antimicrob Chemother 1990; 25(suppl A):83–89.

3. Shepard RM, Fouda HG, Ferraina RA, Mullins MA. Disposition and metabolism of azithromycin in rats, dogs and humans. International Congress for Infectious Diseases. Montreal, Canada. July 15–19, 1990.

4. Foulds G, Shepard RM, Allen RH, Feltcher AM. Transintestinal elimination of azithromycin in dogs. Fifth European Congress of Clinical Microbiology and Infectious Diseases. Oslo, Norway. Sept 9–11, 1991.

5. Foulds G, Chan KH, Johnson JT, et al. Concentrations of azithromycin in human tonsillar tissue. Eur J Clin Microbiol Infect Dis. 1991; 10:853–856.

6. Foulds G, Madsen P, Cox C, et al. Concentration of azithromycin in human prostatic tissue. Eur J Clin Microbiol Infect Dis. 1991; 10:868–871.

7. Krohn K. Gynaecological tissue levels of azithromycin. Eur J Clin Microbiol Infect Dis. 1991; 10:864–868.

8. Bonnet M, Van der Auwera P. In vitro and in vivo intraleukocytic accumulation of azithromycin (CP-62,993) and its influence on ex vivo leukocyte chemiluminescence. Antimicrob Agents Chemother 1992; 36:1302–1309.

9. Shepard RM, Duthu GS, Ferraina RA, Mullins MA. High-performance liquid chromatographic assay with electrochemical detection for azithromycin in serum and tissues. J Chromatogr Biomed Appl 1991; 565:321–337.

10. Avery MJ, Ferraina RA, Shepard RM, Fouda HG. Confirmation and identification of azithromycin metabolites in the dog by HPLC/atmospheric pressure ionization MS/MS. Proceedings of the 40th ASMS Conference on Mass Spectrometry and Allied Topics. Washington, DC. May 31–June 5, 1992.

Distribution of Dirithromycin in Human Respiratory Tissues and Fluids

Eugénie Bergogne-Bérézin

Bichat-Claude Bernard University-Hospital
Paris, France

INTRODUCTION

Dirithromycin, a new oral macrolide, is absorbed rapidly and exhibits an unusually prolonged half-life of 20–50 h. To be active in vivo, sufficient antibiotic concentrations at the site of infection and maintenance of effective concentrations after dosing are required. Thanks to a rapid distribution from the vascular space to tissue, dirithromycin reaches high tissue concentrations, reflecting a large apparent volume of distribution. In fact, following oral administration, dirithromycin is rapidly (30 min), nonenzymatically hydrolyzed to erythromycylamine, which is as active microbiologically as the parent compound. Thus, in in vivo models for the study of tissue distribution of dirithromycin, various human tissue specimens obtained surgically have been analyzed for concentrations of dirithromycin–erythromycylamine corresponding to tissue concentrations of antibiotic activity (4,6) without information as to the respective proportions of each compound.

LUNG PARENCHYMA

In lung parenchyma, dirithromycin and its main metabolite, erythromycylamine, achieved tissue concentrations ranging from 1.58 to 3.81 mg/kg according to the number of doses administered (3,5; Table 1). Significant antimicrobial activity was measured in both healthy and pathological tissue 4, 12, and 24 h after oral administration of dirithromycin, 250 mg once daily (one or five doses; see Table

1). In another study, higher doses of 500 and 750 mg were administered and high-pressure liquid chromatography (HPLC) was used to assay residual erythromycylamine concentrations in tissue samples. The results were similar to those obtained by using bioassay. Further studies have analyzed antimicrobial activity in healthy and pathological lung tissue 12 and 24 h after the last dose of a 5-day regimen of dirithromycin, 500 mg po once daily. The HPLC assay indicated that this activity was related to erythromycylamine, rather than to dirithromycin (see Table 1).

BRONCHIAL MUCOSA

In bronchial mucosa and secretions, data are reported in Table 1; concentrations of dirithromycin in bronchial tissue exceeded 1 mg/kg 4–24 h after a single 250- or 500-mg dose. After multiple doses, at 4, 12, and 24 h, bronchial concentrations ranged from 1.30 to 1.95 mg/kg, indicating sustained antimicrobial postdosing concentrations in bronchial tissues. Bronchial secretions (3 h) contained notable amounts of antimicrobial activity (1.04 mg/L) after a single 250-mg dose; the drug's prolonged half-life resulted in significant concentrations of 1.3 ± 1.6 mg/L in bronchial secretions 12 h after dosing, with a slow decrease, parallel to that in serum. Consecutive administration for 5 days resulted in progressively increasing concentrations of dirithromycin (Fig. 1).

EPITHELIAL LINING FLUID

Epithelial lining fluid (ELF) has also been analyzed for dirithromycin concentration. In 11 patients receiving 500 mg/day of dirithromycin (5 days), bronchoalveolar lavage allowed collection of ELF. Concentrations up to 2.47 mg/L in ELF were measured 24 h postdose, whereas in bronchial mucosa and secretions the levels of dirithromycin were 2.85 mg/L (7). In the three potential sites of infection sustained high concentrations were measured 72 h postdose.

UPPER RESPIRATORY TRACT

In the upper respiratory tract, single and multiple doses of dirithromycin resulted in mean nasal mucosal concentrations of 1.86 ± 0.54 mg/kg and 0.59 ± 0.17, respectively (sampling times: 12 and 24 h). Tissue/plasma concentration ratios were 26.5 and 19.7. Despite poor blood supply in the sinus mucosa, dirithromycin achieved notable tissue concentrations (3; Table 2). In tonsils, dirithromycin concentrations (measured by bioassay) ranged between 1.06 ± 0.48 mg/kg and 5.01 ± 2.91 mg/kg, according to the dose (500 or 1000 mg). These values were about 20-fold higher than those obtained in simultaneous serum samples. Stable

Table 1 Lung Tissue Concentrations of Dirithromycin–Erythromycylamine

Drug	No. patients	Sampling time (h)	Lung tissue[a] Healthy (mg/kg)	Pathologic (mg/kg)	Bronchi[a] (mg/kg)	Plasma (mg/L)
Study 1						
SD	4	4	1.13	0.28	1.03	0.08
SD	5	12	0.89	0.64	0.90	0.11
SD	5	24	0.35	0.26	0.48	0.02
MD	4	4	1.58	1.45	1.83	0.08
MD	4	12	2.03	1.60	1.88	0.05
MD	6	24	1.19	1.67	1.95	0.08
Study 2						
SD	2	4	0.33	0.26		
SD	1	24	0.35	0.18		
MD	4	4	1.68	1.56	0.71	
MD	4	12	2.19	1.50	0.78	
MD	6	24	2.39	3.81	0.40	

Group Study 3	No. patients	Sampling time (h)	Healthy (mg/kg) Bioassay	HPLC	Pathological (mg/kg) Bioassay	HPLC	Bronchi (mg/kg) Bioassay	HPLC
A (SD)	6	12[b]	1.92 ± 0.32	2.24 ± 0.62	2.37 ± 0.56	2.10 ± 0.37	0.92 ± 0.30	1.38 ± 0.48
	6	24	1.67 ± 0.44	1.90 ± 0.68	1.92 ± 0.92	1.40 ± 0.72	0.45 ± 0.11	0.50 ± 0.23
B (SD)	5	12	1.53 ± 0.44	0.94 ± 0.35	1.32 ± 0.27	0.82 ± 0.34	0.66 ± 0.37	0.69 ± 0.29
C (MD)	6	12	2.02 ± 0.36	2.42 ± 0.34	2.05 ± 0.64	1.79 ± 0.45	0.43 ± 0.12	1.31 ± 0.49
D (MD)	5	12	3.78 ± 0.54	3.79 ± 0.45	4.12 ± 0.36	3.85 ± 0.48	1.30 ± 0.16	1.70 ± 0.38
	6	24	2.68 ± 0.57	2.94 ± 0.74	3.40 ± 0.71	2.90 ± 1.22	0.44 ± 0.07	1.00 ± 0.22

[a]Dose dirithromycin: 250 mg po, one dose (SD); 250 mg po qd, five doses (MD).
[b]At all times plasma concentrations were below the low limit of detection (0.05 mg/L) by HPLC. Dose dirithromycin: group A, 750 mg po, one dose (SD); group B, 500 mg po, one dose (SD); group C, 500 mg po qd, two doses (MD); group D, 500 mg po qd, five doses (MD).
Source: After Ref. 3.

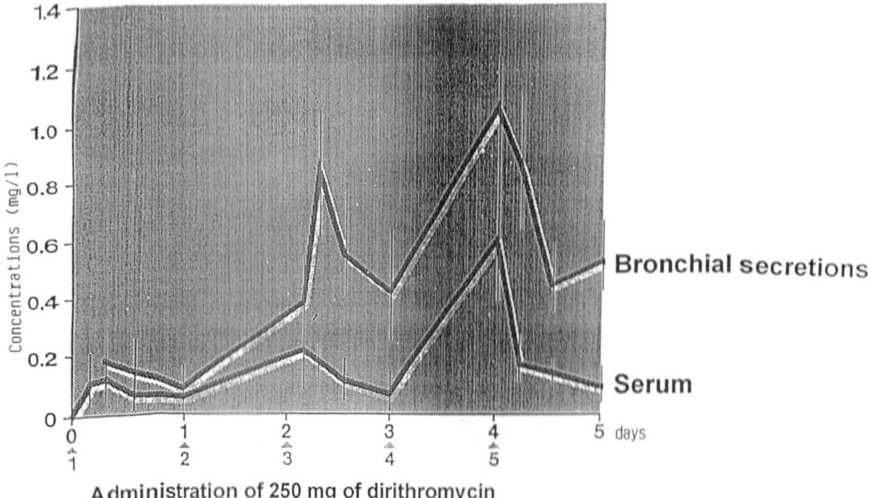

Figure 1   Concentrations of dirithromycin in serum and in bronchial secretions (multiple doses).

tonsil concentrations of 1.37 ± 0.55 mg/kg were maintained at 24 h (see Table 2; 4). The ability of macrolides to penetrate into and distribute within tissues and fluids of the lower respiratory tree has been widely studied (1,2,5) and is confirmed in this study.

Several pharmacokinetic parameters are determinants of the tissue distribution of dirithromycin. Half-life is one of the pharmacokinetic factors that greatly influences the tissue distribution of drugs; those with prolonged half-lives may have improved tissue distribution. Erythromycin has a short half-life; roxithromycin has a longer half-life, ranging from 6.6 to 9.9 h after a single 500-mg dose (2); dirithromycin has the longest half-life of 20–50 h (4). Plasma protein binding of macrolides is variable and is mostly to α_1-acid glycoprotein; protein binding of dirithromycin, evaluated after intravenous (IV) administration, was as low as 19% (range 14.6–32.2), a value favorable for extravascular diffusion of the drug (3). Other pharmacological characteristics of dirithromycin, such as high lipid solubility and low degree of ionization at pH values in blood and tissues, result in free diffusion from serum to extravascular spaces and interstitial fluid.

In respiratory tissues and fluids, high and sustained concentrations of dirithromycin were measured regardless of the protocol of administration and the specific tissue analyzed. In preclinical pharmacological studies in animals, HPLC analysis of in vivo antibiotic concentrations indicated very low concentrations

Table 2 Tissue Concentrations of Dirithromycin in Upper Respiratory Tissues

Tissue	Administration route	Dose[a] (mg)	No. patients	Peak serum (S) concentrations (mean ± SD) (mg/L)	Sampling time (h)	Tissue (T) or fluid (F) concentrations (mean ±SD) (mg/kg or mg/L)	Ratio T/S or F/S
Nasal mucosa	Oral	500 (S)	15	0.03 ± 0.01	24	0.59 ± 0.17	19.7
		500 (M)	15	0.07 ± 0.03	12	1.86 ± 0.54	26.5
		500 (M)	15		24	0.27 ± 0.13	
Tonsils		500 (M)	11	0.18	4	3.6	20
			15	NS	24	1.37 ± 0.55	
		500 (S)	10	0.24 ± 0.10	12	1.06 ± 0.48	4.4
			10	0.05 ± 0.07	24	0.60 ± 0.55	12.0
		500 × 2	6	0.15 ± 0.14	3–5	2.95 ± 2.76	20
		(2 days)	7	0.10 ± 0.05	13–16	5.01 ± 2.91	50

[a](S), single dose; (M), multiple doses; SD, standard deviation.
Source: After Refs. 3,4.

of dirithromycin versus much greater (25- to 170-fold) concentrations of erythromycylamine. In humans, most studies have been carried out by bioassay, which measures antibiotic activity without distinction between the two compounds. However, in human lungs and bronchi the results obtained by using HPLC assay expressed erythromycylamine, rather than dirithromycin. In most human tissue samples only erythromycylamine was present, or any dirithromycin still present in the tissue was likely to be converted to erythromycylamine during the preparation of the thin-layer chromatography of the tissue extracts. Otherwise, in lungs, the presence of an inflammatory exudate, especially the phagocytic component, probably contributes to the increased local concentrations found in pathological tissues. The ability of macrolides to concentrate within phagocytes and alveolar macrophages accounts for the observed high lung tissue concentrations of dirithromycin.

CONCLUSIONS

Dirithromycin exhibits excellent tissue distribution and appears to be rapidly distributed to selected tissues, where it persists for up to 24 h following the last dose of drug. Tissues that have been demonstrated to contain sustained concentrations of antibiotic include lung parenchyma, bronchial mucosa, and secretions. In all plasma and tissue samples collected after administration of dirithromycin, the measurement of antibiotic activity included that of actual erythromycylamine concentrations. A single 750-mg dose was superior to a single 500-mg dose at 12 h after administration. The concentrations of the antibiotic achieved in tissues after multiple doses of dirithromycin and the rate of decrease of tissue concentrations after cessation of administration are consistent with the long terminal half-life of 20–50 h calculated for this compound (6).

REFERENCES

1. Barza M. Principles of tissue penetration of antibiotics. J Antimicrob Chemother 1981; 8(suppl C):7–28.
2. Bergogne-Bérézin, E. The tissue penetration of macrolides with particular reference to the respiratory tract. In: Butzler JP, Kobayashi H, eds. Macrolides: A Review With an Outlook on Future Developments. Amsterdam: Excerpta Medica, 1986:43–53.
3. Bergogne-Bérézin E. Tissue distribution of dirithromycin: comparison with erythromycin. J Antimicrob Chemother 1993; 31(suppl C):77–87.
4. Bozler G, Heinzel G, Lechner U, Schumacher K, Busch U. Pharmacokinetic properties and metabolic behaviour of dirithromycin determine its high tissue penetration in man. 28th Interscience Conference on Antibiotic Agents and Chemotherapy Oct 23–26 Los Angeles, 1988:abstr 924.
5. Brun Y, Forey F, Gamondes JP. Levels of erythromycin in pulmonary tissue

and bronchial mucus compared to those of amoxycillin. J Antimicrob Chemother 1981; 8:459–466.

6. Busch U, Lechner U. Pharmacokinetic behaviour of dirithromycin in human tissues. 28th Interscience Conference on Antimicrobial Agents and Chemotherapy, Oct 23–26, Los Angeles, 1988:abstr 925.

7. Cazzola M, Tufano MA, Polverino M, Catalanotti G, Angrisani M, Varanese L, Rossi F. Pulmonary penetration of dirithromycin in chronic bronchitis. 6th European Congress of Clinical Microbiology and Infectious Diseases, Seville, March 1993:abstr 320.

Distribution of Clarithromycin to Intracellular and Extravascular Sites of Infection: An Overview

F. Scaglione, G. Demartini, and F. Fraschini

University of Milan
Milan, Italy

INTRODUCTION

Antibiotic therapy should not be selected solely on the basis of an agent's in vitro activity or its serum pharmacokinetic parameters. To be effective, an antibiotic should possess activity against invasive microorganisms at the site of infection. Pharmacokinetic parameters such, as T_{max}, C_{max}, and AUC in serum, usually are not predictive of an antibiotic's concentration at the infection site, which can be an extravascular, extracellular, or intracellular compartment, but rarely intravascular. An antibiotic should preferably achieve antibacterial levels in each of these aforementioned compartments. Here we present the results from a series of our published and unpublished studies on the pharmacokinetic behavior of clarithromycin.

PENETRATION OF CLARITHROMYCIN AND 14-OH-CLARITHROMYCIN INTO ORAL AND RESPIRATORY TISSUES AND FLUIDS

Five studies were carried out to determine the penetration of clarithromycin and its 14-hydroxy metabolite into oral and respiratory tissues (1). One hundred twenty-eight patients of both sexes, undergoing dental surgery, rhinoplasty, lung resection, or tonsil resection, or presenting with an acute exacerbation of chronic bronchitis, were administered clarithromycin (generally 250 mg twice daily; 500 mg twice daily for lung resections) for 3 days before sample collection. Serum, tissue, and secretion samples were assayed for clarithromycin and 14-OH-clarithromycin using an agar diffusion bioassay or high-performance liquid chromatography (HPLC). Concentrations were assayed in triplicate, and standard curves were created using computerized linear regression analysis (Table 1).

Blood samples were taken at the time of fluid or tissue collection: both serum and fluid or tissue were frozen immediately after collection and stored at $-20°C$ until assay.

HPLC Analysis

Samples were sonicated for 5 min and extracted with 3 ml of hexame-ethyl acetate 1:1 plus 200 μl sodium carbonate 0.1 M and 0.8 μg of internal standard (erythromycin A 9-*O*-methyloxime). The suspensions were mixed vigorously for 2 min in a vortex and then centrifuged at 1500 rpm for 5 min. The supernatants were collected and evaporated under a nitrogen stream at 45°C. The dry extracts were dissolved in acetonitrile/water 1:1.

The concentrations of clarithromycin and its 14-OH metabolite were evaluated in triplicate in isocratic conditions using acetonitrile/methanol (44 and 10%, respectively) in phosphate buffer, 0.04 M at pH 7.3, as mobile phase and a Bondesil C8 (15-cm) column solution. Serum samples were extracted and assayed using the same procedure (2). The coefficient of variation was 5%, and the detection limit was 0.01 mg/kg^{-1} L^{-1} for both compounds.

Agar Diffusion Bioassay

The agar diffusion bioassay method (3) used *Micrococcus luteus* ATCC 9341 as the test organism in antibiotic medium 11.

The results showed that clarithromycin was rapidly absorbed, with peak serum concentrations of clarithromycin and its 14-hydroxy metabolite occurring 1–3 h after oral administration, and maximum tissue concentrations occurring 4 h after administration of the final dose (Table 2). Both clarithromycin and 14-hydroxy clarithromycin were detectable in tissues 12 h after administration.

From these results it is possible to conclude that clarithromycin and its 14-OH metabolite achieve excellent tissue penetration, with highest levels in lung. Clarithromycin levels are maintained within the therapeutic range in respiratory tissues and fluids and serum for up to 12 h after dosing.

IN VIVO INTRACELLULAR AND EXTRACELLULAR DISTRIBUTION OF CLARITHROMYCIN

Several reports show that β-lactam antibiotics are distributed only in the vascular and extravascular spaces and not intracellularly, whereas other antibiotics, such

Table 1 Patients and Methods

	Study 1	Study 2	Study 3	Study 4	Study 5
Diagnosis/procedure	Acute exacerbation of chronic bronchitis	Oral surgery	Lung resection due to cancer or bronchiectasis	Tonsil resection	Rhinoplasty
No. of patients	12 7 males 5 females	28 16 males 12 females	28 19 males 9 females	30 21 males 9 females	30 17 males 13 females
Mean $\pm$ SD age (yr)	58.0 $\pm$ 8.4	31.6 $\pm$ 5.4	59.0 $\pm$ 12.4	26.0 $\pm$ 10.3	38.0 $\pm$ 9.6
Mean $\pm$ SD wt (kg)	68.0 $\pm$ 9.7	68.0 $\pm$ 12.5	67.0 $\pm$ 9.0	60.0 $\pm$ 10.4	64.0 $\pm$ 8.1
Clarithromycin regimen	250 mg bid 3 days	250 mg bid 3 days	500 mg bid 3 days	250 mg bid 3 days	250 mg bid 3 days
Assay method	HPLC	Bioassay	HPLC	HPLC	HPLC
Samples	Serum, bronchial secretions	Serum, saliva, gingiva, alveolar bone	Serum, lung tissue	Serum, tonsils	Serum, nasal mucosa

Table 2 Peak Concentration (μg/ml or μg/g) of Clarithromycin and 14-OH Clarithromycin in Selected Tissues and Fluids

Tissue/fluid	Clarithromycin	14-OH Clarithromycin
Bronchial secretion[a]	3.98 ± 1.37	1.86 ± 0.67
Lung[b]	13.5 ± 3.30	7.20 ± 0.90
Tonsil[a]	5.34 ± 2.30	3.10 ± 1.10
Nasal mucosa[a]	5.92 ± 2.00	3.20 ± 0.70
Saliva[a]	2.22 ± 0.93	

[a]250 mg bid
[b]500 mg bid

as macrolides, are distributed both intracellularly and extracellularly. To investigate the distribution of antibacterial agents, the serum levels of amoxicillin, clarithromycin, and azithromycin were compared with their bronchial secretion levels, assayed in the intracellular and extracellular compartments, in patients suffering from chronic bronchitis.

Thirty-six patients (mean age = 54 years, range = 42–68), with an acute exacerbation of chronic bronchitis, were enrolled in the study. Antibiotics were administered orally as follows:

amoxicillin, 500 mg tid 12 patients
azithromycin, 500 mg qd 12 patients
clarithromycin, 500 mg bid 12 patients

After 3 days of treatment, samples were collected 2, 4, 8, and 12 h after the morning dose. Bronchial secretion were centrifuged on a gradient of silicon oils to separate cells from fluid. Antibiotic concentrations were measured in both cells and fluid by the HPLC method (2,3). The results are summarized in Table 3.

Amoxicillin achieved good levels in bronchial fluid (extracellularly), with concentrations approximately half of those attained in serum; it was not detectable within bronchial cells. Azithromycin was primarily concentrated within bronchial cells, with very low concentrations achieved in either serum or bronchial (extracellular) fluid. Clarithromycin attained high and balanced concentrations both intracellularly (to levels severalfold higher than serum) and extracellularly (to levels approximately equal to or higher than serum).

INTRACELLULAR AND EXTRACELLULAR DISTRIBUTION AND ACTIVITY OF CLARITHROMYCIN: AN IN VITRO MODEL

The intracellular and extracellular activities of three broad-spectrum antibiotics—amoxicillin, azithromycin, and clarithromycin—were determined by using an improved in vitro model of infection (4).

Table 3 Concentrations (mean ± SD) of Amoxicillin, Azithromycin, and Clarithromycin in Serum and Bronchial Secretions at Different Times After Administration of 500 mg of Each Antibiotic

Time (h)	Amoxicillin			Azithromycin			Clarithromycin		
	Serum (μg/ml)	Bronchial fluid (μg/ml)	Bronchial cells (μg/g)	Serum (μg/ml)	Bronchial fluid (μg/ml)	Bronchial cells (μg/g)	Serum (μg/ml)	Bronchial fluid (μg/ml)	Bronchial cells (μg/g)
2	6.3 ± 2	3.2 ± 1.3	ND	0.4 ± 0.2	0.28 ± 0.5	4.6 ± 1.1	5.2 ± 1.4	1.9 ± 1	4.3 ± 1.2
4	2.8 ± 0.9	1.2 ± 0.8	ND	0.3 ± 0.2	0.3 ± 0.1	11.3 ± 6.2	3.1 ± 0.8	2.8 ± 1.4	9.7 ± 3.4
8	1.0 ± 0.4	0.5 ± 0.2	ND	0.3 ± 0.2	0.2 ± 0.16	12.2 ± 8.4	1.5 ± 1.0	1.8 ± 0.9	8.4 ± 4.1
12	ND	ND	ND	0.3 ± 0.2	0.27 ± 0.2	12.0 ± 7.4	0.7 ± 0.3	1.4 ± 0.4	5.2 ± 2.1

ND, not detectable

An in vitro infection model was created with the use of a suspension of macrophages, polymorphonuclear leukocytes, lymphocytes, fibroblasts, and human serum to which a pathogen and an antibiotic were added. Separate intracellular and extracellular antibiotic activity against *Staphylococcus aureus* and *Legionella pneumophila* was assessed for three antimicrobial agents: amoxicillin, azithromycin, and clarithromycin. Intracellular and extracellular concentrations of the antibiotics were also evaluated using an agar diffusion bioassay (3).

The results showed that amoxicillin was active only extracellularly; it was ineffective intracellularly. In contrast, azithromycin was primarily concentrated and active intracellularly, with little activity in extracellular fluid. Clarithromycin was active both intra- and extracellularly.

Clarithromycin shows balanced penetration and antimicrobial activity against intracellular and extracellular pathogens. Azithromycin shows good intracellular penetration and activity, but poor extracellular activity. Amoxicillin (representing most β-lactams) shows almost no intracellular penetration or activity, but excellent extracellular activity.

REFERENCES

1. Scaglione F, Pintucci JP, Tassi GF, et al. Penetration of clarithromycin into oral and respiratory tissues. Drug Invest 1993; 6:104–109.
2. Ohtake T, Ogura K, Iwatate I, Suwa T. Assay for TE-031 (A-56268) in body fluids (1): high performance liquid chromatography. Chemotherapy 1988; 36:192–197.
3. Chapin-Robertson K, Edberg SC. Measurement of antibiotics in human body fluid: techniques and significance. In: Lorian V, ed. Antibiotics in Laboratory Medicine. Baltimore: Williams & Wilkins, 1991:295–366.
4. Scaglione F, Demartini G, Dugnani S, Fraschini F. A new model examining intracellular and extracellular activity of amoxicillin, azithromycin and clarithromycin in infected cells. Chemotherapy 1993; 39:418–423.

Safety of Clarithromycin in Elderly Patients

E. Spiritus

Pulmonary Consultants of Orange
Orange, California

BACKGROUND

Evaluation of antimicrobial agents is essential in the elderly, a growing subset of the population at increased risk for infection. The physiological changes in this group of patients can affect the pharmacology and disposition of drugs, resulting in higher blood concentration. Consequently, a greater incidence in adverse effects has been observed in elderly patients.

Clarithromycin is a new-generation macrolide, with a broad spectrum of activity against many clinically important gram-positive, gram-negative, and atypical pathogens. Clarithromycin has a broader spectrum of in vitro activity, enhanced serum and tissue kinetics, and improved patient tolerance, compared with erythromycin. Safety and efficacy have been demonstrated in a variety of infections, including bronchitis, pneumonia, pharyngitis, sinusitis, skin and skin structure infections, and lower respiratory tract infections, in which clarithromycin was compared with macrolide and nonmacrolide reference agents.

STUDY OBJECTIVE

Our objective was to compare the safety profile of clarithromycin in elderly patients ($\geq$ 65 years of age) with that observed in patients younger 65 years of age.

"

METHODS

Adverse Events

Adverse events (as assessed by the investigators) are defined as any evidence of drug intolerance or any clinical or laboratory adverse experiences, whether or not they were thought to be drug-related and whether observed by the investigators or reported by the patients. Patients reporting one or more events of the same type were counted only once.

Laboratory Data

Data were typically collected pretreatment, once or twice during treatment, and once or twice following discontinuation of treatment and then assessed for possible clinical significance according to the following criteria:

SGOT, SGPT	$\geq 3 \times H^a$
BUN	$\geq 1.25 \times H$
Creatinine	$\geq 1.3 \times H$
Prothrombin time	>5 sec above baseline or 1.4 × baseline (if %)

[a]H, upper limit of normal.

RESULTS

The results are summarized in Tables 1–5.

Table 1 Age Distribution by Indication

Indication body system	< 65 yr[a] (*n* = 3373) % (*n*)	≥ 65 yr (*n* = 978) % (*n*)
Bronchitis	21 (698)	40 (392)
Pneumonia	13 (426)	15 (148)
Pharyngitis	19 (657)	2 (18)
Sinusitis	13 (445)	2 (20)
Skin and skin structure infections	12 (418)	8 (79)
LRTIs[b]	22 (727)	33 (326)
Other	<1 (2)	0 (0)

[a]Includes five patients of unknown age.
[b]Lower respiratory tract infections.

Table 2 Adverse Events by Body System and Age

Body system	< 65 yr (n = 3373) % (n)	≥ 65 yr (n = 978) % (n)
Body as a whole	5.6 (190)	3.3 (32)
Cardiovascular	0.8 (27)	1.5 (15)
Gastrointestinal	11.8 (399)	8.9 (87)
Other digestive	3.1 (104)	4.5 (44)
Metabolic/nutritional	1.7 (56)	1.5 (15)
Nervous	2.4 (81)	2.6 (25)
Respiratory	1.7 (57)	1.3 (13)
Skin/appendages	2.1 (70)	1.5 (15)
Special senses	3.7 (126)	2.6 (25)
Urogenital	1.6 (55)	0.7 (7)
Overall	25.3 (852)	21.5 (210)

CONCLUSIONS

There were few differences in the incidence of adverse events in patients younger than 65 years versus patients ≥ 65 years or older who received clarithromycin; in fact, older patients had fewer gastrointestinal events compared with younger patients, 8.9 versus 11.8% ($p = 0.01$), respectively.

Notably, neither age group experienced significant effects in SGOT and SGPT, observed with other macrolides. BUN changes were observed in 5% of

Table 3 Gastrointestinal Adverse Events by Age[a]

Event	< 65 yr (n = 3373) % (n)	≥ 65 yr (n = 978) % (n)
Nausea	4.8 (163)	4.0 (39)
Diarrhea	3.9 (130)	2.5 (24)
Abdominal pain	2.4 (82)	1.6 (16)
Dyspepsia	1.7 (59)	1.5 (15)
Vomiting	1.1 (36)	1.6 (16)
Other	0.4 (14)	0.2 (2)
Total patients with GI events	11.8 (399)	8.9 (87)

[a]The majority of gastrointestinal adverse events were mild or moderate in severity; 24 (0.7%) patients younger than 65 years had a severe or adverse event of unknown severity compared with 5 (0.5%) patients 65 years or older.

Table 4 Possibly Clinically Significant Laboratory Values by Age

Laboratory value	< 65 yr S/T[a]	≥ 65 yr S/T[a]
Prothrombin time	26/1595 (2%)	13/410 (3%)
Creatinine	3/2871 (<1%)	7/860 (<1%)
BUN	28/2814 (1%)	41/838 (5%)
SGOT	4/2875 (<1%)	3/860 (<1%)
SGPT	8/2854 (<1%)	3/847 (<1%)

[a]S, number of patients with laboratory values of possible clinical significance; T, total number of patients with a baseline value and on-study value.

Table 5 Premature Withdrawals by Patients Owing to Adverse Events[a] by Body System and Age

Body system	< 65 yr (*n* = 3373) % (*n*)	≥ 65 yr (*n* = 978) % (*n*)
Digestive system	2 (69)	3 (27)
Body as a whole	1 (20)	1 (7)
Skin and appendages	1 (16)	<1 (3)
Nervous system	<1 (14)	1 (5)
Special senses	<1 (9)	<1 (3)
Total patients withdrawn due to AE	3 (111)	5 (44)

[a]Some patients were withdrawn because of adverse events in more than one body system.

the older group compared with 1% of the younger group. This is perhaps not unexpected because the elderly, as a group, have decreased renal function.

Clarithromycin is as well tolerated in elderly patients as in nonelderly patients.

The Kinetics of Erythromycin Stearate During Simultaneous Administration of Oral Nonsteroidal Anti-inflammatory or Nasal Decongestant Drugs

Serafim G. Kastanakis

Chania General Hospital
Chania, Greece

INTRODUCTION

Erythromycin (ERY) is often used for the treatment of respiratory infections. These infections have a variety of symptoms, for which various other drugs, such as analgesics, antipyretics, and nasal decongestants, are used for alleviation. Gastrointestinal absorption of ERY is variable, depending on many known and unknown factors. We decided to study whether some of the most often used "anti-flu" drugs influence the kinetics of ERY.

MATERIALS AND METHODS

The kinetics of ERY, given alone or simultaneously with an anti-flu drug, were studied in 18 patients. All were inpatients of the First Dept. of Medicine, Chania General Hospital and (1) had not received any other antimicrobial for 7 days before or at any stage during the study; (2) weighed between 50 and 100 kg; (3) were between 18 and 75 years old; (4) did not have renal failure, digestive disease, or an infection; (5) were not seriously ill; and (6) had no drug allergy. In women of childbearing age pregnancy was excluded by pregnancy test. All patients gave their informed consent.

Each patient received two doses of ERY stearate, 500 mg orally, at least

3 days apart. On the first occasion, ERY was given alone and a full kinetic profile was performed. On the second occasion ERY was given together with one oral dose of the following: (1) aspirin (ASP) 1 g, six patients; (2) acetaminophen paracetamol; (PAR) 1 g, six patients; or (3) one tablet of Disofrin (DIS), a nasal decongestant combination of dexbrompheniramine (dextrobrompheniramine; 6 mg/tablet) and *d*-pseudoephedrine (D-isoephedrine; 120 mg/tablet), six patients. A second full kinetic profile was then performed. Each patient thus served as his own control.

Concentrations of ERY in serum and urine were measured using a microbiological agar well plate method with *Sarcina lutea* as the indicator organism.

Statistical analysis was performed using a paried *t*-test.

RESULTS

Serum levels of ERY during the two profiles are shown in Table 1, and urine excretion is given in Table 2. Aspirin caused a dramatic decrease of ERY serum levels: the mean peak was reduced from 2.45 to 0.78 mg/L and appeared 30 min later; the mean area under the time–concentration curve (AUC) was reduced from 9.15 to 3.23 mg/L·h ($p < 0.001$) and urine recovery (UR) from 7.95 to 5.06 mg ($p < 0.05$). DIS also had a reducing, but mainly a delaying effect. The peak was reduced from 2.69 to 1.79 mg/L and appeared 140 min later. The AUC was reduced from 10.8 to 6.34 mg/L·h ($p < 0.01$) and UR from 10.06 to 6.16 mg ($p < 0.01$). PAR had the opposite effect: the peak was increased from 1.24 to 3.4 mg/L, appeared 50 min earlier, the AUC rose from 3.91 to 11.19 mg/L·h ($p < 0.001$), and the UR from 4.54 to 14.66 mg ($p < 0.001$).

DISCUSSION AND CONCLUSIONS

The higher serum levels and urinary excretion of ERY caused by PAR may be due to enhancement of absorption of the antimicrobial, but also to displacement of the latter from the plasma proteins. Erythromycin has a high protein-binding capacity, and even small increases of the free portion are important. Increase of the free portion also results in quicker renal excretion, explaining the higher UR. Another mechanism that can explain the observed higher levels is competitive inhibition by PAR at the hepatic enzyme level, resulting in reduced hepatic metabolism and excretion of ERY.

The decrease of oral absorption of ERY by ASP may be due to delayed emptying of stomach through pH reduction of gastric juice by ASP, possible destruction of ERY in the stomach during its prolonged stay there, and delayed arrival of ERY in the small intestine, where its absorption takes place.

The effect of DIS may be due to the sympathomimetic action of

Table 1 Concentrations of Erythromycin (ERY) in Serum of 18 Patients[a]

	Mean levels in milligrams (SD) afterdose												All peaks		Peaking time (h)		AUC (mg/L·h)	
	0.5		1		1.5		2		4		6							
ERY alone	0.11	(0.08)	1.33	(0.42)	1.56	(0.29)	2.45	(0.36)	1.84	(0.30)	0.91	(0.26)	2.45	(0.36)	2.00	(0.00)	9.15	(1.46)
ERY + ASP	0.26	(0.14)	0.56	(0.26)	0.56	(0.26)	0.59	(0.27)	0.67	(0.13)	0.32	(0.09)	0.78	(0.17)	2.50	(1.12)	3.24*	(0.75)
ERY alone	0.00	(0.00)	0.44	(0.34)	0.56	(0.39)	0.64	(0.26)	1.01	(0.64)	0.61	(0.39)	1.24	(0.48)	2.50	(1.08)	3.91	(1.16)
ERY + PAR	1.72	(0.36)	2.31	(0.77)	3.24	(1.19)	2.87	(0.68)	1.56	(0.22)	0.84	(0.11)	3.41	(0.99)	1.67	(0.24)	11.19*	(2.14)
ERY alone	0.24	(0.15)	2.18	(0.99)	2.50	(0.91)	2.61	(0.64)	2.09	(0.51)	0.90	(0.17)	2.69	(0.75)	1.50	(0.29)	10.81	(2.83)
ERY + DIS	0.69	(0.25)	0.80	(0.26)	0.97	(0.29)	1.04	(0.27)	1.29	(0.55)	1.23	(0.80)	1.79	(1.48)	3.83	(1.84)	6.34**	(1.67)

[a]Patients were given 500 mg po ERY either alone or together with 1 g aspirin (ASP; six patients), or 1 g acetaminophen (paracetamol; PAR: six patients, or 1 tablet Disofrin [DIS: 6 mg dexbrompheniramine (dextrobrompheniramine) plus 120 mg d-pseudoephedrine (D-isoephedrine)]; six patients.
*$p < 0.001$, **$p < 0.01$.

Table 2 Excretion of Erythromycin (ERY) in Urine of 18 Patients

	Mean amount in milligrams and (SD) excreted at indicated times (h) after dose				Total excretion (mg)
	0–2	2–4	4–8	8–12	0–12
ERY alone	2.67 (0.80)	2.30 (0.45)	1.68 (0.70)	1.29 (0.72)	7.95 (1.10)
ERY + ASP	0.93 (0.68)	2.19 (0.87)	1.82 (0.70)	0.45 (0.16)	5.06 (2.01)***
ERY alone	1.12 (0.60)	1.90 (0.85)	0.98 (0.57)	0.54 (0.31)	4.54 (0.76)
ERY + PAR	6.16 (0.36)	4.96 (1.24)	2.04 (1.11)	1.50 (1.13)	14.66 (1.86)*
ERY alone	2.48 (1.10)	4.53 (1.30)	1.73 (0.38)	1.33 (0.68)	10.06 (2.96)
ERY + DIS	1.07 (0.68)	2.58 (1.27)	1.81 (0.49)	0.70 (0.22)	6.16 (2.40)**

[a]Patients were given 500 mg ERY stearate po, either alone or together with 1 g aspirin (ASP; six pts), 1 g paracetamol (PAR; six pts), or 1 tablet Disofrin (DIS; 6 mg dextrobrompheniramine plus 120 mg D-isoephedrine; six pts).
*$p < 0.001$, **$p < 0.01$, ***$p < 0.05$.

pseudoephedrine causing delay in stomach emptying followed by the events described in the foregoing.

Concerning the "erythromycin alone" individual data (see Tables 1 and 2), the reason levels are so different in each pair might relate to variations in erythromycin metabolism during its first passage through the liver. Generally the gastrointestinal absorption of drugs is variable among individuals (1–3).

The reduced bioavailability of ERY caused by ASP and DIS is clearly undesirable. On the other hand, the effect of PAR may also be damaging, since overloading the liver detoxifying enzyme system may lead to increased hepatotoxicity, a concern always borne in mind when administering macrolides.

Until further studies define the clinical significance of the observed interactions, we recommend separate administration of ERY and the studied anti-flu drug.

REFERENCES

1. Brodie BB. Physicochemical factors in drug absorption. In: Binns TB, ed. Absorption and Distribution of Drugs. Baltimore: Williams & Wilkins 1964:16–48.
2. Prescott LF, Nimmo WS, eds. Drug Absorption. New York: ADIS Press, 1981.
3. Goodman and Gilman's The Pharmacological Basis of Therapeutics, 8th ed. Pharmacokinetics. 1990:3–32.

Safety and Efficacy of Clarithromycin Compared with Amoxicillin or Cefaclor in Children with Lower Respiratory Tract Infections

J. L. Macklin and S. J. Coles

Abbott Laboratories
Maidenhead, United Kingdom

BACKGROUND

Lower respiratory tract infections (LRTIs), including bronchitis and pneumonia, are commonly seen in children. Bronchitis is typically an acute illness characterized by fever, cough, rhonchi, and other respiratory symptoms. Although many cases of bronchitis are caused by respiratory viruses, *Mycoplasma pneumoniae*, *Bordetella pertussis*, and *Chlamydia pneumoniae* must be considered as aetiologic agents, especially in those with signs and symptoms of bronchitis that persist beyond a week. *Haemophilus influenzae* and *Streptococcus pneumoniae* cause pneumonia with approximately equal frequency in infants, whereas *S. pneumoniae* predominates as the causative pathogen in children older than 3–4 years.

Clarithromycin, an advanced-generation macrolide, offers excellent in vitro activity against most organisms that are responsible for LRTIs in children. In studies conducted in adults, clarithromycin concentrations attained in serum (4.6 μg/ml) (1), bronchial secretions (3.98 μg/ml), and lung tissue (17.5 μg/g) (2) exceed by severalfold the MIC_{90} values for the most prevalent respiratory pathogens (0.5 μg/ml for *S. pneumoniae*; 1 μg/ml for *H. influenzae*; 0.03 mg/ml for *C. pneumoniae*; 0.008 μg/ml for *M. pneumoniae*).

394

STUDY OBJECTIVE

The study was designed to compare the safety and efficacy of clarithromycin with amoxicillin or cefaclor suspensions in the treatment of children with lower respiratory tract infections.

PATIENTS AND METHODS

Study Design

The studies were single (investigator)-blind, randomized and multicenter.

Inclusions

1. Male or nonpregnant/nonlactating female patients 1–12 years old inclusive.
2. Presence of signs and symptoms of LRTI, including cough and two or more of the following: sputum production; change in sputum color or consistency indicative of an acute bacterial infection (e.g., change to yellow or green, increased tenacity of sputum); pyrexia; increased chest discomfort or congestion; development of or increase in dyspnea, rales, rhonchi, or cyanosis; general malaise (one study); chest x-ray films consistent with pneumonia (one study).
3. No use of systemic or long-acting antibiotics within 3–7 days or 4 weeks, respectively, before administration of the study drug.
4. No suspicion of active tuberculosis or neoplasm.
5. No hypersensitivity to macrolide or β-lactam antibiotics.
6. No severe renal or hepatic impairment.
7. Written informed consent.

Drug Administration

Patients were randomized to receive a 5- to 10-day suspension regimen of:

> Clarithromycin 7.5 mg/kg bid (max 500 mg bid), or
> Amoxicillin 125 mg (<25 kg body weight) to 250 mg tid, or
> Cefaclor 20 mg/kg per day tid (max of 1 g/day) for bronchitis, to 40 mg/kg
> per day for pneumonia

EVALUATIONS

	Study day 1	48–72 h[a]	Study days 5–7	≤ 72 h posttreatment
Medical history	X			X
Physical examination	X		X	X
Signs and symptoms	X	X	X	X
Specimen for C and S[b]	X		X	X
Chest x-ray[c]	X			X
Clinical response		X[d]	X[d]	X
Adverse drug events			X	X

[a]After start of therapy; parent or guardian contacted by telephone.
[b]Bronchopulmonary secretions, if available.
[c]If clinically indicated (one study).
[d]One study.

RESULTS

The results are summarized in Tables 1–4.

Table 1 Summary of Demographic Data and Infection Status of Enrolled Patients

	Clarithromycin ($n = 132$)	Amoxicillin ($n = 74$)	Cefaclor ($n = 65$)
Gender			
Female	67	45	32
Male	65	29	33
Age (y)			
Mean	4.8	5.2	5.3
Range	0–12	1.0–12.8	0–12
No. middle ear infections			
in ≤ 12 mo			
Mean	1.5	1.1	1.2
Range	0–5	0–6	0–7
Infection severity			
Mild	11	19	6
Moderate	101	52	34
Severe	20	3	25

Table 2 Clinical Success[a] by Treatment Group and Evaluation Period

Evaluation period	Clarithromycin	Amoxicillin	Cefaclor
Study days 2–3	85% (40/47)	87% (48/55)	
Study days 5–7	100% (53/53)		96% (47/49)
≤ 72 h posttreatment	98% (107/109)	95% (54/57)	96% (52/54)

[a]Clinical cure or improvement.

Table 3 Resolution of Signs and Symptoms of LRTI by Treatment Group

Sign/symptom	Clarithromycin	Amoxicillin	Cefaclor
Sputum production	95% (54/57)	88% (22/25)	86% (25/29)
Sputum appearance	96% (25/26)	100% (3/3)	91% (21/23)
Cough	62% (68/109)	60% (34/57)	74% (40/54)
Dyspnea	94% (62/66)	97% (33/34)	93% (26/28)
Rales/crackles	95% (88/93)	91% (42/46)	92% (45/49)
Rhonchi/wheezes	96% (65/68)	92% (34/37)	100% (26/26)
Pyrexia	94% (93/99)	91% (40/44)	98% (49/50)

Table 4 Summary of Adverse Events[a] by Treatment Group

Adverse event by body system	Clarithromycin ($n = 132$)	Amoxicillin ($n = 74$)	Cefaclor ($n = 65$)
Body as a whole	3% (4)	3% (2)	2% (1)
Digestive	13% (17)	8% (6)	5% (3)
Hematological/lymphatic	2% (2)	0	3% (2)
Nervous	1% (1)	3% (2)	0
Metabolic	1% (1)	0	0
Respiratory	2% (2)	7% (5)	0
Skin	5% (7)	4% (3)	2% (1)
Special senses	1% (1)	1% (1)	2% (1)
GU	1% (1)	0	2% (1)
Overall	23% (31)	20% (15)	12% (8)

[a]Most adverse events were of mild-to-moderate severity across treatment groups.

CONCLUSIONS

Twice daily clarithromycin resulted in high rates of clinical success, comparable with that of three times daily amoxicillin and cefaclor, β-lactam agents often used for the treatment of pediatric LRTIs.

All drugs were well tolerated with no statistically significant difference between groups.

REFERENCES

1. Guay DRP, Craft JC. Overview of the pharmacology of clarithromycin suspension in children and a comparison with that in adults. Pediatr Infect Dis J, 1993; 12(suppl 3):106–111.
2. Fraschini F, Scaglione F, Pintucci G, et al. The diffusion of clarithromycin and roxithromycin into nasal mucosa, tonsil and lung in humans. J Antimicrob Chemother, 1991; 27(suppl A):61–65.

Safety and Efficacy Evaluation of Clarithromycin in Elderly Patients

E. Spiritus

Pulmonary Consultants of Orange
Orange, California

BACKGROUND

The incidence of infection is increased in the elderly, reflecting primarily senescence of the immune system. Advance age also brings about structural and degenerative changes in vital organ systems that may predispose to infection. Physiological changes in the elderly can affect the pharmacology and disposition of drugs, resulting in higher blood concentration and a greater incidence of adverse effects.

Clarithromycin is a new-generation macrolide, with in vitro activity that includes key gram-negative and gram-positive organisms responsible for upper and lower respiratory tract and skin or skin structure infections. The prolonged elimination half-life of clarithromycin (3.5–3.8 h) permits twice-daily dosing. Clarithromycin is well tolerated, with a rate of adverse events equivalent to that of β-lactam agents, and a rate of gastrointestinal adverse events significantly less than that of erythromycin.

OBJECTIVE

The studies' objective was to compare the safety and efficacy of orally administered clarithromycin, 250 or 500 mg bid, with reference agents including ampicillin, amoxicillin, amoxicillin–clavulanate, erythromycin, cefadroxil, cefaclor, cefuroxime axetil, and cefixime, in the treatment of elderly ($\geq$ 65 years) patients with bronchitis, pneumonia, sinusitis, or skin and skin structure infection.

PATIENTS AND METHODS

Enrollment

The patients had a diagnosis of acute bacterial exacerbation of chronic bronchitis, community-acquired pneumonia, acute maxillary sinusitis, or mild to moderate bacterial skin and skin structure infections.

Eligibility

Eligibility criteria included clinical signs and symptoms, confirmed by chest x-ray film for community-acquired pneumonia, or a sinus x-ray film for acute maxillary sinusitis, and positive culture pretreatment.

Evaluation Schedule

Efficacy evaluations were performed within 48 h pretreatment, once during therapy, and once or twice posttreatment. Adverse events were monitored throughout therapy.

Drug Administration

Indication	Clarithromycin	Reference
Bronchitis	250 mg or 500 mg bid	Ampicillin, 250 mg q6h
		Cefaclor, 500 mg tid
		Cefuroxime axetil, 500 mg bid
		Cefixime, 400 mg QD
Pneumonia	250 mg bid	Erythromycin, 250 mg q6h
		Erythromycin, 500 mg q6h
Sinusitis	500 mg bid	Amoxicillin, 500 mg q8h
		Amoxicillin–clavulanate, 500 mg q8h
Skin infection	250 mg bid	Cefadroxil, 500 mg bid
		Erythromycin, 250 mg q6h

RESULTS

The results are summarized in Tables 1–4.

Table 1 Summary of Demographics in All Elderly Patients

	Clarithromycin ($n = 366$)	Reference ($n = 420$)
Gender		
Female	140	165
Male	226	255
Race		
White	335	385
Black	21	20
Asian	2	2
Other	8	13
Age (y)		
Mean ± SD	71.9 ± 5.6	72.0 ± 5.5
Range	65–95	65–93
Weight (kg)		
Mean ± SD	72.1 ± 17.0	71.4 ± 16.2
Range	34–163	34–120

Table 2 Efficacy Results for Evaluable Elderly Patients

	Clarithromycin	Reference
Posttreatment		
Clinical cure	60% (115/191)	53% (109/204)
Clinical improvement	32% (62/191)	40% (82/204)
Clinical success[a]	93% (177/191)	94% (191/204)
Follow-up		
Clinical recurrence	6% (11/177)	5% (10/191)

[a]Cure and improvement.

Table 3 Clinical Success by Indication for Evaluable Elderly Patients

Clinical success	Clarithromycin	Reference
Bronchitis	91% (88/97)	92% (99/108)
Pneumonia	94% (49/52)	93% (53/57)
Sinusitis	100% (9/9)	100% (8/8)
Skin infection	94% (31/33)	100% (31/31)

Table 4 Summary of Safety Profile for All Elderly Patients

	Clarithromycin ($n = 366$)	Reference ($n = 420$)
Adverse events		
Overall	25% (90)	21% (90)
Gastrointestinal	12% (45)	15% (63)
Other digestive	6% (20)	4% (16)
Body as a whole	3% (12)	3% (12)
Special senses	4% (13)	1% (6)
Skin and appendages	2% (8)	1% (4)
Nervous system	1% (5)	2% (7)
Premature termination		
Owing to adverse events	7% (26)	7% (28)

CONCLUSION

Clarithromycin resulted in clinical responses comparable with that of reference agents in elderly patients. The incidence of adverse events was comparable between the two treatment groups.

Overview of the Efficacy and Safety of Roxithromycin Versus Control Antibiotics in the Treatment of Infections in Adults

H. Portier

Hopital du Bocage
Dijon, France

INTRODUCTION

Roxithromycin, an acid-stable, orally administered, macrolide antibiotic, is a derivative of erythromycin. It has an improved pharmacokinetic profile, including an extended half-life of 12 h, enabling twice daily dosage, improved tissue penetration, and the potential for fewer drug interactions. Its spectrum of activity against common pathogens is similar to that of other macrolides.

Clinical efficacy has been confirmed in the treatment of lower respiratory tract infections (LRTI), including community-acquired and atypical pneumonias; upper respiratory tract infections (URTI), including otitis, acute sinusitis, and pharyngitis or tonsillitis; skin and soft tissue infections (SSTI); and sexually transmitted disease (STD).

This overview compares the safety and efficacy of roxithromycin with that of standard treatments for URTI, LRTI, SSTI, and STD, including β-lactams, tetracyclines, and other macrolides (see Table 1).

PATIENTS AND METHODS

Fifteen double-blind and seven open-label studies were reviewed, involving a total of 6204 patients. Male and female patients, 18 years of age or older, with

Table 1 Study Design, Medication, and Dosage

Protocol/ID no. No. patients Site	Study design	Indication	Roxithromycin dose	Comparator	Treatment duration
FFR/83/965/01					
n = 95 France	Phase III OL	LRTI	150 mg bid	None	7–20 days
FF87/965/16					
n = 1573 International	Phase III OL	LRTI URTI SSTI	150 mg bid 300 mg od		10–20 days
DMID 1992, 15:123–129S					
n = 76 Belgium	Phase III DB	LRTI	300 mg od	Doxycycline, 200 mg od	7–14 days
FFR/84/965/03a					
n = 305 France	Phase III DB	LRTI	150 mg bid	Doxycycline, 200 mg od	7–20 days
NZ/90/965/01					
n = 240 New Zealand	Phase III DB	LRTI	150 mg bid	Cefaclor, 250 mg tid	7–14 days
FFR/84/965/04a					
n = 193 France	Phase III DB	LRTI	150 mg bid	Erythromycin, 1 g bid	7–20 days
DMID 1992, 15:91–95S					
n = 96 Belgium	Phase III DB	URTI	150 mg bid	Amoxicillin, 500 mg, + clavulanic acid, 125 mg tid	10 days

UK/84/965/05 $n = 449$ United Kingdom	Phase III DB	URTI	150 mg bid	Amoxicillin, 250 mg tid	7–14 days
FFR/84/965/03e $n = 84$ France	Phase III DB	URTI	150 mg bid	Doxycycline, 200 mg od	4–16 days
FFR/84/965/04b $n = 21$ France	Phase III DB	URTI	150 mg bid	Erythromycin, 1 g bid	4–16 days
ZA/86/965/40 $n = 40$ South Africa	Phase III OB	URTI	150 mg bid	Co-trimoxazole, 960 mg q12h	7–14 days
FFR/84/965/03d $n = 81$ France	Phase III DB	SSTI	150 mg bid	Doxycycline, 200 mg od	
SF/85/965/10 $n = 200$ Finland	Phase III OL	STD	150 mg bid 450 mg od		7–14 days
SF/84/965/01 $n = 300$ Finland	Phase III DB	STD	150 mg bid	Lymecycline, 300 mg bid	7–14 days
FFR/84/965/03c $n = 121$ France	Phase III DB	STD	150 mg bid	Doxycycline, 200 mg od	7–14 days
FF/82/965/03 $n = 28$ Denmark	Phase II OL	LRTI	200 mg bid or 300 mg bid		10 days

(continued)

Table 1 (*continued*)

Protocol/ID no. No. patients Site	Study design	Indication	Roxithromycin dose	Comparator	Treatment duration
FF/82/965/03 $n = 31$ Finland	Phase II OL	LRTI SSTI	200 mg bid 300 mg bid		10 days
F84/965/15 $n = 1208$ International	Phase III OL	LRTI URTI SSTI	150 mg bid	None	7–20 days
DMID 1992, 15:855–89S $n = 490$ France	Phase III OL	LRTI	150 mg bid	Amoxicillin, 500 mg, + clavulanic acid, 125 mg tid	7–14 days
DMID 1992, 15:119–123S $n = 200$ Italy	Phase III OL	URTI	300 mg od	Clarithromycin, 250 mg bid	9 days
FFR/84/965/036 $n = 29$ France	Phase III OL	STD	150 mg bid	None	7–14 days
F84/965/25 $n = 346$ International	Phase III OL	STD	150 mg bid	None	7–14 days

DB, double blind; OB, observer blind; OL, open label; od, once daily; URTI, upper respiratory tract infection; LRTI, lower respiratory tract infection; SSTI, skin and soft tissue infection; STD, sexually transmitted disease.

bacterial infections of mild to moderate severity were recruited. The study design, medication and dosages are shown in Table 1.

Patients who received roxithromycin had a mean age of 40.9 (range 25–68), those receiving other macrolide comparators had a mean age of 50.3 years (range 36–63), and those receiving nonmacrolide comparators had a mean age of 43.9 years (range 27–62).

RESULTS

Among the roxithromycin-treated patients, the clinical and bacteriological success rates were similar, irrespective of the diagnosis or the mode of administration of the 300-mg–daily dose they received. The success rates (cured plus improved), according to indication and treatment group, are given in Table 2.

Adverse events, possibly or probably, related to the study drug were observed in 4% (206/4874) of patients in the roxithromycin group, compared with 12% (12/97) in the macrolide group, and 21% (128/609) in the nonmacrolide group (Table 3). The adverse events most frequently observed were associated

Table 2 Clinical and Bacteriological Success Rates

Indication	Roxithromycin,[a] 150 mg bid or 300 mg od	Macrolide comparator[b]	Nonmacrolide comparator[c]
	(*n* = 4192)	(*n* = 176)	(*n* = 957)
LRTI			
Clin. success rate	1668/1835 (90.9%)	56/73 (76.7%)	446/515 (86.6%)
Bact. success rate	474/502 (84.4%)	11/15 (73.3%)	34/47 (72.3%)
URTI			
Clin. success rate	1298/1402 (92.6%)	72/103 (69.9%)	188/212 (88.7%)
Bact. success rate	384/440 (87.3%)	55/60 (91.7%)	55/60 (91.7%)
SSTI			
Clin. success rate	297/321 (92.5%)		32/39 (82.1%)
Bact. success rate	184/197 (93.4%)		9/11 (81.8%)
STD			
Clin. success rate	584/643 (90.5%)		183/191 (95.8%)
Bact. success rate	447/495 (90.3%)		166/172 (96.5%)

[a]Roxithromycin, 150 mg bid (*n* = 3804); roxithromycin, 300 mg od (*n* = 926).
[b]Erythromycin, 1 g bid (*n* = 104); clarithromycin, 250 mg bid (*n* = 100).
[c]Doxycycline, 200 mg od (*n* = 332); Amoxicillin, 500 mg + clavulanic acid, 125 mg tid (*n* = 292); amoxicillin, 250 mg tid (*n* = 150); lymecycline, 300 mg bid (*n* = 150); cefaclor 250 mg tid (*n* = 119); Co-trimoxazole 960 mg bid (*n* = 20).

Table 3 Adverse Events by Treatment Group

	Roxithromycin[a]	Macrolide comparators	Nonmacrolide comparators
All adverse events possibly or probably related to the study drug	206/4875 (4%)	12/97 (12%)	128/609 (21%)
Adverse events resulting in discontinuation	75/4875 (2%)	2/97 (2%)	34/609 (6%)

[a]10/4875 deaths (0.2%) occurred in the roxithromycin group. None of these were considered to be related to treatment.

with the gastrointestinal system, the most common events in all three groups being nausea, diarrhea, and abdominal pain. Clinically relevant changes in hepatic laboratory parameters were observed in fewer than 1% of patients treated with roxithromycin. No changes were seen in the other groups.

CONCLUSIONS

For the treatment of upper and lower respiratory tract infections, skin and soft tissue infections, and sexually transmitted diseases, the results of these 22 trials clearly demonstrate that roxithromycin in doses of 150 mg twice daily or 300 mg once daily is at least as effective as either macrolide or nonmacrolide comparators. Roxithromycin was also better tolerated than the comparator drugs.

Safety and Efficacy of Clarithromycin in the Treatment of Acute, Mild to Moderate Lower Respiratory Tract Infections

Sawang Saenghirunvattana

Ramathibodi Hospital
Bangkok, Thailand

BACKGROUND

Infections of the respiratory tract are the most common infectious diseases seen by the general practitioner, often resulting in lost days from work or school and medical costs for the patients. Data from a recent, year-plus long study of approximately 10,000 adults in a general practice population showed that acute bronchitis and exacerbation of chronic bronchitis accounted for 88% of the 480 lower respiratory tract infections (LRTIs) seen. The remaining 12% demonstrated changes on chest x-ray films consistent with pneumonia (1). *Streptococcus pneumoniae* followed by *Haemophilus influenzae* are the organisms most frequently isolated from patients with LRTIs, although the spectrum of causative organisms for LRTIs is broad and ever-expanding (2,3). When choosing an antibiotic for the treatment of general practice patients, for whom the infecting pathogen is frequently unknown, one must select an antibiotic with a spectrum of in vitro activity that includes the majority of the pathogens encountered, including not only *S. pneumoniae* and *H. influenzae*, but also *Moraxella catarrhalis*, which almost uniformly produce β-lactamase, *Mycoplasma pneumoniae*, *Chlamydia pneumoniae*, and *Legionella pneumophila* (2–4).

Clarithromycin, an expanded-generation macrolide, possesses potent, broad-spectrum antimicrobial activity that encompasses most clinically relevant respiratory tract pathogens, including those that produce β-lactamase and destroy many β-lactams (5,6). Given the high prevalence of such pathogens in Thailand, we designed a study to evaluate the role of clarithromycin in our general practice population.

PATIENTS AND METHODS

This investigation was designed as an open clinical trial to which male and nonpregnant, nonlactating female adult patients ($\geq$ 15 years old and weighing over 40 kg), with a diagnosis of acute bronchitis, chronic bronchitis with an acute bacterial exacerbation, infected brochiectasis, or mild, community-acquired pneumonia, were enrolled. Eligible patients received clarithromycin, 250 mg every 12 h for 7 days. Chronic bronchitis was defined by a history of recurrent, productive cough present on most days for at least 3 consecutive months in over 2 successive years. The criteria for an acute bacterial exacerbation were one or more of the following: increased cough, increased sputum production, a change in sputum color or consistency indicative of an acute bacterial infection, increased chest discomfort or congestion, and the development of or increase in dyspnea, rales, rhonchi, or cyanosis. The diagnosis of mild, community-acquired pneumonia was supported by a history, physical examination, and a new pulmonary infiltrate on chest x-ray film studies. Patients were required to provide written informed consent to participate in the study.

Patients were excluded if they had pretreatment radiologic evidence of active tuberculosis or pulmonary tumor, documented or suspected bacteremia, or had received recent (within 3 days) systemic antimicrobial therapy.

The initial evaluation included a medical history, physical examination, and an evaluation of the patient's clinical signs and symptoms. Sputum was obtained for Gram stain and culture and susceptibility testing, and a serum sample

Table 1 Summary of Demographic Data, Medical History, and Infection Status for Enrolled Patients

Age (yr)	
Mean	54.5
Range	15–75
Gender	
Male	38
Female	12
Infection type	
Pneumonia	18 (39%)
Acute exacerbation of COPD	10 (20%)
Acute bronchitis	13 (23%)
Bronchiectasis	9 (18%)

Table 2 Clinical Response by Diagnosis

Response	Pneumonia ($n = 18$)	Acute exacerbation of COPD ($n = 10$)	Acute bronchitis ($n = 13$)	Bronchiectasis ($n = 9$)	Total ($n = 50$)
Complete recovery	18	10	12		40 (80%)
Clinical improvement				7	7 (14%)
Failure to improve[a]			1	2	3 (6%)

[a]The infections were caused by antibiotic-resistant organisms: *Acinetobacter calcoaceticus, Pseudomonas aeruginosa,* and *Serratia* species.

was obtained for laboratory analysis. Patients were evaluated twice during therapy, on study day 4 ± 1 and study day 7, and a third time 7 days posttreatment. The evaluations performed at the initial visit were repeated at each of these visits (except laboratory assessment at the posttreatment visit), and the patient's clinical response to therapy was assessed.

RESULTS

Fifty adult patients (mean age of 54.4 years old) were enrolled; approximately three-fourths were men (Table 1). Pneumonia (39% of patients) and acute exacerbations of chronic bronchitis (20% of patients) accounted for over half of the presenting diagnoses for which clarithromycin was prescribed; all patients with these often difficult-to-treat infections were clinically cured of their infection with clarithromycin, 250 mg bid, treatment over 7 days (Table 2). The overall clinical success response across all the mild to moderate LRTIs treated was 94%. The three patients who failed to improve with clarithromycin had infections caused by antibiotic-resistant bacteria—*Acinetobacter calcoaceticus*, *Pseudomonas aeruginosa*, and *Serratia* species. Of note, all strains of *S. pneumoniae* ($n = 32$) and *H. influenzae* ($n = 4$), the most prevalent bacteria causing LRTIs, were eradicated by clarithromycin.

CONCLUSION

Oral clarithromycin, 250 mg bid, is effective therapy for and well tolerated by adult patients with acute bacterial exacerbations of chronic bronchitis, acute bronchitis, bronchiectasis, and community-acquired streptococcal pneumonia.

REFERENCES

1. MacFarlane JT, Colville A, Guion A, MacFarlane RM, Rose DH. Prospective study of aetiology and outcome of adult lower-respiratory-tract infections in the community. Lancet 1993; 341:511–514.
2. Rodnick JE, Gude JK. Diagnosis and antibiotic treatment of community-acquired pneumonia. West J Med 1991; 154:405–409.
3. Meyer RD, Finch RG. Community-acquired pneumonia. J Hosp Infect 1992; 22(suppl A):51–59.
4. File TM Jr. Community-acquired pneumonia. The changing picture. Postgrad Med 1992; 92:197–214.
5. Fernandes PB, Bailer R, Swanson R, et al. In vitro and in vivo evaluation of A-56268 (TE-031), a new macrolide. Antimicrob Agents Chemother 1986; 30:865–873.
6. Hardy DJ, Hensey DM, Beyer JM, Vojtko C, McDonald EJ, Fernandez PB. Comparative in vitro activities of new 14-, 15-, and 16-membered macrolides. Antimicrob Agents Chemother 1988; 32:1710–1719.

Multicenter Study on the Efficacy and Tolerance of Roxithromycin in the Treatment of Respiratory Tract Infections

J. Lorenz

University Hospital
Mainz, Germany

INTRODUCTION

Roxithromycin, the first of the new-generation macrolides, has a spectrum of activity similar to that of erythromycin, but shows an improved pharmacokinetic profile, with good gastrointestinal absorption, high plasma and tissue levels, and a long half-life. The aim of this study was to evaluate the efficacy and tolerance of roxithromycin in the treatment of respiratory tract infections under general practice conditions.

MATERIALS AND METHODS

The efficacy and tolerance of roxithromycin were evaluated in an open, multicenter study in Germany, involving 3411 general practitioners. A total of 16,912 patients were studied as outpatients. The study involved adult patients (older than 18 years), with clinical diagnosis of respiratory tract infection, including tonsillitis, sinusitis, otitis, acute bronchitis, exacerbation of chronic bronchitis, and community-acquired pneumonia. All patients were treated with roxithromycin, 150 mg bid, for 7–10 days.

The results were obtained in an intent-to-treat analysis. A detailed record of all adverse events was maintained to evaluate the safety profile of roxithromycin.

RESULTS

The results are summarized in Tables 1–3.

Table 1 Demographic Characteristics of Patients

Total no. of patients	16,912	(%)
No. of women	8,733	(51.6%)
No. of men	8,030	(47.5%)
Not reported	149	(0.9%)

The mean age was 42 ± 17 years. The final judgment of clinical efficacy is summarized in Figure 1. The demographic characteristics and diagnoses of the 16,912 patients are summarized in Table 1; 25.2% of patients with bronchopulmonary infections, 15.6% of patients with tonsillitis or pharyngitis,

Table 2 Diagnosis on Entry to the Study

Diagnosis[a]	No. patients	(%)
Sinusitis	4899	(29%)
Tonsillitis/pharyngitis	4618	(27.3%)
Otitis media	1500	(8.9%)
Acute bronchitis	5056	(29.9%)
Exacerbation of chronic bronchitis	2001	(11.8%)
Pneumonia	867	(5.1%)

[a]More than one diagnosis was possible.

Table 3 Clinical Success Rates[a]

Tonsillitis/pharyngitis	96.0%
Sinusitis	95.2%
Otitis media	93.8%
Bronchitis and exacerbation of chronic bronchitis and pneumonia	95.3%
Total	95.3%

[a]Disappearance or improvement of clinical symptoms.

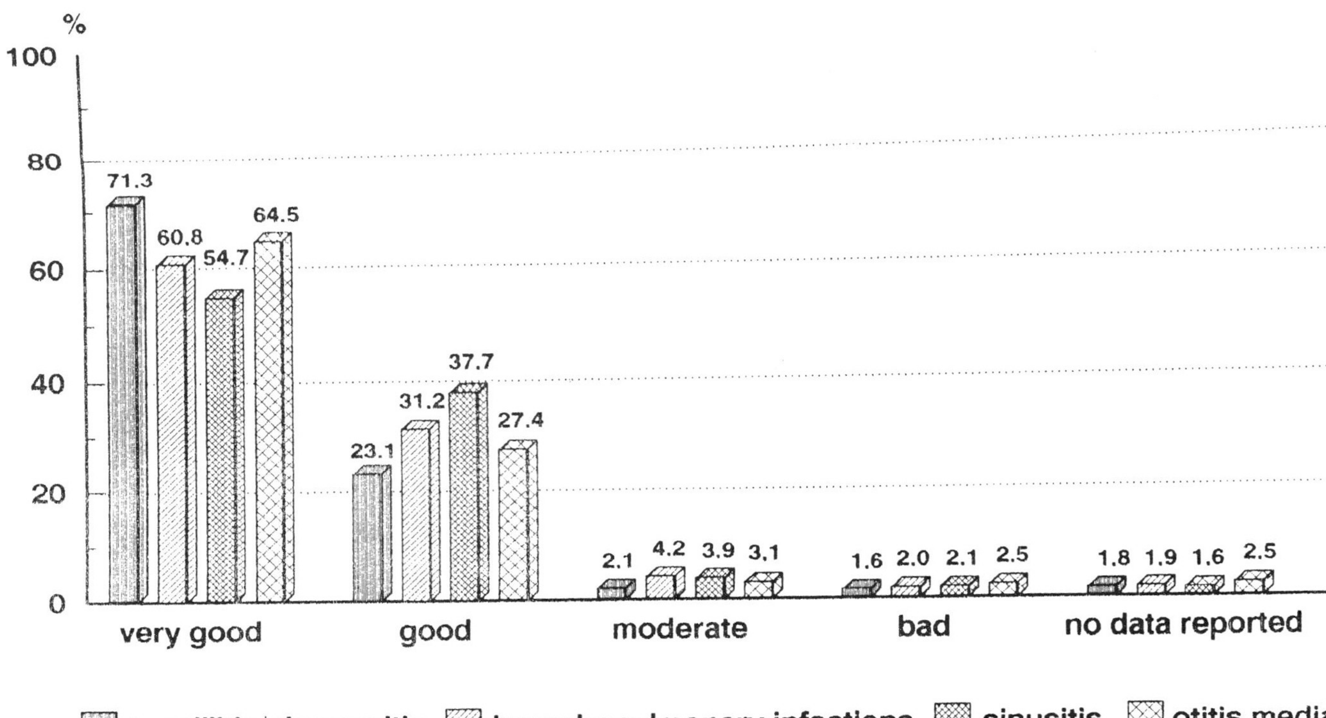

Figure 1 Final judgment of clinical efficacy.

Table 4 Adverse Events Possibly or Probably Related to Roxithromycin

Type	Total no.	Total %
Total	324	1.9
Digestive system[a]	237	1.4
Skin[b]	52	0.3
Nervous system[c]	48	0.3
Others	24	0.15

[a]Nausea, gastrointestinal pain/disorder, diarrhea, vomiting, flatulence, decreased appetite.
[b]Rash, pruritus, sweating increased, urticaria.
[c]Dizziness, headache, sleeping disorder, agitation.

14.7% of patients with sinusitis, and 13% of patients with otitis media had received previous, unsuccessful antibiotic treatment (in most cases penicillin or tetracycline). The percentages of clinical success by diagnosis are shown in Table 2. The final judgment of clinical efficacy in the end of treatment is given in Table 3.

SIDE EFFECTS

Roxithromycin was well tolerated: only 604 (3.6%) reported adverse events. Adverse events with possible or probable relation to roxithromycin were seen in only 324 patients (1.9%). One hundred forty-nine patients (0.9%) stopped treatment owing to adverse events. Side effects consisted mainly of gastric discomfort (Table 4, Fig. 2).

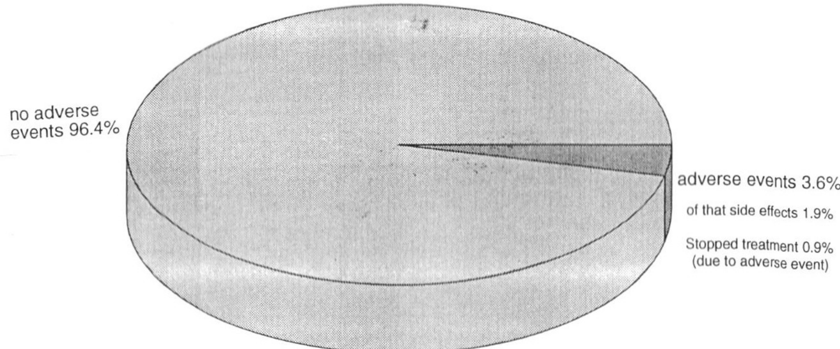

Figure 2 Adverse events.

CONCLUSION

Roxithromycin is in an effective antibiotic in the treatment of all common upper and lower respiratory tract infections in general practice and is well tolerated. The results of this study confirm roxithromycin as a first-line antibiotic in the general practitioner's armamentarium.

Roxithromycin as a Five-Day Empiric Treatment of Respiratory Tract Infections: A Multicenter Study

N. A. Sliman

Jordan University School of Medicine
Amman, Jordan

INTRODUCTION

The choice of antibiotic to be used as a first-line drug for empiric treatment of acute community-acquired respiratory tract infection is made after careful evaluation of the patient's history and a physical examination.

Roxithromycin is a new-generation macrolide, a derivative of erythromycin, which retains the appropriate antibacterial profile of the earlier macrolides used in general practice (1). It has a high and rapid absorption, with a long half-life (2,3), and a high diffusion to the tissues, as demonstrated by concentrations in the lung, prostate, ovary, liver, kidney, and skin (4–6). Its spectrum of activity includes the typical gram-positive and gram-negative organisms responsible for acute community-acquired respiratory tract infection (RTI). In addition, it is effective against such atypical organisms as *Legionella* spp., *Mycoplasma* spp., and *Chlamydia* spp.

Because of these advantages, roxithromycin was chosen to be studied as a first-line drug in the treatment of acute community-acquired respiratory tract infection in Jordan and Cyprus, with a 5-day duration of treatment.

MATERIALS AND METHODS

Twenty-three centers, including university hospitals, community hospitals, and general practices, took part in an open, prospective study undertaken on the basis of everyday general practice.

Exclusion criteria included children; pregnant women; patients with liver, kidney, or heart disease; and patients who had received other antibiotics within 3 days before admission to the study.

A total of 399 patients were admitted to the trial. All patients, except a few with chronic obstructive pulmonary disease, were otherwise healthy, adult, ambulatory patients, who presented with acute respiratory tract infections.

Each patient received 150 mg roxithromycin twice daily for 5 days. Seven patients were lost to follow-up; 392 patients (234 males, mean age 35.1 years (range 15–82) and 156 females, mean age 31.4 years (range 14–94)) completed the study.

Clinical efficacy was assessed on the basis of evolution of functional and physical signs and the time interval before fever began to fall.

RESULTS

Functional signs were eliminated in 243 and improved in 109 patients, and physical signs were eliminated in 252 and improved in 111 patients (Table 1). The overall assessment at the end of treatment was considered to be excellent in 242 (61%) and good in 120 (31%) patients (see Table 1).

Table 1 Changes in Functional and Physical Signs and Overall Assessment After Five Days of Treatment with Roxithromycin

	Bronchopulmonary		Tonsillitis		Sinusitis		Otitis	
	No.	%	No.	%	No.	%	No.	%
Total no. of patients	169		130		37		56	
Functional signs								
Eliminated	75	44	106	81	20	54	42	75
Improved	66	39	18	14	15	40	10	18
Unchanged	26	15	4	3	2	5	4	7
Worsened	2	1	2	1	0	0	0	0
Physical signs								
Eliminated	88	52	102	78	19	51	42	75
Improved	63	17	22	17	16	43	10	18
Unchanged	14	8	3	2	1	3	4	7
Worsened	4	2	3	2	1	3	0	0
Overall assessment								
Excellent	83	49	100	77	18	49	41	73
Good	68	40	24	18	17	46	11	20
Intermediate	13	7	3	2	1	2	3	5
Poor	5	3	3	2	1	2	1	2

Table 2 Overall Assessment for Bronchopulmonary Disease

	Acute bronchitis		Acute exacerbations of chronic bronchitis		Pneumonia	
	No.	%	No.	%	No.	%
No. of patients	116		36		17	
Excellent	63	54	14	39	6	35
Good	44	38	16	44	8	47
Intermediate	7	6	6	17	0	0
Poor	2	2	0	0	3	18

Of the 169 patients with bronchopulmonary disease, the overall assessment was excellent in 8.3 and good in 68 patients (Table 2).

The interval before reduction of fever was longest in cases of pneumonia (2.6 days), followed by acute bronchitis and acute exacerbations of chronic bronchitis (1.9 days), sinusitis (1.7 days), tonsillitis (1.6 days), and was shortest in cases of otitis (1.4 days).

Side effects were seen in 21 cases, most being due to gastric pain (Table 3). Only one patient withdrew from the study because of adverse effects.

CONCLUSIONS

Acute respiratory tract infections are usually treated empirically in everyday clinical practice; therefore it is important that the antibiotic chosen should be both safe for the patient and effective against the most frequent pathogens.

Table 3 Side Effects[a]

Type of event	No. of cases
Diarrhea and fatigue	1
Gastric pain	14
Mouth redness and edema	1
Constipation	1
Vomiting	2
Headache	1
Skin rash	1

[a]In $n = 21$ patients.

In previous studies roxithromycin has been effective and safe in the treatment of acute community-acquired upper and lower respiratory tract infections (7–10), and the twice-daily dosage regimen, which is convenient to patients, improves compliance.

In our multicenter study, we found roxithromycin to be effective in the treatment of respiratory tract infections, even when given at a dose of 150 mg twice daily for only 5 days. A further advantage of roxithromycin is the low incidence (1.8%) of side effects.

Roxithromycin, therefore, would appear to be an appropriate first-line drug for the empiric treatment of acute community-acquired respiratory tract infections.

REFERENCES

1. Barlam T, Neu HC. In vitro comparison of the activity of RU28965, a new macrolide with that of erythromycin against aerobic and anaerobic bacteria. Antimicrob Agents Chemother 1984; 25:529–531.
2. Nilsen OG. Comparative pharmacokinetics of macrolides. J Antimicrob Chemother 1987; 20(suppl B):81–88.
3. Nilsen OG, Aamo T, Zailsen K, Svarva P. Macrolide pharmacokinetics and dose scheduling of roxithromycin. Diagn Microbiol Infect Dis 1991; 15:71S–76S.
4. Bergogne-Berezin E. Tissue distribution of roxithromycin. J Antimicrob Chemother 1987; 20(suppl B):113–120.
5. McLean A, Sutton JA, Salmon J, Chatelet D. Roxithromycin: pharmacokinetic and metabolism study in man. Br J Clin Pract 1987; 41:52–53.
6. Campa M, Zolfino I, Bernardini N, et al. The penetration of roxithromycin into human skin. J Antimicrob Chemother 1990; 26:87–90.
7. Gentry L. Roxithromycin: a new macrolide antibiotic in the treatment of infections in the lower respiratory tract. An overview. J Antimicrob Chemother 1987; 20(suppl B):145–152.
8. Peterslund NA, Hanninen P, Schreiner A, Black FT, Hulten V. Roxithromycin in the treatment of pneumonia. J Antimicrob Chemother 1989; 23:737–741.
9. Champetier de Ribes D, Jockey C, Gadouen G. Etude de l'efficacite et de la tolerance de la roxithromycine dans les infections broncho-pulmonaires. Semin Hop Paris 1989; 65:2819–2821.
10. Dautzenberg B, Scheimberg A, Brambilla C, et al. Comparison of two oral antibiotics, roxithromycin and amoxicillin plus clavulanic acid, in lower respiratory tract infections. Diagn Microbiol Infect Dis 1992; 15:858–898.

Azithromycin Versus Amoxicillin–Clavulanate in Pediatric Acute Otitis Media: Comparative, Randomized, Open Study

N. Principi and P. Marchisio

University of Milan
Milan, Italy

G. Ambrosioni

Maggiore Hospital
Bologna, Italy

G. Caramia and M. Vignini

Children's Hospital
Ancona, Italy

R. Fior and G. Pelos

Children's Hospital
Trieste, Italy

G. Galioto and E. Mavio

University of Pavia
Pavia, Italy

L. Marcucci

Viterbo Hospital
Viterbo, Italy

A. Martini

University of Ferrara
Ferrara, Italy

S. Noce, D. Pavesio, and P. Pecco

University of Turin
Turin, Italy

INTRODUCTION

Azithromycin is a new antimicrobial agent, belonging to the antibiotic class of azalides, which are structurally related to macrolides, characterized by a broad spectrum of activity that includes respiratory pathogens such as *Moraxella catarrhalis*, *Streptococcus pneumoniae*, *Staphylococcus aureus*, and *Haemophilus influenzae* (1). The pharmacokinetic profile of azithromycin is endowed by high and sustained tissue levels and by high concentrations in polymorphonuclear leukocytes, tonsils, respiratory fluids, and pulmonary tissue (2).

By considering the prevalent pathogens related to otitis media in children, *Streptococcus pneumoniae*, *H. influenzae*, and *M. catarrhalis*, the improved spectrum of azithromycin, the activity of which is not reduced by β-lactamase-producing organisms, appears to be of clinical relevance in this disease (3).

Its pharmacokinetic and antibacterial profile makes a short course of therapy with azithromycin as effective as standard 10-day antibiotic therapy in many respiratory bacterial infections (4). The aim of this study was to compare the efficacy of a 3-day regimen of azithromycin with a 10-day regimen of amoxicillin–clavulanate in pediatric patients affected by acute otitis media.

PATIENTS AND METHODS

The study was conducted in four pediatric departments and in four ENT departments situated in Northern and Central Italy. Infants and children 6 months to 12 years old with acute otitis media (AOM) were eligible. Children were enrolled whose parent(s) gave oral informed consent. History and examination findings were recorded on a standardized form. The diagnosis of AOM was based on the presence of specific symptoms of acute infection and the presence of middle-ear effusion determined by pneumatic otoscopy (erythema or white opacification of the tympanic membrane, or both, accompanied by fullness or bulging and impaired mobility) and, when available, by tympanometry (a flat, type B curve).

Children were excluded who had recently received antimicrobial treatment (within the preceding 48 h), who had known hypersensitivity to macrolides or β-lactam antibiotics, or who had potentially complicating or confounding conditions (e.g., chronic diarrhea, or any other gastrointestinal condition) that could affect absorption of the study drug.

Subjects were randomly allocated to receive either azithromycin (10 mg/kg per day once daily for 3 days) or amoxicillin–clavulanate (50 mg/kg per day, based on the amoxicillin component, in two divided doses for 10 days). Antihistamines and decongestants were not prescribed. The use of antipyretics was left to parental discretion.

Patients were evaluated at baseline, at 5 ± 2 days, at 10 ± 2 days, and at 30 ± 2 days, and at each visit clinical responses were assessed, together with signs and symptoms related to the infection. Clinical signs and symptoms, such as fever, otalgia, tympanic hyperemia, and tympanic thickening, were rated as absent, mild, moderate, or severe.

Clinical efficacy was defined as follows: cure (absence of acute signs and symptoms and resolution of otoscopic findings); improvement (partial resolution of acute signs and symptoms); failure (persistence of signs and symptoms of AOM after 3–5 days or need for discontinuation of treatment because of adverse effects); and relapse (improvement followed by reappearance of signs and symptoms).

Occurrence of adverse effects was recorded during treatment and follow-up and scored for severity, duration, and relation to treatment.

Statistical analysis of cure rates for the two treatment groups was performed using two-sided continuity adjusted χ^2 tests. Differences between the two groups were considered to be significant if $p < 0.05$.

RESULTS

Patients' characteristics are summarized in Table 1. A total of 196 children, affected by acute otitis media, were randomized to receive azithromycin ($n = 97$) or amoxicillin–clavulanate ($n = 99$). There were no statistically relevant differences either in demographic characteristics of each group of patients or in severity of clinical symptoms.

Both drugs were effective in the treatment of acute otitis media, and no

Table 1 Patient Characteristics

	Azithromycin	Amoxicillin–clavulanate
Patients treated		
Males	58	55
Females	39	44
Total	97	99
Age (yr)		
Mean ± SD	4.36 ± 3.36	4.56 ± 3.22
Weight (kg)		
Mean ± SD	19.4 ± 11.28	18.69 ± 9.75
Diagnosis of otitis		
Right	31	25
} Unilateral	} 56	} 46
Left	25	21
Bilateral	41	53

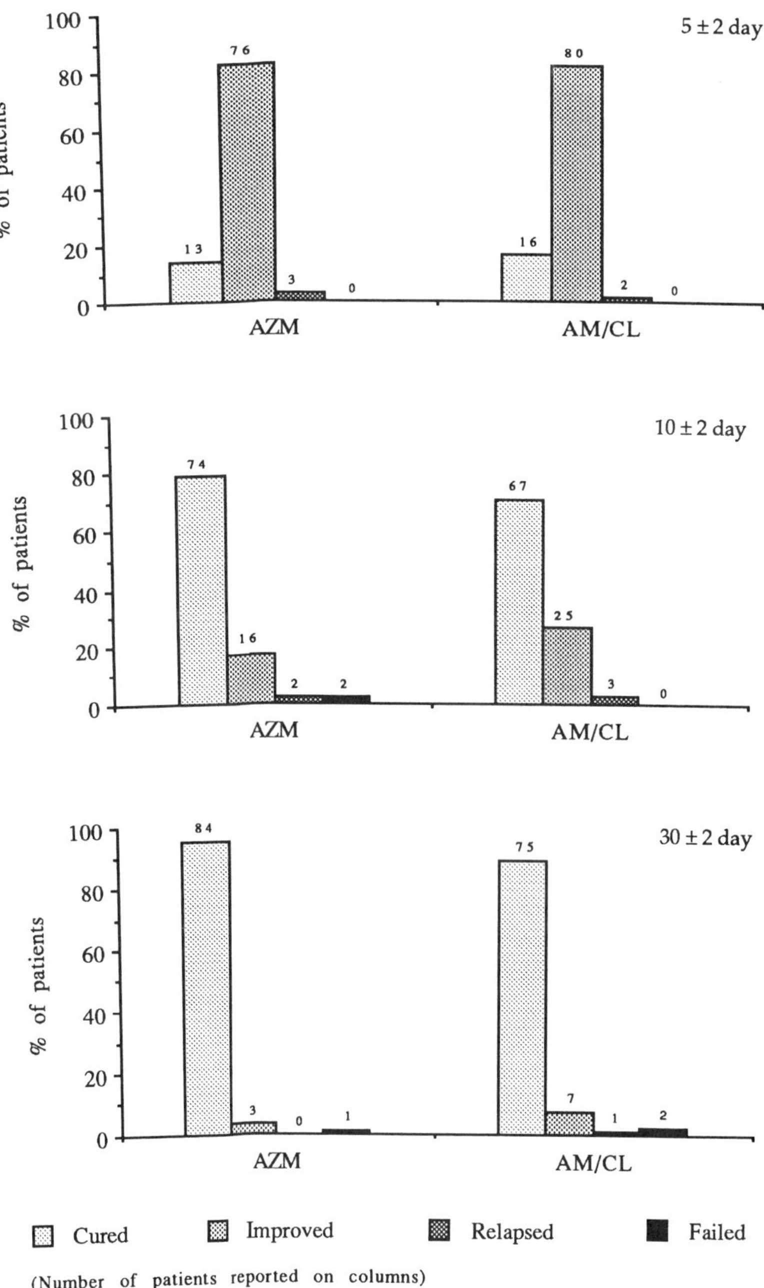

(Number of patients reported on columns)

Figure 1 Clinical response.

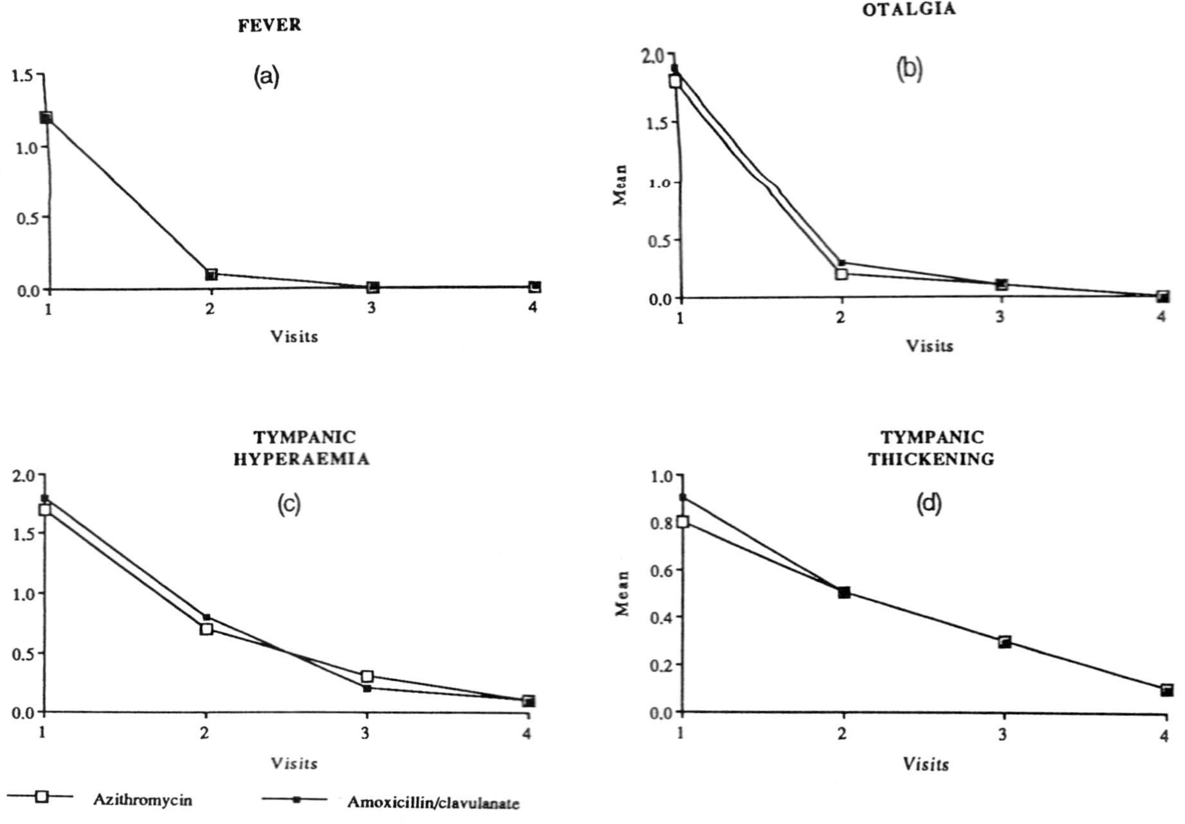

Figure 2   Normalization of pretreatment signs and symptoms.

statistically significant difference appeared between groups relative to clinical cure rate, as shown in Figure 1.

At 5 ± 2 days, 13 patients were cured (14.1%) and 76 (82.6%) improved in azithromycin group, whereas 16 (16.3%) patients were cured and 80 (81.6%) improved in amoxicillin–clavulanate group. At 10 ± 2 days, cured patients were, respectively, 74 and 67 (78.7 vs. 70.5%), and the improved ones 16 and 25 (17 vs. 26.3%).

At follow-up at 30 ± 2 days, the cure rate was 95.5% in azithromycin versus 89.3% in amoxicillin–clavulanate group.

Normalization of pretreatment signs and symptoms was rapid in both groups (Fig. 2), particularly fever, tympanic hyperemia, otalgia, and tympanic thickening.

Side effects were observed in one patient (1%, diarrhea) in the azithromycin group, whereas in the amoxicillin–clavulanate group there were nine (9.1%, five diarrhea, two dyspepsia, two abdominal pain) side effects. The difference between groups in the incidence of side effects was statistically significant ($p = 0.024$).

CONCLUSION

In this study, a short course of therapy with azithromycin resulted in as effective a response as a 10-day course of therapy with amoxicillin–clavulanate in the treatment of acute otitis media in children. Both groups showed a prompt clinical response, with a high rate of clinical success even at 5 ± 2 days of treatment.

The short treatment with azithromycin was better tolerated: this appears to be particularly important in pediatric patients, for whom reduction of therapy duration and frequency of administration can improve patient compliance and final results.

REFERENCES

1. Dunkin KT, Jones S, Howard J. The in vitro activity of CP-62, 993 against *H. influenzae*, *B. catarrhalis*, staphylococci and streptococci. J Antimicrob Chemother 1988; 21:405–411.
2. Schentag JJ, Ballow CH. Tissue-directed pharmacokinetics. Am J Med 1991; 91 (suppl 3A):3–5.
3. Principi N. Azitromicina in pediatria, come, quando, perché. Med Ter 1993; 1(1).
4. Muller O. Comparison of azithromycin versus clarithromycin in the treatment of patients with upper respiratory tract infections. J Antimicrob Chemother 1993; 31 (suppl E):137–146.

Clarithromycin Versus Amoxicillin–Clavulanic Acid in Acute Maxillary Sinusitis in Adults

P. Gehanno

Hôpital Bichat
Paris, France

J. P. Chauvin and J. Hazebroucq

Abbott France
Rungis, France

BACKGROUND

Acute sinusitis is an infection of the paranasal sinuses which, in turn, may be complicated by serious intracranial infections, such as bacterial meningitis, epidural and subdural abscess, and brain abscess. Most cases of acute sinusitis are thought to be a bacterial complication of a viral upper respiratory illness (e.g., common cold). It is thought that the viral infection disrupts the continuous mucociliary cleansing of particulate matter that enters the sinus cavity, thereby setting the stage for secondary bacterial invasion. During acute sinusitis, an exudate, which contains polymorphonuclear leukocytes and high bacterial titers, usually develops in the sinus cavity. From studies that employed direct sinus puncture to attain specimens for culture, the following infectious agents were isolated. *Streptococcus pneumoniae* and *Haemophilus influenzae* (approximately 50% of cases), different anaerobic bacteria (6% of cases), *Staphylococcus aureus* (4%), *Streptococcus pyogenes* and *Moraxella catarrhalis* (2% each), and gram-negative bacteria (9%).

A number of recent studies have examined the role of clarithromycin in the treatment of acute maxillary sinusitis (AMS) in adults. Clarithromycin is a new-generation macrolide with in vitro activity that includes key gram-negative,

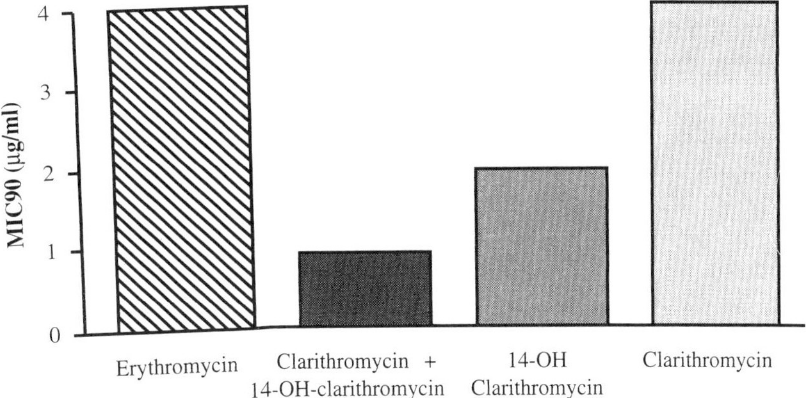

Figure 1 In vitro activity on *Haemophilus influenzae*.

including *H. influenzae*, and gram-positive organisms responsible for upper and lower respiratory tract infections. Clarithromycin and its 14-OH metabolite are highly effective against *H. influenzae* (MIC_{90} of the combination, 1 mg/L; Fig. 1).

Although amoxicillin therapy has resulted in good clinical results in the treatment of acute sinusitis, amoxicillin–clavulanate is often employed based on its increased coverage of anaerobes and gram-negative organisms. This study was designed to compare the safety and efficacy of clarithromycin to that of amoxicillin–clavulanate.

STUDY OBJECTIVE

The study was designed to evaluate the safety and efficacy of orally administered clarithromycin and amoxicillin–clavulanic acid in the treatment of adults with acute maxillary sinusitis.

MATERIALS AND METHODS

Study Design

The study was an open, randomized, comparative clinical trial, and the bacteriological results were kept blind unless clinical failure occurred.

Main Inclusion Criteria

1. Recent facial pain ($<$15 days)

Table 1 Evaluation Criteria for Efficacy

Day 10			
Clinical cure	Resolution of spontaneous facial pain and purulent nasal discharge		
Radiologic cure	Resolution of abnormalities (Sinus wall thickness was not considered pathologic)		
Cure:	Clinical cure	and	radiologic cure
Improvement:	Clinical cure	but	no radiologic cure
Failure:	No clinical cure	and	no radiologic cure
Day 30			
Cure:	Cure or improvement at day 10	and	no recurrence of symptoms at day 30
Failure:	Failure at day 10		
	Cure or improvement at day 10	and	Recurrence of symptoms at day 30

2. Purulent nasal discharge with purulent discharge observed from the middle meatus
3. Radiologic confirmation obtained from x-ray films of the face (total sinus opacity or intrasinus fluid level)

Time Line

Day 1 Inclusion: Clinical and radiological examinations, bacteriological sample; begin study drug administration

Day 2–3: Phone call; assessment of clinical status

Day 8: End of study drug administration

Day 10: Clinical and radiologic examinations (Table 1)

Day 30: Phone call; posttreatment follow-up (see Table 1)

Drug Administration

Patients were randomized to receive clarithromycin, 500 mg po bid, or amoxicillin–clavulanic acid, 500 mg po tid/125 mg po tid for 8 days.

Concomitant Medications

Coprescribed paracetamol (acetaminophen), po, and intranasal oxymetazoline were allowed. Coprescribed corticosteroids and anti-inflammatory agents were excluded.

Microbiology

Sinus punctures are not considered as ethically acceptable in France for acute maxillary sinusitis; hence, sinus fluid aspirations under the middle meatus were performed, as proposed and validated by Savolainen and Wald.

Table 2 Patient Demographic Data

	Clarithromycin	Amoxicillin–clavulanic acid
Patient number	145	139
Males/females	70/75	66/73
Average age (yr)	41.2 ($\pm$14.2)[a]	39.5 ($\pm$15.3)[a]
Average weight (kg)	64.6 ($\pm$10)	66.0 ($\pm$12.4)
Average height (cm)	168.1 ($\pm$7.9)	169.0 ($\pm$8.1)
Smokers	39	34
Nonsmokers	96	95
Former smokers	10	10

[a]Standard deviation in parentheses

Table 3 Patient History (Within Previous Month)[a]

	Clarithromycin ($n = 145$)	Amoxicillin–clavulanic acid ($n = 139$)
Common cold	68% (99)	66% (92)
Swimming in sea or pool	8% (11)	6% (9)
Otitis	6% (8)	7% (10)
Conjunctivitis	2% (3)	6% (9)
Pharyngitis	33% (48)	31% (43)
Bronchitis	11% (16)	15% (21)
Cervical lymph nodes	1% (1)	1% (2)

[a]No significant differences

Table 4 Intranasal Abnormalities

	Clarithromycin ($n = 145$)	Amoxicillin–clavulanic acid ($n = 139$)
Intranasal polyp	5% (7)	3% (4)
Nasal septum deviation	24% (35)	22% (30)
Allergic rhinitis	12% (17)	12% (16)

Table 5 Clinical Symptoms[a]

	Clarithromycin (*n* = 145)	Amoxicillin–clavulanic acid (*n* = 139)
Average temperature (°C)	37.7 (±0.7)	37.7 (±0.6)
Nasal discharge	100% (145)	100% (139)
Spontaneous facial pain	80% (116)	81% (113)
Induced facial pain	85% (123)	84% (117)
Facial congestion	8% (12)	7% (10)
No headache	15% (22)	9% (13)
Moderate headache	58% (84)	53% (73)
Severe headache	27% (39)	38% (53)
Cough	47% (68)	38% (53)

[a]No significant differences

Table 6 Radiologic Signs of Sinusitis[a]

	Clarithromycin (*n* = 145)	Amoxicillin–clavulanic acid (*n* = 139)
Unilateral AMS	63% (91)	69% (96)
Bilateral AMS	28% (41)	26% (36)
Frontal of ethmoidal sinusitis	1% (2)	0% (0)
No RX performed or no radiological sign of maxillary sinusitis	8% (11)	5% (7)

[a]No significant differences

Table 7 Efficacy Analysis (Day 10)

	Clarithromycin (*n* = 134)	Amoxicillin–clavulanic acid (*n* = 129)
Success (cure and improvement)	86% (115)	85% (110)

Table 8 Efficacy Analysis (Day 30)

	Clarithromycin (*n* = 130)	Amoxicillin–clavulanic acid (*n* = 128)
Cure	82% (106)	80% (102)
Failure	18% (24)	20% (26)

Table 9 Clinical Outcome According to Bacteriological Findings[a]

	Clarithromycin		Amoxicillin–clavulanic acid	
Pathogens isolated	No. evaluable patients	Patients with cure	No. evaluable patients	Patients with cure
H. influenzae	38	84% (32)	39	74% (29)
S. pneumoniae	25	88% (22)	26	81% (21)
M. catarrhalis	12	83% (10)	7	86% (6)
Staphylococci	9	67% (6)	19	79% (15)
Streptococci	11	64% (7)	10	60% (6)
Enterobacteriaceae	13	62% (8)	10	80% (8)
Others	2	50% (1)	2	100% (2)

[a]No significant differences

Table 10 Evaluation of Tolerance

	Clarithromycin	Amoxicillin–clavulanic acid
Number of patients reporting one or more adverse events (ADEs)	14% (21/145)	12% (17/139)
Number of treatment interruptions for ADEs	3% (4/145)	4% (5/139)
Number of ADEs	20% (29/145)	19% (26/139)

Methods

Nasal discharge specimens obtained by aspiration under the middle meatus after mucosal retraction

Storage in BioMerieux Portagerm

Shipment by express mail

Culture: Mueller–Hinton broth. Fildes and HTM for *H. influenzae* strains

Disk susceptibility tests of clarithromycin or amoxicillin–clavulanic acid.

RESULTS

The results are summarized in Tables 2–10 and Figure 2.

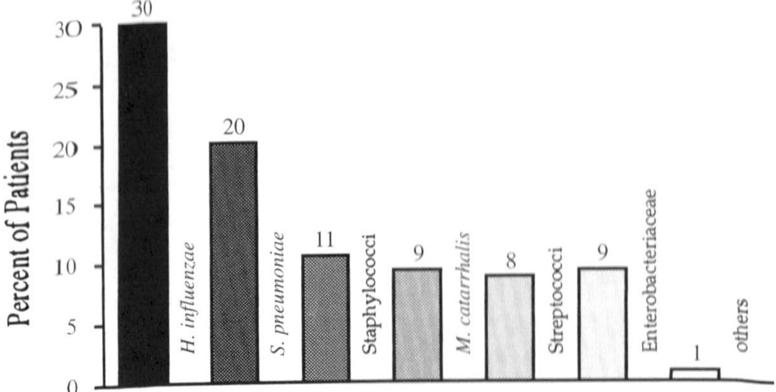

Figure 2   Pathogens isolated.

CONCLUSION

This pragmatic study (with blinded bacteriological results) demonstrates that clarithromycin is at least as effective as amoxicillin–clavulanic acid and is well tolerated for treatment of acute maxillary sinusitis (AMS). Clarithromycin also provides more convenient dosing (bid vs. tid).

Clarithromycin is effective against AMS caused by gram-positive pathogens, including *S. pneumoniae* and against AMS caused by gram-negative pathogens, including *H. influenzae*.

Roxithromycin, 150 mg bid, for Treatment of Sinusitis

A. Saldarriaga

Clinica Internacional
Lima, Peru

INTRODUCTION

The purpose of this study was to evaluate the clinical efficacy and the tolerance of roxithromycin, 150 mg bid, in the treatment of sinusitis in a general practice situation.

PATIENTS AND METHODS

This was an open, noncontrolled, multicenter clinical trial. Patients older than 16 years of both sexes who presented with sinusitis were enrolled for this study. The patients were evaluated in 21 participating centers. The criteria for clinical diagnosis of a sinusitis of bacterial origin was supported by the presence of at least three of the following clinical findings: fever, nasal obstruction, purulent nasal or postnasal drip, local pain, tenderness over the sinusal zone, or radiologic evidence of sinusitis. All the patients had signed an informed consent before entering the study.

The exclusion criteria were the following: history of hypersensitivity to macrolides, evidence of impaired hepatic function, antibiotic therapy in the preceding 3 days, and concomitant therapy with ergot alkaloids.

Treatment

Roxithromycin, 150 mg q12h, per os was for a treatment duration of no fewer than 7 days; the duration of treatment for each patient was chosen by each physician.

"

Assessment of the Efficacy and Tolerance

An exhaustive clinical exploration was performed at the beginning and the end of treatment, and the opinion of the physician concerning the efficacy of treatment was recorded. The patient recorded the time at which the fever dropped. Leukocyte counts, basal and at the end of treatment, and bacteriological examination were performed in 402 patients. For assessment of the general tolerance, any systemic discomfort attributable to the drug and experienced by the patient was closely evaluated during and at the end of treatment.

Data Analysis

Global therapeutic efficacy was defined as the percentage proportion of suppressed symptoms at the end of treatment of the total of initial symptoms. Specific therapeutic efficacy expresses the proportion of patients who having entered the study with fever and purulent rhinorrhea experienced a suppression of such signs at the end of the treatment. Chi-square test and normal proof (Z test) were applied for the estimation of the random probability, when indicated, and binomial confidence intervals were calculated, with the statistical significance set at 0.05.

RESULTS

A total of 366 patients were studied, 61.2% were women. Mean age was 34.7 years ($\pm$ 11.3); mean body weight was 67.6 kg ($\pm$ 7.4; Table 1).

Studied Pathology

The mean time of illness was 8.0 days ($\pm$ 4.5); 15.7% of the patients had received previous antibiotic treatment. The evolution of symptoms is shown in Table 2. Basal cultures were obtained, in 118 cases, with a sterile swab from the meatus of the clinically compromised sinus, mostly middle meatus, after a sterile saline nostril washout.

Table 1 Demographic Data

Data recorded	
Sample size (N)	366
Sex (% females)	61.2
Mean age (yr $\pm$ SD)	34.7 $\pm$ 11.3
Mean time of illness (days $\pm$ SD)	8.0 $\pm$ 4.5
Previous antibiotic treatment (%)	15.7

Table 2 Evolution of Clinical Symptoms
(366 Patients)

Diagnosis	Before inclusion		After end of treatment	
	n	*%*	*n*	*%*
Fever	243	66.3	10	2.7
Spontaneous pain	286	78.2	25	6.8
Local tenderness	224	61.2	27	7.4
Facial tension	204	55.4	18	4.9
Nasal obstruction	196	53.5	32	8.7
Pus exudate	330	90.3	46	12.6

Therapeutic Efficacy

Global therapeutic efficacy was 82.3% (95% confidence interval; CI, 79.2–84.4%) for the whole group and 76.3% (95% CI, 68.2–84.1%) for the *H. influenzae* cases. The specific therapeutic efficacy was 86.9% (CI, 81.1–91.1%).

Mean duration of treatment was 10.4 days (± 2.5). A temperature decrease occurred, on average, by 2.9 days of treatment (± 0.9). Cessation of general discomfort occurred, on average, by 2.7 days of treatment (± 1). In this group, the bacteria most frequently isolated were *Haemophilus influenzae* isolated in 38 cases; *Streptococcus pyogenes*, in 33 cases; *S. aureus*, in 8 cases; and no growth in 39; no patient had more than one bacterial species isolated.

Tolerance

Tolerance to the drug was 97.0% (CI, 94.8–98.9%). A total of 11 adverse reactions were recorded, in 11 patients: nausea, 9 cases, and in 2, epigastralgia. One patient had to discontinue the treatment because of nausea.

DISCUSSION

The antibacterial spectrum of roxithromycin is well suited for the control of the bacteria usually present in acute sinusitis. The pharmacokinetic properties of this macrolide includes high tissue levels in the sinusal mucosa (2).

This study demonstrated that oral roxithromycin, 150 mg bid, reach a clinical cure rate of 82% in sinusitis. These results are supported by the clinical evidence, accumulated worldwide with more than 10,000 patients with acute sinusitis, that report a clinical efficacy between 88 and 96% (1,4–6), in accordance with roxithromycin's pharmacokinetic profile and antimicrobial in vitro effect, which includes bactericidal activity against the usual respiratory pathogens (7,8).

The documented clinical efficacy of roxithromycin, as well as its excellent tolerance (9), as confirmed in our therapeutic trial, allows us to recommend it as a first-choice antibiotic in the treatment of sinusitis of bacterial origin, in which macrolide use is indicated.

REFERENCES

1. Dautzenberg B, Scheimberg A, Brambilla C, et al. Comparison of 2 oral antibiotics, roxithromycin and amoxicillin plus clavulanic acid, in lower respiratory tract infections. 17th International Congress of Chemotherapy, Berlin, June 1991.

2. Dewever M. Determination of roxithromycin concentration in the mucosa of the maxillary sinus. Br J Clin Pract 1988; 42(suppl 55):81.

3. Eissen SA, Miller DK, et al. The effect of prescribed daily dose frequency on patient medication compliance. Arch Intern Med 1990; 150:1881–1884.

4. Fritz J, Fourie E, Pickard I, Reinach G. A randomized controlled study of oral roxithromycin and amoxicillin plus clavulanic acid in the treatment of patients with acute maxillary sinusitis. 17th International Congress of Chemotherapy, Berlin, June 1991.

5. Higuera F, Cooperative Multicentre National Team. Multicentre study on the efficacy and tolerance of roxithromycin in the treatment of respiratory tract infections. 17th International Congress of Chemotherapy, Berlin, June 1991.

6. Marsac J. Ensayo clinico internacional sobre la eficacia y seguridad de roxitromicina en 40,000 pacientes con infecciones agudas del tracto respiratorio adquiridas en la comunidad. 17th International Congress of Chemotherapy, Berlin, June 1991.

7. Shah PM, Schafer V, Metz C, Stille W. Bactericidal activity of roxithromycin compared with that of erythromycin and doxycycline against *Streptococcus pneumoniae*. Br J Clin Pract 42(suppl 55):10–12, 1988.

8. Tome G, Goldberg M, Jugo M, D'andrea EM, Farinati A, Casellas JM. Bacteriostatic and bactericidal activity of roxithromycin against *Haemophilus influenzae*, isolated from patients suffering respiratory tract infections. 18th International Congress of Chemotherapy, Stockholm, 1993.

9. Young RA, Gonzales JP, Sorkin EM. Roxithromycin: a review of its antibacterial activity, pharmacokinetic properties and clinical efficacy. Drugs 1989; 37:8–41.

Roxithromycin in the Treatment of Pharyngotonsillitis

Luis Sanchez

Hospital Arzobispo Loayza
Lima, Peru

INTRODUCTION

Pharyngotonsillitis is a common problem and a significant cause of morbidity. In past years we have learned that besides such well-known pathogens as *Streptococcus pyogenes*, there are other atypical bacteria such as *Chlamydia* and *Mycoplasma* spp. that are cause of throat infections. Therefore, it is important to consider macrolides as first-line agents in therapy for pharyngotonsillitis (1–4).

This study was designed to evaluate the clinical efficacy and tolerance of roxithromycin in patients with pharyngotonsillitis.

PATIENTS AND METHODS

Design

This was a multicenter, open clinical trial, with 21 participating centers. Subjects of both sexes with body weight > 40 kg, with clinical diagnosis of acute pharyngotonsillitis of bacterial origin, who had given informed consent, were eligible for this study. History of hypersensitivity to macrolides, clinical evidence of impaired hepatic function, antibiotic therapy in the 3 days preceding the consultation, and concomitant therapy with ergot alkaloids were considered as exclusion criteria.

Schema of Treatment

Roxithromycin, 150 bid, was given for the minimum treatment duration of 5 days; the maximum duration was decided by each physician.

Assessment of Efficacy and Tolerance

A clinical exploration was performed at the beginning and the end of treatment, and the opinion of the physician concerning the efficacy of treatment was recorded. Additionally, the patient recorded the time at which the fever dropped and the time at which the general discomfort stopped. Bacteriological examination was performed in 296 patients. For the assessment of the general tolerance, any systemic discomfort attributable to the drug and experienced by the patient throughout the study was closely monitored.

Data Analysis

Global therapeutic efficacy was defined as the proportion of patients whose symptoms had all abated by the end of the trial. Specific therapeutic efficacy expresses the proportion of patients who, having entered to the study with fever and tonsil exudate, experienced a suppression of both signs at the end of the trial. Chi-square test and normal proof (Z test) were applied for the estimation of the random probability when it was indicated, and binomial confidence intervals were calculated, with statistical significance set as 0.05 (5).

RESULTS

Sample Description

A total of 638 patients were studied; 55.3% were females. The mean age was 28.4 years (± 10 years); mean body weight was 65.9 kg (± 8.3). Characteristics of the sample by specific diagnosis are shown in Table 1.

Table 1 Characteristics of the Sample

Variables	Pharyngotonsillitis
Sample size (N)	638
Sex (% females)	55.3
Mean age (yr)	28.4 (10.0)
Body weight (kg $\pm$ SD)	66.8 (± 8.4)
Mean time of illness (days $\pm$ SD)	3.9 (± 1.8)

Table 2 Symptom Evolution (638 patients)

Clinical findings	Inclusion		End of treatment	
	n	%	*n*	%
Fever	607	95	11	1.8
Dysphagia	130	20	6	0.9
Odynophagia	618	97	18	2.8
Pus exudate	219	34	6	0.9
General discomfort	567	89	21	3.3

Studied Pathology

The mean time of illness before inclusion in the trial was 3.9 days (± 1.8); 18.1% of the cases had received previous antibiotic treatment, usually short automedication. These 116 patients took the antibiotic 3 days before the inclusion in the trial. The symptomatic spectrum is shown in Table 2.

Therapeutic Efficacy

Global therapeutic efficacy was 94.1% (95% confidence interval, CI 92.1–96.0%) and specific therapeutic efficacy was 96.1% (95% CI, 94.9–97.3%).

The mean duration of treatment was 7.2 days (± 1.0). The decrease in temperature occurred, on average, by the 1.9 day of treatment (± 0.8). Cessation of general discomfort occurred, on average, by the 2.7 day of treatment (± 1). Within the studied subgroup with initial and final leukocytes counts (266), the mean initial leukocyte count was $12{,}422/\mu l$ (± 1.888), and the mean final leukocyte count was $8{,}685/\mu l$ ($\pm 1{,}516$), a statistically significant difference ($Z = 4.08$; $p < 0.001$). Basal throat cultures were done in 296 patients: *Streptococcus pyogenes* was isolated in 181 cases in this group, no other throat pathogen was isolated.

Tolerance

Tolerance to the drug was good in 97.3%. A total of 16 adverse reactions were recorded, in 16 patients: nausea in 11 patients and mild epigastralgia in 5 patients. No patients required treatment discontinuation.

DISCUSSION

Our investigation, performed on a representative sample of patients with amygdalitis, a prevalent bacterial respiratory infection, demonstrated that oral roxithromycin, 150 mg q12 h achieves a cure rate of about 94% efficacy in this disease. These results are supported by the clinical evidence accumulated, worldwide, which has confirmed the efficacy of roxithromycin against pharyngotonsillitis (3–5), in accordance with its pharmacokinetic profile and antimicrobial in vitro effect (4).

In fact, several experimental studies have demonstrated roxithromycin—contrary to other older macrolide antibiotics—is acid-stable, a singular pharmacokinetic property that allows it to maintain antimicrobial activity at the intracellular level: the macrophage and other antigen-producing cells. It also attains high antibiotic concentrations in tissue (1). Several clinical trials have documented high clinical and bacteriological cure rates in this indication for roxithromycin (4–6). The documented clinical efficacy of roxithromycin, as well as its good tolerance (7,8), confirmed in our therapeutic trial, allows us to recommend it as a first-choice antibiotic in the treatment of pharyngotonsillitis.

REFERENCES

1. Bergogne-Berezin E. The tissue penetration of macrolides with particular reference to the respiratory tract. In: Butzler and Kobayashi, eds. Macrolides a Review With an Outlook on Future Developments. Amsterdam: Excerpta Medica, 4353.
2. Bryskier AJ. Newer macrolides and their potential target organism. Curr Opinion Infect Dis 1992; 5:764–772.
3. Prado V, Romero J, Herrera N, Marinkovic K, Bustos R. Actividad comparativa in vitro de azitromicina, laritromicina, roxitromicina, eritromicina y penicilina frente a 120 cepas de *Streptococcus pyogenes*. 6th Congreso Panamericano de Infectologia. Viña Del Mar, Chile, 1993.
4. Philips I, Pechere JC, Davies A, Speller D. Roxithromycin: a new macrolide. J Antimicrob Chemother 1987; 20(suppl B):1–87.
5. Herron J. Roxithromycin in the therapy of *Streptococcus pyogenes* throat infections. Animicrobial Chemother 1987; 20 (suppl B):139–144.
6. Young RA, Gonzales JP, Sorkin EM. Roxithromycin: a review of its antibacterial activity, pharmacokinetic properties and clinical efficacy. Drugs 1989; 37:8–41.
7. Gascon MP. Comparative effects of macrolide antibiotics on liver monoxygenases [abstract]. Clin Pharmacol Ther 1991; 49:158.
8. Neu HC, Young LS, Zinner SH. The New Macrolides, Azalides, and Streptogramin. New York: Marcel Decker, 1993.

Azithromycin (3 or 5 Days) Versus Clarithromycin (7–10 Days) in the Treatment of Adult Patients with Acute Purulent Tracheobronchitis: A Pharmacoeconomic Analysis

J. Sternon

Erasme University Hospital
Brussels, Belgium

RATIONALE

Acute viral or bacterial bronchitis is a frequent illness that affects smokers, young and middle-aged active adults, but also older men with chronic obstructive lung disease (COLD). Its incidence is estimated to be over 2 million cases per year in Belgium (1). About 88% of these cases are seen by the general practitioner, who will prescribe antibiotics in about 80% of those with purulent expectorations. The general symptoms of acute bronchitis often result in the incapacity to work, which generates most of the cost of a bronchitis episode. Measures to reduce the total cost of bronchitis treatment, therefore, should be aimed at shortening the period of work incapacity.

Azithromycin is a novel azalide antibiotic, the antimicrobial spectrum of which covers respiratory pathogens, such as *Streptococcus pneumoniae, Haemophilus influenzae, Moraxella catarrhalis*; and agents of atypical pneumonia, such as *Mycoplasma pneumoniae, Chlamydia pneumoniae*, and *Legionella pneumoniae* (2,3). Azithromycin's long tissue half-life (4) allows a short duration of treatment: 3 or 5 days. Clinical trials have proved that a total dose of 1.5 g of azithromycin is effective in respiratory tract infections (5). If a short treatment can result in faster symptom relief and less absence from work, then azithromycin could be a valuable addition in the treatment of acute bronchitis.

MATERIAL AND METHODS

This open-label, multicenter, randomized trial compared the clinical and economic effect of oral azithromycin and clarithromycin in the treatment of acute purulent bronchitis. The study was conducted by 17 general practitioners. Clarithromycin, 250 mg bid, was given for 7–10 days. Azithromycin was administered for 3 days (500 mg od) or 5 days (500 mg od on the first day, 250 mg od during the next 4 days); the investigators were free to choose between the azithromycin 3-day or 5-day dosage scheme.

The diagnosis of acute purulent tracheobronchitis was based on the presence of purulent sputum and rhonchi on auscultation. Patients were excluded if they had received any antibiotic during the past 2 weeks. Pregnant women, or women of childbearing age without reliable means of contraception, were excluded from this investigation. Written informed consent was obtained from all patients.

Clinical and economic data were collected at baseline and after 7 ± 2 days of follow-up. Clinical status was assessed by means of a scoring system, which graded signs and symptoms as absent (0), mild (1), moderate (2), or severe (3). Patients kept track of all bronchitis-related medical expenses and filled out questionnaires at days ± 5 and days 15–20. These questionnaires dealt with quality of life issues, time spent for medical services, the perceived efficacy of treatment, and its rapidity of action.

Because of the economic aspect of the trial, only persons with an employment income were included. Revenue was estimated by proposing net monthly income brackets. We used these data to calculate gross annual income, total burden to the employer, and the cost of 1 productive workday for the employer. The length of working disability (LWD), which is an estimate of the indirect cost, was obtained at follow-up by asking the patient how many days he or she had been absent from work. Net LWD was calculated by excluding weekends and holidays from the period of working disability. The direct cost of an acute tracheobronchitis episode was obtained by adding expenditure for medical services and drug consumption (self-administered or prescribed). The cost of the antibiotic was not included in the analysis, since azithromycin did not yet have an official price in Belgium. Data were analyzed using the SPSS 5.0 software package. All statistical tests were two-tailed.

RESULTS

A total of 132 patients (63 azithromycin, 69 clarithromycin) were evaluable. Two more patients were lost to follow-up after the first visit. There were no

Table 1 Outcome of Treatment as Assessed by Physician

Outcome	Azithromycin	Clarithromycin	Total
Cure (%)	44 (70%)	38 (55%)	82
Improvement (%)	15 (24%)	24 (35%)	39
Failure, relapse, indeterminate outcome (%)	4 (6%)	7 (10%)	11
Total	63	69	132

significant differences in the baseline characteristics of the treatment groups relative to demographic parameters, clinical status, duration of current infection, use of medication before visit 1, or medical antecedents.

Sixty percent of azithromycin-treated patients received a 3-day prescription. Most clarithromycin-treated patients received treatment for 8 days or more. Treatment duration was mainly related to the choice of the physician, rather than to the severity of the infection.

Both treatments were of equivalent efficacy, as assessed by the physician (Table 1).

No significant difference in clinical response could be observed between the two groups ($p = 0.215$). However, time to clinical improvement (as assessed by the patient) was significantly shorter for the azithromycin group (mean, 3.1 days), than for the clarithromycin group (mean, 4.2 days): log rank test: $p = 0.002$. No such difference was observed between the two azithromycin dosage regimens (log rank test: $p = 0.703$). Comparable incidences of side effects, mostly mild and of gastrointestinal origin, were found in both treatment groups, with the possible exception of nausea, which occurred in 2 azithromycin patients and 13 clarithromycin patients ($p = 0.013$). Since this is a post hoc finding, it must be interpreted with caution.

One serious adverse event occurred during the study: one azithromycin-treated patient with a history of allergic asthma was hospitalized because of dyspnea. The patient recovered uneventfully.

Seventy-seven percent of azithromycin patients and 78% of clarithromycin patients had at least 1 day of working incapacity. When considering patients with working disability, both crude ($p = 0.003$) and net ($p = 0.014$) LWD were significantly shorter for the azithromycin group (mean, 4.4 and 3.6 days) than for the clarithromycin group (mean, 5.9 and 4.5 days). The economic effect of this difference on the whole group disappears when all patients (with or without working disability) are taken into account ($p = 0.074$ by t test). The mean cost of 1 day of working disability was 146 and 140 U.S. dollars for azithromycin and clarithromycin-treated patients, respectively ($p = 0.649$). The mean indirect cost of a bronchitis episode was estimated at 438 U.S. dollars (all groups compounded). The direct costs of an episode of tracheobronchitis were calculated from the consumption of drugs and ancillary services.

DISCUSSION

Both antibiotic treatments were of equal clinical efficacy. Time to improvement of symptoms, however, was 1 day shorter in the azithromycin group (3.1 days), when compared with the clarithromycin group (4.2 days). This difference in time to improvement was reflected in the crude LWD, which was significantly shorter for azithromycin-treated patients (median of 3 days versus 5 days for clarithromycin-treated patients). This difference in crude LWD could not be explained by a worse clinical status at the beginning of the study.

Side effects were less common in the azithromycin group than in the clarithromycin group, but not significantly so ($p = 0.062$).

The indirect costs, mainly generated by loss of productive working days, accounted for 95% of the total cost of a bronchitis episode.

REFERENCES

1. IMS data, Belgium.
2. Maskell JP, Sefton AM, Williams JD. Comparative in-vitro activity of azithromycin and erythromycin on gram-positive cocci, *Haemophilus Influenzae* and anaerobes. J Antimicrob Chemother 1990; 25(suppl A):19–24.
3. Renaudin H, Bebear C. Comparative in vitro activity of azithromycin, clarithromycin, erythromycin and lomefloxacin against *Mycoplasma pneumoniae*, *Mycoplasma hominis* and *Ureaplasma urealyticum*. Eur J Microb Infect Dis 1990; 9:838–841.
4. Girard AE, Girard D, Retsema JA. Correlation of the extravascular pharmacokinetics of azithromycin with in vivo models of localized infection. J Antimicrob Chemother 1990; 25(suppl A):61–71.
5. Hoepleman AIM, Sips AP, van Helmond JLM, et al. A single-blind comparison of three-day azithromycin and ten-day co-amoxiclav treatment of acute lower respiratory tract infections. J Antimicrob Chemother 1993; 31(suppl E):147–152.

Josamycin in Comparison with Clarithromycin and Roxithromycin in the Treatment of Bronchitis

J. Mühlbacher, W. Ridl, B. Sárffy-Panosch, and W. Moser

Biochemie Gesellschaft mbH
Kundl, Austria

INTRODUCTION

The aim of the study was to investigate the efficacy and tolerance of josamycin, clarithromycin, and roxithromycin in acute bronchitis or acute exacerbation of chronic bronchitis.

Acute bronchitis is an inflammatory condition of the tracheobronchial tree that is usually associated with generalized respiratory infection (1). Although this disease is mainly caused by common cold viruses, secondary bacterial invasion is of importance.

Chronic bronchitis is a condition associated with excessive tracheobronchial mucus production, sufficient to cause cough with expectoration for at least 3 months of the year for more than 2 consecutive years (2). Prognosis is poor (5-year survival rate of blue bloater patients is 30%), especially with secondary infection of the respiratory tract (3). Therefore, in both diseases antibiotic treatment seems to be indicated.

The most important bacteria in this context are *Mycoplasma pneumoniae*, *Streptococcus pneumoniae*, *Staphylococcus aureus*, *Haemophilus influenzae*, and *Bordetella pertussis* (1,6). Each of them is included in the spectrum of the macrolides tested.

Macrolide antibiotics inhibit protein synthesis by binding reversibly to 50S ribosomal subunits of sensitive microorganisms. Josamycin has a 16-membered

Table 1 Demographic Data

Data	Josamycin	Clarithromycin	Roxithromycin
Age (yr)			
Mean	45.58	50.24	35.71
Medium	37.0	52.0	34.0
Minimum	17.0	19.0	17.0
Maximum	85.0	80.0	69.0
Temperature at start			
of therapy (°C)			
Mean	37.66	37.51	37.6
Medium	37.7	37.5	37.45
Minimum	36.0	36.5	36.7
Maximum	38.9	39.2	39.0
Temperature control (°C)			
Mean	36.98	36.94	36.92
Medium	36.95	36.9	36.9
Minimum	36.0	36.2	35.2
Maximum	39.2	38.2	38.2
Temperature at end			
of therapy (°C)			
Mean	36.67	36.57	36.58
Medium	36.7	36.7	36.7
Minimum	36.1	36.0	36.1
Maximum	38.9	37.2	37.2
Sex (%)			
Male	46.3	50	52.4
Female	53.7	50	47.6
Smoker (%)			
Yes	35.1	38.9	33.3
No	64.9	61.1	66.7

lactone ring, with an amino and a neutral sugar; clarithromycin and roxithromycin are 14-membered macrolides (5).

MATERIAL AND METHODS

In an open, multicenter, randomized clinical study, including a total of 115 patients, 40 patients were given 2 × 750 mg josamycin, 37 patients 2 × 250 mg clarithromycin, and 38 patients 2 × 150 mg roxithromycin for 12 days.

The nine study centers were considered from general practitioners in Tyrol, Austria.

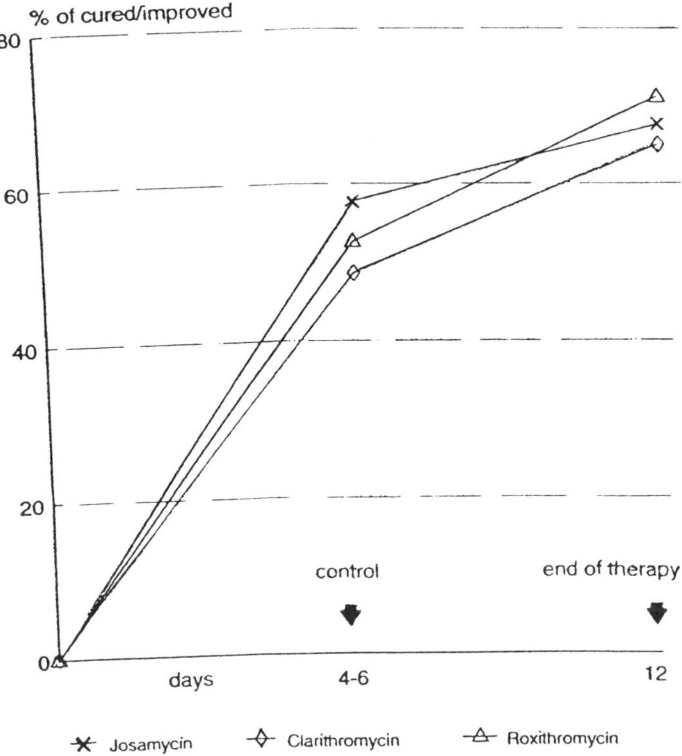

Figure 1 Results.

Patient Data

The following patient data (sex, age, temperature, and smoking customs (Table 1) can be compared in all the three groups of treatment.

A clinical investigation of patients was carried out on days 1, 4–6, and 12–14 after admission to the study. At the same time a sputum sample was obtained: the bacteriological results of this sample could not be used for an evaluation of the study because of frequent contamination by bacterial flora of the pharynx. Therefore, efficacy of treatment was assessed by following clinical parameters: temperature, cough, dyspnea, expectoration, and rhonchi.

Efficacy was classified as cured or improved and not improved. Cured or improved was defined as temperature $\leq$ 37°C and an improvement of at least two of four residual clinical parameters. Patients with a temperature of $>$ 37°C after 4–6 days were considered treatment failures, regardless of improvement or clearance of clinical symptoms and signs. This was because patients who respond to the antibiotic (or whose bacteria are sensitive) should be free from fever after 4–6 days of antibiotic treatment according to our clinical experience.

Since no identification of the causative organisms was carried out, bronchitis of a viral origin cannot be excluded.

RESULTS

At the end of therapy, 67.5% of patients were assessed cured or improved in the josamycin group, 64.9% in the clarithromycin group, and 71% in the roxithromycin group. No statistically significant difference was observed ($p >$ 0.05). For the controls after 4–6 days of treatment, 57.7% were considered cured or improved for josamycin, 48.6% for clarithromycin, and 52.6% for roxithromycin (Fig. 1).

CONCLUSIONS

The study showed that all three macrolides are equally well tolerated and effective in bronchitis. However, at the 4–6 day follow-up visit a trend toward a more rapid improvement was observed for josamycin and a higher incidence of side effects for roxithromycin (data not presented).

REFERENCES

1. Mandell, Douglas, Bennett. Principles and Practice of Infectious Diseases, 3rd ed. New York: Churchill Livingstone, 1990:529.
2. Harrison's Principles of Internal Medicine 2, 11th ed. New York: McGraw-Hill, 1987:1087.
3. Hope RA, Longmore JM, et al. Oxford Handbuch der Klinischen Medizin. Bern: Verlag Hans Huber, 1990:334.
4. Goodman Gilman A, et al. Goodman and Gilman's The Pharmacological Basis of Therapeutics, 8th ed. New York: Pergamon Press, 1985:1131.
5. Simon C, Stille W, Wilkinson PJ. Antibiotic Therapy in Clinical Practice, 2nd ed. Stuttgart: Schattauer Verlag, 1993:159–161.
6. Fraschini F. Clinical efficacy and tolerance of two new macrolides, clarithromycin and josamycin, in the treatment of patients with acute exacerbations of chronic bronchitis. Int Med Res 1990; 18:171–176.

Clarithromycin Versus Amoxicillin Suspensions in the Treatment of Acute Otitis Media in Children

S. J. Coles and J. L. Macklin

Abbott Laboratories
Maidenhead, United Kingdom

M. B. Addlestone

Abbott Laboratories
Leeds, United Kingdom

M. K. Kamdar

Abbott Laboratories
Canvey Island, Essex, United Kingdom

BACKGROUND

Next to upper respiratory infection, acute otitis media is the most common acute infection of childhood (1). Approximately two-thirds of children experience one or more episodes by the age of 3 (2). Perhaps more important than the immediate effects of otitis media on the well-being of the affected child are the medical sequelae that must be considered: perforation of the ear drum, cholesteatoma (often requiring multiple surgical procedures), acute mastoiditis, atelectasis of the eardrum (3), as well as a number of rare secondary events (e.g., hydrocephalus, meningitis, lateral venous sinus thrombosis) (4,5). Young children may also experience hearing loss that affects the development of speech, language, cognition, and behavior (6,7).

The microbial etiology of acute otitis media has been well defined by the examination of middle ear exudate obtained by tympanocentesis. *Streptococcus pneumoniae* accounts for approximately one-third of all infections. *Haemophilus influenzae* is the second most important pathogen: the majority are nontypable, and between 10 and 30% are β-lactamase producers. *Moraxella catarrhalis* has been increasingly recognized as a cause of acute otitis media, with most of strains exhibiting β-lactamase production (8). Other less common causes of acute otitis media include *Chlamydia trachomatis*, especially in early infancy (9).

Clarithromycin, an advanced-generation macrolide, offers excellent in vitro and in vivo activity against most organisms that are responsible for acute otitis media in children. Clarithromycin concentrations attained in the middle ear exudate (mean = 2.5 μg/g) of children (10) exceed by severalfold the MIC_{90} values for the most prevalent otic pathogens (0.5 μg/ml for *S. pneumoniae*; 1 μg/ml for *H. influenzae*; 0.25 μg/ml for *M. catarrhalis*).

STUDY OBJECTIVE

The study was designed to compare the safety and efficacy of clarithromycin (125–250 mg bid) with amoxicillin (125–250 mg tid) suspensions in the treatment of acute otitis media in children.

PATIENTS AND METHODS

Study Design

The study was a single (investigator)-blind, randomized, multicenter study.

Inclusions

1. Male or nonpregnant, nonlactating female patients 1–12 years old inclusive.
2. Presence of signs and symptoms of acute otitis media, including two or more of the following: otalgia; fever; acute hearing loss; tugging or rubbing of the ear; or upper respiratory tract infection with one or more of the following: hyperemia; decreased mobility or bulging of the tympanic membrane; loss of tympanic membrane "landmarks"; acute otorrhea not caused by external otitis.
3. Otologic examination and tympanometry (if done) were consistent with the presence of fluid in the middle ear.
4. No use of systemic or long-acting antibiotics within 3 days or 4 weeks, respectively, before study drug administration.
5. No evidence of chronic, suppurative otitis media.
6. No evidence of perforated typanum.
7. No hypersensitivity to macrolide or β-lactam antibiotics.
8. No severe renal or hepatic impairment.
9. Written informed consent.

Drug Administration

Patients were randomized to receive either clarithromycin; 125 or 250 mg bid, or amoxicillin, 125 or 250 mg tid (125 mg for patient weighing less than 25 kg), suspensions for 5 days.

Evaluations

	Study day 1	Study days 6–8	Study days 28–32
Medical history	X	X	X
Physical examination	X	X	X
Signs and symptoms	X	X	X
Clinical response		X	X
Adverse drug events		X	X

RESULTS

The results are summarized in Tables 1–4.

Table 1 Summary of Demographic Data and Infection Status of Enrolled Patients

Data	Clarithromycin ($n = 132$)	Amoxicillin ($n = 127$)
Gender[a]		
Female	78	57
Male	54	70
Age (yr)		
Mean ± SD	5.8 ± 3.1	5.3 ± 2.8
Range	1.0–12.5	1.0–11.7
Weight		
<25 kg	92	94
≥25 kg	40	33
No. middle ear infections in ≤12 months		
Mean ± SD	1.6 ± 1.1	1.8 ± 1.4[b]
Range	0–6	0–7
Days since onset of infection		
Mean ± SD	2.2 ± 1.4[c]	2.4 ± 1.8[b]
Range	1–7	1–14
Infection severity		
Mild	23	24
Moderate	100	96
Severe	9	7

[a]Significantly different distribution of males and females between the groups for all patients ($p < 0.05$, Chi-square test with Yates correction), but not for evaluable patients.
[b]$n = 126$.
[c]$n = 131$.

Table 2 Clinical Response (Clinically Evaluable Patients)

Response	Clarithromycin	Amoxicillin
Clinical cure	80%* (91/114)	68% (71/105)
Clinical improvement	16% (19/114)	28% (30/105)
Clinical success	96% (110/114)	96% (101/105)
Recurrence	5% (6/114)	4% (5/105)

*$p = 0.057$, Chi-square test with Yates correction.

Table 3 Resolution of Signs and Symptoms of Acute Otitis Media (Clinically Evaluable Patients)

Sign/symptom	Clarithromycin	Amoxicillin
Otalgia	94% (103/110)	91% (89/98)
Tympanic hyperemia	82% (80/98)	78% (78/100)
Irritability	97% (87/90)	94% (80/85)
URTI	89% (76/85)	87% (71/82)
Acute otorrhea	84% (21/25)	86% (12/14)
Tympanic bulging	92% (54/59)	93% (52/56)
Tympanic mobility	88% (42/48)	80% (37/46)
Tympanic landmarks	80% (72/90)	73% (59/81)
Ear pain subside $\leq$48 h	79% (90/114)	74% (78/105)

Table 4 Summary of Adverse Events[a] (Excluding Those Not Related to the Study Drug)

Adverse event	Clarithromycin ($n = 132$)	Amoxicillin ($n = 127$)
Vomiting	1	4
Diarrhea	2	3
Nausea	0	1
Wheezing	1	0
Coughing	0	1
Taste perversion	1	0
Overall	4 (3%)	8 (6.3%)

[a]Number of patients with one or more adverse events.

Four clarithromycin-treated patients experienced five (none severe) adverse drug-related events, and eight amoxicillin-treated patients experienced nine (two severe) adverse drug-related events. Three (2%) amoxicillin and no (0%) clarithromycin patients discontinued therapy because of an adverse event.

CONCLUSIONS

Clarithromycin suspension is at least as well tolerated and as effective as amoxicillin suspension in pediatric patients. Given the need to treat acute otitis media to prevent suppurative complications, clarithromycin provides an alternative to β-lactam antibiotics, which are increasingly being rendered ineffective by β-lactamases elaborated from some of the important pathogens that cause acute otitis media.

REFERENCES

1. Shah N. Otitis media and its sequelae. J R Soc Med 1991; 84:581–586.
2. Teele DW, Klein JO, Rosner B, the Greater Boston Otitis Media Study Group. Epidemiology of otitis media during the first seven years of life in children in greater Boston: a prospective, cohort study. J Infect Dis 1989; 160:83–94.
3. Farrior J. Complications of otitis media in children. South Med J 1990; 83:645–648.
4. Facione N. Otitis media: an overview of acute and chronic disease. Nurse Pract 1990; 104:949–951.
5. O'Connell JE. Lateral sinus thrombosis: a problem still with us. J Laryngol Otol 1990; 104:949–951.
6. Bluestone CD, Klein JO, Paradise JL. Effects of otitis media on the child. Pediatrics 1983; 83:639–652.
7. Teele DW, Klein JO, Chase C, et al. Otitis media in infancy and intellectual ability, school achievement, speech, and language at age 7 years. J Infect Dis 1990; 162:685–694.
8. Kovatch A, Wald E, Michaels RH. beta-Lactamase-producing *Branhamella catarrhalis* causing otitis media in children. J Pediatr 1983; 102:261–264.
9. Tipple MA, Beem MO, Saxon EM. Clinical characteristics of the afebrile pneumonia associated with *Chlamydia trachomatis* infection in infants less than six months of age. Pediatrics 1979; 63:192–197.
10. Sundberg L. Penetration of clarithromycin into middle ear effusion. 1st International Conference on the Macrolides, Azalides and Streptogramins. Santa Fe, NM, January 1991: abstr 203.

Roxithromycin Versus Amoxicillin–Clavulanic Acid for Community-Acquired Lower Respiratory Tract Infection: A Pharmacoeconomic Study

W. G. Scott and H. M. Scott

Wellington, New Zealand

B. C. Cooper

Delpharm Limited
Auckland, New Zealand

N. C. Karalus

Waikato Hospital
Hamilton, New Zealand

INTRODUCTION

Roxithromycin, the first of a new generation of macrolide antibiotics, has an improved pharmacokinetic profile, with a long half-life, good tissue penetration, and a spectrum of activity encompassing all pathogens encountered in community-acquired lower respiratory tract infection (LRTI). It has been demonstrated to be an effective and particularly well-tolerated antibiotic in multiple clinical trials (1).

Amoxicillin–clavulanic acid has a well-established safety and efficacy profile (2) and is an antibiotic of choice for the treatment of LRTI. As such, it represents one of the standards against which other treatments should be evaluated.

A multicenter, open-label, centrally randomized, investigator-blind trial was undertaken to compare the efficacy, safety, and cost-effectiveness of roxithromycin, 150 mg bid, with amoxicillin–clavulanic acid, 500/125 mg tid, in the treatment of community-acquired LRTI, including pneumonia, exacerbations of chronic bronchitis, exacerbations of bronchiectasis, and acute bronchitis (3).

A limited, but clearly definable set of costs, was measured. The economic evaluation considered only the direct medical costs from the societal perspective of Australia. Incremental analysis was used. Only those costs that changed or differed between the treatment options were relevant to the analysis.

PATIENTS AND METHODS

From September 1991 until February 1993, 242 patients were enrolled by 40 general practitioners in New Zealand and Australia. Seven patients had illnesses unsuitable for treatment with the antibiotics in the trial and eight patients were lost to follow-up. Therefore, 227 patients were evaluable on an intention-to-treat basis. Of these, 117 patients received roxithromycin and 110 received amoxicillin–clavulanic acid.

Patients older than 16 years of age (mean age 42 years) were required to have a productive cough and signs on examination consistent with LRTI. A chest x-ray film was required at inclusion; sputum was cultured, and blood collected for serological testing and routine hematological and biochemical assessment. Sputum and blood tests were repeated at the end of therapy, which was initially set at 7 days. If more prolonged treatment was required, a further 7 days of the same antibiotic was dispensed.

Primary medicine costs were obtained by combining the average treatment duration, the average daily dose, and the listed price per unit of the medicine. All prices for additional medicine (for treatment failures and side effects) were generic-dispensed prices, and cost was calculated by multiplying the dispensed price per unit by the number of units dispensed. Details were provided by general practitioners using a standardized form. The difference in costs (apart from primary medicine used) between treatment options was manifest in terms of treatment failure, withdrawal, or adverse effects. The relevant exchange rate was US\$0.68762 = A\$1 (as at December 1992; National Australia Bank).

RESULTS

The two treatment groups were comparable at baseline for age, gender, and underlying disease. The majority were ethnically Caucasian or Polynesian. The average duration of illness before enrollment was 1 week, and most cases were of mild to moderate severity.

The results of the clinical study are summarized in Table 1. Clinical efficacy at 7 days was significantly better for roxithromycin (69 vs. 56%; $p = 0.05$). There was no significant difference in efficacy at study end, but significantly fewer patients assigned roxithromycin required an extended course of treatment

Table 1 Results of Clinical Efficacy of Roxithromycin and Amoxicillin–Clavulanic Acid (Intention-to-Treat Analysis)

	Roxithromycin		Amoxicillin–clavulanic acid		Significance
	n	%	n	%	p
Patient evaluable	117		110		
Average treatment duration (days)	8.29		9.34		NS
Efficacy at 7 days	81	(69)	62	(56)	0.05
Efficacy (at end of study)	106	(91)	100	(91)	NS
Patients requiring extended course of treatment	30	(26)	42	(38)	0.04
Patients withdrawn from study (side effects or treatment failure)	5	(4)	3	(3)	NS
Side effects possibly/probably related to treatment	12	(10)	19	(17)	0.12

NS, no significant difference.

($p = 0.04$). The average treatment length was 1.05 days shorter for patients assigned roxithromycin, and fewer of these patients had side effects considered to be possibly or probably related to treatment.

Comparison of the direct incremental costs of roxithromycin and amoxicillin–clavulanic acid on a per patient basis showed that the primary medicine cost was less for roxithromycin (Table 2). In addition, the number and cost of additional medicines and of further diagnostic tests was less in the roxithromycin group. Roxithromycin patients generated less cost for additional consultations than did amoxicillin–clavulanic acid treated patients (see Table 2).

The direct incremental benefits of roxithromycin versus amoxicillin–clavulanic acid are summarized in Table 3. The total incremental net benefit per clinical success was A\$16.73, and the benefit per 100,000 episodes of LRTI would be A\$1.673 million.

CONCLUSIONS

In contrast with many trials, the study on which this economic analysis was based was specifically designed to emulate general practice diagnostic and assessment methods. However, the variation in treatment length between the artificial minimum of this trial and day-to-day clinical experience should be noted.

Direct medical cost savings were based on the actual trial use of the primary

Table 2 Comparison of Direct Incremental Costs

	Total costs for trial (A\$)[a]	Per patient evaluable for treatment (A\$)[a]
Number of patients evaluable for treatment		
Roxithromycin 117		
Amoxicillin–clavulanic acid 110		
Antibiotic direct cost		
Roxithromycin	2250	19.23
Amoxicillin–clavulanic acid	3288	29.89
Net cost: roxithromycin less amoxicillin–clavulanic acid	–1037	–10.66
Additional medicines to treat side effects and treatment failures		
Roxithromycin (23 medicines)	403	3.44
Amoxicillin–clavulanic acid (23 medicines)	442	4.02
Net cost: roxithromycin less amoxicillin–clavulanic acid	–39	–0.58
Additional diagnostic tests		
Roxithromycin (1 test)	38	0.32
Amoxicillin–clavulanic acid (2 tests)	77	0.70
Net costs: roxithromycin less amoxicillin–clavulanic acid	–39	–0.38
Additional consultations		
Roxithromycin (33 consultations)	792	6.77
Amoxicillin–clavulanic acid (48 consultations)	1152	10.47
Net cost: roxithromycin less amoxicillin–clavulanic acid	–360	–3.70
Total		
Roxithromycin	3483	29.77
Amoxicillin–clavulanic acid	4959	45.08
Net cost: roxithromycin less amoxicillin–clavulanic acid	–1476	–15.31

Notes: Individual items may not add exactly to the totals shown because of rounding. A negative net cost (e.g., –15.31) is a cost avoided by roxithromycin (a benefit).
[a] 1 A\$ = 0.69 US\$

Table 3 Summary of Direct Incremental Benefits: Roxithromycin Versus Amoxicillin–Clavulanic Acid

Benefits (or costs avoided) per patient	A$[a]
Primary antibiotic medicine dispensed	10.66
Medicines to treat side effects and treatment failures	0.58
Diagnostic tests	0.38
Consultations	3.70
Total direct incremental cost avoided = incremental benefit	15.31
Incremental benefit per clinical success (roxithromycin 90.6%, amoxicillin–clavulanic acid 90.9%)	16.73

Notes: Individual items may not add exactly to the totals shown because of rounding.
[a] 1 A$ = 0.69 US$

antibiotics by general practitioners, but the numbers of additional medications, consultations and diagnostic tests may have been higher in the trial than in day-to-day medical practice. The economic analysis took into consideration only those additional diagnostic tests, general practitioner visits, and pharmaceutical costs that resulted from inadequate treatment of the initial infection at study end or from adverse effects of trial treatments. The study did not subsume these costs; therefore, they are representative of costs that might normally result from the treatments offered.

As a result of the very small number of additional tests undertaken in the trial, small variations in numbers and unit costs could result in comparatively big changes in diagnostic test costs. As the latter make up a relatively small proportion of total costs, this would not alter the overall results.

Information on nonmedical and intangible costs and benefits, such as increased production and the effect of treatment on quality of life, were not available. The savings calculated, therefore, represent an underestimate to society, as there were fewer side effects and treatment failures at 7 days with roxithromycin.

Sensitivity analysis was applied to determine the breakdown point at which the incremental benefit per clinical success fell to zero. This point was achieved by increasing the average treatment time for roxithromycin by 6.5 days or by increasing the price per tablet for roxithromycin by 79%.

The results of this economic analysis are consistent with a previous comparative study of roxithromycin versus cefaclor (5), in which roxithromycin was shown to be a more cost-effective treatment of general practice LRTI. The observed differences in requirement for additional therapy and the occurrence of adverse events in favor of roxithromycin in this study are translated into actual cost savings.

REFERENCES

1. Young RA, Gonzales JP, Sorkin EM. Roxithromycin: a review of its antibacterial activity, pharmacokinetic properties and clinical efficacy. Drugs 1989; 37:8–41.
2. Todd P, Benfield P. Amoxycillin/clavulanic acid: an update of its antibacterial activity, pharmacokinetic properties and therapeutic use. Drugs 1990; 39:264–307.
3. Karalus N, Garret J, Land SDR, et al. Roxithromycin 150 mg bid versus amoxycillin 500 mg/clavulanic acid 125 mg tid for the treatment of lower respiratory tract infections in general practice. Infection 1994 (submitted).
4. Mandell GL, Douglas RG, Bennett JE. Principles and Practice of Infectious Disease, 3rd ed. London: Churchill, 1990.
5. Scott WG, Tilyard MW, Dovey SM, Cooper B, Scott HM. Roxithromycin vs. cefaclor in lower respiratory tract infection. A general practice pharmacoeconomic study. Pharmacoeconomics 1993; 4:122–130.

Evaluation of the Efficacy and Safety of Roxithromycin Versus Erythromycin in the Treatment of Community-Acquired Pneumonia

C. Brambilla, the International Study Group

Centre Hospitalier Regional et Universitaire de Grenoble
Grenoble, France

INTRODUCTION

Identification of the causative pathogens of community-acquired pneumonia from blood, respiratory secretions, or serology is often difficult and requires specialized and invasive methods that are not always available in general practice. Nevertheless, community-acquired pneumonia is a disease that requires prompt and effective treatment. Roxithromycin, one of a new generation of macrolides, has a greatly improved pharmacokinetic profile (1,2); its long half-life of 10–12 h enables convenient once-daily administration and its spectrum of activity is similar to that of erythromycin against both typical and atypical pathogens. Roxithromycin is acid-stable and is reliably absorbed, producing serum concentration up to four times that of erythromycin at as low as one-fifth the dose. Good penetration of phagocytes (3) and effective intraphagocyte bioactivity (4,5) have been demonstrated, which is particularly important in the treatment of infections involving atypical organisms, such as *Mycoplasma pneumoniae* (6).

A randomized, double-blind, double-dummy, comparative, multicenter study was conducted in Sweden, Finland, France, and South Africa to compare the efficacy and safety of roxithromycin, 300 mg once daily, with erythromycin, 500 mg twice daily, in the treatment of community-acquired pneumonia.

MATERIALS AND METHODS

Fifty-two adult patients, presenting to private clinics or hospital outpatients with confirmed or presumptive community-acquired bacterial pneumonia, were admitted to the trial. Patients were randomly assigned to a 10-day course of either roxithromycin or erythromycin ethylsuccinate.

At the initial visit a medical history was taken and physical examination performed. A chest x-ray was performed within 24 h of inclusion into the trial. Serological investigations were also performed, and pretreatment sputum cultures obtained. Susceptibility of the organisms to the study drugs was determined by disk sensitivity method. If a resistant pathogen was isolated at baseline, the patient was considered not evaluable for clinical efficacy in the per protocol analysis. At the discretion of the investigator, the patient was either eliminated from the study or, if clinical improvement was observed, allowed to continue. These patients were included in the intention-to-treat analysis.

Clinical assessments were performed at the second visit (day 3–5) and again at the third visit (day 11–14) that took place after the end of the drug treatment period and also included serological investigations, chest x-ray films, and posttreatment cultures.

Clinical Efficacy

Clinical response was satisfactory if the patient was cured or if radiologic signs had not worsened. Clinical response was unsatisfactory if the clinical signs persisted or worsened, or new signs developed that were consistent with active infection.

Bacteriological Efficacy

Response was satisfactory if the causative pathogen was eradicated, or if a new pathogen was present, but with no clinical evidence of a new infection, or if the patient was unable to produce sputum. Response was unsatisfactory if the causative pathogen persisted, or if a new pathogen was cultured, with clinical evidence of a new infection.

Intention-to-Treat Analysis

Response was satisfactory if clinical signs cleared or improved, and was unsatisfactory if clinical signs were unchanged or worse at the end of treatment, or if further antibiotic therapy was required.

RESULTS

Of the 52 patients enrolled in the study, 28 received roxithromycin and 24 received erythromycin. The two groups were well matched demographically (Table 1).

Table 1 Demographic Data

Characteristics	Roxithromycin	Erythromycin
No. of patients	28	24
Sex		
Male	21	13
Female	7	11
Race		
African	9	6
Caucasian	19	18
Age (yr)		
Mean ± SD	42.6 ± 17.31	41.1 ± 17.68
Range	18–76	18–83
Weight (kg)		
Mean ± SD	71.3 ± 14.18	66.9 ± 13.62
Range	47.5–104	50–102
Height (cm)		
Mean ± SD	168.4 ± 9.09	167.5 ± 8.91
Range	150–190	150–183

Approximate duration of symptoms before the start of treatment was 4.3 ± 3.8 days (range 1–21 days) in the roxithromycin group and 4.5 ± 3.4 days (range 1–14 days) in the erythromycin group. Severity of infection and the general condition of patients at inclusion are summarized in Table 2.

In ten patients resistant pathogens were isolated at baseline; therefore, at the end of treatment 24 patients in the roxithromycin and 18 patients in the erythromycin group were evaluable for clinical efficacy. The satisfactory response rate was 91.6% (22/24) and 94.4% (17/18), respectively. No statistically

Table 2 Severity of Infection and General Status of the Patient at Inclusion

	Roxithromycin	Erythromycin
No. of patients	28	24
Severity of infection		
Mild	5 (18%)	4 (17%)
Moderate	22 (79%)	18 (75%)
Severe	1 (4%)	2 (8%)
General condition		
Good	19 (68%)	17 (71%)
Fair	9 (32%)	6 (25%)
Poor	0	1 (4%)

Table 3 Assessment of Clinical and Bacteriological Efficacy (per Protocol Analysis)

	Roxithromycin	Erythromycin
Clinical (*n* = 42)		
Satisfactory	91.6% (22/24)	94.4% (17/18)
Unsatisfactory	8.3% (2/24)	5.5% (1/18)
Not evaluable	14.3% (4/28)	25.0% (6/24)
Bacteriological (*n* = 12)		
Satisfactory	87.5% (7/8)	75.0% (3/4)
Unsatisfactory	12.5% (1/8)	25.0% (1/4)
Not evaluable	71.4% (20/28)	83.3% (20/24)

Fifty-two patients initially enrolled; 42 more evaluable for clinical efficacy, 10 were not evaluable; 12 were evaluable for bacteriological efficacy, 40 were not evaluable.

significant differences were observed between the two treatment groups (Table 3).

In the intention-to-treat analysis, which included patients who had received at least one dose of study medication and who had had a pre- and posttreatment evaluation, satisfactory response rates were 88.8% (24/27) in the roxithromycin and 90.5% (19/21) in the erythromycin group. There was no statistically significant difference between the two groups.

A total of 23 organisms were identified in the pretreatment sputum cultures: *Streptococcus pneumoniae* (11), *S. pyogenes* (1), *Haemophilus parainfluenzae* (2), *H. influenzae* (4), *Branhamella (Moraxella) catarrhalis* (4), and *Staphylococcus aureus* (1). Fourteen organisms were found in the roxithromycin group and nine in the erythromycin group. Two organisms (both *S. pneumoniae*) were resistant to both regimens; two organisms (*B. catarrhalis* and *H. influenzae*) were resistant to roxithromycin, and two organisms (*H. parainfluenzae* and *H. influenzae*) were resistant to erythromycin.

Twelve patients were evaluable for biological efficacy. Satisfactory response rates were 87.5% (7/8) in the roxithromycin and 75% (3/4) in the erythromycin group. Two patients receiving roxithromycin had a superinfection after eradication of the initial pathogen. There was no statistical difference between the two groups (see Table 3).

Following serological investigations, eight atypical organisms were identified as causative pathogens: *Mycoplasma pneumoniae* (6/9), *Legionella* (1/9), and *Chlamydia* TWAR (1/9); in one patient respiratory syncytial virus was isolated. Of the seven evaluable patients, four were in the roxithromycin and three in the erythromycin group.

Eight of the 52 patients (15%) experienced adverse events, 4 in each group.

The 4 in the roxithromycin group presented with abdominal distension and dry mouth (1), headache (1), pruritus (1), and sneezing (1). In the erythromycin group, five side effects were reported by four patients, all of which were gastrointestinal, including nausea and vomiting.

CONCLUSIONS

These results show that roxithromycin, 300 mg once daily, is as effective as erythromycin, 500 mg twice daily, in the treatment of community-acquired pneumonia. No serious side effects have been observed, and the once-daily administration is convenient. The results suggest that roxithromycin at a dose of 300 mg once a day is suitable and effective for empiric use in community-acquired pneumonia.

REFERENCES

1. Nilsen OG. Comparative pharmacokinetics of macrolides. J Antimicrob Chemother 1987; 20(suppl B):81–88.
2. Puri SK, Lassman HB. Roxithromycin: a pharmacokinetic review of a macrolide. J Antimicrob Chemother 1987; 20(suppl B):89–110.
3. Carlier MB, Zenebergh A, Tulkens PM. Cellular uptake and subcellular distribution of roxithromycin and erythromycin in phagocytic cells. J Antimicrob Chemother 1987; 20(suppl B):47–56.
4. Anderson R, van Rensburg CEJ, Joone G, Luckey PT. An in vitro comparison of the intraphagocytic bioactivity of erythromycin and roxithromycin. J Antimicrob Chemother 1987; 20(suppl B):57–68.
5. Tulkens PM. Intracellular pharmacokinetics and activity of antibiotics. 29th Interscience Conference on Antibiotic Agents and Chemotherapy, Houston, September 1989.
6. Hara Y, Suyama N, Yamaguchi K, Sohno S, Saito A. Activity of macrolides against organisms responsible for respiratory infection with emphasis on mycoplasma and legionella. J Antimicrob Chemother 1987; 20(suppl B):73–80.

Antibiotic Utilization and Cost Analysis in Hospitalized Patients with Community-Acquired Pneumonia

Gary E. Stein and Sandra L. Mantz

Michigan State University
East Lansing, Michigan

INTRODUCTION

The treatment of hospitalized adult patients with community-acquired pneumonia (CAP) continues to be a substantial challenge. Despite newer diagnostic tests and potent, broad-spectrum antibiotics, at least 50,000 deaths per year in the United States are attributed to this illness (1). Choosing appropriate empiric treatment of CAP is difficult because of the diversity of potential pathogens, as well as their everchanging susceptibility patterns. The initial choice of an antimicrobial should be based on several factors that include: the medical history, physical examination, sputum evaluation, chest radiograph, and local trends in antimicrobial resistance (2).

A wide range of organisms are now known to cause CAP. These etiologic agents commonly include typical (*Streptococcus pneumoniae, Haemophilus influenzae, Staphylococcus aureus*) and atypical (*Mycoplasma pneumoniae, Chlamydia pneumoniae, Legionella* spp.) pathogens (3). Unfortunately, a sputum is often unobtainable or nondiagnostic, and cultures identify a pathogen in only 35–50% of cases of CAP (4). Consequently, the treatment of hospitalized patients with CAP often requires antimicrobials with broad-spectrum activity. Common choices include newer cephalosporins, penicillins, aminoglycosides, and macrolides (5).

In this investigation, we performed a medical chart review of hospitalized adult patients with CAP. The purpose of this study was to identify cost-effective antimicrobial regimens for the treatment of CAP in our hospital.

PATIENTS AND METHODS

The medical records of all adult patients admitted to Sparrow Hospital, a large community and teaching medical center, with presumptive CAP during the first 6 months of 1993 were reviewed. This study was approved by the hospital institutional review board.

Patients with clinical findings, such as cough, sputum production, fever, chills, dyspnea, or pleuritic chest pain, and a new pulmonary infiltrate on chest radiograph, were included in our review. Those patients admitted with pulmonary embolus, septic shock, cystic fibrosis, or with a history of acquired immunodeficiency syndrome (AIDS) were excluded from this study.

Demographic, clinical, and laboratory information for each patient was recorded. A cost analysis of antibiotic use was performed for each patient, based on drug(s), dosage, duration of therapy, and acquisition cost to the hospital.

RESULTS

During the 6-month study period, 172 medical charts were reviewed and 67 (39%) cases of acute CAP were identified. Patient age ranged from 20 to 90 years old. The majority of patients (73%) were older than 60 years old. Five patients had a history of lung cancer and two patients were receiving oral steroids. Fifteen (22%) patients were taking an oral antibiotic before hospital admission.

Empiric parenteral antibiotics were initiated in all but two patients. The most common agents were cefuroxime (42%), ampicillin–sulbactam (28%), and ceftriaxone (14%). Parenteral therapy was given for a mean of 5.2 days (range, 1–23 days; median, 4 days). The mean therapy cost for these drugs was highest for ceftriaxone (1.0 g q12h) and lowest for cefuroxime (0.75 g q8h). The cost of therapy with these regimens is listed in Table 1. Concomitant erythromycin or clarithromycin was prescribed in 42% of these patients.

A pathogen was isolated from only 18 (27%) patients. These organisms included *S. pneumoniae* (7), *S. aureus* (3), *H. influenzae* (3), *K. pneumoniae* (2), *H. parainfluenzae* (2), and *E. coli* (1). All but one isolate, a methacillin-resistant *S. aureus*, was sensitive to a generic oral antibiotic, but sequential oral therapy usually reflected the empiric regimen. Only 10 (56%) of these isolates were treated with a generic oral antibiotic. The other 40 patients discharged from the hospital on an oral antibiotic regimen received a new broad-spectrum agent. Three of these patients received both cefuroxime and erythromycin. The mean duration of outpatient antibiotic therapy was 8.6 days (range, 5–21 days; median, 7 days). Cefuroxime (32%), clarithromycin (20%), and amoxicillin–clavulanate

Table 1 Cost of Parenteral Antibiotic Therapy

Parenteral antibiotics	Dose/schedule	No. of patients (%)	Mean cost/ per patient ($)
Cefuroxime	0.750 mg q8h	10 (15)	69.50
	1.5 g q8h	17 (26)	123.63
Ampicillin– Sulbactam	1.5 g q6h	10 (15)	87.72
	3.0 g q6h	8 (12)	179.45
Ceftriaxone	1.0 g qd	3 (5)	170.31
	1.0 g q12h	6 (9)	271.69
Other Agents		11 (17)	

(20%) were most commonly prescribed. The mean cost of these regimens are listed in Table 2.

The duration of hospitalization of patients in this study ranged from 2 to 37 days (mean, 8.3 days; median, 6.0 days). Five (7.5%) patients died during hospitalization. These patients were elderly and had comorbid conditions, such as chronic pulmonary disease, chronic renal failure, and congestive heart failure. All other patients had a successful clinical outcome, and no serious side effects were associated with antimicrobial therapy.

DISCUSSION

This medical record review of hospitalized patients with acute CAP revealed several interesting findings. Virtually all patients were placed on a broad-spectrum parenteral antimicrobial for empiric therapy. A newer cephalosporin or ampicillin–sulbactam were most commonly prescribed. A high dose of these antibiotics was used over 50% of the time in this study, even though clinical trials do not support greater efficacy with higher doses (6). Low-dose cefuroxime (0.75 g q8h) is effective therapy for CAP (7) and was less expensive than other common regimens used in this investigation.

Almost one-half of our study population were also initially treated with a macrolide antibiotic. This trend reflects the enhanced awareness of atypical pathogens causing CAP and an increased understanding of the clinical findings suggestive of atypical pneumonia (2). New macrolides, such as clarithromycin, are now being used in place of erythromycin when a greater spectrum, improved pharmacokinetics, or better tolerance is warranted (8). Clarithromycin was used as initial therapy in ten (15%) of our study patients.

Recent studies of hospitalized patients with CAP have found atypical

Table 2 Cost of Outpatient Antibiotic Therapy

Antibiotics	Dose/schedule	No. of patients (%)	Mean cost per patient ($)
Cefuroxime	500 mg q12h	10 (20)	85.19
	250 mg q12h	6 (12)	35.72
Clarithromycin	500 mg q12h	10 (20)	39.24
Amoxicillin – Clavulanate	500 mg q8h	8 (16)	45.37
	250 mg q8h	2 (4)	
Erythromycin	500 mg q6h	4 (8)	4.00
Ofloxacin	400 mg q12h	4 (8)	53.13
Cephalexin	500 mg q6h	4 (8)	6.20
Others		2 (4)	

pathogens in 25–50% of cases and atypical pathogens in 10–30% of cases (4). Identification of a respiratory pathogen was infrequent in this investigation. An organism was definable in only 27% of our study patients. No atypical pathogens were identified at the time of hospital discharge. The low frequency of pathogen identification observed in this and other studies hinders step-down therapy to narrow-spectrum antibiotics. Patients in this review were routinely converted to broad-spectrum oral antibiotics that had a spectrum similar to the empiric parenteral regimen. Moreover, newer oral antibiotics were used in several cases when a generic or narrow-spectrum antibiotic could have been used to treat a particular pathogen. Of the newer oral antibiotics prescribed to patients to complete their treatment, clarithromycin had the broadest spectrum and lowest cost in this study. A recent drug usage evaluation also found clarithromycin to be cost-effective as sequential therapy for patients with CAP (9).

CONCLUSION

Numerous antibiotics are used to treat CAP owing to the variability in the clinical presentation, difficulty in obtaining a precise etiological diagnosis, and the seriousness of this illness. In this review, we found that low-dose cefuroxime, with or without erythromycin, was the least costly empiric regimen for hospitalized patients with CAP. A generic antibiotic could usually be selected as sequential therapy when an organism was identified. When the causative pathogen of the pneumonia was not identified, clarithromycin was the least expensive broad-spectrum oral antibiotic. The use of clarithromycin would also obviate the need for oral cephalosporin–erythromycin combinations.

REFERENCES

1. Lynch JP. Community-acquired pneumonia: what new trends mean in practice. J Respir Dis 1992; 13:1619–1643.
2. Neu HC, Sabath LD. Criteria for selecting oral antibiotic therapy for community-acquired pneumonia. Infect Med 1993; (suppl):33–40.
3. Fass RJ. Aetiology and treatment of community-acquired pneumonia in adults: an historical perspective. J Antimicrob Chemother 1993; 32(suppl A):17–27.
4. Fang G, Fine M, Orloff J, et al. New and emerging etiologies for community-acquired pneumonia with implications for therapy. Medicine 1990; 69:307–316.
5. Grasela TH, Welage LS, Walawander CA, et al. A nationwide survey of antibiotic prescribing patterns and clinical outcomes in patients with bacterial pneumonia. DICP Ann Pharmacother 1990; 24:1220–1225.
6. Cade JF, Presneill J, Sinickas V, Hellyar A. The optimal dosage of ceftazidime for severe lower respiratory tract infections. J Antimicrob Chemother 1993; 32:611–622.
7. Zeisler JA, McCarthy JD, Richelieu WA, Nichol MB. Cefuroxime by continuous infusion: a new standard of care? Infect Med 1992; (Nov):54–60.
8. Stein GE, Havlichek DH. The new macrolide antibiotics. Postgrad Med 1992; 92:269–282.
9. Dempsey CL, Kaley TC, Zenkel J. Drug usage evaluation: clarithromycin as sequential therapy. Hosp Formul 1993; 28:999–1001.

Clarithromycin in the Treatment of Community-Acquired Pneumonia in Young Adult Noncompromised Patients

M. Sutti, S. Raschi, F. Inversi, and M. V. Lavorato

IRCCS San Raffaele
Milan, Italy

INTRODUCTION

Pneumonia is a severe, frequent illness that needs prompt and effective treatment. Community-acquired pneumonia in young adult (age younger than 40 years), noncompromised patients is caused most commonly by gram-positive strains, especially *Streptococcus pneumoniae*, and by *Mycoplasma pneumoniae*. Other etiologic agents have been described, such as *Chlamydia pneumoniae* (1,2).

Microbiological investigations for targeted therapy, even when feasible, usually take several days; hence, an empiric antibiotic treatment is generally needed (2,3). As empirical antibiotic therapy in this group of patients we used a macrolide that is effective against gram-positive and intracellular microorganisms (4).

MATERIALS AND METHODS

Between December 1990 and May 1993, in an open multicenter study of empirical antibiotics in pneumonias, 78 young, noncompromised patients with community-acquired pneumonia were treated with oral or intravenous clarithromycin at the dose of 500 mg twice a day. Non-responders after 72 h were given second-line therapy with parenteral cefazolin, at the dose of 1 tid. The patients were hospitalized and received therapy for at least 1 week.

Table 1 Community-Acquired Pneumonia in Young Adult (<40), Noncompromised Patients: Microbiological Data from 22% (17/78) Patients

Microorganism	No. patients
Mycoplasma pneumoniae (antibody titer)	12
Legionella pneumophila (antibody titer)	2
Staphylococcus aureus (sputum)	1
Streptococcus spp.	1
Branhamella (*Moraxella*) *catarrhalis*	1

RESULTS

The clinical complete response rate was high, 97.7% (Fig. 1). Only three patients failed to respond to first-line therapy. One of these recovered with cefazolin; a second one did not respond to either cefazolin or ceftriaxone and eventually recovered with oxacillin plus netilmicin; the third patient had a sputum that was culture-positive for *Staphylococcus aureus*, resistant to macrolide and sensitive to cefazolin (the patient was treated with ciprofloxacin, since he had a β-lactam allergy, and he responded). The tolerance was good and no patients had to stop therapy.

DISCUSSION

The high success rate confirms the effectiveness of clarithromycin in the empiric treatment of community-acquired pneumonia. We believe that this antibiotic

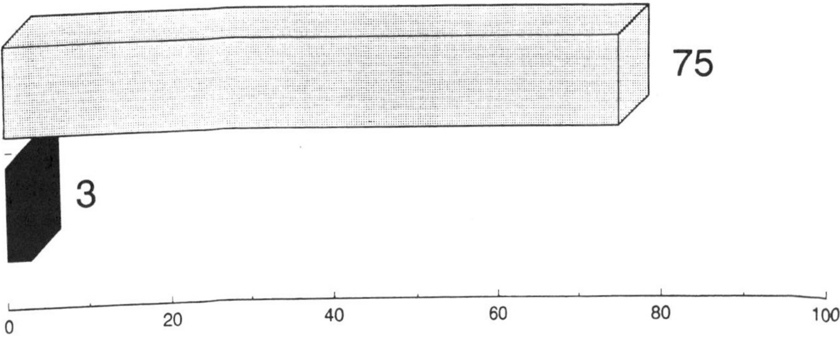

Figure 1 Community-acquired pneumonia in young adult (< 40 years), non-compromised patients. The clarithromycin efficacy was 97.7% (75/78 patients).

represents a good choice, particularly because of its activity against new, emerging pulmonary pathogens, such as *Mycoplasma pneumoniae* and *Chlamydia pneumoniae*, which are not sensitive to penicillin and its derivatives (2–4). In our study the etiological agent was identified in only 17 of 78 cases (Table 1).

Clarithromycin is different from other macrolides, since it is very well tolerated and has a low incidence of adverse reactions, especially gastrointestinal effects, which are very common with erythromycin. In fact, none of our patients had to withdraw treatment because of side effects.

REFERENCES

1. Research Committee of the British Thoracic Society. Community-acquired pneumonia in adults in British Hospitals in 1982–83: a survey of aetiology, mortality, prognostic factors and outcome. Q J Med 1987; 62:195–220.
2. MacFarlane J. Community-acquired pneumonia. Br J Dis Chest 1987; 81:116–127.
3. Fang GD, Fine M, Orloff J, et al. New and emerging etiologies for community-acquired pneumonia with implications for therapy. Medicine 1990; 69:307–316.
4. Neu HC. New macrolide antibiotics. Azithromycin and clarithromycin. Ann Intern Med 1992; 116:517–519.

Treatment of Community-Acquired Atypical Pneumonia with Roxithromycin: Preliminary Results of an Open Study

Bruno C. Palombini, Carlos A. Villanova, and Daiana Stolz

Pavilhão Pereira Filho
Santa Casa, Porto Alegre, Brazil

INTRODUCTION

In the "Guidelines for Initial Management of Adults with Community-Acquired Pneumonia", it is stated that an initial approach to managing patients with community-acquired pneumonia involves a determination of three factors (1): (1) Should the patient be treated in the hospital or as an outpatient? (2) Does the patient have a serious coexisting illness or advanced age (older than 60 years)? (3) How severely ill is the patient at the time of initial evaluation? Once this assessment has been made, initial antimicrobial therapy can be selected according to some recommendations. The choices should cover the most common pathogens.

The most common causes of comorbidity include chronic obstructive pulmonary disease (COPD), diabetes mellitus, renal insufficiency, congestive heart failure, chronic liver disease, and other equivalent medical conditions.

Community-acquired pneumonia may be typical or atypical. Atypical pneumonia has been recognized for at least four decades as a clinical syndrome characterized by a less severe clinical course than typical bacterial pneumonia. Atypical pneumonias are caused by a variety of different organisms, including *Mycoplasma pneumoniae*, chlamydiae, rickettsiae, viruses, and *Legionella pneumophila* (2,3). Of the chlamydiae, *Chlamydia pneumoniae* is now considered the most important pathogen.

Pennington (5) states that "precise diagnosis of etiologic categories for community-acquired pneumonia is also impossible." The difficulty in obtaining a good quality sputum specimen for microscopic and bacteriological examination or, for that matter, the difficulty in obtaining any sputum in some patients; the lack of sensitivity of sputum smears or cultures; the logistic difficulties in obtaining acute and convalescent viral titers, mycoplasmal, *Legionella* spp., or *Chlamydia pneumoniae* serological examinations; plus the nonavailability of cultures for these agents in many laboratories, are all important reasons that the true incidence of specific etiologies cannot be determined in most cases of atypical pneumonia.

However Fang et al. (4) studying 359 cases of CAP in a prospective multicenter survey, demonstrated that the four most common etiologic agents were *Streptococcus pneumoniae* (15.3%), *Haemophilus influenzae* (10.9%), *Legionella* spp. (6.7%), and *Chlamydia pneumoniae* (6.1%). *Mycoplasma pneumoniae* was the agent in 2.0%; unknown etiology: 32.9%. Therefore, 44% of the most frequent agents of the four main causes of CAP may belong to the atypical types.

Recently, new macrolide antibiotics have been developed. Among them roxithromycin (ROX) has improved microbiological and pharmacological properties. It is better absorbed from the gastrointestinal tract than erythromycin and produces higher concentrations in tissue and cells. Although the activity of this drug against group A streptococci, *S. pneumoniae*, and viridans streptococci is similar to erythromycin, it inhibits *M. pneumoniae*, *Legionella* spp., *C. pneumoniae*, and *Moraxella catarrhalis* at lower concentrations than erythromycin.

The efficacy and safety of ROX was evaluated in the first-line therapy of moderate to severe community-acquired atypical pneumonia.

For the purpose of this project we recognized additional conditions of comorbidity, such as smoking, chronic use of steroids, asthma, sinusitis, alcoholism, osteoporosis, essential cryoglobulinemia, bronchiectasis, lung cancer, cardiac arrhythmias and breast cancer.

PATIENTS AND METHODS

Study Design

The study included 12 inpatients presenting with CAP, who were admitted from January 1 to August 18, 1993. It was an open, unicenter study.

Inclusion Criteria

At least 18 years or older
Men or nonpregnant, nonlactating women

Diagnosis of atypical CAP suggested by intense nonproductive cough, or slightly productive of mucopurulent sputum
Fever (usually low grade)
Prostration or headache
Chest x-ray film: patchy infiltration without significant consolidation; thickening of the bronchial walls; no pleural effusion; no areas of lung abscess.
Slight leukocytosis or left deviation.
No response to β-lactam antibiotics

Exclusion Criteria

Allergy to macrolides or penicillin
Presence of liver diseases or renal insufficiency
Severe cardiovascular or GI diseases
Immunodeficiency (AIDS and selective IgA deficiency)
Contraindication to use of macrolides

Comorbidity

The comorbidities included smoking (Smok), six cases; chronic use of steroids (Ster), three cases, because of essential cryoglobulinemia, atopic dermatitis and asthma; asthma (Asth), two cases; sinusitis (Sinus) two cases; and one case of each of the following conditions: alcoholism, osteoporosis, essential cryoglobulinemia, bronchiectasis, lung cancer, cardiac arrhythmias, and breast cancer.

Serological Tests

Specific antibodies were measured in eight patients (IgM, IgG, and cryoagglutinins), and were considered positive with a titer lower than 1:16. Mycoplasma serology was positive in five cases; legionella serology was positive in two cases; and simultaneously chlamydial and mycoplasmal serologies were positive in one case.

Drug Administration

Approximately 75% had used a β-lactam antibiotic during a mean period of 4.6 days. Each patient was given 150 mg ROX bid for 7–30 days (six patients, 14 days; two patients, 7 days; two patients, 30 days; one patient, 11 days; and one patient, 21 days). The mean duration of treatment was 15.8 days; for patients with positive serological results, the duration was 14.4 days. Efficacy was evaluated on a clinical basis, including evolution of functional and physical signs.

RESULTS

The overall clinical efficacy rate, at the end of treatment, was 91.6%. The only case (8.3%) presenting partial improvement was due to legionella. Side effects probably related to ROX (mild gastrointestinal complaints, not requiring discontinuation of therapy) were present in only one patient.

CONCLUSION

We believe that this study reinforces that ROX is effective and well tolerated in the empiric treatment of community-acquired atypical pneumonia, even when comorbid conditions are present.

REFERENCES

1. American Thoracic Society. Guidelines for the initial management of adults with community-acquired pneumonia: diagnosis, assessment of severity, and initial antimicrobial therapy. Am Rev Respir Dis 1993; 148:1418–1426.
2. Bates JH, Campbell GD, Barron AL, McCracken GA, Morgan PN, Moses EB, Davis CM. Microbial etiology of acute pneumonia in hospitalized patients. Chest 1992; 101:1005–1012.
3. British Thoracic Society Research Committee and the Public Health Laboratory Service. The aetiology, management and outcome of severe community-acquired pneumonia in the intensive care unit. Respir Med 1992; 86:7–13.
4. Fang GD, Fine M, Orloff J, Arisumi D, Yu VL, Kapoor W, Grayston JT, Wang SP, Kohler R, Muder RR, Yee YC, Rihs JD, Vickers RM. New and emerging etiologies for community-acquired pneumonia with implications for therapy; a prospective multicenter study of 359 cases. Medicine 1990; 69:307–316.
5. Pennington JE. Community-acquired and hospital-acquired pneumonia in adults. In: Simmons DH. Current Pulmonology, vol 7. Chicago: Year Book Medical Publishers, 1986.
6. Schlick W. The problems of treating atypical pneumonia. J Antimicrob Chemother 1993; 31(suppl 6):111–120.

Clinical Study of Intravenous Azithromycin

S. Schönwald and B. Baršić

University Hospital of Infectious Diseases "Dr. Fran Mihaljević"
Zagreb, Croatia

I. Francetić

School of Medicine, University of Zagreb
Zagreb, Croatia

I. Klinar

PLIVA, Pharmaceutical, Chemical, Food and Cosmetic Industry
Research Institute
Zagreb, Croatia

INTRODUCTION

Azithromycin is a prototype of the novel class of macrolide antibiotics known as the azalides. Structurally, it differs from macrolides in having a methylated nitrogen atom incorporated in an expanded, 15-membered lactone ring. A notable antibacterial advantage of azithromycin over erythromycin is greater activity against many gram-negative and several other pathogens, notably *Haemophilus influenzae*, *H. parainfluenzae*, *Moraxella catarrhalis*, *Neisseria gonorrhoeae*, *Ureaplasma urealyticum*, and *Borrelia burgdorferi* (1). Pharmacokinetic advantages include improved acid stability, rapid and extensive uptake from the circulation into intracellular compartments, and longer elimination half-lives. These properties enable very high tissue concentrations of azithromycin to be sustained for several days, leading to once-daily dosing and short duration of therapy (2). The efficacy of azithromycin has been demonstrated in several respiratory tract and skin and soft-tissue infections as well as in chlamydial or gonococcal urethritis or cervicitis (1). Azithromycin is associated with less gastrointestinal adverse effects than erythromycin (3) and has lower drug interaction potentials (1).

Oral dosage of azithromycin is well established in clinical practice. An intravenous form has recently been developed, and the present study was designed to assess the efficacy and safety of intravenously administered azithromycin in the treatment of respiratory tract and skin and soft-tissue infections in patients who could not receive peroral therapy.

PATIENTS AND METHODS

A total of 54 adult hospitalized patients with acute bacterial respiratory tract or skin and soft-tissue infections were enrolled in the study. Diagnosis was established on the basis of clinical history, physical findings, chest radiograph, and microbiological or serological data. Exclusion criteria were known hypersensitivity to macrolide antibiotics, pregnancy or lactation, renal or hepatic disorders (creatinine > 130 μmol/L, aminotransferases more than two times higher than normal values), and the use of systemic antibiotics in a period shorter than 72 h before study entry. The study was approved by the review boards of each of the participating institutions.

Azithromycin (supplied by Pliva Pharmaceuticals, Zagreb, Croatia) was given for 3–5 consecutive days at a dose of 250 mg daily, as a 30 min infusion in 250 ml of infusion solution (5% glucose or normal saline). Patients were monitored every day, but the results of physical examination were assessed at baseline (before therapy) and on days 3, 6, and 11. Clinical response was classified as follows: very good, resolution of main clinical symptoms within 48 h after the initiation of therapy; good, resolution of clinical symptoms within 5 days of treatment; and failure, persistence of symptoms after the fifth day of treatment. Bacteriological eradication was defined as elimination of the causative pathogen by day 11. Blood for serological tests was taken before starting therapy and 15–21 days after. Side effects were recorded and samples for hematology, serum chemistry, and urine analysis were obtained at the time of efficacy assessment.

RESULTS

Among the 54 patients included in the study, 50 (29 women and 21 men) were evaluable for efficacy analysis, 4 patients were excluded (3 because of the violation of the protocol and 1 because of missed visit at the end of therapy). None of the patients withdrew because of treatment-related side effects or clinically significant laboratory abnormalities. Clinical response was very good in 43 patients (86%), good in 7 (14%), and there were no treatment failures (Table 1). Significant temperature curve decreases were recorded within first 48 h after the initiation of therapy ($p < 0.0001$, two tailed t-pair test; Fig. 1).

Table 1 Clinical Response to Intravenous Azithromycin

		Clinical Response	
Diagnosis	No. of patients	Very good	Good
Tonsillitis/pharyngitis	4	3	1
Acute sinusitis	1	1	—
Pneumonia	25	20	5
Atypical pneumonia	5	5	—
Erysipelas	15	14	1
Total	50	43 (86%)	7 (14%)

Causative microorganisms were isolated in 16 of 50 patients (most frequent *Streptococcus pyogenes*). Bacteriological response was achieved in all examined patients. Seven patients had positive serological findings for atypical pneumonia.

Side effects were recorded in 2 of 50 patients and were considered to be of mild severity, not requiring treatment discontinuation. In one patient, during administration of azithromycin on the second day of therapy, sweating and nausea with tachycardia occurred. It was most probably due to underlying heart disease and intolerance of increased preload caused by infusion. Subsequent doses of azithromycin were infused over 1 h without any side effects. In the other patient, mild and transient elevation of aminotransferases was registered.

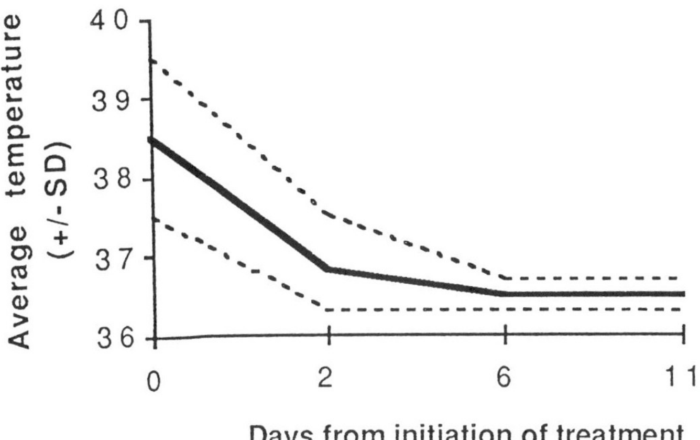

Figure 1 Body temperature during treatment with intravenous azithromycin.

CONCLUSION

Intravenously administered azithromycin seems to be very safe and effective in the treatment of respiratory tract and skin and soft-tissue infections. An absence of major side effects or severe abnormalities in laboratory parameters make it acceptable for the treatment when the oral route is contraindicated.

REFERENCES

1. Peters DH, Friedel HA, McTavish D. Azithromycin. A review of its antimicrobial activity, pharmacokinetic properties and clinical efficacy. Drugs 1992; 44:750–799.
2. Foulds G, Shepard RM, Johnson RB. The pharmacokinetics of azithromycin in human serum and tissues. J Antimicrob Chemother 1990; 25(suppl A):73–82.
3. Hopkins S. Clinical toleration and safety of azithromycin. Am J Med 1991; 91(suppl 3A):40S–45S.

Clarithromycin for the Treatment of Disseminated *Mycobacterium avium* Infection in AIDS: Bacteriological and Clinical Assessment in 25 Cases

D. Merrien, E. Billaud, V. Reliquet, D. Moinard, and F. Raffi

University Hospital
Nantes, France

INTRODUCTION

Mycobacterium avium infection (MAI) is the most common bacterial systemic infection in the acquired immunodeficiency syndrome (AIDS; 1,2). Although this infection occurs at a late stage of human immunodeficiency virus (HIV) infection, it is considered to have a poor prognosis (3,4) and contributes significantly to patient morbidity and decreased survival, compared with matched controls without MAI (5). New therapeutic agents have recently been shown to reduce bacteremia, to improve patient morbidity, and to prolong survival, to time periods comparable with non–*M. avium*-infected AIDS patients (6). Clarithromycin in monotherapy has demonstrated a good efficacy in MAI, with a clinicobacteriological correlation of improvement. The onset of resistance with a treatment duration between 2 and 7 months with clarithromycin monotherapy requires a combination of other antimycobacterial agents (7,8).

We conducted a retrospective study to determine bacteriological and clinical responses and survival in AIDS patients with MAI who were treated with clarithromycin-containing regimens.

METHODS

Twenty-five patients (20 men and 5 women; mean age, 31 years) were retrospectively studied. They were treated with clarithromycin and various other antimycobacterial agents. Twenty-one patients had positive smear culture from a sterile site (blood or bone marrow). For 4 patients, positive smears from a nonsterile site (stools or bronchial secretions) were considered when symptoms were suggestive of MAI and no other etiology was found. Clinical and bacteriological assessments were made every month. Survival time was calculated from the time of MAI diagnosis.

RESULTS

The most frequent HIV risk factor among the 25 patients was homosexual activity in 11 cases. *Mycobacterium avium* was the first opportunistic infection (OI) in 10 patients, and HIV seropositivity was unknown in 2 patients at the time of diagnosis. Thirteen patients had one or many other diseases at the time of MAI (three associated diseases for 2 patients, two associated diseases for 2 other patients, and one for 9 patients). The mean time between the diagnosis of AIDS and MAI was 6 months (range, 0–44) and the mean CD4 cell count was $19/mm^3$ (range; 4–50). All patients had impaired general health status, with weight loss in 25 patients, fever in 22, diarrhea in 13, pulmonary signs in 16, hepatic dysfunction in 14, and pancytopenia in 12 patients.

Mycobacterium avium was isolated from blood ($n = 21$), bronchial secretions ($n = 13$), stools ($n = 6$), and bone marrow ($n = 3$). Blood was the only positive specimen in 9 patients.

Minimum inhibitory concentrations (MIC) were determined using the Bactec system, and only 1 of the 17 tested strains was resistant in vitro to clarithromycin (MIC > 8 mg/L).

Patients received clarithromycin (mean dose, 1.7 g/day), with a mean of 2.6 antibiotics. The most frequent combination was clarithromycin–ethambutol–rifampin–ciprofloxacin ($n = 11$). Others antibiotics used in combination were: amikacin, clofazimine, and minocycline. Treatment was modified in five patients owing to digestive ($n = 3$) or hepatic ($n = 1$) intolerance or to in vitro resistance ($n = 1$).

Among 22 bacteriologically evaluable patients, 16 had complete eradication of *M. avium* within a mean of 47 days (range, 1–120 days). There was no significant difference concerning improvement of general health status, diarrhea, pulmonary signs, or hepatic dysfunction between the group of 16 patients for whom bacteriological eradication was obtained and the group of 6 patients for whom no such bacteriological effect was obtained. Moreover, mean survival between the two groups was not significantly different (7.2 months when

Table 1 Bacteriological Eradication

Parameter	Yes ($n = 16$)	No ($n = 6$)
Improvement of fever	8/16 (50%)	3/4 (75%)
General health status in a	8/16 (50%)	4/6 (66.6%)
mean delay of	1.5 mo	1.7 mo
Diarrhea	4/8 (50%)	2/3 (66.6%)
Pulmonary signs	4/11 (36.3%)	2/3 (66.6%)
Hepatic Disorder	4/10 (40%)	1/2 (50%)
Mean survival	7.2 mo	8.4 mo
Survival >10 mo	3/16 (18.7%)	2/6 (33.3%)

bacteriological eradication was obtained and 8.4 months for the other group; Table 1). Therefore, the survival course was comparable in the two groups (Fig. 1).

When we compare five patients whose survival was up to 10 months with the other patients, we note no difference in CD4 cell count, antiretroviral therapy, and prophylaxis of *Pneumoncystis carinii* pneumonia. However, 60% of patients with short survival (i.e., less than 10 months) had other opportunistic infections at the time of diagnosis when compared with only 20% in the group with more prolonged survival (Table 2).

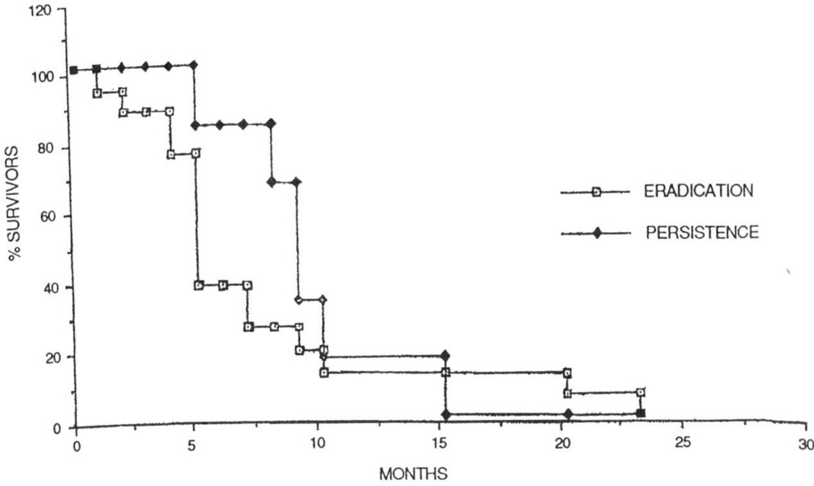

Figure 1 Course of survival.

Table 2 Survival Parameters

Parameter[a]	Survival >10 mo (n = 5)	Survival <10 mo (n = 20)
CD4 cell count	18/mm^3	19/mm^3
Antiretroviral therapy	3/5 (60%)	13/20 (65%)
PCP Prophylaxis	4/5 (80%)	16/20 (80%)
AIDS before	5/5 (100%)	11/20 (55%)
Others OI	1/5 (20%)	12/20 (60%)
Bacteriological eradication	2/5 (40%)	14/20 (70%)

[a]PCP, *Pneumocystis carinii* pneumonia; OI, opportunistic infection.

Bacteriological eradication during treatment was rapid in eight patients by 2 months, but mean survival was not significantly improved in these patients (mean survival was 8 months, compared with 6 months for the eight other patients with slower bacteriological eradication).

Early treatments (less than 8 days after samples) were performed before obtaining bacteriological confirmation of the disease in four patients because of severe symptomatology and impaired general health status (survival of 6 months). Therefore, no improvement of survival was observed in these patients compared with patients for whom therapy was begun later (more than 2 months; survival of 9.6 months).

DISCUSSION

Clarithromycin-containing regimens are active treatments of disseminated MAI in AIDS patients. Bacteriological eradication from blood and other cultured samples was obtained in 72% of the cases, and survival for longer than 10 months was achieved in 20% of the patients.

The absence of a correlation between bacteriological eradication and clinical improvement or survival in our study should be interpreted with caution owing to the small number of patients, the retrospective nature of the evaluation, and the absence of standardized follow-up. Furthermore, we found that concurrent opportunistic infections were very frequent in this severely immunosuppressed population, were associated with increased mortality, and could have interfered with the clinical assessment of anti-MAI treatments.

Despite prolonged treatment (up to 32 months in one patient), none of the patients with bacteriological eradication had a bacteriological or clinical relapse.

CONCLUSIONS

These results confirm that clarithromycin is useful in the treatment of disseminated MAI in AIDS and that with combination regimens, long-term treatment can improve symptoms and survival of a significant number of patients. Early diagnosis and empiric therapy with clarithromycin-containing regimen should further improve the prognosis of this frequent infection in severely immunosuppressed AIDS patients.

REFERENCES

1. Coker RJ, Hellyer TJ, Brown IN, Weber JN. Clinical aspects of mycobacterial infections in HIV infection. Res Microbiol 1992; 143:377–381.
2. Young LS. *Mycobacterium avium* complex infection. J Infect Dis 1988; 157:863–867.
3. Ellner JJ, Goldberger MJ, Parenti DM. *Mycobacterium avium* infection and AIDS: a therapeutic dilemma in rapid evolution. J Infect Dis 1991; 163:1326–1335.
4. Horsburgh CR. *Mycobacterium avium* complex infection in the acquired immunodeficiency syndrome. N Engl J Med 1991; 324:1332–1338.
5. Horsburgh CR Jr, Havlik JA, Ellis DA, et al. Survival of patients with acquired immune deficiency syndrome and disseminated *Mycobacterium avium* complex infection with and without antimycobacterial chemotherapy. Am Rev Respir Dis 1991; 144:557–559.
6. Craft JC. Survival in AIDS patients treated with clarithromycin for disseminated MAC infection. Poster presentation ICMAS, 1993.
7. Dautzenberg B, Salnt Marc T, Meyohas MC, Eliaszewitch M, Hanlez F, Rogues AM, De Wit S, Cotte I, Chauvin JP, Grosset J. Clarithromycin and others antimicrobial agents in the treatment of disseminated *Mycobacterium avium* infections in patients with acquired immunodeficiency syndrome. Arch Intern Med 1993; 153:368–372.
8. Ruf B, Schürmann D, Mauch H, Jautzke G, Fehrenbach FJ, Pohle HD. Effectiveness of the macrolide clarithromycin in the treatment of *Mycobacterium avium* complex infection in HIV-infected patients. Infection 1992; 20:267–272.

Treatment of Nontuberculosis Mycobacteria. The French Experience with Clarithromycin

B. Dautzenberg

GH Pitie Salpetriere
Paris, France

J. P. Chauvin, The French Clarithromycin Group

Abbott France
Paris, France

INTRODUCTION

The very first clinical trial that demonstrated the efficacy of clarithromycin in disseminated *Mycobacterium avium* disease in acquired immunodeficiency syndrome (AIDS) patients was conducted in France in 1990. Since that time, clarithromycin has been studied worldwide for this infection. We report some aspects of various studies conducted in France.

MYCOBACTERIUM AVIUM INFECTION IN AIDS PATIENTS

Study I. Randomized Phase II Pilot Study to Demonstrate Clarithromycin Activity

Methods

Twenty-three patients were enrolled between October 1988 and November 1989 in a double-blind, randomized, placebo-controlled, crossover study that evaluated the bacteriological efficacy of clarithromycin. Fifteen men with late-stage AIDS and positive blood cultures for *M. avium* at study entry were assessed. For the first 6 weeks of the study (Phase I), patients were randomized to receive oral clarithromycin, 1000 mg bid, or placebo. During the following 6 weeks (Phase II), patients who received clarithromycin were crossed over to placebo plus a combination of rifampin, 10 mg/kg daily; isoniazid, 5 mg/kg daily; ethambutol, 20 mg/kg daily; and clofazimine, 100 mg daily. The patients who received placebo during Phase I were crossed over to clarithromycin, 1000 mg bid, plus the same four-drug combination. Efficacy was measured bacteriologically by serial quantitative blood cultures of *M. avium*, which were determined at baseline and every 2 weeks thereafter.

Results

After Phase I, the mean count (colony-forming units; CFU/ml; Fig. 1) of *M. avium* decreased by 2.65 log in eight evaluable patients who were randomized to receive clarithromycin (in six cases, CFU decreased to an undetectable level) and progressively increased in five patients who were randomized to receive placebo (Fig. 2). After Phase II of treatment, CFU counts of *M. avium* decreased

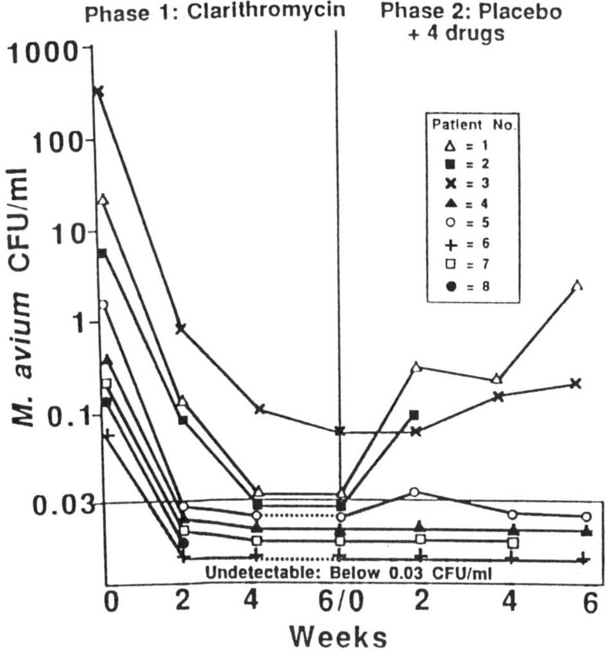

Figure 1 Log changes in CFUs of *M. avium* in blood cultures of patients receiving clarithromycin during phase I of the trial and placebo plus a four-drug combination (rifampin, isoniazid, ethambutol, and clofazimine) during phase II.

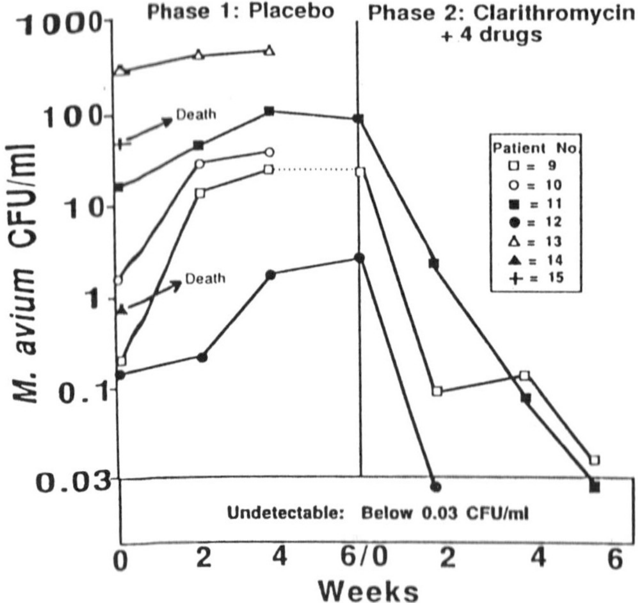

Figure 2 Log changes in CFUs of *M. avium* in blood cultures of patients receiving placebo during Phase I of the trial and clarithromycin plus a four-drug combination (rifampin, isoniazid, ethambutol, and clofazimine) during Phase II.

by a mean of 1.34 log for three patients who were crossed over to clarithromycin and the four-drug combination; the colony count was unchanged or increased in the seven patients who were crossed over to placebo and the associated antimycobacterial drugs.

Study II. Randomized Phase II Study to Determine Optimal Clarithromycin Dosage

Methods

A randomized, prospective, 6-week study was designed to compare the tolerance and efficacy of clarithromycin, 1000 mg bid (high dose) and 1000 mg qd (low dose), in HIV-positive patients with disseminated *M. avium* infection. Patients who weighed less than 50 kg (body weight) received 750 mg bid or qd. Clinical symptoms, tolerance, and quantitative blood cultures were assessed on study days 0, 14, 28, and 42.

Results

Of the 55 patients (48 men and 7 women; 36.6 ± 9.7 years old; 11.2 ± 14.3 $CD4/mm^3$) who were enrolled, 27 were randomized to receive the bid regimen, and 28 were randomized to receive the qd regimen. Twenty-seven patients were not bacteriologically evaluable owing to negative blood cultures at baseline (4 and 6 in the bid and qd groups, respectively), early death (3 and 1), early toxicity (3 and 1), and absence of quantitative blood cultures (4 and 5). The CFU count decreased by 3.13 ± 0.82 log in the bid group ($n = 13$) and 2.67 ± 1.8 log in the qd group ($n = 15$) after 6 weeks [no significant (NS) difference between groups]. The median time to conversion was 16 and 24 days, respectively (NS). Improvement in clinical symptoms was similar between the two dosage groups. Among the 55 enrolled patients, side effects led to premature discontinuation of study drug in 3 and 1 patients in the bid and qd groups, respectively; 2 and 1 patients experienced increases in liver enzyme values; 8 and 7, abdominal pain; 4 and 1, hearing disturbance; and, 1 and 2, alteration of taste.

Conclusion

A trend toward better bacteriological eradication and lower patient tolerance was observed with the high-dose (bid) group compared with the low-dose (qd) group. These results suggest that the clarithromycin dosage be reduced from 1000 mg bid to 1000 mg qd in patients who experience side effects during therapy.

Study III. Compassionate Use of Clarithromycin

Methods

The activity of clarithromycin in 173 AIDS patients with disseminated *M. avium* infection was assessed during a compassionate use program. Clinical symptoms, quantitative blood cultures, and safety were assessed.

Results

Initial bacteriological eradication of *M. avium* from blood was observed in 136 of 147 (92%) of evaluable patients. Acquired resistance to clarithromycin, which was associated with relapse, appeared to develop after 2–7 months of drug therapy in 31 of the 136 (23%) patients who had initial bacteriological eradication. The relapse rate was twofold lower in patients who also received ethambutol, but was identical in those who received other antimycobacterial agents. Side effects led to premature discontinuation of clarithromycin in 14 cases (8%) and modification of treatment in 8 cases (5%). The main side effects were elevated liver enzyme levels and hearing impairment.

Conclusions

This study provided evidence for the activity of clarithromycin in disseminated *M. avium* infection and underscored the need for the identification of associated drugs to prevent the development of resistance during therapy.

Summary

The French studies in AIDS patients with disseminated *M. avium* infection have

> Demonstrated the bacteriological efficacy of clarithromycin for the treatment of *M. avium* disease in AIDS patients
> Shown the clinical benefit associated with bacteriological eradication
> Described the relapse and acquired resistance phenomenon with monotherapy
> Suggested a protective effect of ethambutol on relapse rate
> Demonstrated that the 1000 mg bid dose can be reduced to 1000 mg qd in cases of intolerance

In vitro studies have raised the issue of controlling pH for accurate MIC assessment (Grosset).

NONTUBERCULOSIS MYCOBACTERIAL INFECTION IN NON-AIDS PATIENTS

Mycobacterium avium Lung Infection

Before the availability of clarithromycin, the treatments for *M. avium* lung infection in non-AIDS patients were generally ineffective.

Methods

A clarithromycin-containing regimen was evaluated among 45 HIV-negative patients with *M. avium* lung infection. Eleven patients were immunocompromised, and 21 had preexisting lung disease. Clarithromycin 1622 ± 428 mg/day was given alone ($n = 15$) or in association with other drugs: rifampin ($n = 7$), aminoglycoside ($n = 1$), quinolone ($n = 9$), clofazimine ($n = 15$), isoniazid ($n = 3$), ethambutol ($n = 7$), pyrizinamide ($n = 1$), or minocycline ($n = 5$) or some combination thereof.

Results

After 3 months of therapy, 27 patients were culture-negative, 11 had bacteriological results pending, 1 was culture-positive, 2 discontinued their treatment, and 3 were dead. After 6 months, 15 patients remained culture-negative, 5 patients became culture-positive, and 5 had bacteriological results pending.

Twelve patients with successful treatment had therapy discontinued (mean duration of 228 ± 129 days); there were no relapses at 147 ± 158 days after treatment cessation. Adverse events included minor hearing impairment ($n = 4$), increases in liver enzyme levels ($n = 5$), and GI pain ($n = 10$), leading to discontinuation of therapy in 2 patients who received high doses of clarithromycin (> 40 mg/kg).

Conclusions

Clarithromycin-containing regimens produced bacterial eradication in 97% of evaluable HIV-negative patients with *M. avium* lung infection; relapse occurred in 25%. The 30-mg/kg–daily dose of clarithromycin was effective and well tolerated. Concomitant drugs must be evaluated.

Mycobacterium avium Node Infection

Eleven patients (six adults, five children) with *M. avium* node infection were treated with a clarithromycin-containing regimen. Of the eight patients who were assessed after 3 and 6 months of therapy, seven were cured. One, a 72-year-old woman, had a relapse, with acquired resistance, and the infection persisted 1 year later.

Mycobacterium chelonei Infection

Methods

Ten patients (four men and six women) with *M. chelonei* infections received clarithromycin, 500 mg bid ($n = 9$) or 1000 mg bid ($n = 1$) for skin ($n = 6$), lung ($n = 3$), nodes ($n = 1$), or bone ($n = 1$) infections (one or two sites).

Results

The six *M. chelonei* skin infections (due to iatrogenic puncture) were treated with clarithromycin 500 mg bid for 27–40 days after failure of other antimycobacterial or aminoglycoside therapy (Fig. 3). In four cases, clinical regression and bacteriological eradication occurred (Fig. 4); after 1–3 months, the skin lesion reappeared in two of the four patients while cultures remained negative. Two patients had no follow-up.

The patient with *M. chelonei* bone infection was culture-negative after 18 months of treatment. One patient with *M. chelonei* lung infection (Fig. 5) remained culture-negative 6 months after receiving 5 months of postoperative clarithromycin. One patient with *M. chelonei* node and lung infection initially experienced lesion regression, which was followed by clinical relapse. Sputum remained positive for *M. chelonei*, and susceptibility to clarithromycin measured after 8 months was decreased.

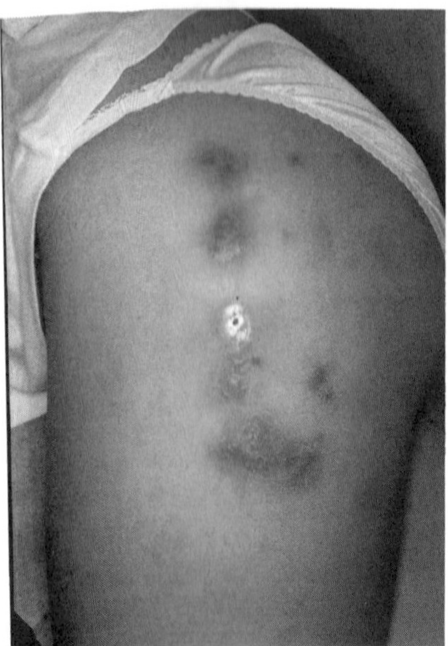

Figure 3   Cutaneous infection with *M. chelonei* before treatment.

One HI V-infected patient (CD4 = $36/mm^3$) with *M. chelonei* lung infection became culture-negative and remained so until death 3 months after the initiation of therapy.

Conclusions

Clarithromycin is effective in the treatment of *M. chelonei* infections, but relapse with acquired resistance may occur when given as a single agent. Optimal dosage, duration of treatment, and associated drugs remain to be investigated.

Mycobacterium xenopi Lung Infection

There is no standardized regimen for *M. xenopi* infections. Clarithromycin shows in vitro activity against *M. xenopi* (MIC = 0.5 mg/L).

Sixteen patients (54 years old ± 13 years, 2 HIV-positive) received clarithromycin-containing regimens. Among the 14 HIV-negative patients, 2 with osteoarticular disease had a favorable outcome. The 12 remaining patients had *M. xenopi* lung infection. One patient who discontinued treatment had sputum cultures that remained positive 18 months later. Nine of 11 (82%) HIV-negative patients who received > 6 months of clarithromycin therapy were culture-negative after 3 months and sputums remained negative at 6 months. One patient relapsed after completing 1 year of treatment (MIC determination pending).

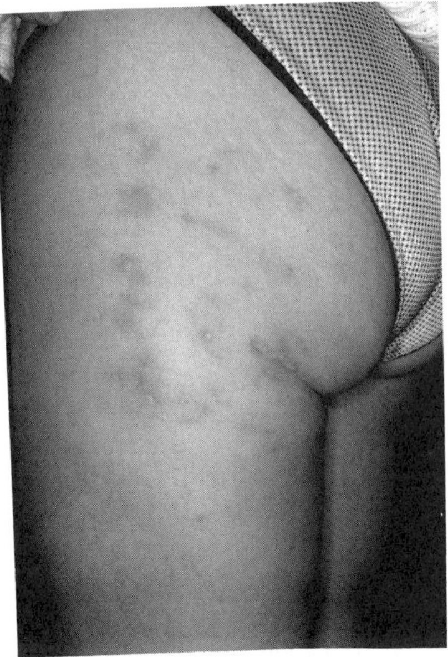

Figure 4 Cutaneous infection with *M. chelonei* after treatment.

Conclusions

The combination of clarithromycin (30 mg/kg) with ofloxacin (8 mg/kg) and ethambutol or clofazimine appears to be safe and effective for the treatment of *M. xenopi* lung disease in HIV-negative patients. Long-term follow-up and larger study populations are warranted.

Mycobacterium marinum Skin Infection

Mycobacterium marinum is a nontuberculosis mycobacteria that causes rare cutaneous disease, the treatment for which has not been established. Clarithromycin shows activity against *M. marinum* (MIC = 0.25 mg/L).

In France from December 1990 to December 1991, five HIV-negative patients (four men and one woman; 25–55 years old; 60–84 kg body weight) with *M. marinum* infection were treated with clarithromycin, 1000 mg bid (750 mg bid for the patient who weighed 44 kg), alone ($n = 3$) or in combination with other antimycobacterial drugs. Clinical improvement was observed within 1 week in all patients, including four who had failed previous treatment with other antibiotics. One patient who had pain for 6 months experienced well-being after the third dose of clarithromycin. After 1 month of therapy, the disease was

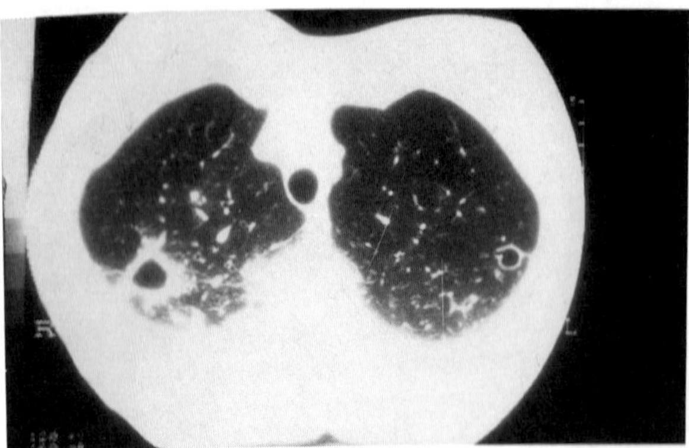

Figure 5   Computed tomography scan of lung infection caused by *M. chelonei*.

cured in all patients. No relapses were observed after discontinuation of treatment (follow-up 6 ± 6 months). The treatment was well tolerated by all patients.

Conclusion

A clarithromycin-containing regimen is highly effective for *M. marinum* skin infection.

SUMMARY

Several studies conducted in non-AIDS patients have demonstrated that clarithromycin is safe and effective in the treatment of *M. avium*, *M. xenopi*, *M. chelonei*, and *M. marinum* infections. The optimal regimen, including the companion drug(s) to clarithromycin, must be established.

Use of an Influence Diagram to Determine Outcome-Based Guidelines for *Mycobacterium avium* Complex Prophylaxis: What Agent(s) Should Be Used?

Herman Chmel

St. Francis Medical Center
Trenton, New Jersey
and
UMDNJ/Robert Wood Johnson Medical School
East Brunswick, New Jersey

INTRODUCTION

Mycobacterium avium complex (MAC) causes disseminated disease in as many as 40% of human immunodeficiency virus (HIV)-infected patients with advanced disease and CD4 lymphocyte cell counts below $100/mm^3$ (1–8). Disseminated MAC infections are characterized by fever, weight loss, night sweats, and anemia. The duration and quality of life for HIV-infected patients with MAC infections could probably be improved with more effective therapy and earlier effective intervention or prevention. Several newer antimicrobial agents are active against MAC (rifabutin, azithromycin, and clarithromycin). Recently, rifabutin has been approved and recommended for the prevention of MAC infections (8). The morbidity and decreased survival associated with disseminated *M. avium* complex infection is substantial (1–8). Concerns have arisen whether an adequate amount of direct evidence exists justifying the prophylactic use of antimicrobials against *M. avium* complex. Some of these issues include the development of drug resistance, potential adverse or toxic effects of the drug, and costs.

Most clinicians would favor direct evidence in linking an intervention

"

(MAC prophylaxis) with an outcome (prevention of MAC infections and, theoretically, a positive effect on quality and length of life). To assist clinicians in making these types of decisions, influence diagrams have been suggested and developed (9). This preliminary report describes our efforts to develop such an approach.

MATERIALS AND METHODS

All patients admitted to St. Francis Medical Center between January 1, 1993 and December 13, 1993, who had cultures of various bodily substances (blood, bone marrow, sputum, stool, or other) submitted for mycobacterial cultures were reviewed, and only those who were positive for *M. avium* complex were studied. The following data were collected (in patients with significant disease): age, sex, primary illness, CD4 lymphocyte counts, sites positive for MAC, length of hospital stay, and costs associated with hospital stay.

Patients with significant disease were defined as individuals who had symptoms suggestive of infection; those with positive cultures for MAC from blood, bone marrow, or tissue; and those with MAC organisms demonstrated on pathological examination in tissue. The medical literature was also reviewed to generate indirect evidence to support the modes generated in the influence diagram.

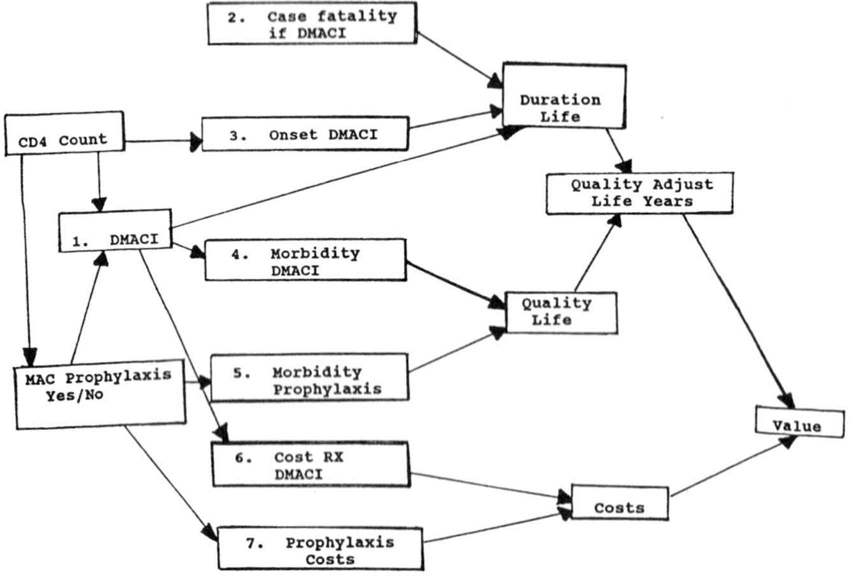

Figure 1   Influence diagram for *Mycobacterium avium* complex prophylaxis.

An influence diagram was developed (Fig. 1) using the CD4 lymphocyte count for setting the threshold for initiating prophylaxis that might be controversial.

RESULTS

Sixty-six patients had 90 cultures positive for MAC from various body sites. Twenty-six patients (39%) were defined as having significant cultures and disease (20 with positive blood cultures, 2 positive bone marrow aspirates, and 4 tissue biopsies). Table 1 demonstrates the demographic data collected. All patients had advanced HIV disease, with CD4 lymphocyte cell counts of fewer than $100/mm^3$ (average 15, range 100–0). Fever, weight loss, fatigue, and anemia were present in 94% of the patients. The average hemoglobin was 8.3 g/dl (range 5.8–11). Eighty-nine percent of the patients had a history of intravenous drug administration (IVDA); 58% had a history of another opportunistic infection (OI), most

Table 1 Demographic Data

Patients	26
Age[a]	46 (range 19–86)[a]
Sex	4.5 men/1 woman
HIV+	26
CD4 lymphocytes cells/mm^3)	15 (100–0)[a]
Sites positive for MAC	
Blood	20
Bone marrow	2
Tissue	4
Symptoms	
Fever	26
Weight loss	24
Fatigue	24
Anemia	26
Risk Factors	
IVDA	23
Other	3
Average length of stay[b]	29.8 (2–122)
HIV to Onset DMACI[c]	39 (1–120)
Costs	$35,275.33 ($2,794.62–$123,062.96)

[a]Average (range).
[b]Average length of hospital stay.
[c]Average in months (range).

commonly *Pneumocystis carinii* pneumonia (PCP); and 80% were receiving antiretroviral therapy. HIV disease had been present for an average of 39 months (range 1–120 months). The average length of stay was 29.8 days (range 2–122 days). The average cost for diagnosis and treatment was 35,275.33 dollars (range 2,794.62–123,062.96 dollars). Table 2 lists the information derived from the literature review.

Table 2 Available Evidence for Use in an Influence Diagram

Number (see Fig. 1)	Necessary information	Example	Ref.
1	Probability of DMAC based on CD4 count with/without MAC prophylaxis	% DMAC[a] by 12 mo with CD4 count <100 varies 15–40% % DMAC breakthrough on prophylaxis varies approximately 8.5%; 50% with positive blood cultures	1–7
2	Case fatality for episode of DMACI	Variable; average 4 mo after DX[b] with RX[c], 8 mo after RX, 100% at 2 yr.	
3	Probability of onset DMACI if it occurs based on CD4 count	Variable; 12–30% within 1–2 yr	
4	Morbidity DMACI	Variable	
5	Drug-related morbidity	Side effects depend on drugs: (rifabutin, clarithromycin, azithromycin; primarily GI)	
6	Cost RX, DMACI	Variable depending on hospital system. Average based on our system $7782 (ALOS 29.8 days)	
7	Prophylaxis costs	Project 1 yr (based on Red Book information) Rifabutin 300 mg/day $2,352/yr[d] Clarithromycin 1 g/day $1800 (projected cost/use)[e] Azithromycin 1200 mg/wk $1000 (projected cost/use)[e]	

[a]DMACI, Disseminated *Mycobacterium avium* complex infection.
[b]DX, diagnosis.
[c]RX, therapy.
[d]Currently approved for prophylaxis.
[e]Currently investigational for prophylaxis.

DISCUSSION

The use of an influence diagram employing indirect evidence gathered from literature reviews and a review of our experience at St. Francis Medical Center for 1 year in patients with disseminated MAC infections, leads us to feel that a strong argument can be made for the use of preventative therapy in the HIV patient with CD4 cell counts of fewer than 100/mm^3. The latter is based on the fact that it costs St. Francis Medical Center an average of 35,275.33 dollars to treat HIV patients who develop disseminated MAC infections. Considering this and that prophylaxis with rifabutin 300 mg/day (the only currently approved drug) costs 2352 dollars a year, if clarithromycin at 1 g/day (1800 dollars a year) or azithromycin at 1200 mg/week (1100 dollars a year) are approved for prophylaxis in the future, great cost savings and reduction in hospital admissions could be achieved. The quality of life could also improve with the absence of symptoms associated with the development of disseminated MAC infections, although the length of life may or may not change owing to other factors. However, concern would still exist about the development of drug resistance and adverse reactions to the prophylactic medications. This is a preliminary report, and further research in this area is currently ongoing.

ACKNOWLEDGMENT

This investigation was supported in part by an unrestricted research grant from Roerig/Pfizer Pharmaceuticals and Pfizer International. Thanks to Carol M. Fachet for secretarial assistance.

REFERENCES

1. Ellner JJ, Goldberger MJ, Parenti DM. *Mycobacterium-avium* infection and AIDS: a therapeutic dilemma in rapid evaluation. J Infect Dis 1991; 163:1326–1335
2. Inderlied CB, Kemper CA, Bermudez LEM. The *Mycobacterium-avium* complex. Clin Microbiol Rev 1993; 6:266–310
3. Benson CA, Ellner JJ. *Mycobacterium avium* complex infection and AIDS: advances in theory and practice. Clin Infect Dis 1993; 17:7–21
4. Jacobson MA, Hopewell PC, Yajko DM, et al. Natural history of disseminated *Mycobacterium avium* complex infection in AIDS. J Infect Dis 1991; 164:994–998
5. Nightingale SD, Byrd LT, Southern PM, et al. Incidence of *Mycobacterium avium–intracellulare* complex bacteremia in human immunodeficiency virus-positive patients. J Infect Dis 1992; 165:1082–1085
6. Young LS. Mycobacterial diseases and the compromised host. Clin Infect Dis 1993; 17(suppl 2):S436–S441
7. Nightingale SD, Cameron DW, Gordin FM, et al. Two controlled trials of

rifabutin prophylaxis against *Mycobacterium avium* complex infection in AIDS. N Engl J Med 1993; 329:828–833

8. Masur H, Public Health Service Task Force on Prophylaxis and Therapy of *Mycobacterium avium* Complex. Recommendations on prophylaxis and therapy for disseminated *Mycobacterium avium* complex disease in patients infected with human immunodeficiency virus. N Engl J Med 1993; 329:898–904

9. Howard RA, Matheson JE. Influence diagrams. In: Howard RA, Matheson JE, eds. The Principles and Applications of Decision Analysis. Menlo Park, CA: Strategic Decisions Group, 1984:719–762

A Retrospective Study of Clarithromycin as Primary Prophylaxis for MAC Disease

D. L. Payne

Desert Samaritan Medical Center
Mesa, Arizona

BACKGROUND

Disseminated *Mycobacterium avium* infection occurs in 15–24% of patients with acquired immunodeficiency syndrome (AIDS; 1–3). Overall survival is significantly reduced for AIDS patients with disseminated *M. avium* complex (MAC) disease. In two studies from the Centers for Disease Control, median survival for AIDS patients with disseminated nontuberculous mycobacterial disease was 7.4 and 4.1 months, respectively, versus 12.7 and 11.1 months, respectively, for AIDS patients with other opportunistic infections (4–6).

Disseminated MAC infection occurs late in the course of human immunodeficiency virus (HIV) infection, diagnosed a mean of 4–15 months from the time of first diagnosis of AIDS (2,7). The major risk factor for this infection is the level of immune dysfunction, as reflected by the CD4 cell count. The mean number of CD4 cells in patients with disseminated MAC infection is fewer than $60/mm^3$, and infection is rare in patients with more 100 CD4 cells per cubic millimeter (2,8,9).

Colonization with MAC in HIV-infected patients has not been well defined, as a consequence, its incidence is unknown. In one retrospective study, investigators concluded that disseminated MAC disease may occur in the absence of prior detectable respiratory or gastrointestinal (GI) tract colonization with MAC, and that MAC may be isolated from the respiratory or GI tract without the occurrence of disseminated disease during up to 9 months of observation

(10). In the absence of prospective analyses, more precise estimates of the relation between colonization and disease are not possible.

Clarithromycin is a macrolide antimicrobial agent that is highly potent against a variety of aerobic and anaerobic gram-positive and gram-negative organisms, with activity equal to or greater than erythromycin for most strains tested. It has also demonstrated in vitro and in vivo activity against MAC.

The ability of clarithromycin to inhibit multiplication of *M. avium* within human macrophages has also been evaluated in an in vitro system (11). Normal human-derived macrophage monolayers were infected with clinical isolates of MAC and incubated in the presence or absence of clarithromycin or one of three other antimicrobial agents. Clarithromycin was the most effective agent in inhibiting the intracellular replication of *M. avium* (11). Combinations of clarithromycin–rifabutin and clarithromycin–sulfisoxazole, also tested in this model, demonstrated activity that was not significantly different from that of clarithromycin alone in reducing replication of *M. avium* (11).

Clinical study experience treating AIDS patients with clarithromycin for disseminated MAC disease is limited. In a Phase II, double-blind, randomized, placebo-controlled crossover study carried out by Dautzenberg et al. in France, equal numbers of patients were randomized to receive clarithromycin, 1000 mg bid (group 1) or placebo bid (group 2) for 6 weeks (12). After the initial 6 weeks, group 1 patients were crossed over to receive an additional 6 weeks of therapy with placebo plus a combination of isoniazid (5 mg/kg per day), ethambutol (20 mg/kg/per day), rifampin (600 mg/day), and clofazimine (100 mg/day); group 2 patients were crossed over to receive 6 weeks of therapy with clarithromycin, 1000 mg bid, plus the same four drug regimen (12). Of 13 patients, 7 were evaluable in group 1 and 6 were evaluable in group 2. Patients treated with clarithromycin alone had a marked decrease in colony counts of *M. avium* in blood over the initial 6-week–treatment period, with 4 of 7 patients having growth reduced to undetectable levels (12). When these patients were crossed over to placebo plus the four-drug regimen, 3 of 7 patients showed an increase in MAC colony counts in the blood. Conversely, patients in group 2 had dramatic increases in MAC growth in blood during initial placebo treatment followed by marked decreases in colony counts when crossed over to receive clarithromycin plus the four-drug regimen, with 3 of 5 patients having undetectable growth of MAC during clarithromycin treatment (12). Tolerance of clarithromycin was good; 2 patients reported nausea and 2 had subclinical hearing loss demonstrated by audiogram during drug treatment, effects that were reversed with drug discontinuation (12).

Preliminary data obtained from a Phase II, dose-ranging, double-blind study indicate clarithromycin is 80–84% effective in eradicating or partially eradicating *M. avium* from the blood of AIDS patients when treated for 12 weeks at doses of 500 mg, 1000 mg, and 2000 mg bid (13).

Accumulating evidence supports the contention that the presence of disseminated MAC disease contributes to morbidity and adversely affects survival of patients with AIDS. Persons with advanced HIV infection, particularly AIDS, are at risk for the development of disseminated MAC disease. Clarithromycin has been shown to decrease and eradicate *M. avium* from the blood of AIDS patients (12,13). Successful prophylaxis of this opportunistic infection would reduce morbidity significantly.

STUDY OBJECTIVE

This retrospective study reviews the results of patients put on a clarithromycin regimen for prophylaxis of MAC disease.

METHODS

Charts were reviewed for
1. Date clarithromycin was started
2. Approximate CD4 lymphocyte count at the time prophylaxis was started
3. Length of time the patients remained disease-free
4. Patients discontinued owing to side effects

Exclusions included

1. Patients treated for active MAC disease before being placed on a prophylaxis regimen
2. Patients taking clarithromycin and clofazamine

RESULTS

A total of 14 patients were found who had received clarithromycin for MAC prophylaxis without having been treated for active MAC disease. The clarithromycin dosage was 500 mg bid in all but 2 patients, who preferred to take 500 mg qd.

Of these 14 patients, none discontinued clarithromycin because of intolerable side effects, although one patient did complain of some GI distress.

The average CD4 lymphocyte count at onset of prophylaxis was 77, with a range of 3–241. The average disease-free interval was 8.14 months, with an average of 8.5 months in those still alive. None of the patients in the study developed MAC disease while receiving clarithromycin.

CONCLUSION

Although this is a small retrospective study and many patients died of other complications, it did appear that clarithromycin kept the patients in this small group free from MAC disease and the gradual debilitation it causes.

Clarithromycin is generally well tolerated and seems to be quite effective in preventing MAC disease in severely immunocompromised patients. It should be considered a good potential agent for MAC prophylaxis.

REFERENCES

1. Hawkins CC, Gold JWM, Whimbey E, Kiehn TE, Brannon P, Cammarata R, Brown AE, Armstrong D. *Mycobacterium avium* complex infections in patients with the acquired immunodeficiency syndrome. Ann Intern Med 1986; 105:184–188.

2. Hoy J, Mijch A, Sandland M, et al. Quadruple-drug therapy for *Mycobacterium avium–intracellulare* bacteremia in AIDS patients. J Infect Dis 1990; 161:801–805.

3. Bessesen MT, Berry CD, Johnson MA, Klaus B, Blaser MJ, Ellison RT. Site of origin of disseminated MAC infection in AIDS [abstract]. In: Program and Abstracts of the 30th Interscience Conference on Antimicrobial Agents and Chemotherapy, Atlanta, Georgia, October 21–24, 1990. Washington, DC: American Society of Microbiology, 1990:297.

4. Whimbey E, Kiehn TE, Armstrong D. Disseminated *Mycobacterium avium–intracellulare* disease: diagnosis and therapy. Curr Clin Top Infect Dis 1986; 7:112–133.

5. Horsburgh CR, Selik RM. The epidemiology of disseminated nontuberculous mycobacterial infection in the acquired immunodeficiency syndrome (AIDS). Am Rev Respir Dis 1989; 139:4–7.

6. Horsburgh CR, Havlik JA, Thompson SE. Survival of AIDS patients with disseminated *Mycobacterium avium* complex (DMAC): a case–control study. 5th International Conference on AIDS, San Francisco, CA, 1990: abstr Th.B. 516.

7. Benson CA, Pottage JC Jr, Kessler HA. Treatment of AIDS-related disseminated *Mycobacterium avium* complex disease (D-MAC) with a multiple drug regimen including amikacin. 6th International Conference on AIDS, San Francisco, CA June 1990: Th.B. 517.

8. Chiu J, Nussbaum J, Bozzette S, et al. Treatment of disseminated *Mycobacterium avium* complex infection in AIDS with amikacin, ethambutol, rifampin and ciprofloxacin. Ann Intern Med 1990; 113:358–361.

9. Metroka C. Prophylaxis for *Pneumocystis carinii* pneumonia and other opportunistic infections. AIDS Target Inf News 1990; 4(6):1–2.

10. Benson C, Kerns E, Sha B, et al. Relationship of respiratory and GI tract colonization with *Mycobacterium avium* complex (MAC) to disseminated MAC disease in HIV-infected patients. 6th International Conference on AIDS, San Francisco, CA, June 1990: Th.B. 514.

11. Gikas A, Perrone C, Truffot C, et al. Inhibition of *Mycobacterium avium–intracellular* (MAIC) by antimicrobials in human macrophages. Abstracts of the 29th Interscience Conference on Antimicrobial Agents Chemotherapy, Houston, TX. September, 1989: abstr 885A.

12. Dautzenberg B, Legris S, Truffot C, Grosset J. Double blind study of efficacy of clarithromycin versus placebo in *Mycobacterium avium–intracellulare* infection in AIDS patients. Abstracts of the 1990 World Conference on Lung Health, Boston, MA, 1990. J Am Thorac Soc 1990; 141:A615.

13. Data on file, Abbott Laboratories, Abbott Park, IL.

Combined Therapy with Roxithromycin and Co-trimoxazole in Lyme Disease

R. Gasser, I. Wendelin, E. Reisinger, J. Berglöff, B. Feigl,
I. Schafhalter, B. Eber, M. Grisold, and W. Klein

Medizinische Universitätsklinik
Graz, Austria

INTRODUCTION

Lyme disease is due to a complex systemic infection with the spirochete *Borrelia burgdorferi*. It is a potentially lethal disorder, especially when the cardiac or central nervous systems are involved. The literature clearly evidences major therapeutic problems, particularly in later stages of the disease. In vitro, azithromycin, clarithromycin, erythromycin, and roxithromycin have shown excellent efficacy against *B. burgdorferi* (1,2). In vivo studies have shown dissenting results on oral macrolides in the treatment of early Lyme disease (2–5).

Late stages of spirochetal infection are more complex and difficult to treat. Both in late syphilis and chronic Lyme disease the gold standard treatment with IV penicillin or cephalosporins has shown a failure rate of 20–60% (3). Oral macrolides have not been recommended for the treatment of *late* manifestations of Lyme disease (3,4).

COMBINED THERAPY WITH ROXITHROMYCIN AND CO-TRIMOXAZOLE OF *BORRELIA BURGDORFERI* INFECTION

Despite negative reports on oral roxithromycin (RX) even in early Lyme disease, we showed that a combination of roxithromycin and co-trimoxazole (CT) was successful in treating chronic Lyme disease in a patient who did not respond to

IV penicillin and IV ceftriaxone (6). These results were confirmed by similar findings of Pedersen and Friis-Möller (7), as well as by Bózsik et al. (8), ourselves and Dr. Drulle (personal communication, 1993).

On one hand, it has clearly been shown that RX alone is completely ineffective in vivo, even in early stages of Lyme disease (5). On the other hand, *B. burgdorferi* is known for its poor susceptibility to CT, the latter being sometimes used to keep borrelia cultures free from contamination. Thus, the mechanism underlying the synergism between RX and CT is of considerable interest. However, it has not yet been elucidated (11).

Here, we present data on the in vitro and in vivo efficacy of a combination of roxithromycin and co-trimoxazole against *B. burgdorferi*.

METHODS

In Vitro Study

The checkerboard technique was performed as a macrodilution broth method in 24-well tissue culture clusters (Costar, Cambridge, MA). Roxithromycin was obtained from Roussell Uclaf (Paris, France) and sulfamethoxazole and trimethoprim from Hoffmann-La Roche (Basel, Switzerland). Sulfamethoxazole and trimethoprim were mixed 5:1 (co-trimoxazole). The inoculum used was a 4-day old culture of *B. burgdorferi* strain B31 (type strain ATCC 35210) in modified Barbour–Stoenner–Kelly medium (BSK II), with a cell density of approximately 10 /ml. Antibiotics were diluted 1:2, thus obtaining a dilution for RX from 2 to 0.004 μg/ml and for CT 256, 4 μg/ml. Plates were incubated at 36°C after preparation with BSK II medium, antibiotics and *B. burgdorferi* inoculum. On day 4 the number of motile borrelia were counted (resolution 400×; volume 10 μl, covered with 18 × 18-mm glass; 20 fields per well). Subcultures were grown in fresh BSK II medium and controlled weekly for 21 days.

The minimal inhibitory concentration (MIC) was defined as the lowest antimicrobial concentration of each drug—single or in combination—with fewer than or equal to 5×10^5 motile borrelia per milliliter. The minimal bactericidal concentration (MBC) was defined as the lowest antimicrobial concentration of each drug—single or in combination—that completely inhibited growth in the subcultures. For each experiment $n = 4$.

In Vivo Study

Of 105 patients who have been referred to our specific clinic for *B. burgdorferi*-associated disorders within 1 year, 68 exhibited clinically documented borreliosis. Patients who had objective evidence of late Lyme borreliosis were offered admission to this open, noncomparative, pilot trial. After explaining to them

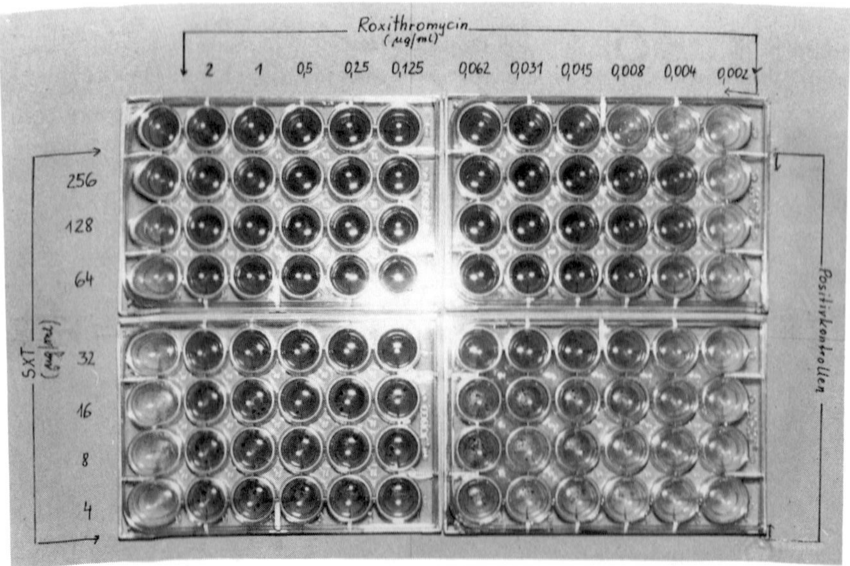

Figure 1   Typical experiment with *B. burgdorferi* in a modified BSK II medium. SxT stands for co-trimoxazole, concentrations are given in micrograms per milliliter (µg/ml); on the right, last row shows positive controls. Dark color, no living borrelia; slightly dark, reduced metabolism and reduced motility; bright color, metabolically active borrelia.

risks and possible side effects, especially because of the high doses used, 18 patients agreed to participate in the study; one of those, however, did not return to our clinic after having agreed to participate.

All patients had involvement of at least two organ systems, as seen in typical stage II/III Lyme disease. Other disorders that can produce similar symptoms had to be excluded. The patients received RX (300 mg bid po) and CT (trim./sulf. 120/600 mg bid po) over 5 weeks. Patients were seen before, directly at the end of treatment, and 3 and 6 months, as well as 1 year after treatment was completed.

RESULTS

In Vitro Study

MIC

In vitro we found an excellent efficacy of RX against *B. burgdorferi* (MIC, 0.031 µg/ml); activity was seen for CT. However, the combination of both antibiotics

Table 1 Typical Experiment[a]

RX (μg/ml)	2	1	0.5	0.25	0.125	pc	0.062	0.031	0.015	0.008	0.004	0
CT (μg/ml)												
256	0	0	0	0	0	>200	0	0	**2**	*20*	*150*	*>200*
128	0	0	0	0	0	>200	0	0	**2**	*150*	*200*	*>200*
64	0	0	0	0	0	>200	0	0	**3**	*150*	*200*	*>200*
32	0	0	0	0	0	>200	0	0	**10**	*100*	*150*	*>200*
16	0	0	0	0	0	>200	0	0	**10**	*80*	*200*	*>200*
8	0	0	0	0	0	>200	0	*1*	**10**	*50*	*200*	*>200*
4	0	0	0	0	0	>200	0	**1**	*20*	*100*	*>200*	*>200*
0	0	0	0	0	0	>200	0	**1**	*40*	*100*	*>200*	*>200*

[a]Number of motile borrelia per field (day 4); MIC $\leq$ 10 (= 5×10^5 cells per ml); italics, *B. burgdorferi* with reduced motility; bold, MIC. MIC for roxithromycin decreased by 1 titer at concentrations of CT from 256 to 8 μg/μl when MIC is determined as less than or equal 5×10^5 borrelia per milliliter. pc, positive controls for viability; contains no antibiotic.

Table 2 Subcultures (day 21) from Foregoing Experiment[a]

RX (µg/ml)	2	1	0.5	0.25	0.125	pc	0.062	0.031	0.015	0.008	0.004	0
CT (µg/ml)												
256	0	0	0	0	0	>200	**0**	20	200	>200	>200	>200
128	0	0	0	0	**0**	>200	1	80	200	>200	>200	>200
64	0	0	0	0	**0**	>200	2	30	200	>200	>200	>200
32	0	0	0	0	**0**	>200	2	30	200	>200	>200	>200
16	0	0	0	0	**0**	>200	1	80	>200	>200	>200	>200
8	0	0	0	0	**0**	>200	1	30	>200	>200	>200	>200
4	0	0	0	0	**0**	>200	1	40	>200	>200	>200	>200
0	0	0	0	**0**	5	>200	70	100	150	>200	>200	>200

[a]Number of motile borrelia per field. Italics, *B. burgdorferi* with reduced motility; bold, MBC; MBC, lowest antimicrobial concentration that completely inhibited growth in the subcultures. MBC on day 21 of RX alone was 0.25, in combination with CT, MBC of RX was 0.125 even at very low concentrations of CT, thus being decreased by one titer. Motility markedly reduced at very low concentrations of ROX and CT. pc, positive controls for viability; contains no antibiotic.

led to a minor synergistic effect, decreasing the MIC for roxithromycin by 1 titer at concentrations of CT from 256 to 8 μg/μl, when MIC is determined as less than or equal 5×10^5 borrelia per milliliter, which equals ten motile borrelia per field. In addition, a clearly reduced growth of microorganisms was seen at concentrations of RX as low as 0.015 μg/ml in combination with 256–4 μg/ml CT, when compared with the positive controls (Table 1). However, the motility of *B. burgdorferi* was markedly reduced even at very low concentrations when the two drugs were combined: In Table 1 reduced motility is indicated by an italic number for motile borrelia. It can be seen that in the presence of RX without CT there is no reduced motility of *B. burgdorferi*.

MBC

The MBC was defined as the lowest antimicrobial concentration that completely inhibited growth in the subcultures. It can be seen that the MBC on day 21 of RX alone was 0.25, in combination with CT, the MBC of RX was 0.062 at higher CT concentrations and was still one titer lower even at very low concentrations of CT (Table 2). Noteworthy is that motility was extremely reduced in subcultures at RX concentrations of 0.031 when combined with CT and still was slow in many borrelia at 0.015, although the number of motile borrelia was more than 10^7. In RX without CT, motility was normal at concentrations of 0.031 and 0.015 μg/ml (see Table 2).

In Vivo Study

In the present nonrandomized, open, prospective pilot study, we found that of 17 patients with clinically documented late Lyme borreliosis (stage II/III) who were treated with combined roxithromycin (RX; 300 mg bid) and co-trimoxazole (CT; 120/600 mg bid), 13 (76%) recovered completely and 4 continued to have symptoms. These 4 patients received IV penicillin G (3×10 million IU/day) over 18 days. Two of these patients recovered, and 2 continued to show persistent symptoms after 1 year follow-up. In these latter 2 patients, a further treatment with IV ceftriaxone (2 g bid) also failed. The success rate seen under the combination of RX and CT is similar to the rate reported on IV penicillin and ceftriaxone in the literature (3,4,12). Adverse effects were minor: two patients developed mild, reversible leukopenia at the end of treatment when treated with RX/CT. Two patients had a transient, reversible rise in GOT and GPT. Three patients noticed mild gastrointestinal symptoms within the first few days. None of these effects required interruption of therapy.

DISCUSSION

Oral treatment for late Lyme borreliosis would most certainly be desirable for two reasons: administration would be easy and hospitalization avoided. This would be of major importance, especially in countries where facilities for IV treatment either inhospital or with appropriate home care are not available. In late Lyme disease oral treatment has not been recommended because of the high failure rate reported (3,4,11).

Oral treatment with roxithromycin alone seemingly has not brought about the results expected, as reported by Hansen et al. (5). However, this is the only report on failure of treatment with oral macrolides in early Lyme disease. There are other reports in the literature of excellent results with RX, azithromycin, clarithromycin, and erythromycin (1–3). Possibly the dose as well as the duration of treatment were not sufficient in Hansen's study.

The form of synergy and the reason for the observed in vivo effectiveness of the combined treatment with RX and CT are not entirely clear. The observation that the combination of RX and CT largely reduced the motility of surviving borrelia in vitro could be of interest in this context. Sadziene et al. suggested that the motility of *B. burgdorferi* could play a key role in the invasion of the spirochete in human tissues (13,14). This observation derived from observations on a flagellaless, nonpathogenic mutant of *B. burgdorferi* that was unable to penetrate layers of endothelial cells. Furthermore, less motile borrelia will be more accessible to the host immune system. That a combination of CT with RX is able to reduce the MIC and MBC by one titer step, has already been shown for the macrolide clarithromycin combined with CT in the treatment of *Pneumocystis carinii* infection in rats (15). It is also noteworthy that therapeutic concentrations of roxithromycin enhance the phagocytosis and killing activity of human neutrophils (PMN), and induce a significant increase in PMN chemotaxis, oxidative metabolism, and phagocytic killing ex vivo (16).

In summary, oral treatment of early Lyme borreliosis is effective in many cases, whereas later stages are treated effectively with oral antibiotics. However, the combined use of macrolides with CT has shown promising results that have been consolidated by our laboratory findings in *B. burgdorferi* strain B31.

ACKNOWLEDGMENT

We thank Prof. G. Stanek, Vienna for providing *Borrelia burgdorferi* strain B31.

REFERENCES

1. Kirst HA, Sides GD. New directions for macrolide antibiotics: pharmacokinetics and clinical efficacy. Antimicrob Agents Chemother 1989; 33:1419–1422.
2. Johnson RC, Kodner C, Russel M, Girard D. In vitro and in vivo susceptibility of *Borrelia burgdorferi* to azithromycin. J Antimicrob Chemother 1990; 25(suppl A):33–38.

3. Sigal LH. Current recommendations for the treatment of Lyme disease. Drugs 1992; 43:683–699.

4. Gasser R, Reisinger E, Feigl B, Pongratz S, Grisold M, Klein W. Current views on antimicrobial treatment of Lyme disease. Consent of the Vth International Conference on Lyme Borreliosis. Lyme Dis Update 1992; 11:1–3.

5. Hansen K, Hovmark A, Lebech AM, Lebech K, Olsson I, Sorensen L. Roxithromycin in Lyme borreliosis: discrepant results of an in-vitro and in-vivo animal susceptibility study and a clinical trial in patients with erythema migrans. Acta Derm Venerol 1992; 72:297–300.

6. Gasser R, Dusleag J. Oral treatment of late Lyme borreliosis with roxithromycin plus co-trimoxazole. Lancet 1990; 336:1189–1190.

7. Pedersen LM, Friis-Möller A. Late treatment of chronic Lyme arthritis. Lancet 1991; 337:241.

8. Bózsik BP, Timmer M, Esztro K. Combined antibiotic treatment of Lyme borreliosis. Vth International Conference on Lyme Borreliosis, Arlington, 1992:abstr A12.

9. Fruhwald FM, Gasser R, Dusleag J, Feigl B, Pongratz S, Klein W. Reversal of dilated cardiomyopathy by long-term oral roxithromycin in a patient with late Lyme-borreliosis. Int J Angiol 1993; (in press).

10. Gasser R, Dusleag J, Reisinger E, Stauber R, Grisold M, Pongratz S, Furian C, Feigl B, Klein W. A most unusual case of a whole family suffering from late Lyme borreliosis for over 20 years. Angiology 1993; (in press).

11. Gasser R, Dusleag J, Klein W. Oral treatment of early and late Lyme borreliosis. Lyme Dis Update; 1992; 6:1–3.

12. Dattwyler RJ, Halperin JJ, Volkman DJ, Luft BJ. Treatment of late Lyme borreliosis—randomized comparison of ceftriaxone and penicillin. Lancet 1988; 1:1191–1194.

13. Sadziene A, Thomas DD, Bundoc VG, Holt SC, Barbour AG. A flagella-less mutant of *Borrelia burgdorferi*. Structural, molecular and in vitro functional characterization. J Clin Invest 1991; 88:82–92.

14. Ma Y, Sturnock A, Weis JJ. Intracellular location of *Borrelia burgdorferi* within human endothelial cells. Infect Immun 1991; 59:671–678.

15. Alder J, Mitten M, Hernandez L, Clement J. Synergy between clarithromycin and sulfomethoxazole in the treatment of *Pneumocystis carinii* in rats. First International Conference on the Macrolides, Azalides and Streptogramins. Santa Fe, NM, 1992: abstr 40.

16. Labro MT, El Benna J, Barre J. Effect of roxithromycin and erythromycin on human neutrophil function in vivo. First International Conference on the Macrolides, Azalides and Streptogramins. Santa Fe, NM, 1992: abstr 39.

Macrolides in Prophylaxis for Endocarditis

R. Rahn, H. J. Linde, C. Riffel, C. Dornauf, and P. M. Shah
Universitätsklinik Frankfurt am Main
Frankfurt, Germany

INTRODUCTION

Bacterial endocarditis still remains a serious disease, with significant morbidity and mortality. In patients with known valvular heart disease, most cases are caused by oral viridans streptococci (2). Transient bacteremia with viridans streptococci can occur during dental treatment, such as dental extraction or subgingival scaling. The incidence of these bacteremias depends on factors, such as oral hygiene and the kind of treatment, and may rise to 90% (5–8). High-risk conditions that provoke endocarditis following bacteremias include previous history of infective endocarditis and prosthetic heart valves. As bacteremias of oral origin cannot totally be prevented, prophylaxis of endocarditis during dental procedures in patients with known valvular heart disease should be aimed at reducing the number of bacteria entering the blood stream and eliminating those that do invade. The prevention of bacterial endocarditis following dental surgery in susceptible patients is usually attempted with antibiotics. Any antibiotic used must be highly active against oral viridans streptococci. It must also be present in the blood in adequate concentrations throughout the bacteremic period. As it is not practical for the dentist to give parenteral antibiotics, oral antibiotics are usually given for most routine procedures. Penicillin V is recommended in such settings, and for patients allergic to penicillin, clindamycin or erythromycin is an alternative (1,2). Erythromycin is highly active against viridans streptococci and most oral microorganisms, but has a great variability in absorption (3).

The present study was undertaken to compare a new macrolide—roxithromycin—with erythromycin in reducing the bacteremia incidence after dental procedures. Erythromycin and roxithromycin have different pharmacokinetic profiles. Roxithromycin has higher serum concentrations and a longer elimination half-life (3,4).

METHODS

In a randomized, controlled study, erythromycin (ethylsuccinate, 1g) or roxithromycin (150 mg) or no drug (control group) were given 1 h before a dental procedure with a projected high incidence of bacteremia (dental extraction or intraligamentary injection). A total of 150 healthy adults were enrolled, 50 in each group. The antibiotics were administered, under supervision, 1 h before the dental treatment.

Blood cultures were collected 3, 6, and 9 min after extraction or intraligamentary injection. Five milliliters of blood was added directly to each aerobic and anaerobic blood culture bottle (BACTEC 6 A and 7 A). All bottles were subcultured, the microorganisms were identified by published methods.

RESULTS

Incidence of Bacteremia Caused By Aerobes and Anaerobes

Both antibiotics reduced the incidence of bacteremia following dental procedures (Table 1). Dental organisms, either aerobes or anaerobes, or both, were isolated from the blood of 29 of the 50 control patients (58%), 4 of the 50 erythromycin-treated patients (8%), and 4 of the 50 roxithromycin-treated patients (8%).

The difference between the numbers of bacteremias in the control group compared with the two antibiotic groups was highly significant (χ^2 test, $p = 0.001$).

Incidence of Streptococcal Bacteremia

Streptococci were isolated from the blood cultures of 21 of the 50 control patients (42%), none of the 50 erythromycin-treated patients, and none of the 50 roxithromycin-treated patients.

Table 1 Incidence of Bacteremia Following Dental Procedures ($N = 150$)

	Erythromycin	Roxithromycin	Control
Total	4/50	4/50	29/50
Aerobes (excluding viridans streptococci)	4/50	3/50	27/50
Anaerobes	0/50	1/50	11/50
Viridans streptococci	0/50	0/50	21/50

Incidence of Aerobic Bacteremia

Aerobes—nonstreptococcal—were isolated from blood cultures of 27 of the 50 from the control group (54%), 4 of the 50 erythromycin-treated patients (8%), and 3 of the 50 roxithromycin-treated patients (6%).

Incidence of Anaerobic Bacteremia

Anerobes were isolated from blood cultures of 11 of 50 from the control group (22%), none of the 50 erythromycin-treated patients, and 1 of the 50 roxithromycin-treated patients (2%).

DISCUSSION

For the prevention of bacterial endocarditis following dental procedures, penicillin is recommended in the Federal Republic of Germany. For penicillin-allergic patients, erythromycin is an alternative agent. In the present study bacteremia was detected in 29 of 50 control patients and in 4 out of 50 patients receiving erythromycin 1 g or roxithromycin 150 mg 1 h before a dental procedure. The viridans streptococci were found in 21 of the control patients and in none of the erythromycin- or roxithromycin-treated patients. Roxithromycin at 150 mg is as effective as erythromycin 1 g for the prevention of transient bacteremia following dental procedures.

CONCLUSION

Roxithromycin seems to be a promising alternative agent for endocarditis prophylaxis during dental surgery, especially in patients with allergy to penicillin.

REFERENCES

1. Baltch A, Pressman HL, Hammer CM, Sutphen NC, Smith RP, Shayegani M. Bacteremia following dental extractions in patients with and without penicillin prophylaxis. Am J Med Sci 1982; 283:129–140.
2. Glauser MP, Francioli P. Successful prophylaxis against experimental streptococcal endocarditis with bacteriostatic antibiotics. J Infect Dis 1982; 146:806–810.
3. Nilsen OG. Comparative pharmacokinetics in macrolides. J Antimicrob Chemother 1987; 20:81–88.
4. Puri, SK, Lassman HB. Roxithromycin: a pharmacokinetic review of a macrolide. J Antimicrob Chemother 1987; 20:89–100.
5. Rahn R, Shah PM, Schäfer V, Frenkel G, Halbherr K. Bakteriämie nach Zahnentfernung—Einfluß verschiedener Faktoren. Zahnärztl Welt 1986; 95:822–826.

6. Rahn R, Frenkel G, Atamni F, Shah PM, Schäfer V. Bakteriämie nach intradesmodontaler Anästhesie. Schweiz Monatsschr Zahnmed 1987; 97:859–863.

7. Rahn R, Shah PM, Schäfer V, Frenkel G, Seibold K. Bakteriämie nach chirurgisch-endodontischen Eingriffen. Zahnärztl Welt 1987, 96:903–907.

8. Rahn R, Shah PM, Schäfer V, Muggenthaler F, Frenkel G, Knothe H. Orale Endokarditis-Prophylaxe bei zahnärztlich-chirurgischen Eingriffen. Schweiz Monatsschr Zahnmed 1986; 98:478–481.

Lansoprazole Plus Roxithromycin and Metronidazole for Eradication of *Helicobacter pylori:* Results of a Pilot Study

A. Burette

Nouvelle Clinique de la Basilique
Brussels, Belgium

Y. Glupczynski and C. Deprez

Brugmann University Hospital
Brussels, Belgium

D. Jacobs

Roussel-Uclaf
Brussels, Belgium

BACKGROUND

The currently accepted standard triple therapy (bismuth–metronidazole–amoxicillin or tetracycline) eradicates *Helicobacter pylori* in 80–90% of the treated patients (1), but is accompanied by side effects in 20–30% of them. To diminish the side effects rate while maintaining a high eradication rate, a new triple therapy using a proton pump inhibitor and a macrolide in combination with metronidazole was tested.

AIM OF THE STUDY

The study's aim was to assess the efficacy of a triple-drug therapy, including lansoprazole, roxithromycin, and metronidazole for eradication of *H. pylori* in patients with duodenal ulcer.

METHODS

Study Design

The study was an open, noncomparative, pilot study performed in one center.

Drug Regimen

All patients received the same triple therapy consisting of:

Lansoprazole, 30 mg once a day (od), for 4 weeks
Roxithromycin, 300 mg once a day (od), for the first 2 weeks
Metronidazole, 500 mg twice a day (bid), for the first 10 days

Patients

The inclusion criteria were as follows:

Active duodenal ulcer patients
Older than 18 years of age
Male or nonlactating, nonpregnant female patients
Helicobacter pylori-positive by histology and culture
Voluntary oral witnessed or written informed consent

Standard exclusion criteria were used with a 1-month washout period for specific *H. pylori* treatment.

Diagnostic Methods

The following endoscopic biopsies were taken at pretreatment visit and at follow-up visit, 4–6 weeks after treatment:

At least four antral biopsies (two or more for histological examination, one for culture, one for rapid urease test at endoscopy)
At least three corporeal (body) biopsies (two or more for histological examination, one for culture)

Histological examination of biopsies included

All biopsies reviewed by one experienced pathologist (CD)
Hematoxylin–eosin plus Giemsa stain
Histological assessment of gastritis and intensity of *H. pylori* colonization according to the Sydney system (2)

For *Helicobacter pylori* culture and susceptibility testing biopsies were cultured according to standard procedures (selective blood agar incubated at 37°C for 3–7 days under humid, atmospheric conditions). Susceptibility testing to roxithromycin and metronidazole were performed by disk diffusion and MIC agar dilution technique. Organisms with MIC $\geq$ 2 μg/ml for roxithromycin or MIC $\geq$ 8 μg/ml for metronidazole were considered resistant.

The sensitivity and specificity of the diagnostic methods used for *H. pylori* assessment were as follows: biopsy urease test, sensitivity 89%, specificity 98%; histology (H&E + Giemsa), sensitivity 91%, specificity 98%; culture, sensitivity 95%, specificity 100%.

Compliance with Study Drug Regimen

Compliance was verified by counting the number of tablets or capsules remaining in the bottles, recording the date that the last dose was taken, and questioning the patient about any discrepancies. Patients were considered compliant if they had taken 90% or more of the prescribed treatment.

Study Procedures

A full clinical examination and an endoscopy with biopsies collection were performed within 72 h before treatment. Four to six weeks posttreatment, a control endoscopy with biopsies was done. At least 3 months posttreatment, the eradication of *H. pylori* was confirmed by a [^{14}C] urea breath test.

RESULTS

Disposition of Patients

Twenty-two patients were enrolled. Two patients were excluded from analysis (one patient for noncompliance to study drug regimen; one patient was lost to follow-up). Twenty patients were evaluable for efficacy analysis (15M/5F; mean age 46 years). All of these patients were considered compliant with the study drug regimen.

Susceptibility of *Helicobacter pylori* to Roxithromycin and Metronidazole

Resistance to roxithromycin did not occur in any of the strains either before, or after failed eradication. Initial (pretreatment) resistance to metronidazole occurred in 3 of 20 strains. Development of resistance to metronidazole after treatment occurred in 3 of 17 strains.

Eradication of *Helicobacter pylori*

Sixteen of the 20 evaluable patients (80%) became *H. pylori*-negative 4 weeks posttreatment; *H. pylori* was eradicated in two of three patients with strains resistant to metronidazole.

Duodenal Ulcer Healing

Healing of duodenal ulcer was observed in all patients 4–6 weeks posttherapy, except for one patient with linear duodenal ulcer and failed eradication.

Long-Term Results

Up to now, 15 patients with eradication of the organism at 4–6 weeks after treatment were available for further examination by endoscopy or [^{14}C]urea breath test at least 3 months after treatment. All except one (with persistent slight active antral gastritis 4 weeks after therapy) remained free of *H. pylori*.

Adverse Events

No patient discontinued treatment because of adverse events. Three patients reported minor adverse events possibly related to the study drugs (one cutaneous eruption; one transient GOT/GPT increase in a patient with an ongoing history of gallstones; one nausea).

CONCLUSIONS

Lansoprazole, 30 mg od, for 4 weeks plus roxithromycin, 300 mg od, for 2 weeks and metronidazole, 500 mg bid, for 10 days eradicated *H. pylori* in 80% (16 of 20) of all evaluable patients 4–6 weeks after treatment, and up to now, 93% of them (14 of 15) remained free of *H. pylori* at least 3 months after treatment.

Resistance to roxithromycin did not occur before therapy or after failed eradication. Pre- or posttreatment resistance to metronidazole was documented in all treatment failures. *Helicobacter pylori* was eradicated in two of three patients with strains that had primary resistance to metronidazole. Duodenal ulcer was healed in all patients, except one (95%), 4–6 weeks after treatment. The drug regimen tested was well tolerated and resulted in a high compliance rate.

REFERENCES

1. Chiba N, et al. Am J Gastroenterol 1992; 87:1716–1727.
2. Misiewicz JJ, et al. In: Working Party Reports of the World Congresses of Gastroenterology. Melbourne: Blackwell Scientific Publications, 1990:1–10.

The Effect of Azithromycin Given as a Single Oral Dose of 1 Gram in Men and Women with Uncomplicated Gonorrhea: A Retrospective Comparison Between Capsules and Tablets

A. Okkerse, R. L. P. Lijnen, and E. Stolz

Academic Hospital Rotterdam-Dijkzigt
Rotterdam, The Netherlands

E. Prooy

Pfizer B.V.
Capelle a/d IJssel, The Netherlands

INTRODUCTION

Azithromycin is a new azalide antibiotic. A single high dose of this drug is effective against uncomplicated gonococcal infections (1–3). A single 1-g dose is as effective as doxycycline (100 mg given orally twice daily for 7 days) for the treatment of chlamydial infections (4). In vitro, it has good activity against *Ureaplasma urealyticum* (5). We evaluated the efficacy and tolerance of azithromycin given as a single 1-g dose to men and women with uncomplicated gonorrhea. Azithromycin was given orally in two different forms. One group of 33 patients received 4 × 250-mg capsules. The other group of 53 patients received 2 × 500-mg tablets. The study is still ongoing with the latter form.

Treatment with capsules had a cure rate of 93%, but was less effective compared with tablets, which had a cure rate of 98%.

MATERIALS AND METHODS

We recruited 99 patients with either a positive gonococcal culture or gram-negative diplococci in their smear. Only those subsequently determined to have a positive gonococcal culture were evaluated. Urethral, rectal, pharyngeal, and cervical samples were taken for culture of *Neisseria gonorrhoeae*, *Chlamydia trachomatis*, *Mycoplasma hominis*, and *Ureaplasma urealyticum*.

Samples for culture were taken at the baseline visit, and 1 week and 4 weeks after therapy. Laboratory tests (hematological, biochemical, urine analysis, and syphilis serology) were also conducted. Patients were instructed to abstain from sexual intercourse for the time of the study. Bacteriological response was classified as elimination (*N. gonorrhoeae* absent posttreatment), persistent (*N. gonorrhoeae* present posttreatment), and indeterminate (unevaluable or reinfection possible). All adverse events were carefully assessed and recorded.

RESULTS

A total of 99 patients were treated. Thirteen patients were not evaluated for various reasons: 11 lost to follow-up, 1 vomited her capsules, and 1 could not swallow the capsules. We evaluated 86 patients (75 men and 11 women); 33 patients had received capsules and 53 patients had received tablets. Gonococcal infection persisted in 2 patients treated with capsules (elimination rate = 93%) and in 1 patient treated with tablets (elimination rate = 98%). One patient treated with capsules and 2 patients treated with tablets became reinfected (Table 1). Concomitant chlamydial infections were all cured (9/9). Four patients were infected with a third pathogen. The outcome of all mixed infections, including

Table 1 Elimination of *N. gonorrhoeae* from Different Sites (Capsule and Tablet Trial Separately), Results from all Evaluable Male and Female Patients

	Urethra		Cervix		Rectum		Pharynx	
	Capsule	Tablet	Capsule	Tablet	Capsule	Tablet	Capsule	Tablet
Elimination	29 (90%)	42 (98%)	2	7	4	6	2	2
Persistence	2	1	—	—	—	—	—	—
Indeterminate	1[a]	2[b]	—	—	—	—	—	—

[a]First visit positive culture for *N.gonorrhoeae* and a negative culture for chlamydia. Second visit negative culture for *N. gonorrhoeae*, positive smear for gram-negative diplococci and positive culture for chlamydia.

[b]In one case there was eradication after 1 week; 2 weeks later a new infection with the same strain. In the second case there was reinfection resulting from sexual intercourse with untreated partner.

Table 2 Cure of Mixed Infections with a Single Dose of 1 g Azithromycin (Capsule and Tablet Separately)

Baseline pathogens	Capsules cured	Tablets cured
N. gonorrhoeae + *C. trachomatis*	2	3
N. gonorrhoeae + *C. trachomatis* + *U. urealyticum*	1	2
N. gonorrhoeae + *U. urealyticum*	3	5 (4 cured)
N. gonorrhoeae + *C. trachomatis* + *M. hominis*	—	1

those with *U. urealyticum* and *M. hominis*, is shown in Table 2. Postgonococcal urethritis was observed more often after treatment with capsules (6/30) than after treatment with tablets (2/50). Adverse events were all mild, but were more frequently observed in the group treated with tablets (Table 3). The mean MICs for *N. gonorrhoeae* were 0.20 μg/ml in the tablet group and 0.18 μg/ml in the capsule group (range for both groups; 0.06–0.25 μg/ml).

DISCUSSION

It is generally accepted that the ideal treatment for gonorrhea is a single dose of antibiotic, which is safe and will cure chlamydial infections simultaneously. Azithromycin is a new antibiotic that belongs to the group of azalides (15-membered lactone ring), a subclass of the macrolides (16-membered ring). The

Table 3 Adverse Events in Patients After a Single Dose of 1 g Azithromycin in Capsules or Tablets

Adverse events	Capsules (no. of patients)	Tablets (no. of patients)
Diarrhea	10	11
Gastrodynia	—	3
Dyspepsia	—	2
Abdominal pain	—	1
Nausea	—	2
Vomiting	1	—
Exanthema	—	1
Dizziness	1	2
Pollakiuria	—	1

pharmacokinetic profile is characterized by low serum levels and sustained, high tissue levels (6,7). In a Phase I bioequivalence study in which 250-mg capsules were compared with 500-mg tablets, it was not possible to confirm the bioequivalence of both dosage forms (mean AUC 0–96 μg h^{-1} ml^{-1}) values 4.45 (2 × 250-mg capsule) and 5.20 (1 × 500-mg tablet) (unpublished data). In vitro, azithromycin is effective against *U. urealyticum* (5). In a controlled trial a single 1-g dose was as effective as a 7-day course of doxycycline for the treatment of uncomplicated chlamydial infection (4). Treatment of gonorrheal infections with a single 1-g dose of azithromycin (capsules) had a cure rate of 96% (2,3). To date in our study, in which a single 1-g dose was used, we have achieved successful cure rates of 93% using capsules (4 × 250 mg) and 98% using tablets (2 × 500 mg). Adverse events were mild. All concomitant chlamydial infections were cured as well.

From the results we conclude that further investigations into the usefulness of azithromycin to treat uncomplicated gonorrheal infections would be justified.

REFERENCES

1. Handsfield HH, Siegal NA, Verdon MS. Single-dose azithromycin vs ceftriaxone for the treatment of uncomplicated gonorrhea. 28th Interscience Conference on Antimicrobial Agents and Chemotherapy, Chicago, IL. Washington, DC: American Society for Microbiology, 1991:abstr 79.
2. Waugh M. Open study of the safety and efficacy of a single oral dose of azithromycin for the treatment of uncomplicated gonorrhea in men and women. J Antimicrob Chemother 1993; 31(suppl E):193–198.
3. Steingrimsson O, Olafsson JH, et al. Single dose azithromycin treatment of gonorrhea and infections caused by *C. trachomatis* and *U. urealyticum* in men. Sexually Transmitted Dis 1994; 21:43–46.
4. Martin DH, Mroczkowski TF, Dalu ZA. A controlled trial of a single dose of azithromycin for the treatment of chlamydial urethritis and cervicitis. N Engl J Med 1992; 327:921–925.
5. Ryan RW, Kwasnik I, Tilton RC. In vitro activity of the macrolide CP 62993-XZ450 against selected microorganisms. 26th Interscience Conference on Antimicrobial Agents and Chemotherapy, New Orleans. Washington, DC: American Society for Microbiology, 1986:267.
6. Krohn K. Gynaecological tissue levels of azithromycin. Eur J Clin Microbiol Infect Dis 1991; 10:864–871.
7. Foulds G, Shepard RM, Johnson RB. The pharmacokinetics of azithromycin in human serum and tissues. J Antimicrobial Chemother 1990; 25(suppl A):73–82.

Index

8a-AZA-8a-homoerythromycin A 6,9-cyclic imioether, 204
9a-Aza-9a-homoerythromycin A 6,9-cyclic iminoether, 204
Acinetobacter, 209
AIDS, atypical mycobacteria associated with, 126
Amoxicillin, 216, 217, 218
Antilegionella activity of Roxithromycin and use of E test to determine potency, 267–270
Antirickettsial activity of azithromycin and clarithromycin in in vitro systems, 291–296
ATCC 9341, *micrococcus luteus*, 198
Azalides, 206
    14-membered ring, 7, 7, 8t
    15-membered ring, *4–5*, 4–7, 5-6t
    classifications, 7–9, *9*
    defined, 4–7
    gastrointestinal reactions, 62–63, 63–64t
    macrolides, with different antibacterial properties, 203–211
    molecular-modeling study, and macrolides with different antibacterial properties, 203–211
Azithromycin, 204, 208, 268, 273, 343, 344, 345
    intestinal bacterial flora, 341–346

Bacillus cereus ATCC 11778, 198
Bacillus pumilus NCTC 8241, 198
Bacillus subtilis NCTC 8236, 198
Bacillus suis VB, 199
Bacteroides fragilis group, 228
Borrelia burgdorferi, 229
Branhamella (Moraxella) catarrhalis, 199
Brucella abortus VB, 199

Candida albicans, 281
Cefaclor, 216, 217, 218
Cefamandole, 253
Cefprozil, 216, 217, 218
Ceftriaxone, 273
Cefuroxime axetil, 216, 217, 218
Chlamydia
    macrolides, 98–99
    pneumonia, 227
    trachomatis, 281
Chlamydia psittaci, antibiotic agents against, 288–290
Chloramphenicol, 194
Ciprofloxacin, 236–246, 253, 268, 273
    erythromycin, on *Staphylococcus epidermidis*, 255–259
    on *Staphylococcus epidermidis* in Biofilm, 255–259
    and vancomycin, antipneumococcal activity of, 236–246

Clarithromycin, 216, 217, 218, 343, 344, 345
  14-hydroxyclarithromycin, respiratory pathogens, 212–219
  14-OH, 216, 217, 218
  15-μg, 214
  Mycobacterium avium complex determined in Bactec Broth: Effect of pH, 302–305
  14(*R*)-hydroxy metabolite against *Haemophilus influenzae* isolated in 1993 in New York City, 220–224
Clindamycin, 194, 253, 268
Clostridium spp., 228
Comefloxacin, 268
Congenital toxoplasma infection, macrolides, 134
Corynebacterium, 199, 226
Cotrimoxazole, and roxithromycin, in Lyme disease, combined therapy with, 508–515
Cycloheximide, 195

9-Deoxo-9a-aza-9a-homoerythromycin A, 204
Dirithromycin, 188, 268, 308, 309
  cell-free inhibition of protein synthesis, 187–190
  erythromycin, and roxithromycin on neutrophil functions, 311–313
  erythromycylamine uptake by human neutrophils in vitro, 307-310
Doxycycline, 268, 276, 281, 282, 289
Drug–drug interactions, azalides, 64-65, 65t

Enterococcus, 209
Epidirithromycin, 188
Erythromycin, 188, 194, 236–246, 268, 269, 273, 276, 281, 282, 289, 317
  15-μg, 214
  on neutrophil functions, 311–313
  sparfloxacin, ciprofloxacin, and vancomycin, antipneumococcal activity of, 236–246
  on *Staphylococcus epidermidis*, 255–259

Erythromycylamine, 188, 308
  on neutrophil functions, 311–313
Escherichia coli ATCC 10596, 199

Fleroxacin, 268
Fluoroquinolones, 268
Fusobacterium spp., 228

Gardnerella vaginalis, 281
Giardia lamblia, 229
Gonorrhea, macrolides, 148–149

Haemophilus ducreyi in Rwanda, antimicrobial susceptibility of, 271–274
Haemophilus influenza, 193, 199, 214, 217, 227, 230
  β-lactamase, 213
  roxithromycin, with respiratory tract infection, 231–235
Helicobacter pylori, 229, 230
14-hydroxyclarithromycin, respiratory pathogens, 212-219

Intracellular killing of chlamydiae by clarithromycin and erythromycin, 284–287

Josamycin, 195, 281, 282, 289

Klebsiella pneumoniae P, 199

Lankacidin C, 194, 195
  bacterial ribosomal-binding site for, characterization of, 191–195
Legionella, 95–119, 96-99, 97t, 227, 230
  antimicrobial agents, activity against, 96–99
Lincomycin, 281, 282, 317
Listeria monocytogenes, 226
Lyme disease
  cotrimoxazole, and roxithromycin, combined therapy with, 508–515
  early, macrolide antibiotics, treatment with, 141–146, 142–143t

Macrolides
  aglycone, 11, *11–12*
  as antibacterial agents, 9–21, *10*
  as antifungal agents, 21–22, 23t
  as anti-inflammatory agents, 22–24,
    24t
  as antimycobacterial agents, 121–129
  as antiparasitic agents, 22
  and azalides, structure–activity relation-
    ship of, 3–30
  as cardiovascular agents, 24–25
  chemical modifications on aglycone ring,
    10, 10–11
  chlamydia, sexually transmitted diseases,
    147–154
  D-desosamine, 18–21, *20*
  defined, 4
  derived pharmacokinetic characteristics,
    54–56, 55t
  with different antibacterial properties,
    203-211
  efflux genes, 38-39
  elimination, modes of, 57t, 57–58
  EM-523, 26, *27*
  erm genes, spread of, 36-38
  erythromycylamine derivatives, 13-15,
    16, 17t
  9-ether oxime derivatives, 12–13, 14t,
    15
  gastrointestinal prokinetic agents, 25–
    28
  in gram-positive infections, 83–93
  with human neutrophils in vitro, interac-
    tion, 306–314
  hypotensive activity of, 24–25, *25*
  L-cladinose, 21, *21*
  lincosamine-streptogramins, 268
  LY 267108, 26, *27*
  migrating motor complex in human gas-
    trointestinal tract, 25
  motilides, 26
  motilin, 26
  for *Mycobacterium leprae*, 125–126
  newer, pharmacokinetics of, 51–60
  pharmacokinetics, in children, 56
  position 6, modifications in, 12, 13t

[Macrolides]
  position 8, modifications in, 15–
    16, *18*, 18t
  position 9, modifications in, *12*, 12–15
  position 11, modifications in, 16–18,
    19t, *19–20*
  position 12, modifications in, 16–18,
    19t, *19–20*
  potential class III antiarrhythmic agents,
    24
  rationale to develop prokinetic
    macrolidelike agents, 26
  resistance, 31–40
    clinical epidemiology of, 41–49, 42t,
      43–44, 46
    genetic basis of, 31–36, 33t, *33–35*,
      36–37t
  safety, 61–69
  serum pharmacokinetics, 52–54, 53-54t
  structure–activity relations, 26–28
  substituents, 12-21
  in toxoplasmosis, 131–140
Methicillin, 326–332, 329, 330, 331
11-*O*-Methylazithromycin, 204
Minocycline, 253, 281, 282, 289
Moraxella catarrhalis, 213, 227, 230
Multiple dose pharmacokinetics and phar-
    macodynamics of RP 57669–RP
    54476 in preinfected Fibrin clots,
    323–333
Mycobacterium
  rapidly growing, effect of macrolides
    against, 125
  in vitro testing of macrolides against,
    122, 122–123
Mycobacterium avium complex
  clarithromycin, *122*, 124–125
  macrolides, 123–125
Mycobacterium avium–intracellulare, 228
Mycobacterium catarrhalis, 214, 217, 218
Mycobacterium chelonae, 228
Mycobacterium fortuitum, 228
Mycobacterium hominis, 227
Mycobacterium kansasii, 228
Mycobacterium leprae, 228
Mycobacterium paratuberculosis, 228

Mycobacterium tuberculosis, 126, 228
Mycobacterium flavus ATCC 10420, 198
Mycoplasma, macrolides, 98
Mycoplasma hominis, and *Ureaplasma urealyticum*, virginiamycin, 279–283
Mycoplasma pneumoniae, 199, 227

Neisseria gonorrhoea, 227
New antimicrobial properties of clarithromycin, 225–230
Nongonococcal infections, macrolides, 150t, 150–153, 152t
Novobiocin, 253

Ofloxacin, 268, 269, 281, 282, 289
Oxacillin, 253

Pasteurella haemolitica L-314, 199
Pefloxacin, 289
Penicillin G, RP 59500, erythromycin sparfloxacin, ciprofloxacin, and vancomycin by time–kill methodology, 236-246
Peptostreptococcus spp., 228
Plasmodium falciparum, 229
Pneumocystis carinii, 229
Prevotella spp., 228, 281
Pristinamycin, 281, 282, 289, 317
Proprionibacterium spp., 228
Protective effect, of roxithromycin on endotoxin-mediated microvascular leakage and leukocyte recruitment in airways, 347–352

Respiratory infections, macrolides in, clinical activity of, 103-113, 104–108t, 110–111t
Rifampin, 253, 268, 269
Roxithromycin, 268, 269, 276, 289, 337, 338, 355
    against haemophilus influenzae, 231–235
    against mycobacterium avium complex, 297-301
    neutrophil functions, 311–313

RP 59500, 236–246, 253, 268
    antipneumococcal activity of, 236–246
    ciprofloxacin, on *Staphylococcus epidermidis* in Biofilm, 255–259

Safety profiles, macrolides, 62–65
Salmonella, 209
    enteritidis 5 Z, 199
Shigella sonnei 34 Z, 199
Sparfloxacin, 236–246
Spiramycin, 289, 317
Staphylococcus, 193
    agalactiae, 198, 226, 230
    aureus, 226
        500 KR, 198
        ATCC 6538, 198
        macrolides, 83–86, 84–85t
        (MRSA), 230
        (MSSA), 230
    epidermidis, 226
        ATCC 12228, 198
    epidermidis 322KR, 198
    pneumoniae, 198, 214, 216, 226
        penicillin, 213
    pyogenes, 214, 218, 230
    suis SS-48, 199
Strephylococcus, 209
Streptococcus
    A, 198
    B, 199
    pneumoniae, 209, 230
        macrolides, 86–87
    pyogenes, 193, 213, 226
    suis SS-27, 199
Streptogramin, 194
    A, 317
    B, 317
    resistance by acetylation among streptogramin-resistant staphylococcal clinical isolates in France, 315–322
    RP 59500, against methicillin-sensitive and -resistant staphylococci, 251–254

Suppression of pseudomonas aeruginosa-induced Biofilm formation on epithelial cells by Roxithromycin, 260–266
Synergism of Roxithromycin and Pyrimethamine or Sulfadiazine against *Toxoplasma gondii* 334–340
Syphilis, macrolides, 149–150

Teicoplanin, 253
Tetracycline, 194, 276, 289
Tissue penetration, macrolides, 58–59
TMP/SMX, 268
Toxoplasma gondii, 229
Toxoplasmic chorioretinitis, 135
Toxoplasmic encephalitis
    in immunocompromised hosts, 135–136
    macrolides, 134

Toxoplasmosis, in pregnancy, 134–135
Trichomonas vaginalis, 281
Trimethoprim, 273
Trimethoprim-sulfamethoxazole, 273
Tylosin, 194, 195, 197
    polyhydro derivatives of, 196–202
Tysolin, 200

Ureaplasma urealyticum, 199, 227
    antibiotic susceptibility of, 275–278
    virginiamycin, 279–283

Vancomycin, 236–246, 253
    antipneumococcal activity of, 236–246
Virginiamycin, 281, 282

About the Editors

Harold C. Neu is Chief of the Division of Infectious Diseases, Professor of Medicine, and Professor of Pharmacology at the Columbia University College of Physicians & Surgeons, New York, New York, as well as an Attending Physician and Hospital Epidemiologist at the Columbia Presbyterian Medical Center, New York, New York. The author or coauthor of over 800 journal articles, reviews, and book chapters and the editor or coeditor of over 20 books, Dr. Neu is a Fellow of the American Academy of Microbiology, the New York Academy of Medicine, and the New York Academy of Sciences, a master of the American College of Physicians, and a member of several other societies. He received the A.B. degree (1956) from Creighton University, Omaha, Nebraska, and the M.D. degree (1960) from the Johns Hopkins University, Baltimore, Maryland.

Lowell S. Young is Director of the Kuzell Institute for Arthritis and Infectious Diseases, Medical Research Institute of San Francisco; Chief of the Division of Infectious Diseases at the California Pacific Medical Center, San Francisco; and Clinical Professor of Medicine at the University of California, San Francisco. He is also Adjunct Professor of Pharmacy at the University of the Pacific, San Francisco. The author or coauthor of more than 250 articles and an editorial board member of numerous journals, Dr. Young is a Fellow of the American College of Physicians and the Infectious Diseases Society of America and a member of the American Society for Clinical Investigation, among others. He received the A.B. degree (1960) from Princeton University, Princeton, New Jersey, and the M.D. degree (1964) from Harvard Medical School, Boston, Massachusetts.

Stephen H. Zinner is Professor of Medicine, interim Chairman of the Department of Medicine, and Director, Division of Infectious Diseases, Department of Medicine, Brown University, Providence, Rhode Island; Head, Division of Infectious Diseases, Roger Williams Medical Center, Providence; Head of the Division of Infectious Diseases at Rhode Island Hospital, Providence; Consultant in Infectious Diseases at Women and Infants Hospital of Rhode Island, Miriam Hospital, and the Veterans Administration Medical Center; and a Lecturer in Medicine at Harvard Medical School, Boston, Massachusetts. The author or coauthor of over 200 articles, book chapters, and abstracts, Dr. Zinner is a Fellow of the American College of Epidemiology, the Infectious Diseases Society of America, the American College of Physicians, and the American Heart Association, and a member of the American Society for Clinical Investigation and many other organizations. He received the B.A. degree (1961) from Northwestern University, Evanston, Illinois, and the M.D. degree (1965) from the University of Pennsylvania School of Medicine, Philadelphia.

Jacques F. Acar is Professor of Microbiology, Université de Paris VI, Pierre et Marie Curie, Head of the Department of Clinical Microbiology and Infectious Diseases, Hôpital, Saint-Joseph, and Head of the Laboratory of Clinical Microbiology, Broussais Hospital, all in Paris, France. The author or coauthor of more than 400 articles, Dr. Acar also serves as an editorial board member for several journals and is the Editor-in-Chief of *Clinical Microbiology and Infection*, the official journal of the European Society of Clinical Microbiology and Infectious Diseases. A consultant at the World Health Organization, he is a member of the Infectious Diseases Society of America, the American Society for Microbiology, the Société Française de Microbiologie, and the Société de Pathologie Infectieuse de Langue Français. He is also a former President of the International Society of Infectious Diseases and the European Society of Clinical Microbiology and Infectious Diseases. Dr. Acar received the M.D. degree (1954) from the University of Paris, France. He was a Fellow at Harvard Medical School, Boston, Massachusetts, and an invited lecturer at several American universities.